Dietary Reference Intakes (DRIs): Recommended Dietary Allowances and Adequate Intakes, Vitamins
Food and Nutrition Board, Institute of Medicine, National Academies

LIFE STAGE GROUP	VITAMIN A (µg/d)[a]	VITAMIN C (mg/d)	VITAMIN D (µg/d)[b,c]	VITAMIN E (mg/d)[d]	VITAMIN K (µg/d)	THIAMIN (mg/d)	RIBOFLAVIN (mg/d)	NIACIN (mg/d)[e]	VITAMIN B6 (mg/d)	FOLATE (µg/d)[f]	VITAMIN B12 (µg/d)	PANTOTHENIC ACID (mg/d)	BIOTIN (µg/d)	CHOLINE (mg/d)[g]
Infants														
0 to 6 mo	400*	40*	10	4*	2.0*	0.2*	0.3*	2*	0.1*	65*	0.4*	1.7*	5*	125*
6 to 12 mo	500*	50*	10	5*	2.5*	0.3*	0.4*	4*	0.3*	80*	0.5*	1.8*	6*	150*
Children														
1-3 y	300	15	15	6	30*	0.5	0.5	6	0.5	150	0.9	2*	8*	200*
4-8 y	400	25	15	7	55*	0.6	0.6	8	0.6	200	1.2	3*	12*	250*
Males														
9-13 y	600	45	15	11	60*	0.9	0.9	12	1.0	300	1.8	4*	20*	375*
14-18 y	900	75	15	15	75*	1.2	1.3	16	1.3	400	2.4	5*	25*	550*
19-30 y	900	90	15	15	120*	1.2	1.3	16	1.3	400	2.4	5*	30*	550*
31-50 y	900	90	15	15	120*	1.2	1.3	16	1.3	400	2.4	5*	30*	550*
51-70 y	900	90	15	15	120*	1.2	1.3	16	1.7	400	2.4[h]	5*	30*	550*
> 70 y	900	90	20	15	120*	1.2	1.3	16	1.7	400	2.4[h]	5*	30*	550*
Females														
9-13 y	600	45	15	11	60*	0.9	0.9	12	1.0	300	1.8	4*	20*	375*
14-18 y	700	65	15	15	75*	1.0	1.0	14	1.2	400[i]	2.4	5*	25*	400*
19-30 y	700	75	15	15	90*	1.1	1.1	14	1.3	400[i]	2.4	5*	30*	425*
31-50 y	700	75	15	15	90*	1.1	1.1	14	1.3	400[i]	2.4	5*	30*	425*
51-70 y	700	75	15	15	90*	1.1	1.1	14	1.5	400	2.4[h]	5*	30*	425*
>70 y	700	75	20	15	90*	1.1	1.1	14	1.5	400	2.4[h]	5*	30*	425*
Pregnancy														
14-18 y	750	80	15	15	75*	1.4	1.4	18	1.9	600[j]	2.6	6*	30*	450*
19-30 y	770	85	15	15	90*	1.4	1.4	18	1.9	600[j]	2.6	6*	30*	450*
31-50 y	770	85	15	15	90*	1.4	1.4	18	1.9	600[j]	2.6	6*	30*	450*
Lactation														
14-18 y	1,200	115	15	19	75*	1.4	1.6	17	2.0	500	2.8	7*	35*	550*
19-30 y	1,300	120	15	19	90*	1.4	1.6	17	2.0	500	2.8	7*	35*	550*
31-50 y	1,300	120	15	19	90*	1.4	1.6	17	2.0	500	2.8	7*	35*	550*

NOTE: This table (taken from the DRI reports, see www.nap.edu) presents Recommended Dietary Allowances (RDAs) in **bold type** and Adequate Intakes (AIs) in ordinary type followed by an asterisk (*). An RDA is the average daily dietary intake level; sufficient to meet the nutrient requirements of nearly all (97-98 percent) healthy individuals in a group. It is calculated from an Estimated Average Requirement (EAR). If sufficient scientific evidence is not available to establish an EAR, and thus calculate an RDA, an AI is usually developed. For healthy breastfed infants, an AI is the mean intake. The AI for other life stage and gender groups is believed to cover the needs of all healthy individuals in the groups, but lack of data or uncertainty in the data prevent being able to specify with confidence the percentage of individuals covered by this intake.

As retinol activity equivalents (RAEs). 1 RAE = 1 µg retinol, 12 µg β-carotene, 24 µg α-carotene, or 24 µg β-cryptoxanthin. The RAE for dietary provitamin A carotenoids is two-fold greater than retinol equivalents (RE), whereas the RAE for preformed vitamin A is the same as RE.

As cholecalciferol. 1 µg cholecalciferol = 40 IU vitamin D.

Under the assumption of minimal sunlight.

As α-tocopherol. α-Tocopherol includes RRR-α-tocopherol, the only form of α-tocopherol that occurs naturally in foods, and the 2R-stereoisomeric forms of α-tocopherol (RRR-, RSR-, RRS-, and RSS-α-tocopherol) that occur in fortified foods and supplements. It does not include the 2S-stereoisomeric forms of α-tocopherol (SRR-, SSR-, SRS-, and SSS-α-tocopherol), also found in fortified foods and supplements.

As niacin equivalents (NE). 1 mg of niacin = 60 mg of tryptophan; 0-6 months = preformed niacin (not NE).

As dietary folate equivalents (DFE). 1 DFE = 1 µg food folate = 0.6 µg of folic acid from fortified food or as a supplement consumed with food = 0.5 µg of a supplement taken on an empty stomach.

Although AIs have been set for choline, there are few data to assess whether a dietary supply of choline is needed at all stages of the life cycle, and it may be that the choline requirement can be met by endogenous synthesis at some of these stages.

Because 10 to 30 percent of older people may malabsorb food-bound B12, it is advisable for those older than 50 years to meet their RDA mainly by consuming foods fortified with B12 or a supplement containing B12.

In view of evidence linking folate intake with neural tube defects in the fetus, it is recommended that all women capable of becoming pregnant consume 400 µg from supplements or fortified foods in addition to intake of food folate from a varied diet.

It is assumed that women will continue consuming 400 µg from supplements or fortified food until their pregnancy is confirmed and they enter prenatal care, which ordinarily occurs after the end of the periconceptional period—the critical time for formation of the neural tube.

SOURCES: Dietary Reference Intakes for Calcium, Phosphorous, Magnesium, Vitamin D, and Fluoride (1997); Dietary Reference Intakes for Thiamin, Riboflavin, Niacin, Vitamin B6, Folate, Vitamin B12, Pantothenic Acid, Biotin, and Choline (1998); Dietary Reference Intakes for Vitamin C, Vitamin E, Selenium, and Carotenoids (2000); Dietary Reference Intakes for Vitamin A, Vitamin K, Arsenic, Boron, Chromium, Copper, Iodine, Iron, Manganese, Molybdenum, Nickel, Silicon, Vanadium, and Zinc (2001); Dietary Reference Intakes for Water, Potassium, Sodium, Chloride, and Sulfate (2005); and Dietary Reference Intakes for Calcium and Vitamin D (2011). These reports may be accessed via www.nap.edu.

Dietary Reference Intakes (DRIs): Acceptable Macronutrient Distribution Ranges Food and Nutrition Board, Institute of Medicine, National Academies

	RANGE (PERCENT OF ENERGY)		
MACRONUTRIENT	CHILDREN, 1-3 y	CHILDREN, 4-18 y	ADULTS
Fat	30-40	25-35	20-35
n-6 polyunsaturated fatty acids[a] (linoleic acid)	5-10	5-10	5-10
n-3 polyunsaturated fatty acids[a] (α-linolenic acid)	0.6-1.2	0.6-1.2	0.6-1.2
Carbohydrate	45-65	45-65	45-65
Protein	5-20	10-30	10-35

Approximately 10 percent of the total can come from longer-chain n-3 or n-6 fatty acids.

SOURCE: Dietary Reference Intakes for Energy, Carbohydrate, Fiber, Fat, Fatty Acids, Cholesterol, Protein, and Amino Acids (2002/2005). The report may be accessed via www.nap.edu.

Dietary Reference Intakes (DRIs): Acceptable Macronutrient Distribution Ranges Food and Nutrition Board, Institute of Medicine, National Academies

MACRONUTRIENT	RECOMMENDATION
Dietary cholesterol	As low as possible while consuming a nutritionally adequate diet
Trans fatty Acids	As low as possible while consuming a nutritionally adequate diet
Saturated fatty acids	As low as possible while consuming a nutritionally adequate diet
Added sugars[a]	Limit to no more than 25% of total energy

[a]Not a recommended intake. A daily intake of added sugars that individuals should aim for to achieve a healthful diet was not set.

SOURCE: Dietary Reference Intakes for Energy, Carbohydrate, Fiber, Fat, Fatty Acids, Cholesterol, Protein, and Amino Acids (2002/2005). The report may be accessed via www.nap.edu.

(Cont'd on inside back cover)

Nutritional Foundations and Clinical Applications

A NURSING APPROACH

Sixth Edition

Michele Grodner, EdD, CHES
Professor
Department of Public Health
William Paterson University
Wayne, New Jersey

Sylvia Escott-Stump, MA, RD, LDN
President, Academy of Nutrition and Dietetics, 2011-2012
Director, Dietetic Internship
East Carolina University
Greenville, North Carolina

Suzanne Dorner BSN, RN, CCRN
Clinical Nurse
Medical Intensive Care Unit
Tampa General Hospital
Tampa, Florida

ELSEVIER
MOSBY

3251 Riverport Lane
St. Louis, Missouri 63043

NUTRITIONAL FOUNDATIONS AND CLINICAL APPLICATIONS: ISBN: 978-0-323-24210-3
A NURSING APPROACH

Notice

Knowledge and best practice in this field are constantly changing. As new research and experience broaden our knowledge, changes in practice, treatment and drug therapy may become necessary or appropriate. Readers are advised to check the most current information provided (i) on procedures featured or (ii) by the manufacturer of each product to be administered, to verify the recommended dose or formula, the method and duration of administration, and contraindications. It is the responsibility of the practitioner, relying on their own experience and knowledge of the patient, to make diagnoses, to determine dosages and the best treatment for each individual patient, and to take all appropriate safety precautions. To the fullest extent of the law, neither the Publisher nor the Authors assume any liability for any injury and/or damage to persons or property arising out or related to any use of the material contained in this book.

Previous editions copyrighted 1996, 2000, 2004, 2007, 2012

Library of Congress Cataloging-in-Publication Data
Grodner, Michele.
    Nutritional foundations and clinical applications: a nursing approach / Michele Grodner, Sylvia Escott-Stump, Suzanne Dorner. — 6th ed.
        p. ; cm.
    Rev. ed. of: Nutritional foundations and clinical applications: a nursing approach / Michele Grodner, Sara Long, Bonnie C. Walkingshaw. 5th ed. c2014.
    Includes bibliographical references and index.
    ISBN 978-0-323-24210-3 (pbk. : alk. paper)   1. Diet therapy.   2. Nutrition.   3. Nursing.
I. Escott-Stump, Sylvia.   II. Dorner, Suzanne   III. Grodner, Michele. Foundations and clinical applications of nutrition.   IV. Title.
    [DNLM: 1. Diet Therapy—methods—Nurses' Instruction.   2. Nutritional Physiological Phenomena—Nurses' Instruction. WB 400]
    RM216.G946 2012
    615.8′54—dc22

                                                                    2010035542

Director, Traditional Education: Kristin Geen
Sr. Content Development Specialist: Lisa P. Newton
Publishing Services Manager: Deborah L. Vogel
Project Manager: Pat Costigan
Design Direction: Brian Salisbury

Printed in China

Last digit is the print number: 9 8 7 6 5 4 3 2

To my multigenerational household … Jared, Judith, Adam, and granddaughters Ruby and Lily
… thanks for keeping my life balanced and always interesting!
Michele Grodner

I wish to dedicate this text to my husband, Russ, my children, Matt and Lindsay,
and the wonderful nurses in my family and network of friends.
Sylvia Escott-Stump

To my amazing parents, Becky and Dan, for your everlasting love, encouragement, and support.
And to the rest of my family, best friends, and my many mentors,
I am so grateful to have you all in my life!
Suzanne Dorner

ACKNOWLEDGMENTS

To the individuals who shared their stories with us in the *Personal Perspective* boxes, our gratitude for your willingness to educate nursing professionals through your experiences. We acknowledge Gregory Annese, Yetta Kaemmer, and Tanya Popovetsky.

SPECIAL ACKNOWLEDGMENTS

One of the perks of working on a new edition is working again with the staff of Elsevier. Under the guidance of Yvonne Alexopoulos, Senior Education Content Strategist, we approached the sixth edition motivated to restructure content to promote ease of use of the material presented for instructors and their students. Kristin Geen, Director of Education Content, took over for Yvonne part way through the revision and we recognize her contributions as we continued through the process. We are delighted to again work with Lisa Newton and John Gabbert. Lisa Newton, Senior Content Development Specialist, cheerfully supervised our progress with the many layers of revisions while we shared weather reports during a particularly cold and snowy winter. Special thanks to John Gabbert, Project Manager, whose production and organizational skills allow for clarity of process and ease of publication; and with whom we share travel stories. We are grateful to Pat Costigan, Project Manager, who cheerfully completed the production of this edition. We look forward to working with him on the next edition. Thanks to Brian Salisbury, Senior Design Manager, for the fresh design concept of this edition.

In addition, we want to acknowledge the work of the Nursing Marketing Department for understanding what's special about our concept and for continuing to communicate this to instructors here in North America and internationally.

Writing is a solitary act. With projects such as this continually revised textbook, the process becomes a private aspect of self that cannot be shared. To family, friends, and colleagues who are unavoidably inconvenienced by this lengthy process, our apologies. We vow to discover strategies for easing the burden on others while we proceed with this important and recurring process.

We symbolize a collaboration of expertise in nutrition education, dietetics, and nursing. As we each become more sensitive to the multilayered responsibilities of nurses, we fine-tune our answers to the questions of "What do nurses need to know about nutrition?" and "How would they apply this knowledge to their patients and clients?" Or as one of us (SE-S) asks, "Need to know? Or nice to know?" This edition reflects our ever-evolving responses to these questions.

Michele Grodner
Sylvia Escott-Stump
Suzanne Dorner

REVIEWERS

Daniel G. Graetzer, PhD
Northwest University,
Department of Natural Science and Mathematics
College of Arts and Sciences,
Health and Sciences Center
Kirkland, Washington

Jean Markie, BSN, MSN, RN, APRN-BC
Assistant Professor of Nursing
Jeanette C. Rudy School of Nursing
Cumberland University
Lebanon, Tennessee

Carolyn McCune, RN, MSN, CRNP
Columbiana County Career & Technical Center
LPN Director
Lisbon, Ohio

Cindy Neff, RN MSN
Allegany College of Maryland
Professor of Nursing
Cumberland, Maryland

Every day, more information is revealed about the links between our personal behavior patterns and our level of health. But which study results or "healthiest" dietary patterns should be adopted for ourselves and, more so, for our patients? As health professionals, we need to be aware of our own dietary patterns as well as those of our patients. Changing food behavior patterns can be difficult even if we are knowledgeable of the benefits to be accrued. So many distractions of contemporary life keep us from achieving our goals. *Nutritional Foundations and Clinical Applications*, sixth edition, continues to recognize the role of nurses to support healing and wellness.

This nutrition text takes into account the personal nutrition needs of nurses to nourish themselves and their families as well as their demanding professional responsibilities to educate patients and clients (and their families) to follow prescribed therapeutic nutrition to maintain or improve health. This approach unites the worlds of nutrition and nursing. The role of nurses expands from the medical clinic into the community, thereby having a significant influence on the health promotion of individuals and the communities in which they work. Consequently, the need for nurses to have a thorough background in both personal and clinical nutrition applications becomes paramount.

This edition represents a major evolution of *Nutritional Foundations and Clinical Applications: A Nursing Approach*. This evolution comes from the addition of two new authors and a significant reorganization of content.

Michele Grodner, EdD, CHES, Professor, Department of Public Health, William Paterson University, continues as the author of nutrition and health content (Chapters 1-10). **Sylvia Escott-Stump, MA, RD, LDN,** Dietetic Internship Director, East Carolina University and former President, Academy of Nutrition and Dietetics, has rewritten and restructured the nutrition therapy content (Chapters 11-20). **Suzanne Dorner, BS, BSN, RN,** Critical Care Rotation Program, Tampa General Hospital, has updated The Nursing Approach feature of all chapters.

Significant reorganization of content has been achieved in several ways. First, chapters have been streamlined by combining similar content areas, resulting in 20 chapters. Health and wellness nutrition content is present in Chapters 1-10. Chapter 9 **Energy, Weight, and Fitness** encompasses previously separate chapters on energy supply, fitness, and management of body composition. Chapter 10 **Nutrition Across the Life Span** covers content of former chapters on health promotion during pregnancy, lactation, infancy, childhood, adolescence, and adulthood. The content related to nutrition therapy appears in Chapters 11-20. Second, reorganization of subject matter allowed for the addition of two new chapters: Chapter 12 **Food-Related Issues** and Chapter 19 **Nutrition for Neuro-Psychiatric Disorders.** Chapter 12 Food-Related Issues organizes concerns such as modified diets, food allergies, food poisoning, and potential interactions between drugs, nutrients, and/or herbs. Chapter 19 **Nutrition for Neuro-Psychiatric Disorders** addresses nutrition interventions for neurologic disorders including Alzheimer's disease, Parkinson's disease, amyotrophic lateral sclerosis, and migraine, and the chapter addresses psychiatric disorders such as eating disorders, bipolar spectrum, depression, and schizophrenia. The addition of this chapter recognizes the importance of nutrition for a healthy brain.

AUDIENCE

Nursing students are the primary audience for this book as they explore and apply basic nutrition and therapeutic nutrition. Secondary audiences include public health and health science majors. Useful in a variety of health care settings, the text provides an excellent reference for nurses, nurse practitioners, and other health care professionals.

The book consists of four parts, allowing for selective use within a one-semester course. For instance, Part I, *Wellness, Nutrition, and the Nursing Role;* Part II, *Nutrients, Food, and Health;* and Part III, *Health Promotion Through Nutrition and Nursing Practice* can be used for a basic, one-semester nutrition course, whereas Part IV, *Overview of Nutrition Therapy,* may be used as a future course or reference related to applications of nutrition therapy. Or all parts may be covered within a one-semester course.

APPROACH

Our main focus is on the nursing professional, concentrating on the nutrition skills applicable to nursing practice. The method of this text tailors nutrition and therapeutic nutrition to the unique perspective of the nursing profession. Most other nutrition texts attempt to meet the needs of dietetic and nutrition majors in addition to nursing majors. Information needed by dietetic majors but not by nurses is omitted. We appreciate that nurses do not prescribe or develop "diets" as nutrition therapy for patients. Instead, skills essential for nursing professionals are emphasized regarding implementation of diet orders and education of patients and clients about their prescribed dietary patterns.

FEATURES AND CONTENT

The nursing profession is multifaceted. While health promotion and clinical care are primary concerns, nurses have other factors to consider when providing care. These are addressed in every chapter of this sixth edition of *Nutritional Foundations and Clinical Applications.* Consider these features:

- **Cultural diversity of populations served**
  Food and health customs and concerns are analyzed specific to an array of ethnic groups. Students become

sensitized and respectful of culturally defined food differences and are then able to approach, interview, and assess patients from diverse backgrounds. Each **CULTURAL CONSIDERATIONS** box includes a section called, "Application to Nursing," to highlight how to use the knowledge in daily practice. As an added resource, Chapter 12 Food-Related Issues provides resources about cultural dietary patterns of different ethnic and religious groups, allowing nurses to focus on the specific population with whom they work.

- **Controversial health issue explorations**
  Health care professionals and the public-at-large have access to an abundance of health-related information through the many forms of media. Consequently, differing opinions or controversies about food, nutrition, and health concerns emerge. Students are encouraged to develop their own beliefs. As applicable, some chapters have **HEALTH DEBATE** boxes.

- **Awareness of the personal perspective of individuals**
  Content throughout this text is expressed in a human personal way. This approach, which underlies the philosophy of this text, is reflected by first-hand accounts of the ways in which nutrition affects the lives of both nursing professionals and everyday people. Powerful images of patients and their families emerge as individuals describe in their own words their experiences pursuing health and healing. Each chapter offers a **PERSONAL PERSPECTIVES** box on a related experience.

- **Comprehension of societal issues that impact health status**
  SOCIAL ISSUES boxes emphasize ethical, social, and community concerns on local, national, and international levels to reveal the various influences on health and wellness. It is imperative for nursing health care professionals to understand the potential effects of societal issues on the lives and health status of populations served.

- **Recognition of the educational role of nursing**
  Nursing professionals have a primary role in supporting clients as they strive to achieve compliance of prescribed therapeutic dietary modifications or just attempt to improve their nutrient intake. *TEACHING TOOL* boxes in every chapter provide strategies for teaching clients about optimum dietary patterns and therapeutic nutrition recommendations.

  When appropriate, specific issues of literacy, such as strategies for enhancing patient education for those with low literacy skills, are also presented in *TEACHING TOOL* boxes.

- **Recognition of psychosocial strategies for behavior change to achieve wellness**
  The **TOWARD A POSITIVE NUTRITION LIFESTYLE** section in each chapter within Parts I, II, and III presents psychosocial strategies to support health behavioral changes for individuals wishing to adopt healthier lifestyles. This section recognizes the multidisciplinary skills needed to apply lifestyle changes for oneself and one's clients/patients.

- **Focus on the Nursing Process**
  THE NURSING APPROACH boxes analyze a realistic nutrition case study from the perspective of the nursing process. By creating situations that may be encountered in clinical practice, the chapter's nutrition subject matter is consistently refocused into a nursing perspective. Discussion questions based on the case study enhance critical thinking and application skills. These can be used for class discussions or as homework assignments. Responses are included for instructors. They are written from a professional nursing perspective and case studies have been written or revised by author Suzanne Dorner, who brings a fresh perspective and experience in clinical nursing, dietetics, and patient education.

TEACHING AND LEARNING RESOURCES

For Instructors

Instructor Resources on Evolve, available at http://evolve.elsevier.com/Grodner/foundations provides a wealth of material to help you make your Nutrition instruction a success. In addition to all of the Student Resources, the following are provided for Faculty:

- *TEACH for Nurses* **Lesson Plans**, based on textbook chapter Learning Objectives, serve as ready-made, modifiable lesson plans and a complete roadmap to link all parts of the educational package. These concise and straightforward lesson plans can be modified or combined to meet your particular scheduling and teaching needs.

- **PowerPoint Presentations** are organized by chapter with approximately 30 slides per chapter for in-class lectures. These are detailed and include customizable text and image lecture slides to enhance learning in the classroom or in Web-based course modules. If you share them with students they can use the note feature to help them with your lectures.

- **Audience Response Questions for i>clicker and other systems** are provided with 1 to 3 multiple-answer questions per chapter to stimulate class discussion and assess student understanding of key concepts.

- The **Test Bank** has more than 650 test items, complete with the correct answer, rationale, cognitive level of each question, corresponding step of the nursing process, appropriate NCLEX; Client Needs label, and text page reference(s).

For Students

Student Resources on Evolve, available at http://evolve.elsevier.com/Grodner/foundations.

Students will find a wealth of valuable learning resources on Evolve. The Evolve Resources page in the front of the book gives login instructions and a description of each resource.

- **Virtual Case Studies (Online):** Video clips of six fictitious patients—including one with type 2 diabetes mellitus, one with a respiratory infection, and one with HIV/AIDS wasting syndrome—are accompanied by written case studies; short answer and essay questions; NCLEX-formatted, multiple-choice, examination-style questions; and Internet assignments. This exciting feature provides students with realistic clinical practice.

- *Applying Content Knowledge* **Questions (Online):** One case and question per chapter are provided online, in addition to the cases and questions contained within the foundation and life-span chapters of the textbook (Chapters 1-10).
- *Critical Thinking: Clinical Applications* **Questions (Online):** *One case study with accompanying application questions is provided online for each of the clinical chapters (Chapters 11-20), in addition to the cases and questions contained within those same textbook chapters.*
- *Quick Review* **Questions (Online):** Approximately 5 to 10 short-answer questions per chapter are supplied online.

- *Nutritrac Nutrition Analysis Program, Version 5.0* **(Online):** The new edition of this popular tool is designed to allow the user to calculate and analyze food intake and energy expenditure, taking the guesswork out of nutrition planning. The new version features comprehensive databases containing more than 5000 foods organized into 18 different categories and more than 175 common/daily recreational, sporting, and occupational activities. The *Personal Profile* feature allows users to enter and edit the intake and output of an unlimited number of individuals, and the *Weight Management Planner* helps outline healthy lifestyles tailored to various personal profiles. In addition to foods and activities, new program features include an ideal body weight (IBW) calculator, a Harris-Benedict calculator to estimate total daily energy needs, and the complete *Exchange Lists for Meal Planning.*

CONTENTS

x

CHAPTER 1

Wellness Nutrition

Nutrients are substances in foods required by the body for energy, growth, maintenance, and repair. Some nutrients are essential; they cannot be made by the human body and must be provided by foods.

http://evolve.elsevier.com/GRODNER/FOUNDATIONS

LEARNING OBJECTIVES

- Define health and wellness.
- Describe health promotion.
- State the purpose of *Healthy People 2020* (*HP2020*).
- Describe health literacy.
- Identify the six nutrient categories.
- List the functions of essential nutrients.

ROLE IN WELLNESS

Nourishing our bodies seems so simple. Just eat food. But which food? How much food? How prepared? Which foods to promote or maintain health? Which foods are "best" during illness or trauma? Who shops for food? How much should we spend on food or, rather, nourishment? Should we buy ready-made (or "order in") or cook from scratch? Who cooks? Who do we eat with or do we eat alone? Who cleans the kitchen? Not so simple after all.

The intent of this nutrition textbook is twofold. The first is to educate about the nutrients, foods, and related issues for our personal health and wellness goals. The second is to prepare nursing health professionals who understand the function and context of nutrition care prescribed for nutritional intervention for the prevention and treatment of diseases and conditions that may be alleviated or treated through specific dietary recommendations. Nutrition care is diagnosed and/or prescribed by Registered Dietitian/Nutritionists (RDNs) as part of multidisciplinary health care teams. Although nurses do not develop dietary treatment regimens, nurses often educate patients about prescribed dietary treatment. Nurses may reinforce the dietary recommendations within the context of an overall nursing care plan. Therefore in every chapter, *The Nursing Approach* box addresses related issues of implementation of dietary therapy and case management.

This chapter starts by considering the question, what are the concepts of health and wellness for which we strive?

DEFINITION OF HEALTH

In the past, health was defined as the absence of disease or illness. Modern medicine has conquered many life-threatening diseases, such as smallpox and polio. Public health measures such as pasteurization and sanitation have reduced the risk of foodborne and environmental hazards. As concern about the physical status of the human body has lessened, we have been able to consider other aspects of the qualities of health.

One of the first expanded definitions of *health* was provided by the World Health Organization (WHO, 1946): "Health is a state of complete physical, mental, and social well-being and not merely the absence of disease and infirmity." Although this definition addresses the concern that health is more than just the absence of disease, health is presented as a static concept that individuals achieve.

A more expanded definition of health was presented by Rene Dubos (1968), biologist and philosopher, who wrote, "Health is a quality of life involving social, emotional, mental, spiritual, and biologic fitness on the part of the individual, which results from adaptations to the environment." This view leads to our present understanding of health as a complex concept best represented by physical and psychologic dimensions, as follows:

Physical health: The efficiency of the body to function appropriately, to maintain immunity to disease, and to meet daily energy requirements

Intellectual health: The use of intellectual abilities to learn and to adapt to changes in one's environment

Emotional health: The capacity to easily express or suppress emotions appropriately

Social health: The ability to interact with people in an acceptable manner and sustain relationships with family members, friends, and colleagues

Spiritual health: The cultural beliefs that give purpose to human existence, found through faith in the teachings of organized religions, in an understanding of nature or science, or in an acceptance of the humanistic view of life

Environmental health: The external factors that affect our health and well-being, including the physical context within which one lives and works as affected by determinants of ethnicity, education, income, and occupation; and extending to the larger environment of safeguarding natural resources to reduce exposure to preventable hazards.

This holistic view incorporates many aspects of human existence. Using this definition of health allows more individualized assessment of health status. As our own health and the health of our clients are evaluated in relation to each dimension, some dimensions will be stronger than others (see the *Teaching Tool* box Dimensions of Health).

✳ TEACHING TOOL

Dimensions of Health

To broaden a patient's understanding of health, use the six dimensions of health. Describe the dimensions and then discuss with the patient each that pertains to his or her nutrition and health situation. By exploring aspects of health other than physical health, a person can then use all resources to restore the overall level of well-being.

Wellness through the Six Dimensions of Health
Physical health: Efficient body functioning
Intellectual health: Use of intellectual abilities
Emotional health: Ability to control emotions
Social health: Interactions and relationships with others
Spiritual health: Cultural beliefs about the purpose of life
Environmental health: External factors that impact living and work settings

Role of Nutrition

Nutrition is the study of nutrients and the processes by which they are used by the body. Nutrients are substances in foods required by the body for energy, growth, maintenance, and repair. Some nutrients are essential; they cannot be made by the human body and must be provided by foods.

Because the primary role of nutrients is to provide the building blocks for efficient functioning and maintenance of the body, nutrition may appear to belong only within the physical health dimension. However, the effects of nutrients and their sources on the other health dimensions are far reaching. Nutrition is the cornerstone of each health dimension.

Physical health depends on the quantity and quality of nutrients available to the body. The human body, from skeletal bones to minute amounts of hormones, is composed of nutrients in various combinations.

Intellectual health relies on a well-functioning brain and central nervous system. Nutritional imbalances can affect intellectual health, as occurs with iron-deficiency anemia. Although milk is an excellent source of protein, calcium, and phosphorus, it provides a negligible amount of iron. Some young children drink so much milk that it diminishes their appetite for other foods such as meats, chicken, legumes, and leafy green vegetables, all of which are good sources of iron. As a result, iron deficiency may occur in children with nutritional imbalances. The cognitive abilities of iron-deficient children may be affected, which could lead to possible learning problems.

Emotional health may be affected by poor eating habits, resulting in hypoglycemia or low blood glucose levels. Low blood glucose occurs normally in anyone who is physically hungry. When the body's need for food is ignored (e.g., when we miss meals because of poor planning or are too busy to eat), feelings of anxiety and confusion and trembling may occur. Emotions may be harder to control when we feel this way. Although blood glucose levels may affect our emotions, there are, of course, other factors that influence emotional health.

Social health situations often center on food-related occasions, ranging from holiday feasts to everyday meals. Nutritional status is sometimes affected by the quality of our relationships with family and friends. Are family meals an enjoyable experience or a tense ordeal? How might this issue affect a person's dietary intake?

Spiritual health often has ties to food. Several religions prohibit the consumption of specific foods. Many followers of Islam and Judaism adhere to the dietary laws of their religions. Both forbid consumption of pork products. Seventh Day Adventists follow an ovo-lacto vegetarian diet in which they consume only plant foods and dairy products. In India cows are viewed as sacred, not to be eaten but to be revered as a source of sustenance (milk), fuel (burning of feces), power (as a work animal), and fertilizer (manure).

Environmental health includes access to adequate meal-preparation facilities, knowledge about preparation, and financial and physical access to food stores within one's community. In major cities in the United States, some residents may live in "food deserts" within which large grocery stores are not easily accessible, thereby limiting access to fresh and reasonably priced foods. The environmental health of such a community is compromised.

DEFINITION OF *WELLNESS*

Wellness is a lifestyle (pattern of behaviors) that enhances our level of health. It occurs through development of each of the six dimensions of health. Individuals engaged in wellness lifestyles feel a sense of competency and achievement in their ability to modify their behaviors to increase or maintain positive levels of health.

Hectic contemporary schedules may seem to interfere with efforts to achieve wellness. The aim is to strive for wellness

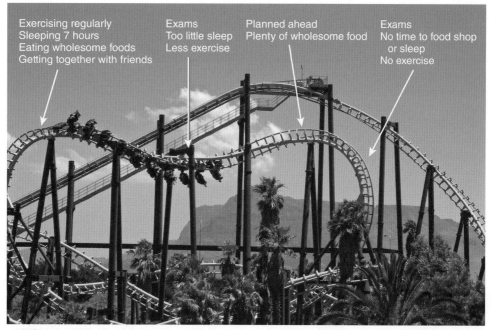

Exercising regularly
Sleeping 7 hours
Eating wholesome foods
Getting together with friends

Exams
Too little sleep
Less exercise

Planned ahead
Plenty of wholesome food

Exams
No time to food shop
or sleep
No exercise

FIG 1-1 Wellness effort roller coaster. (Modified from www.thinkstockphotos.com.)

even if the path may seem more like a roller coaster than a smooth uphill climb (Figure 1-1). At times, clients may falter in their efforts, but the key is to renew positive behaviors as soon as possible.

Role of Nutrition

"Wellness nutrition" approaches food consumption as a positive way to nourish the body. This approach focuses on ways to organize our lives so we can more easily follow an eating pattern designed to enhance health status. Consuming a diet based on lower fat and higher fiber (increase in plant-based foods such as fruits, vegetables, and whole grains) as well as moderate caloric consumption is then not a chore but rather an affirmation of our competency to care for ourselves. Conveying this approach to clients is a nursing challenge (see the *Personal Perspectives* box Getting Back to "Great" Again).

PERSONAL PERSPECTIVES

Getting Back to "Great" Again

This section in each chapter features an individual's viewpoint about a nutrition or health issue. Sometimes the viewpoint may represent a composite of opinions on a topic. Here, a recent university graduate shares his story of getting back to the feeling of "great" again.

I was a very athletic kid in high school. I played sports, worked out, and played drums (my favorite cardio activity) all the time. I wasn't the biggest or best at anything, but I felt great every day. I didn't drink or smoke much; I just liked to have fun and play sports. At the end of my senior year, I was in the greatest shape of my life. I was at my best.

Let's fast-forward to May of my senior year of college. I drank a lot every weekend. I smoked more in a week than most have in a lifetime. I never got up to do anything other than go to class or eat. Now I knew little by little throughout college I was losing that feeling of "great" I had in high school. I was out of it all the time, eating crap food and simply not caring about my body. I'm a thin guy, so it wasn't showing on the outside, but it sure as hell was showing on the inside. I always had a sore throat from smoking, and my stomach was constantly hurting from the munchies and eating junk food. My back actually

started to hurt my senior year; it was seriously from sitting on my butt and not moving for hours every day.

By graduation, I felt like crap. How was I ever going to stop? Shortly before graduation, I said to myself, "Self, you can keep this up until you go home. When you go home, it's time to cut the crap. No more smoking and no more eating junk foods every day. You are going to be living with your parents, and you are going to have a job. You have to be at your best again." And it was really weird, too, because that night I had a dream where I looked at myself in the mirror and I was all cut and muscular.

Now I am at my best again. It's August. I made a 100% turnaround since May. I only eat six or seven small meals a day of healthy foods and lift weights, exercising almost daily. The feeling of "great" is back.

It takes a lot of mental toughness to change. Just listen to my message. Cut out the negative stuff and bring in the good stuff, and YOU WILL BE AT YOUR BEST, yet again.

Greg Annese
Westwood, N.J.

HEALTH PROMOTION

Health promotion consists of strategies used to raise the level of the health of individuals, families, groups, and communities. In community and occupational health settings, health-promotion strategies implemented by nurses often focus on lifestyle changes that will lead to new, positive health behaviors. Development of positive behaviors may depend on knowledge, techniques, and community supports, as follows (see the *Teaching Tool* box Literacy and Health later in the chapter):

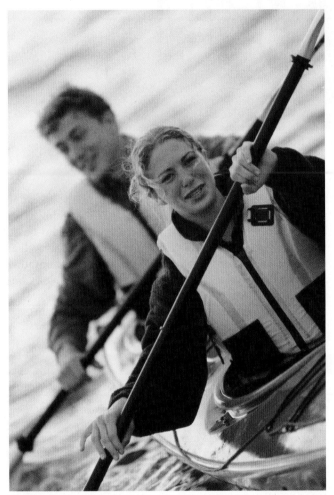

Physical health benefits from a good diet. (From www.thinkstockphotos.com.)

Knowledge: Learning new information about the benefits or risks of health-related behaviors

Techniques: Applying new knowledge to everyday activities; developing ways to modify current lifestyles

Community supports: Availability of environmental or regulatory measures to support new health-promoting behaviors within a social context

Role of Nutrition

For almost 40 years, national health targets have been set. In 1979 the first initiative, the Surgeon General's report titled *Healthy People,* laid out life-stage targets that continue to be tracked today. Since then, health targets have been updated every 10 years through collaboration among the government, voluntary, and professional health associations, businesses, and individuals under the direction of the secretary of the U.S. Department of Health and Human Services (USDHHS). The objectives focus on the decisions and policies that affect prevention efforts and create a standard against which to later assess the performance of meeting these goals. In addition, the interrelatedness of the health of communities and individuals is emphasized. The health status of an individual depends on the health supports accessible within the community. (This concept is also discussed in Chapter 2 under the heading Community Nutrition.)

The target results of the previous report are used to develop the next set of target goals. Data generated by *Healthy People 2010* (*HP2010*) were used to develop the next set of national health targets, *Healthy People 2020* (*HP2020*).

HP2020 is guided by a framework based on the vision of "a society in which all people live long, healthy lives" (USDHHS, n.d.). The mission is "to improve health through strengthening policy and practice." Four overarching goals present pathways by which to achieve the vision and mission. Details of the *HP2020* framework are listed in Box 1-1.

The approach to identifying national health objectives of *Healthy People 2020*'s overarching goals considers that the overlapping of environmental and social determinants of health affects health outcomes (Figure 1-2). Continued focus is on population disparities in determinants of health, such as living, working, and socioeconomic conditions, as well as individual behaviors as affected by the traits of individuals, such as age, gender, sexual orientation, race/ethnicity, and biological and geographic factors. The implementations of strategies to affect these factors are assessed by their outcomes. The outcomes are then evaluated, distributed, and used to create additional interventions. These actions will bring us as a nation closer to achieving the goals by 2020.

Nutrition Monitoring

The nutritional status of the American population is monitored through several ongoing surveys. The National Nutrition Monitoring Act of 1990 provides for partnerships among government organizations that conduct national surveys of the nation's health and nutritional status. This collaboration supports the use of similar standards and research methods so the surveys' findings can be compared.

The major survey that focuses on nutritional and health status of Americans is the National Health and Nutrition Examination Survey (NHANES), in that a program within the NHANES focuses on data from the dietary intake, medical history, biochemical evaluation, physical examinations, and measurements of American population groups who are carefully chosen to represent the total population. The dietary intake portion of the NHANES is called What We Eat in America (WWEIA). Records of food intake for 2 days are kept. These nutrient values are then compared with recommended dietary standards. NHANES and WWEIA are

BOX 1-1   Healthy People 2020 *Framework*

Vision

A society in which all people live long, healthy lives.

Mission

Healthy People 2020 strives to:

- Identify nationwide health-improvement priorities.
- Increase public awareness and understanding of the determinants of health, disease, and disability and the opportunities for progress.
- Provide measurable objectives and goals that are applicable at the national, state, and local levels.
- Engage multiple sectors to take actions to strengthen policies and improve practices that are driven by the best available evidence and knowledge.
- Identify critical research, evaluation, and data-collection needs.

Overarching Goals:

- Attain high-quality, longer lives free of preventable disease, disability, injury, and premature death.
- Achieve health equity, eliminate disparities, and improve the health of all groups.
- Create social and physical environments that promote good health for all.
- Promote quality of life, healthy development, and healthy behaviors across all life stages.

From HealthyPeople.gov: *Healthy People 2020: Framework: The vision, mission, and goals of Healthy People 2020,* n.d.. Accessed June 3, 2013, from www.healthypeople.gov/2020/Consortium/HP2020Framework.pdf/.

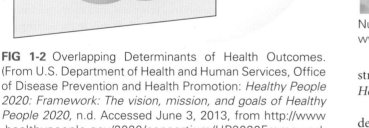

Healthy People 2020

A society in which all people live long, healthy lives

FIG 1-2 Overlapping Determinants of Health Outcomes. (From U.S. Department of Health and Human Services, Office of Disease Prevention and Health Promotion: *Healthy People 2020: Framework: The vision, mission, and goals of Healthy People 2020,* n.d. Accessed June 3, 2013, from http://www.healthypeople.gov/2020/consortium/HP2020Framework.pdf/, page 3.)

Nutrition is an integral part of health care education. (From www.thinkstockphotos.com.)

conducted as a collaboration between the U.S. Department of Agriculture (USDA), USDHHS, and the Centers for Disease Control and Prevention (CDC), National Center for Health Statistics (USDA et al, 2012).

DISEASE PREVENTION THROUGH NUTRITION

Disease prevention is the recognition of a danger to health that could be reduced or alleviated through specific actions or changes in lifestyle behaviors. The hazard may be caused by disease, lifestyle, or genetic factors or by an environmental threat. The three classifications of disease prevention are primary, secondary, and tertiary. Disease prevention has

strong ties to nutrition (see the *Cultural Considerations* box *Healthy People* and Culturally Competent Care).

Primary prevention consists of activities to avert the initial development of a disease or poor health. A primary disease prevention approach is to eat a variety of foods to avert nutrient deficiencies. Adopting a low-fat, high-fiber (plant-based) eating style before diet-related health problems develop is a form of primary prevention.

Secondary prevention involves early detection to halt or reduce the effects of a disease or illness. Some diseases cannot be prevented, but early detection can minimize negative health effects. Secondary prevention strategies are useful to reduce the effects of chronic diet-related diseases. Controlling the intake of certain nutrients can decrease the severity of some disorders. Some individuals with high blood pressure (hypertension) are sodium sensitive, and simply reducing the amount of sodium they consume can decrease their blood pressure levels and thus bring the disorder under control. Because hypertension is a risk factor for coronary artery disease, stroke, and renal disease, reduction of blood pressure

CULTURAL CONSIDERATIONS
Healthy People and Culturally Competent Care

Lifestyle and behavior are central to the maintenance of health and wellness. To influence lifestyle and behavior, health professionals need to take into account the values, attitudes, culture, and life circumstances of individuals. Changes in health status, particularly of minority populations, require professionals to take into account the increasing ethnic/cultural diversity of Americans. There are four recognized minority groups in the United States: Asian/Pacific Islanders, African Americans, Hispanic Americans, and Native Americans. Currently, it is estimated that one in five Americans belongs to a minority group. Minority populations are projected to grow to constitute one third of the population by the year 2050.

Healthy People reports document that the number of premature and excess deaths of ethnic minority populations far outweighs those of Caucasian majority groups. Research shows that the factors contributing to this difference are complex and have multiple elements. Socioeconomic status among minority groups is generally lower than among the majority groups. Socioeconomic status is measured by the combination of occupation, income, and educational attainment. A second major factor is the use of and access to health care programs by minorities. Many of the available health programs are not culturally relevant or sensitive to the minority populations they serve. There is a paucity of bilingual and bicultural health professionals, and health education materials are generally not culturally specific.

Application to Nursing
Diet and nutrition assessment is imperative to provide culturally competent care. Efforts to understand dietary patterns of clients need to go beyond relying on their membership in a defined group. For example, by learning the assimilative practices of an individual, nurses can assist dietitians in developing the most effective and culturally sensitive nutrition recommendations. Together they can develop a treatment regimen that does not conflict with the cultural food practices of the client.

through decreased sodium consumption is a secondary prevention strategy.

Tertiary prevention occurs after a disorder develops. The purpose is to minimize further complications or to assist in the restoration of health. These efforts may involve continued medical care. Often, learning more about the disorder is helpful for patients and their families. Tertiary prevention frequently involves diet therapy. Direct treatments of many disorders have a dietary component. Some of these disorders are ulcers, diverticulitis, and coronary artery disease; they usually occur during the middle and older years of adulthood. Other disorders may affect food intake and the ability of the body to absorb nutrients. For example, chemotherapy for cancer may have the side effects nausea and loss of appetite. Nutrition counseling during and after these treatments is necessary so patients are as well nourished as possible to aid the healing process. The six dimensions of health can be an excellent teaching tool in promoting health and preventing diseases related to nutrition.

HEALTH LITERACY

Health literacy is the ability to acquire and comprehend basic health concepts, such as nutrition, and apply them to one's own health decisions (CDC, 2011).

So how does health literacy develop? It is not the same as literacy of the printed word, although it is related. Health literacy develops through education on topics related to health promotion and illness. This process of education occurs in three different forms: formal, nonformal, and informal. *Formal education* is purposefully planned for implementation in a school setting. *Nonformal education* takes place through organized teaching and learning events in hospitals, clinics, and community centers. *Informal education* encompasses a variety of educational experiences that occur through daily activities. The informal experiences include watching television, reading newspapers and magazines, browsing the Internet, and conversing with other people. Health information from many sources becomes part of an individual's database of knowledge. Some information may be valid, some may be partially true, and some may be completely false. Our goal is to ensure that health decisions are based on accurate information.

Health literacy allows for education to be most effective, resulting in behavior changes. Nurses, through formal, nonformal, and informal educational interactions, can introduce knowledge and strategies for personal lifestyle choices that consider the health context of patients' lives. *Health context* takes into account the influence of cultural, social, and individual factors on the acquisition of health literacy. Cultural factors may encompass ethnic, religious, and racial traditions surrounding health issues. Social factors create the settings in which members of a community receive support or lack support for health-promoting behaviors. Individual factors reflect on the choices people make regarding willingness to acquire and then apply health knowledge. *Health literacy actualization* means being able to use acquired health knowledge and skills. The extent to which this occurs within health care settings is influenced by the level to which health care providers are supportive of literate health populations seeking greater involvement in their health care (Figure 1-3).

Nurses are involved with the development of client health literacy (see the *Teaching Tool* box Literacy and Health). Formal education may be conducted by school nurses who teach health courses; topics can be approached through the health and nutrition issues of the ethnic and cultural groups of the particular school's population. Nonformal education occurs when associations such as the American Heart Association or hospital wellness programs teach courses on risk-reducing lifestyle changes; these courses are usually open to the community. Informal education takes place when a nurse chats with a patient and his or her family, explaining the purpose of the dietary modifications recommended for the patient's particular disorder.

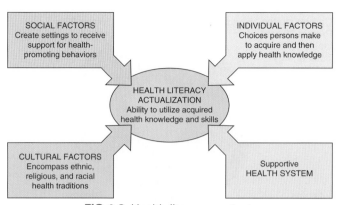

SOCIAL FACTORS
Create settings to receive support for health-promoting behaviors

INDIVIDUAL FACTORS
Choices persons make to acquire and then apply health knowledge

HEALTH LITERACY ACTUALIZATION
Ability to utilize acquired health knowledge and skills

CULTURAL FACTORS
Encompass ethnic, religious, and racial health traditions

Supportive
HEALTH SYSTEM

FIG 1-3 Health literacy context.

✳ TEACHING TOOL

Literacy and Health

Although health professionals may take their high level of literacy for granted, many clients do not have command of basic literacy skills. Limited literacy skills often equate with even more limited health literacy (the ability to use health information to make appropriate health decisions) and with limited numeracy (the ability to understand simple math concepts and apply them in everyday life situations). In fact, low reading skills are associated with poor health and greater use of health services. The implications of these limitations are important because they may limit the effectiveness of a nurse's efforts to educate clients to improve their knowledge and compliance.

Health literacy affects patient care in many ways (only a few are mentioned here). Simply filling out medical history and consent forms can leave patients struggling. Patients may also have difficulty explaining their symptoms because of limited vocabulary. They may not understand the medical terminology health care providers use to discuss health conditions but may be too uncomfortable to ask for clarification. Even if understood, the recommendations given to clients may be difficult to implement because their ability to decode or understand food labels is limited. Following cooking directions may be hard, and serving sizes may be misinterpreted. If clients are to track carbohydrate or sodium consumption, their reading literacy level and numeracy limitations may hinder accuracy and may foster discouragement or worsening of symptoms.

Throughout this textbook, strategies are provided for working with low-literacy clients, discussing the cultural connection, and evaluating and writing health education materials—all with the goal of enhancing health outcomes.

Never before have we had so much information about the effects of our personal behavior patterns on our level of health. Changing (or maintaining) our patterns of behaviors—and therefore our lifestyles—is the key to achieving wellness. Many social, community, and occupational forces affect our ability to change. Strategies and techniques ease our ability to modify our personal behaviors.

Modifying behaviors means changing lifestyles. Patterns of behaviors affecting the foods we choose to eat constitute our nutrition lifestyles. Not all of us have the same nutrition lifestyles. Some of us are caught up in extremely hectic work, college, or sports schedules; we are lucky to find time to eat at all. Others find our families of origin still at the center of our eating patterns; our families, however, may not have adopted recent recommendations to decrease the risks of diet-related diseases. Many of us are part of new social settings on campus and need to adjust to rigid schedules and school cafeteria menus. Yet, despite these variances, we have in common the ability to improve wellness through our nutrition lifestyles.

As health care professionals, we need to be concerned with our own nutritional patterns as well as those of our clients. To reflect a health-promotion perspective, individuals cared for by health professionals to maintain health are called *clients.* Those who are ill or recuperating from illness are called *patients.*

Enhancing personal health provides the stamina and well-being to fulfill the rigorous demands of the nursing practice. A fundamental responsibility of nursing is client education. When teaching clients about nutritional wellness, nurses also function as role models for the positive effects of enhanced nutrition lifestyles.

OVERVIEW OF NUTRIENTS WITHIN THE BODY

Which nutrients are the cornerstones of health and disease prevention? What do they do that makes them so important? Why can't we just take a nutrient pill?

Nutrient Categories

Nutrients can be divided into the following six categories:
1. Carbohydrates
2. Proteins
3. Lipids (fats)
4. Vitamins
5. Minerals
6. Water

Nutrients may be either essential or nonessential, depending on whether the body can manufacture them. When the body requires a nutrient for growth or maintenance but lacks the ability to manufacture amounts sufficient to meet the body's needs, the nutrient is *essential* and must be supplied by the foods in our diet. Table 1-1 lists the essential nutrients needed in our diet. Other nutrients that the body can make are called *nonessential.* Some nutrients have very specific functions, whereas others are diverse in their impact. Overall the functions of essential nutrients in the body include the following:

- *Providing energy:*
  - Carbohydrates, proteins, and lipids provide energy.
  - Vitamins and minerals have indirect roles as catalysts for the body's use of energy nutrients.
- *Regulating body processes:*
  - Proteins, lipids, vitamins, minerals, and water are required.

TABLE 1-1 Known Essential Nutrients

NUTRIENT	SOURCE
Carbohydrates	Glucose
Lipids (fats)	Linoleic acid, linolenic acid
Protein	Amino acids: histidine, isoleucine, leucine, lysine, methionine, phenylalanine, threonine, tryptophan, valine
Vitamins	Fat-soluble vitamins: A (retinol), D (cholecalciferol), E (tocopherol), K
	Water-soluble vitamins: thiamin, riboflavin, niacin, pantothenic acid, biotin, B_6 (pyridoxine), B_{12} (cobalamin), folate, C (ascorbic acid)
Minerals	Major minerals: calcium, phosphorus, sodium, potassium, sulfur, chlorine, magnesium
	Trace minerals: chromium, cobalt, copper, fluorine, iodine, iron, manganese, selenium, zinc
Water	Water

Carbohydrates 152 kcal
Protein 28 kcal
Lipids 18 kcal
Total energy 198 kcal

Carbohydrates 38 g

Water 23 g

Protein 7 g

Vitamins
 Thiamin (B_1) .26 mg
 Riboflavin (B_2) .20 mg
 Niacin (B_3) 2.4 mg

(3.5" diameter)

Lipids 2 g

Minerals
 Calcium 29 mg
 Phosphorus 46 mg
 Iron 1.8 mg
 Potassium 50 mg
 Sodium 245 mg

FIG 1-4 Most foods contain a mixture of nutrients; a food's kcal content is based on the energy-yielding nutrients it contains. (Photo from www.thinkstockphotos.com; data from U.S. Department of Agriculture, Agricultural Research Service, Nutrient Data Laboratory: *USDA national nutrient database for standard reference* [Release 26], 2012. Accessed June 13, 2014, from www.ars.usda.gov/ba/bhnrc/ndl/.)

- Each vitamin serves a specific function related to regulation.
- *Aiding growth and repair of body tissues:*
  - Proteins, lipids, minerals, and water are essential for growth and repair.

FOOD, ENERGY, AND NUTRIENTS

Although the discussion to this point has focused on nutrients, we must remember that nutrients are found in foods. Because foods usually contain a mixture of nutrients, we often categorize a food on the basis of the predominant nutrient it contains. A bagel is a carbohydrate food and contains mostly complex carbohydrates, although it also contains protein, water, small amounts of vitamins and minerals, and an even smaller amount of lipids or fat (Figure 1-4). The gold mine of nutrients found in whole foods (foods that are minimally processed) is one of the reasons why taking a nutrient-specific pill will not provide for all the necessities of the human body.

Energy

Let's consider the energy-containing nutrients of carbohydrates, protein, and lipids. These contain energy because they are organic. Being *organic* means they are composed of a structure that consists of hydrogen, oxygen, and carbon. Living or once-living things, including plants and animals, produce organic compounds. The carbon-containing structure identifies these nutrients as being organic. When these nutrients are oxidized (burned in the body), energy is released and available for use by the cells. Although vitamins are also organic, they do not provide energy for the human body. Only carbohydrates, proteins, and lipids are energy-yielding nutrients.

TABLE 1-2 Kilocalorie Values of Types of Food

NUTRIENT	KCAL VALUE PER GRAM
Carbohydrates	4
Protein	4
Lipids (fats)	9
Alcohol	7

The energy released from food is measured in kilocalories (thousands of calories) or calories. Technically, a *calorie* is the amount of heat necessary to raise the temperature of a gram of water by 1° C (0.8° F). When someone asks how much energy is in an 8-ounce glass of skim milk, the correct response is 90,000 calories or 90 kilocalories. For numeric simplicity, we commonly refer to the calories in a food rather than using the correct term, *kilocalories*. To ensure accuracy, the term *kilocalories* (kcal) is used throughout this text.

Energy-yielding nutrients provide different amounts of energy (Table 1-2). Carbohydrates and proteins each provide 4 kcal per gram. Lipids contain more than twice as much energy as carbohydrates or protein, providing 9 kcal per gram. The kcal content of a specific food—for example, a bagel—is based on the amount of carbohydrate, lipid, and protein energy contained in the food (see Figure 1-4). When we consume energy-yielding foods, we usually ingest other nutrients as well, including vitamins, minerals, and water.

Another energy-yielding substance is alcohol. Alcohol provides 7 kcal per gram. Although alcohol provides energy, it is not considered a nutrient because the body does not need it. In fact, when alcohol is consumed in excess, the body treats it as a toxin. Breaking down or metabolizing alcohol not only is stressful to the body but also uses essential nutrients that could be better used to nourish the body. Moderate consumption of alcohol, however, may be protective for heart disease. The beneficial components of alcohol-containing beverages such as red wine are alcohol plus phytochemicals—nonnutritive plant substances found in the ingredients (red grapes) used to produce the alcoholic beverages.

Moderate use of alcohol is defined as two servings or fewer per day for men and one serving for women. One serving of alcohol equals 12 ounces *beer*, 5 ounces *wine*, or 1.5 ounces 80-proof *spirits*. Alcohol should be avoided if any of the following apply: driving a vehicle, being pregnant or breastfeeding, taking certain medications, and having certain medical conditions.

Although proteins, lipids, and carbohydrates provide energy, they—along with the other three nutrient categories, vitamins, minerals, and water—have other important functions. A brief introduction to each nutrient category follows.

Carbohydrates

Carbohydrates are a major source of fuel. They consist of simple carbohydrates, often called sugars, and complex carbohydrates that include starch and most fiber. Simple carbohydrates are found in fruits, milk, and all sweeteners, including white and brown sugar, honey, and high-fructose corn syrup. Complex carbohydrates are found in cereals, grains, pastas, fruits, and vegetables. All, except fiber, are broken down to units of glucose, which is one of the simple carbohydrates. Glucose provides the most efficient form of energy for the body, particularly for muscles and the brain.

Most fiber cannot be broken down by the human digestive system; therefore, it provides little, if any, energy. However, consuming fiber is necessary for good health. Dietary fiber has several beneficial effects on the digestive and absorptive systems of the body. These effects range from preventing constipation to possibly reducing the risk of colon cancer and heart disease.

Proteins

Proteins, in addition to providing energy, perform an extensive range of functions in the body. Some of these functions are roles in the structure of bones, muscles, enzymes, hormones, blood, the immune system, and cell membranes. The linking of amino acids in various combinations forms proteins. Twenty amino acids are required to create all the necessary proteins to maintain life. Some amino acids are formed by the body, whereas others, called *essential amino acids,* must be consumed in foods. The nine essential amino acids are found in animal and plant sources. Animal sources include meat, fish, poultry, and some dairy products, such as milk and cheeses. Plant sources include grains, legumes (peas and beans that contain protein), seeds, nuts, and many vegetables (albeit in small amounts).

Although protein is important nutritionally, eating too much of it can be a problem. Eating substantially more than the recommended amounts of protein does not produce superhumans. Instead, our physical systems can become overworked. Excess protein is broken down to amino acids. The amino acids are then used for energy or broken down further in metabolic processes and are either stored as body fat or excreted through the kidneys in urine.

Lipids (Fats)

Fats are the densest form of energy available in foods and as stored energy in our bodies. Fats, or lipids, serve other purposes, such as functioning as components of all cell structures, having a role in the production of hormones, and providing padding to protect body organs. Essential fatty acids and the fat-soluble vitamins, A, D, E, and K, are found in food lipids. It is the fats in certain foods that make them taste so appealing.

Lipids are divided into three categories: triglycerides, phospholipids, and sterols. Triglycerides are called *saturated, monounsaturated,* or *polyunsaturated fats* according to the types of fatty acids they contain. Fatty acids are carbon chains of varying lengths and degrees of hydrogen saturation. The most common phospholipid is lecithin; among sterols, we hear most about cholesterol. Although we consume lecithin and cholesterol in food, our bodies manufacture them as well.

Fats and cholesterol are often in the news. Saturated fats or triglycerides found in some fat-containing foods, *trans* fats from processed fats, and dietary cholesterol are associated with increased blood lipid levels. Elevations of blood lipids, whether formed by our bodies or consumed in dietary sources, make up a risk factor for the development of coronary artery disease. Saturated fats, and to a certain extent polyunsaturated fats, also have been associated with increased risk for certain cancers. Coronary artery disease and cancer are serious public health diseases that affect millions of North Americans. Consequently, medical and health professionals emphasize the need to reduce intake of foods that contain fats and cholesterol.

Vitamins

Vitamins are compounds that indirectly assist other nutrients through the complete processes of digestion, absorption, metabolism, and excretion. Thirteen vitamins are needed by the body, and each has a specific function. As noted earlier, vitamins provide no energy but assist in the release of energy from carbohydrates, lipids, and proteins.

Vitamins are divided into two classes on the basis of their solubility (i.e., ability to dissolve). The water-soluble vitamins include the B vitamins (thiamin, niacin, riboflavin, folate, cobalamin [B12], pyridoxine [B6], pantothenic acid, and biotin) and vitamin C. The fat-soluble vitamins, which dissolve in fats, are vitamins A, D, E, and K.

Vitamins are found in many foods; fruits and vegetables are particularly good sources. Because some foods are better sources of specific vitamins, eating a variety of foods is the best way to consume sufficient amounts.

Minerals

Minerals serve structural purposes (e.g., bones and teeth) in the body and are found in body fluids. Minerals in body fluids affect the nature of the fluids, which in turn influences muscle function and the central nervous system. The 16 essential minerals are divided into two categories: major minerals and trace minerals. Although this distinction is based on the quantity of minerals required by the body, all are equally important.

Minerals are plentiful in fruits, vegetables, dairy products, meats, and legumes. Although minerals are indestructible, some may be lost through food processing. For example, when whole-wheat flour is processed or refined to white flour, minerals such as phosphorus and potassium are lost and not replaced.

Water

Water is a major part of every tissue in the body. We can live only a few days without water. Water functions as a fluid in which substances can be broken down and reformed for use by the body. As a constituent of blood, water also provides a means of transportation for nutrients to and from cells.

The need for water is more urgent than the need for any other nutrient. (From www.thinkstockphotos.com.)

Many of us probably do not drink enough water or liquids to best meet the needs of our bodies. We should consume the equivalent of about 9 to 13 cups of water a day from foods and beverages (National Research Council [NRC], 2006). Awareness of the value of water consumption is growing as bottled water companies heavily advertise their products to the public. Bottled waters have become a fashionable alternative to other beverages. These products seem to offer convenience and status against which tap water cannot compete. Although more money may be spent on bottled water than is necessary, the health benefits are still achieved. Unflavored, plain water, whether purchased bottled or drunk from public

water supplies, provides the best value; waters fortified with vitamins, minerals, and herbs are not necessary.

DIETARY STANDARDS

Simply knowing which nutrients are essential to life is not sufficient. We need to know how much of each nutrient to consume to be assured of basic good health. Similarly, eating foods without awareness of their nutrient value does not ensure an adequate intake of nutrients. Dietary standards provide a bridge between knowledge of essential nutrients and food consumption. They also provide a guide to adequate nutrient intake levels against which to compare the nutrient values of foods consumed.

Dietary Reference Intakes

In the United States, past dietary standards were based on providing nutrients in amounts that would prevent nutritional deficiency diseases. The current set of nutrient standards, Dietary Reference Intakes (DRIs), combines the classic concerns of deficiency diseases that were the original focus of nutrient recommendations with the contemporary interest of reducing the risk of chronic diet-related diseases such as coronary artery disease, cancer, and osteoporosis. The DRIs also take into account the availability of nutrients, food components, and the use of dietary supplements. They are designed to apply to various individuals and population groups.

Responsibility for dietary standards lies with the Standing Committee on the Scientific Evaluation of Dietary Reference Intakes of the Food and Nutrition Board, Institute of Medicine, and National Academy of Sciences, along with the participation of Health Canada. The DRIs are now the nutrient recommendations for the United States and Canada.

The DRIs are based on (1) reviewing the available scientific data about specific nutrient use, (2) assessing the function of these nutrients to reduce the risk of chronic and other diseases and conditions such as coronary artery disease and cancer, and (3) evaluating current data on nutrient consumption levels among U.S. and Canadian populations.

Dietary Reference Intakes Lingo

The DRIs consist of the Estimated Average Requirement (EAR), the Recommended Dietary Allowance (RDA), Adequate Intake (AI), the Tolerable Upper Intake Level (UL), and Acceptable Macronutrient Distribution Ranges (AMDRs).

The Estimated Average Requirement (EAR) is the amount of a nutrient needed to meet the basic requirements of half the individuals in a specific group that represents the needs of a population. The EAR considers issues of deficiency and physiologic functions. Public health nutrition researchers and policymakers primarily use the EARs to determine the basis for setting the RDAs.

The Recommended Dietary Allowance (RDA) is the level of nutrient intake sufficient to meet the needs of almost all healthy individuals of a life-stage and gender group. The aim is to supply an adequate nutrient intake to decrease the risk of chronic disease. The RDA is based on EARs for that nutrient, plus an additional amount to provide for the particular need of each group. Some nutrients have not an RDA but an AI.

Adequate Intake (AI) is the approximate level of an average nutrient intake determined by observation of or experimentation with a particular group or population that appears to maintain good health. The AI is used when there are insufficient data to set an RDA.

The Tolerable Upper Intake Level (UL) is the level of nutrient intake that should not be exceeded to prevent adverse health risks. This amount includes total consumption from foods, fortified foods, and supplements. The UL is not a recommended level of intake but a safety boundary for total consumption. ULs exist only for nutrients for which adverse risks are known.

Acceptable Macronutrient Distribution Ranges (AMDRs) are daily percentage energy intake values for the macronutrients fat, carbohydrate, and protein. For these energy-yielding nutrients, the following daily intake ranges are set to provide adequate energy and nutrients while offering reduced risk of chronic disorders:
- 45% to 65% of kcal intake from carbohydrate
- 20% to 35% of kcal intake from fat
- 10% to 35% of kcal intake from protein

The DRIs are designed to meet the needs of most healthy individuals. Individuals generally use the RDAs and AIs when assessing their nutrient intakes. People with special nutritional needs, such as those suffering from disease, injury, or other medical conditions, may have nutrient needs that are higher than the DRIs.

Use of Dietary Reference Intakes

The DRIs are widely used throughout the U.S. food systems, for example, in the following activities:
- Planning meals for large groups, such as the military
- Creating dietary standards for governmental food assistance programs, such as the Special Supplemental Nutrition Program for Women, Infants and Children (WIC) and Supplemental Nutrition Assistance Program (SNAP)
- Interpreting food consumption information on individuals and populations

Although originally intended only for analysis of the diets of large groups of people, DRIs can be used for individuals if compared with an average intake over a period of time. The intake of a single day does not have to meet the recommended levels. A comparison with the DRIs does not determine nutritional status but is only one of several measurements used to assess nutritional status, as follows:
- Meeting national nutrition goals such as those listed in *HP2020*
- Developing new food products, such as imitation products, that duplicate the nutrient values of the original

However, the DRI standards are not the basis of the nutrient information that appears on food and supplement products. The Daily Value (DV) is used for nutrition labeling and is based on dietary standards from 1968—when nutrition labeling was first implemented. When the current food labeling standards were revised in 1994, the U.S. Food and Drug Administration (FDA) did not update the nutrient values. (See Chapter 2, under the heading Consumer Information and Wellness, for a detailed discussion of food labeling.)

Additional Standards

The Estimated Energy Requirement (EER) is the DRI for dietary energy intake. The EER aims to maintain good health by providing energy intake levels to maintain individuals' body weights within specific age, gender, height, weight, and physical activity categories. These energy intake recommendations are an average of the need for each category. To avoid recommending potentially excessive intakes of energy, a margin of safety is not added; consuming too much energy may be a primary cause of obesity, a major public health issue that increases chronic disease risk.

Global Standards

Other countries have developed dietary standards on the basis of energy needs, food supply, or environmental factors that affect their populations. In addition, organizations such as the Food and Agriculture Organization of the United Nations, along with the WHO, have developed dietary standards that meet the practical needs of healthy adults worldwide.

Why aren't nutrient recommendations the same for every country or population? After all, the needs of the human body must be the same around the world. The difference lies in the definitions and purposes of nutrient recommendations.

Standards may be designed to provide the basic amount of a nutrient to prevent deficiency symptoms or to supply sufficient amounts for basic good health. These amounts may differ substantially according to the nature of the nutrient, such as whether it is stored in the body. In addition, health professionals of a nation or organization may interpret the same scientific data differently, arriving at various recommended amounts.

Whether a standard is set to provide for only basic nutrient needs may depend on the availability of food. In the United States, where access to food is easy and the supply plentiful, the setting of nutrient recommendations higher than minimum levels is reasonable; most citizens have access to foods to meet those levels. In parts of the world where the food supply is more limited, the immediate goal is to supply as many individuals as possible with basic needs to prevent deficiencies.

Some values differ from the U.S. standards, on the basis of the most common sources of nutrients worldwide. For example, most of the world relies heavily on plant protein sources, whereas North Americans use mainly animal sources. Recommended protein levels reflect this difference.

Ultimately, all standards are simply guidelines. Standards represent a range of the nutrient requirement, even when set at a specific amount. Individual needs may vary, so consuming enough food to meet the basic amounts should be each person's nutritional goal.

ADEQUATE EATING PATTERNS

Knowing the DRIs makes nutrition seem simple. Just eat enough of the DRI nutrients, and good health seems ensured. However, we don't eat nutrients; we eat foods. For an eating pattern to be considered adequate, the foods we eat must provide all the essential nutrients plus fiber and energy. An adequate eating pattern takes into account assortment, balance, and nutrient density.

Assortment addresses the value of eating a variety of foods from every food group. Eating the same foods every day may be convenient but may not serve health and nutrient needs. The limited selection of foods may not contain sufficient amounts of essential nutrients and dietary fiber or may be high in some nutrients, such as fat, and low in others, such as vitamin A. As shown in Figure 1-5, eating a ham and cheese sandwich every day may seem like a quick lunchtime solution, but an assortment of selections over a 5-day period

MONDAY

600 kcal
33 g Fat
100 mg Cholesterol
1480 mg Sodium

TUESDAY

300 kcal
11 g Fat
19 mg Cholesterol
708 mg Sodium

WEDNESDAY

453 kcal
19 g Fat
50 mg Cholesterol
1400 mg Sodium

THURSDAY

535 kcal
30 g Fat
96 mg Cholesterol
1200 mg Sodium

FRIDAY

418 kcal
18 g Fat
0 mg Cholesterol
1400 mg Sodium
(310 mg unsalted peanut butter)

FIG 1-5 An adequate eating pattern incorporates an assortment of foods. Eating the same sandwich every day may be convenient, but an assortment of foods over a 5-day period provides a daily average of fewer calories and a greater variety of nutrients. (Data from U.S. Department of Agriculture, Agricultural Research Service, Nutrient Data Laboratory: *USDA national nutrient database for standard reference* [Release 26], 2012. Accessed June 13, 2014, from www.ars.usda.gov/ba/bhnrc/ndl/.)

FIG 1-6 A balance of nutrients in the diet helps ensure adequacy. (From www.thinkstockphotos.com.)

FIG 1-7 The more nutrients and the fewer kcal a food provides, the higher its nutrient density. (From www .thinkstockphotos.com.)

provides a daily average of fewer calories, less fat, less cholesterol, and less sodium. A good strategy is to adopt a habit of selecting different foods for lunch or, at the least, rotating food choices throughout the week.

An eating pattern exhibiting *balance* will provide foods from all the food groups in quantities so essential nutrients are consumed in proportion to one another, thus achieving a balance among the levels of nutrients eaten. The USDA's food guidance system MyPlate represents this concept by taking into account different food groups and numbers of servings. Balance also ensures that energy plus nutrient needs will equal the intake of energy and nutrients to satisfy adequacy (Figure 1-6).

Nutrient density assigns value to a food on the basis of a comparison of its nutrient content with the kcal the food contains. The more nutrients and the fewer kcal a food provides, the higher its nutrient density. Figure 1-7 demonstrates that a 12-ounce glass of orange juice contains many more nutrients than a 12-ounce soda, which contains "empty" kcal. The orange juice is nutrient dense compared with the soda. Although both may quench your thirst and taste sweet, the orange juice supplies so much more for similar kcal.

No single food contains all the nutrients essential for optimum health. An adequate eating pattern incorporates an assortment of foods.

Undernutrition, Overnutrition, and Malnutrition

Estimates of food consumption are often used to determine the nutritional status of individuals and populations. Sometimes, if the dietary intake is imbalanced, undernutrition, overnutrition, or malnutrition may be diagnosed.

Undernutrition is the consumption of not enough energy or nutrients in comparison with DRI values. This means either not eating enough food to take in all the essential nutrients or eating enough food for energy but choosing foods that lack certain nutrients. In the United States, some women do not consume enough of the vitamin folate, although the rest of their nutrient intake is adequate. Folate

is very important during the childbearing years, as discussed in Chapter 7.

Overnutrition is consumption of too many nutrients and too much energy in comparison with DRI values. North Americans generally over-consume saturated fats, which is a risk factor for the development of heart disease.

Malnutrition is a condition resulting from an imbalanced nutrient and/or energy intake. Malnutrition is both undernutrition and overnutrition—consumption of too few nutrients or too low an energy intake and excess nutrient or energy consumption. An obese man who consumes an excessive amount of kcal is malnourished because his intake is out of balance. His intake does not equal his energy output. A nutrient overdose is malnutrition. In contrast, a college student who constantly diets for slimness or sports, consuming less than the DRI for nutrients and energy, is also malnourished.

TOWARD A POSITIVE NUTRITION LIFESTYLE: *SELF-EFFICACY*

Achieving wellness is an ongoing process. We all experience times when meeting our personal dietary goals is easy and other times when it seems as if we will never regain a sense of control over our nutrition lifestyles. These ups and downs are all part of the process of achieving wellness.

To support our pathway toward achieving wellness, this section in each chapter will feature psychosocial strategies to enhance positive self-efficacy. *Self-efficacy* is our perception of our ability to have power over our lives and behaviors. Positive self-efficacy means believing that personal behaviors can be changed and one has control over one's life. Negative self-efficacy refers to feeling as if one is powerless, with little control over circumstances. A sense of positive self-efficacy is essential to attaining and then maintaining nutrition lifestyles for optimum health. These strategies may be applicable in our own life situations and are useful for our clients as they, too, strive for enhanced self-efficacy.

SUMMARY

- Health is the merging and balancing of the six physical and psychological: physical, intellectual, emotional, social, spiritual, and environmental. Wellness is a lifestyle that enhances our level of health, resulting in a sense of competency and achievement to modify behaviors to increase or maintain positive levels of health.
- Health promotion consists of strategies used to increase the level of the health of individuals, families, groups, and communities. Development of positive behaviors may depend on knowledge, techniques, and community supports.
- *Healthy People 2020 (HP2020)* is a set of national health goals and objectives for the United States that considers the overlapping of environmental and social determinants of health as affecting health outcomes.
- Health literacy is the ability to acquire and comprehend basic health concepts, such as nutrition, and apply them to one's own health decisions.
- Health context takes into account the influence of cultural, social, and individual factors on the acquisition of health literacy.

- Nutrition, the study of nutrients and the processes by which they are used by the body, uses six nutrient categories: carbohydrates, proteins, lipids (fats), vitamins, minerals, and water.
- The functions of essential nutrients are providing energy, regulating body processes, and aiding growth and repair of body tissues.
- Dietary Reference Intakes (DRIs) are a set of dietary standards intended to prevent nutrient deficiency diseases and to reduce the risk of chronic diet-related disorders.
- The DRIs include Estimated Average Requirement (EAR); Recommended Dietary Allowance (RDA), Adequate Intake (AI), Tolerable Upper Intake Level (UL), and Acceptable Macronutrient Distribution Ranges (AMDRs).
- An adequate eating pattern takes into account assortment, balance, and nutrient density. If dietary intake is imbalanced, undernutrition, overnutrition, or malnutrition may occur.

◎ THE NURSING APPROACH

Nurses Assisting with Nutrition—Using the Nursing Process

The Nursing Approach boxes can be found at the end of every chapter of this book. Most boxes include a patient case study (an individualized nurse-patient scenario). As you read each case study, note how the nursing process is used to help a patient improve his/her nutrition status. The nursing process is a systematic method of thinking used widely by nurses to organize the care of individuals, groups, and/or communities. It is similar to the problem-solving method. The nursing process is cyclical, and it is constantly being updated and revised as the patients' needs change. The nursing process components usually follow the sequence of assessing, diagnosing, planning, implementing, and evaluating. Nurses are held legally accountable by their licenses and scopes of practice to assess the patient's health care status, make a judgment about patient responses to actual or potential health problems, design plans to meet identified needs, deliver specific nursing interventions, and evaluate patient outcomes.

Steps of the Nursing Process

The steps of the nursing process can be remembered with the acronym *ADPIE:* assessment, diagnosis, planning, implementation, and evaluation. Following is a more detailed explanation of each step.

Assessment

Definition: Collecting, organizing, and recording patient information obtained through interview, physical assessment, and reading patient charts.

Example: The nurse asks a patient about his/her appetite and how the patient's culture may affect personal food choices. The nurse also obtains the patient's height and weight, records fluid intake and urinary output, and monitors laboratory results.

Assessment may be comprehensive or focused, depending on the situation. The data recorded may be objective (obtained through physical examination and direct laboratory and radiologic studies) and/or subjective (from patients' statements about their history and what they are experiencing). Objective data are sometimes referred to as *signs*—for example, vomiting, grimacing, and moaning. Subjective data are sometimes referred to as *symptoms*—for example, nausea and pain.

Diagnosis

Definition: A clinical judgment about patient responses to actual or potential health problems.

The North American Nursing Diagnosis Association International (NANDA-I) publishes a list of nursing diagnoses, with

◉ THE NURSING APPROACH—cont'd

common causes and evidences. "A nursing diagnosis provides the basis for selection of nursing interventions to achieve outcomes for which the nurse has accountability" (NANDA-I, 2012, p. 515). Four types of nursing diagnoses have been developed by NANDA-I: actual, health promotion, risk, and syndrome, as summarized in the following table (NANDA-I, 2012,

pp. 61-62). The association no longer recognizes "wellness diagnosis" as a nursing diagnosis because this area is encompassed within the health-promotion nursing diagnosis category. You will find examples of each type of nursing diagnosis in the case studies in this book, the most commonly used type being the actual nursing diagnosis.

TYPES OF NURSING DIAGNOSES	DESCRIPTION	EXAMPLES OF NURSING DIAGNOSES RELATED TO NUTRITION
Actual	Problem present at the time of assessment	Imbalanced nutrition: less than body requirements Impaired swallowing Excess fluid volume Deficient knowledge (specify)
Health promotion	Behavior related to desire to increase well-being and actualize health potential	Readiness for enhanced nutrition
Risk	A problem that does not exist, but is likely to develop	Risk for imbalanced nutrition: more than body requirements Risk for constipation
Syndrome	A cluster of nursing diagnoses that occur together and are best addressed through similar interventions together	None present at this time

After assessing the patient, the nurse selects a nursing diagnosis from an established NANDA-I list. Then the nurse identifies and constructs a nursing diagnosis statement for the specific individual patient. The statement may have two or three parts. You will see examples of these statements in the case studies.

Example: Imbalanced nutrition: less than body requirements

Planning

Definition: (1) Establishing priorities; (2) setting realistic, measurable patient outcomes; and (3) deciding which nursing interventions are best.

Example: The patient will gain one pound by August 31.

The plan of care should be developed by a team composed of health care professionals and in cooperation with the patient. The nursing interventions may be prescribed by the physician or nurse practitioner, directed by the registered dietitian/nutritionist, or designed independently by the nurse.

Examples of nursing interventions to support nutrition:
• Provide snacks and supplements in between meals
• Give medicine to counteract nausea, vomiting, and/or pain
• Teach the patient guidelines for following the new diet
• Assist the patient to choose appropriate selections from the hospital menu
• Assist with eating because of weakness or other physical problems

Independent nursing interventions are planned according to the nursing diagnosis and the causes or contributing factors identified. When developing nursing interventions, the nurse must have an understanding of nutrition care for patients with a variety of health conditions. They must be able to support the interventions they select for individual patients with scientific rationale. You will see examples of these rationales in the case studies. Nurses are responsible for evidence-based practice,

choosing interventions on the basis of proven nursing research results.

Implementation

Definition: Carrying out the plan and documenting the care provided. The registered dietitian is the expert in food and nutrition. However, it is usually the nurse who interacts most often with the patient throughout the day and night and is therefore in a position to provide and coordinate the care plan developed by the interdisciplinary team.

Example: Provided 8 fluid ounces of a nutritional supplement twice a day between meals.

Evaluation

Definition: Assessing to what extent the patient outcomes were met and revising the care plan as needed.

Example of a patient outcome: The patient gained one-half pound within 5 days. Goal partially met.

Using *The Nursing Approach* Boxes

The Nursing Approach boxes describe nurses from a variety of settings and levels, including: nurse practitioners and nurses from the hospital, the clinic, home health, occupational health, and schools. Regardless of the setting, the nurse is in a unique position to assess and help improve an individual's nutritional status. The nurse who has practical knowledge of basic nutrition will appreciate the importance of dietary intake in maintaining the patient's good health and in facilitating the patient's recovery from disease or injury. By ensuring that the patient receives adequate nutrition and hydration, the nurse acts as the patient advocate for health, healing, and well-being.

While going through each *The Nursing Approach* box, answer the discussion questions at the end of each case study by using critical thinking skills. A few boxes contain a student learning activity, such as a nutrition teaching project.

APPLYING CONTENT KNOWLEDGE

Health promotion strategies often involve lifestyle changes. Bob needs to reduce his dietary fat intake because he is at risk for coronary vascular disease. He lives in a suburban community and takes a train into New York City, where he works. Although it is only a half mile to the train station, he usually drives his car there to save time. Breakfast is often coffee, with a midmorning break that consists of a Danish and more coffee. He obtains lunch from street vendors who sell hot dogs and sausage sandwiches. Bob usually eats dinner with his family, but it often features meat and potatoes, his favorites. Because he leaves early in the morning and returns tired in the evening, he says he doesn't know how to change his behavior.

Using the strategies of knowledge, techniques, and community supports, describe the education care plan that could be developed with Bob.

WEBSITES OF INTEREST

Academy of Nutrition and Dietetics

www.eatright.org

A resource about nutrition, health, wellness, and dietetic professionals.

Healthy People

www.healthypeople.gov

The official website of Healthy People 2020.

Nutrient Data Laboratory

www.ars.usda.gov/nutrientdata

A nutrient database of food items commonly consumed in the United States.

REFERENCES

Centers for Disease Control and Prevention (CDC): *Health literacy: Accurate, accessible and actionable health information for all*, 2011. From www.cdc.gov/healthliteracy/. Accessed June 1, 2013.

Dubos R: *So human the animal*, New York, 1968, Scribner's.

National Research Council (NRC): *Dietary reference intakes: The essential guide to nutrient requirements*, Washington, DC, 2006, The National Academies Press.

North American Nursing Diagnosis Association International: *Nursing diagnoses: Definition and classifications, 2012-2014*, Ames, IA, 2012, Wiley-Blackwell.

U.S. Department of Agriculture, Agricultural Research Service, Beltsville Human Nutrition Research Center, Food Surveys Research Group (Beltsville, MD) and U.S. Department of Health and Human Services, Centers for Disease Control and Prevention, National Center for Health Statistics (Hyattsville, MD): *What we eat in America*, National Health and Nutrition Examination Survey, 2012. From www.ars.usda.gov/Services/docs.htm?docid=13793. Accessed June 1, 2013.

U.S. Department of Health and Human Services, Office of Disease Prevention and Health Promotion: *Healthy People 2020: Framework: The vision, mission, and goals of Healthy People 2020*, n.d.. From http://www.healthypeople.gov/2020/consortium/HP2020Framework.pdf/. Accessed June 3, 2013.

World Health Organization: *Preamble to the Constitution of the World Health Organization as adopted by the International Health Conference, New York, 19-22 June, 1946; signed on 22 July 1946 by the representatives of 61 States (Official Records of the World Health Organization, no. 2, p. 100) and entered into force on 7 April 1948*. From: www.who.int/about/definition/en/print.html. Accessed June 1, 2013.

CHAPTER 2

Personal and Community Nutrition

The nutritional status of our communities is a reflection of our individual nutritional health.

http://evolve.elsevier.com/GRODNER/FOUNDATIONS

LEARNING OBJECTIVES

- Identify factors that influence food selection.
- Describe the *Dietary Guidelines for Americans, 2010* (*Dietary Guidelines*).
- Discuss the relationship between *Dietary Guidelines*, MyPlate, and Daily Food Plan.

- List the information required on the Nutrition Facts panel.
- Explain the purpose of food label descriptors and health claims.

Have you ever thought about who is responsible for your health? Perhaps you thought of your parents, spouse, or significant other. Or possibly you have always taken your health for granted, not as something to actively work toward improving or maintaining. What influences your health behaviors? What about the health of the community in which you live or work? Have you ever considered the health status of the residents of your town or college community?

The U.S. Department of Health and Human Services (USDHHS) program *Healthy People 2020* approaches these questions through several levels of health determinants:

> Health and health behaviors are determined by influences at multiple levels, including personal (i.e., biological, psychological), organizational/institutional, environmental (i.e., both social and physical), and policy levels. Because significant and dynamic inter-relationships exist among these different levels of health determinants, interventions are most likely to be effective when they address determinants at all levels. Historically, many health fields have focused on individual-level health determinants and interventions. *Healthy People 2020* should therefore expand its focus to emphasize health-enhancing social and physical environments. Integrating prevention into the continuum of education—from the earliest ages on—is an integral part of this ecological and determinants approach. (USDHHS, n.d.)

The health of the individual is tied to the overall health of the population or community. Likewise, the health status of the community is influenced by the shared attitudes and actions of those who reside in it. To support promotion of good health, we must take responsibility for our personal health and the health of communities at large. This chapter considers strategies to improve our health by taking charge of our personal nutrition and becoming aware of the nutrition issues of our communities.

ROLE IN WELLNESS

As presented in Chapter 1, wellness is a lifestyle through which we continually strive to enhance our level of health. Health is the merging and balancing of physical, intellectual, emotional, social, spiritual dimensions, and environmental dimensions. Considering these dimensions in relation to personal and community nutrition broadens our understanding. The *physical health* dimension is represented by the food guides presented in this chapter. By following the recommendations of the food guides, we may reduce the risk of diet-related diseases. Consumer decisions about food purchases and application of food safety recommendations depend on reasoning abilities that reflect the *intellectual health* dimension. The *emotional health* dimension may affect a person's ability to be flexible when adopting suggested guideline changes. If we (or our clients) have problems doing so, will we view ourselves as "failures"? *Social health* dimension is tested as we (and our clients) interact with family and friends while we attempt to follow the guidelines. Can we be role models for others without being perceived as threats? Many religions stress personal responsibility for caring for one's body, which embodies the *spiritual health* dimension. Part of that responsibility includes the foods we choose to eat. The *environmental health* dimension considers access to safe and conducive settings to support preparation and consumption of nutritious meals.

The decisions individuals make about the food they eat determine their health and wellness. Health professionals frequently give advice about appropriate foods for clients to consume. Therefore, it is important for nurses in institutional and community settings to understand how personal factors and community issues that affect food availability, consumption and expenditure trends, consumer information, and food safety can influence a person's food behaviors. The effects of these personal and community factors on consumers' food decisions are some of the major topics of this chapter.

PERSONAL NUTRITION

As an adult, each of us is ultimately responsible for the quality of our dietary intake. Although external forces may affect our everyday food choices, we can decide to have the internal self-awareness to consciously modify those forces. Being accountable for our nutritional status and health may require adjustment of some personal goals to allow time to work on achieving a wellness lifestyle.

Food Selection

Our food preferences, food choice, and food liking affect the foods we select to eat. Although these terms reflect similar food-related behaviors, they are different (Logue, 2004). Food preferences are those foods we choose to eat when all foods are available at the same time and in the same quantity. Factors affecting preferences include genetic determinants and environmental effects. Genetic factors include inborn desires for sweet and salty flavors. Studies of taste receptors note that because of variations in genetic taste markers, some people are "super tasters." Super tasters may experience the taste of vegetables such as broccoli and Brussels sprouts as bitter and therefore avoid such foods, whereas other people find this flavor enjoyable (Negri, et al, 2012). Consumption of cruciferous vegetables, such as broccoli and Brussels sprouts, may be associated with a decreased risk for development of certain cancers. If some people avoid them because of perceived bitter taste, will they be more at risk for cancers?

Environmental effects are learned preferences that are the result of cultural and socioeconomic influences. We often adjust our choices to match those around us. Because we are around our families the most, their influence is the most significant factor in the choices we make; therefore, the dietary patterns we experience as children affect us throughout our lives (Howard, et al, 2012). In fact, even the food a mother eats prenatally affects the preferences of her child in the future (Mennella and Beauchamp, 2001).

An indirect influence on food preferences is the media. Television advertising in particular is a potent force that influences the foods we prefer and buy. Programs spread messages about the food and lifestyle preferences of different socioeconomic groups. A TV show about a working-class family presents images of food intake associated with those of a lower socioeconomic status; dinner might be hot dogs and beans. In another TV show, an upper socioeconomic family might sit down to a meal of baked salmon and salad. Each unintentionally sends messages about appropriate food intake for individuals belonging to the socioeconomic group.

Health promotion issues are tied to food preferences. If recommendations call for changes in foods for which preference is rooted in genetic determinants, the motivation for change needs to be different from when the food preference

is environmentally learned. New preferences can be learned; genetic preferences are more difficult to change.

Food choice concerns the specific foods that are convenient to choose when we are actually ready to eat; rarely are all our preferred foods available at the same time to satisfy our preferences. Food choices are restricted by convenience. As a result of our hectic lifestyles, we tend to avoid foods that take long to prepare. Instead, we often repeatedly choose foods that are easy to prepare and eat, regardless of their nutritional value. Cost is also a factor. We sometimes weigh cost benefits against time benefits. If a food costs more but saves time, we may choose it. We may decide that a food item, even if nutrient dense, costs too much money for the benefits received. Again, nutritional value may not be a prime concern that affects food choice.

Food liking considers which foods we really like to eat. We may want to eat foods that enhance our health, but we like to eat chocolate cake, for example. We constantly weigh all the factors of preference, choice, and liking when we select the foods we eat. Ultimately, these three types of food behaviors greatly affect individual nutritional status (Logue, 2004).

These three food behaviors may be covertly manipulated when the food industry develops and markets foods that appeal to our biological preferences for sugar, salt, and fat. We may become "hooked" into craving processed food products that contain high levels of added sugar, salt, and fat. Physiologic changes that occur create an addiction-like response. These preferences are reinforced by repeated consumption and through advertising promoting the taste of and "having the fun" of consuming these processed products. Marketing strategies of major food corporations have powerful means to mold our food taste preferences (Moss, 2013). Media promotions and product availability may influence selection by consumers because of convenience, including accessibility, cost, and time saving, often with no consideration of nutritional value. Food liking evolves from, and may be the result of, repeated exposures. Although some people are able to moderate their consumption of less nutrient-dense food products, others cannot, thereby impacting their nutritional status and health determinants.

It is the small steps we take that eventually lead to cumulative change. As we study different aspects of food and nutrition, suggestions will be presented that move us and our clients toward significant change. These suggestions will lead to the formation of new personal food habits.

COMMUNITY NUTRITION

The nutritional status of our communities is a reflection of our individual nutritional health. Perhaps the most significant factor affecting the nutritional status of communities is economics. Having sufficient funds to purchase adequate food supplies is a necessity. Public health nutrition efforts to prevent nutrient deficiencies include two federal government programs. The Supplemental Nutrition Assistance Program (SNAP), formerly known as The Food Stamp Program, provides individuals and families whose income are below certain levels with nutrition assistance. Another program is the Special Supplemental Nutrition Program for Women, Infants, and Children (WIC). The WIC program provides nutrition counseling, supplemental foods, as well as referrals to other health care and social services to women who are pregnant or breastfeeding and to infants and children up to the age of 5 who are at nutritional risk. Both programs are provided through the Food and Nutrition Service of the United States Department of Agriculture (USDA) and have a significant impact on improving the nutritional status of those who participate. Additional government programs are discussed in Chapter 10.

Another level of public health nutrition is aimed at the nutrient excesses of our dietary intake. In the late 1970s, a new era in nutrition recommendations began in the United States. Rather than focusing on nutrient deficiencies as a cause of poor health, health professionals began to notice that the cause of an increasing amount of chronic illness was possibly tied to excessive intake of certain nutrients, such as saturated fats, cholesterol, sodium, and sugars. As knowledge of diet-related diseases (e.g., heart disease, hypertension, cancer, diabetes, osteoporosis, and obesity) has improved, sets of dietary recommendations from different government agencies and voluntary health and scientific associations have evolved to address this issue.

Each set of recommendations serves a different purpose. For example, recommendations from the American Heart Association focus on lifestyle and dietary factors that affect risk factors of coronary artery disease, whereas those of the American Cancer Society center on issues related to cancer development. Despite differences in the focus of the recommendations, consensus exists on the guidelines for maintaining general good health. These recommendations are incorporated into our national goals. All recommendations suggest reducing intake of saturated fat, *trans* fat, total fat, cholesterol, sodium, sugar, and excessive kcal and increasing our intake of fiber, complex carbohydrates, fruits, and vegetables. These goals form the basis of health promotion efforts to implement primary, secondary, and tertiary prevention strategies. Education at the community level that reaches as many individuals and families as possible continues to be a challenge for health professionals.

The recommendations are still needed because four of the ten most common leading causes of death in the United States are diet-related disorders—heart disease, cancers, stroke (cerebrovascular disease), and diabetes mellitus (a disorder of carbohydrate metabolism) (Hoyert and Xu, 2012).

Dietary Guidelines for Americans

In response to the dietary recommendations, the USDA and the USDHHS developed the *Dietary Guidelines for Americans,* which were first released in 1980. These guidelines are updated every 5 years and are intended for healthy Americans more than 2 years of age. The *2015-2020 Dietary Guidelines for Americans* are based on the latest scientific knowledge about diet, physical activity, and other health issues. This knowledge is used to formulate lifestyle and dietary pattern recommendations that will contain adequate nutrients, promote health, maintain active lifestyles, and decrease the risk of chronic diseases. As such, the *Dietary Guidelines* serve as the foundation of federal nutrition policy and education (USDA and USDHHS, 2016).

The American public consumes insufficient amounts of certain nutrients, such as vitamin D, calcium, potassium, and dietary fiber, but an excess of solid fats and added sugars (SoFAS), refined grains, sodium, and saturated fat. This combination has resulted in an excessive energy intake that has led to a majority of Americans' being overweight or obese (Figure 2-1).

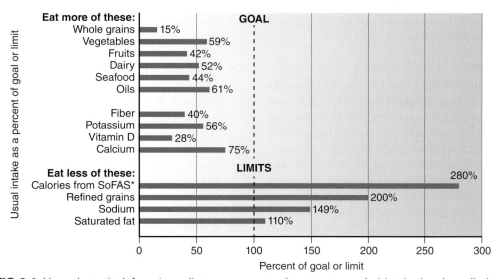

FIG 2-1 How do typical American diets compare to the recommended intake levels or limits? (From U.S. Department of Agriculture and U.S. Department of Health and Human Services: *Dietary Guidelines for Americans, 2010,* ed 7, Washington, DC, 2010, U.S. Government Printing Office. Accessed July 11, 2013, from www.health.gov/dietaryguidelines/dga2010/DietaryGuidelines2010.pdf/.)

The current *2015-2020 Dietary Guidelines for Americans* (hereafter referred to simply as *Dietary Guidelines*), focuses on the goals of "good health and optimal functionality across the life span" with consideration of the malnutrition (deficiency of nutrient intake) and weight issues of the population at large (USDA and USDHHS, 2016). Consequently, to attain these goals, a lifestyle (behavioral) approach is suggested. This approach centers on a total diet concept. To implement a total diet concept that is balanced in energy and nutrient content, dietary patterns would emphasize portion size and greater consumption of plant foods such as vegetables, beans, fruits, whole grains, and nuts and seeds, increased intake of low-fat dairy products, and moderate amounts of poultry, lean meats, and eggs. In addition, lower intake of foods with added sugars and solid fats supports energy balance goals.

To sustain this endeavor, community support will be critical, so that on a population level, individuals and families can adopt these guidelines whether eating at home, at school or work, or in restaurants. Local food availability is a concern to ensure that more nutrient-dense foods are affordable and accessible in all settings from the neighborhood supermarket to fast food restaurants. The techniques to prepare simple home cooked meals and strategies of food safety are prerequisites for achieving the goals of the *Dietary Guidelines*. These techniques and strategies can be taught in nonformal and formal educational settings, including health care clinics, public health departments, faith-based organizations, and print and electronic media.

Box 2-1 lists the five major guidelines that if implemented would assist everyone to practice health-promoting nutrient consumption.

Additional details of the *Dietary Guidelines* are available at health.gov/dietaryguidelines/2015.

As nurses work within communities and/or hospital settings, the *Dietary Guidelines* provide nutrient and health recommendations on which community programming and patient education can be based.

Lifestyle Applications

Your clients and patients would certainly like to follow the *Dietary Guidelines,* but how should they do this? Their busy schedules barely allow time to eat much of anything. Ask them to consider the following nutrition-related suggestions:

- In the morning, choose dry cereals and bread products (e.g., English muffins) that contain whole grains, and alternate or mix these with less-fiber favorites. If no time can be found for breakfast, stock up on portable juices and portable fruit, such as apples, bananas, dried fruits, or a handful of nuts, which can be eaten on the way to class or work. Bring fruit and nuts in backpacks or briefcases for a quick snack.
- Be creative with vending machine selections. Choose healthier-fat and lower-sugar selections such as raisins, bagel chips, pretzels (rub off the excess salt), popcorn, and nuts or trail mix. Some vending machines stock small cans of tuna fish, yogurt, and fruit. Contact the staff responsible

---

BOX 2-1   The Dietary Guidelines for Americans 2015-2020

1. Follow a healthy eating pattern across the lifespan. All food and beverage choices matter. Choose a healthy eating pattern at an appropriate calorie level to help achieve and maintain a healthy body weight, support nutrient adequacy, and reduce the risk of chronic disease.
2. Focus on variety, nutrient density, and amount. To meet nutrient needs within calorie limits, choose a variety of nutrient-dense foods across and within all food groups in recommended amounts.
3. Limit calories from added sugars and saturated fats and reduce sodium intake. Consume an eating pattern low in added sugars, saturated fats, and sodium. Cut back on foods and beverages higher in these components to amounts that fit within healthy eating patterns.
4. Shift to healthier food and beverage choices. Choose nutrient-dense foods and beverages across and within all food groups in place of less healthy choices. Consider cultural and personal preferences to make these shifts easier to accomplish and maintain.
5. Support healthy eating patterns for all. Everyone has a role in helping to create and support healthy eating patterns in multiple settings nationwide, from home to school to work to communities.

From U.S. Department of Agriculture and U.S. Department of Health and Human Services: *2015-2020 Dietary Guidelines for Americans—Executive Summary*, Washington, DC, Accessed on April 10, 2016, from http://health.gov/dietaryguidelines/2015/resources/DGA_Executive-Summary.pdf

---

for filling the vending machines to request healthier selections.

- If lunch and dinner are on the run and fast-food drive-throughs are the only option, select lower-fat items such as grilled chicken sandwiches or plain hamburgers without the sauce. Don't order French fries or milkshakes every time, but instead alternate them with salads and low-fat milk, juice, or water.
- Perhaps lunch and dinner are in a college or employee cafeteria. Try to select turkey, chicken (without the skin), fish, and lean beef dishes. Include whole-grain bread, a grain (rice or pasta), several vegetables, and salad. Try fruit for dessert; it is good with frozen low-fat yogurt, if available.
- Maybe your clients don't really eat "meals" but eat snacks throughout the day. This is called *grazing*. It is possible to graze and follow the *Dietary Guidelines* by choosing wholesome foods instead of candy bars and soda. High-quality grazing foods often available include bagels (with a little cream cheese), yogurt, fruit, pretzels, pizza (but not daily because of the high-fat content of the cheese), and dry cereals with milk. Care must be taken to control for overall calorie intake.

Encourage your clients, the next time they are food shopping or grabbing a snack or meal, to stop a moment and consider the best choices available (Box 2-2).

BOX 2-2 **Implementing Dietary Guidelines: Easier Said Than Done**

As most of us become familiar with the *Dietary Guidelines for Americans* recommendations and MyPlate, we probably reflect on the different food choices available to us and what changes we could most easily implement. But many low-income and unemployed individuals and families don't have the luxury of deciding among a variety of available foods. Instead, their problem is one of food insecurity.

Food insecurity is the limited access to safe, nutritious food, and it may be measured as a marker of undernutrition among people who are also poor and isolated from mainstream society. Retarded growth and iron deficiency along with food insecurity may lead to health disparities because of income, race, and ethnicity. The available financial resources of the households of such individuals and families may not stretch far enough to provide sufficient quantities of high-quality foods. A recurring strain for these families is to provide enough food for their children and themselves; sometimes they may all experience hunger.

In this context, the definition of hunger is not just the physiologic need for food. Instead, a social definition of hunger is the inability to access enough food to feel nourished and satisfied.

Although government programs like food stamps and the Women, Infants, and Children's Program (WIC) and private nonprofit food banks do fill hunger gaps, they are often insufficient to provide enough food for all of those in need. When clients struggle to adopt new dietary guidelines, the nurse should keep in mind the range of food choices easily available to them.

FOOD GUIDES

When we are armed with the latest nutrient recommendations, we can easily apply this knowledge to the way we eat every day. Because we think about what *food* to eat rather than what *nutrients* we need, these nutrient recommendations are most useful when translated into real food. To help us do this, food guides have been developed.

MyPlate

How do we and our clients implement the recommendations of the *Dietary Guidelines* on an everyday basis? In the past, the Food Guide Pyramid filled this purpose, but it has been replaced by the MyPlate food guidance system, which is designed to guide us through our food selections to meet the goals of the *Dietary Guidelines* (USDA/CNPP, 2012). The creation of MyPlate took into account the current patterns of consumption of Americans plus the recommendations of the *Dietary Guidelines* and the Dietary Reference Intakes (DRIs). The result is a total diet that meets the nutrient needs from foods while limiting dietary components that are often eaten in excess. A tool to use in conjunction with MyPlate is the Nutrition Facts labels on food products.

MyPlate is an Internet-based interactive tool providing recommendations based on a person's age, sex, and activity level. Individuals can go directly to the website and enter their own data to receive personalized guides to the food group servings to meet their needs. The food groups on the MyPlate visual are grains, vegetables, fruits, and protein plus dairy (Figure 2-2). MyPlate is intended for adults. Resources can be found at www.ChooseMyPlate.com that focus on other specific target groups, such as preschoolers, children, college students, dieters, pregnant and breastfeeding women, as well as educators/teachers and health care professionals. For individuals who do not have a computer or access to one, or don't have computer skills, hard-copy print materials are available.

By following the interrelated recommendations of MyPlate, the following results can be expected (USDHHS, n.d.):

- Increasing intake of vitamins, minerals, dietary fiber, and other essential nutrients, especially those often consumed at low levels in typical diets
- Lowering intake of saturated fats, *trans* fats, and cholesterol and raising intake of fruits, vegetables, and whole grains, thereby decreasing risk for some chronic diseases
- Balancing intake with energy needs, thereby preventing weight gain and/or promoting a healthy weight

The recommendations represent the following four themes (Figure 2-3):

Variety: Eat foods from all food groups and subgroups.

Proportionality: Eat more of some foods (fruits, vegetables, whole grains, fat-free or low-fat milk products) and less of others (foods high in saturated or *trans* fats, added sugars, cholesterol, salt, and alcohol).

Moderation: Choose types of foods that limit intake of saturated or trans fats, added sugars, cholesterol, salt, and alcohol.

Activity: Be physically active every day.

The simple MyPlate symbol reminds us and our clients to make healthy food choices and to be physically active. The significant concepts of the symbol are highlighted in Figure 2-2.

Other Food Guides

Not all health professionals view the recommendations of MyPlate as the most sound to improve and maintain health. Some cite the rising incidence of diet-related disorders as evidence that MyPlate recommendations do not meet our health goals. These disorders include type 2 diabetes, obesity, and metabolic syndrome (MetS or syndrome X), a group of heart disease risk factors including abdominal obesity, insulin resistance, high blood pressure, and abnormal blood lipid levels. It is also possible that MyPlate is not being followed correctly, resulting in continuing diet-related disorders. As

Getting Started with MyPlate

Choose**MyPlate**.gov

MyPlate Icon

- MyPlate is part of a larger communications initiative based on *2010 Dietary Guidelines for Americans* to help consumers make better food choices.
- MyPlate is designed to *remind* Americans to eat healthfully; it is not intended to change consumer behavior alone.
- MyPlate illustrates the five food groups using a familiar mealtime visual, a place setting.

ChooseMyPlate.gov

- The website features practical information and tips to help Americans build healthier diets.

- It features selected messages to help consumers focus on key behaviors. Selected messages include:

  - ○ **Balancing Calories**
    - ▪ Enjoy your food, but eat less.
    - ▪ Avoid oversized portions.

  - ○ **Foods to Increase**
    - ▪ Make half your plate fruits and vegetables.
    - ▪ Make at least half your grains whole grains.
    - ▪ Switch to fat-free or low-fat (1%) milk.

  - ○ **Foods to Reduce**
    - ▪ Compare sodium in foods like soup, bread, and frozen meals—and choose foods with lower numbers.
    - ▪ Drink water instead of sugary drinks.

- Choose**MyPlate**.gov includes much of the consumer and professional information formerly found on MyPyramid.gov.

USDA
U.S. Department of Agriculture
Center for Nutrition Policy and Promotion   Revised August 2012

FIG 2-2 Getting Started with MyPlate. (From U.S. Department of Agriculture, Center for Nutrition Policy and Promotion: *Getting started with MyPlate,* revised 2012. Accessed June 17, 2013, from www.choosemyplate.gov/downloads/GettingStartedWithMyPlate.pdf/.)

noted earlier, the dietary intake of most Americans is unbalanced in comparison with the recommendations of MyPlate. Intake of meats and grains is higher than recommendations, and consumption of dairy, fruits, and vegetables is lower (Centers for Disease Control and Prevention [CDC], 2010).

One of the first alternative plates to address these concerns was developed by The Nutrition Source of the Department of Nutrition, Harvard School of Public Health (HSPH). Compared with MyPlate, the Healthy Eating Plate provides more guidance as to which types of food in each category to choose on a daily basis. Based on accumulated scientific research, the Healthy Eating Plate includes only whole-grain sources, with limited intake of refined grains, and also highlights plant sources of protein, such as nuts and legumes, and identifies sources of healthful plant oils (Figure 2-4). Fish, poultry, beans, and nuts are listed as protein sources that are lower in saturated fat and dietary cholesterol. Red meat is to be used sparingly or infrequently. Rather than suggesting, as MyPlate does, dairy as a beverage or food to be consumed at every meal, the Healthy Eating Plate recommends water or nonsugary beverages. In addition, the Healthy Eating Plate includes recommendations for daily exercise and weight control (HSPH, 2013) (see Figure 2-4).

Alternative and ethnic food guides are also available, providing specific food selections that conform to the general MyPlate categories. These guides recognize that dietary patterns other than the standard American diet (SAD) offer opportunities to decrease the risk of diet-related disorders. An alternative food guide is represented by The Power Plate, created by the Physicians Committee for Responsible Medicine (PCRM, 2009) (Figure 2-5). A vegan dietary pattern is

Consumer Resources

Let's Eat for the Health of It
The 2010 Dietary Guidelines Brochure

This brochure contains practical strategies to make healthy food choices. The Brochure highlights themes from the Guidelines such as *Balancing Calories, Foods to Reduce,* and *Foods to Increase.* This resource is available online as a PDF.

10 Tips Nutrition Education Series

The 10 Tips Nutrition Education Series provides consumers and professionals with easy-to-follow tips in a convenient, printable format. Educators can use them to support existing lessons, and consumers can choose one or more of these tip sheets to start making small changes toward healthier eating. These and many other printable items are also available in Spanish.

Also on the Web

- Sample Menus for a Week
- Food Group-Based Recipes
- Historical Development of Food Guidance
- Nutrition Communicators Network for Partners – Application Forms
- All print-ready content

MyPlate Style Guide

USDA encourages the use of the MyPlate icon in a variety of applications, including textbooks and other educational materials. Any educator or consumer interested in using the image should refer to this Guide for all appropriate information.

FIG 2-2, cont'd

based on a plant-based dietary intake that eliminates animal-derived foods and nutrients, thereby significantly reducing saturated fat and dietary cholesterol. (Discussed further in Chapter 6.)

Ethnic food guides applicable to North America include Asian, Latino, and African Heritage Diet Pyramids developed by the Oldways Preservation Trust (Oldways) (Figure 2-6). These pyramids differ from MyPlate in the number of servings of animal foods, legumes, varieties of fruits and vegetables, nuts, and seeds recommended (Oldways, 2013). Other countries and commonwealths have food guides reflecting their national food supply, food consumption patterns, and nutritional status. Although the shapes of the guides may differ from MyPlate of the United States, all recommend similar distributions of food category servings. Ethnic and national food guides may be useful to nurses caring for clients from other countries.

"FRUITS & VEGGIES—MORE MATTERS"

Perhaps you have noticed banners and brochures in your local supermarket that proclaim "Fruits & Veggies—More

My Daily Food Plan

Based on the information you provided, this is your daily recommended amount for each food group.

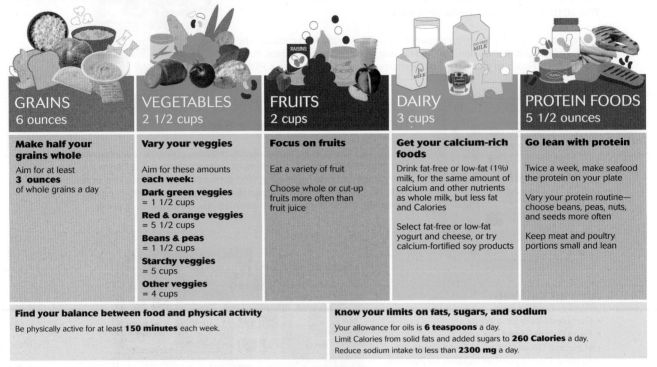

GRAINS 6 ounces	VEGETABLES 2 1/2 cups	FRUITS 2 cups	DAIRY 3 cups	PROTEIN FOODS 5 1/2 ounces
Make half your grains whole Aim for at least **3 ounces** of whole grains a day	**Vary your veggies** Aim for these amounts **each week:** **Dark green veggies** = 1 1/2 cups **Red & orange veggies** = 5 1/2 cups **Beans & peas** = 1 1/2 cups **Starchy veggies** = 5 cups **Other veggies** = 4 cups	**Focus on fruits** Eat a variety of fruit Choose whole or cut-up fruits more often than fruit juice	**Get your calcium-rich foods** Drink fat-free or low-fat (1%) milk, for the same amount of calcium and other nutrients as whole milk, but less fat and Calories Select fat-free or low-fat yogurt and cheese, or try calcium-fortified soy products	**Go lean with protein** Twice a week, make seafood the protein on your plate Vary your protein routine— choose beans, peas, nuts, and seeds more often Keep meat and poultry portions small and lean

Find your balance between food and physical activity	**Know your limits on fats, sugars, and sodium**
Be physically active for at least **150 minutes** each week.	Your allowance for oils is **6 teaspoons** a day. Limit Calories from solid fats and added sugars to **260 Calories** a day. Reduce sodium intake to less than **2300 mg** a day.

Your results are based on a 2000 Calorie pattern.   **Name:** _____

This Calorie level is only an estimate of your needs. Monitor your body weight to see if you need to adjust your Calorie intake.

FIG 2-3 My Daily Food Plan. Visit www.ChooseMyPlate to access your own customized My Daily Food Plan. The plan is created on the basis of the information you provide after clicking on "Get a Personalized Plan." The Daily Food Plan shown meets the needs of a person requiring 2000 kcal per day. (Accessed June 17, 2013, from www.choosemyplate.gov/food-groups/downloads/results/MyDailyFoodPlan_2000_18plusyr.pdf/.)

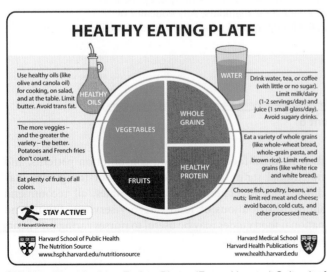

FIG 2-4 The Healthy Eating Plate. (From Harvard School of Public Health: *The nutrition source: Healthy Eating Plate*, Cambridge, MA, 2013, Author. Accessed June 29, 2013, from www.hsph.harvard.edu/nutritionsource/.)

FIG 2-5 The Power Plate. (From Physicians Committee for Responsible Medicine: *The Power Plate*, Washington, DC, 2009, Author. Accessed July 18, 2013, from pcrm.org/health/diets/pplate/power-plate-lose-weight-lower-cholesterol-diabetes/.)

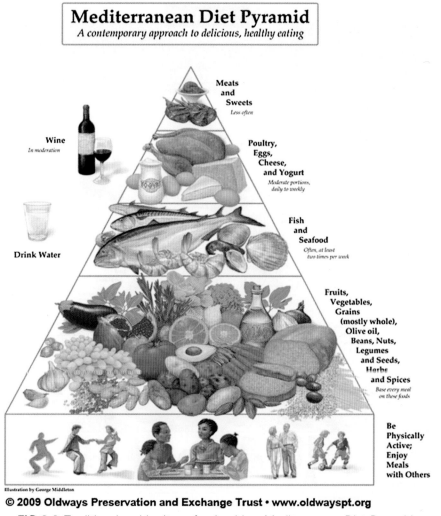

Mediterranean Diet Pyramid
A contemporary approach to delicious, healthy eating

Meats
and
Sweets
Less often

Wine
In moderation

Poultry,
Eggs,
Cheese,
and Yogurt
*Moderate portions,
daily to weekly*

Fish
and
Seafood
*Often, at least
two times per week*

Drink Water

Fruits,
Vegetables,
Grains
(mostly whole),
Olive oil,
Beans, Nuts,
Legumes
and Seeds,
Herbs
and Spices
*Base every meal
on these foods*

Be
Physically
Active;
Enjoy
Meals
with Others

Illustration by George Middleton

© 2009 Oldways Preservation and Exchange Trust • www.oldwayspt.org

FIG 2-6 Traditional and heritage food guides. Mediterranean Diet Pyramid.

Continued

Matters" and other posters advising increased consumption of fruits and vegetables (Figure 2-7). This program represents the first partnership of government, not-for-profit agencies, and private industry to improve the health of Americans. By increasing consumption of fruits and vegetables by all age groups, the program may reduce the risk of certain cancers, diabetes, stroke, and high blood pressure (Produce for Better Health Foundation, 2013).

The CDC is the federal agency leading this public health initiative to encourage and motivate consumers to adopt strategies that result in the consumption of 2 to 6½ cups (4 to 13 servings) of fruits and vegetables as recommended daily. If consumers do so, the goals of the *Dietary Guidelines for Americans, Healthy People,* and other dietary recommendations may be achieved.

Research shows that for American adults the median intake of fruits a day is about 1.1 times a day, compared with the recommended four servings (2 cups); for vegetables, the median intake is about 1.6 times a day, compared with the recommended five servings (2½ cups). Overall, about 50%

of Americans adults report consuming *less than one fruit or vegetable daily* (CDC, 2013). Therefore, most Americans do not meet the recommended five servings (about 2 to 2½ cups each) of fruits and vegetables a day, even though this amount is the minimum amount recommended by MyPlate.

By focusing on only fruits and vegetables, the "Fruits & Veggies" campaign becomes an easy way to decrease intake of fats because fruits and vegetables are naturally low in fat. Consumption of fiber, vitamin C, and beta carotene will increase. These nutrients, in addition to their functions as essential nutrients, are recognized as having the potential to reduce the risk for development of heart disease and certain cancers. Fruits and vegetables are also excellent sources of antioxidants and phytochemicals, for which potential health benefits are continually being uncovered.

Although it may be difficult to determine the percentage of daily dietary fat consumed, it is easy to count the number of servings of fruits and vegetables. If more fruits and vegetables are eaten every day, cravings for high-fat foods will tend to decrease.

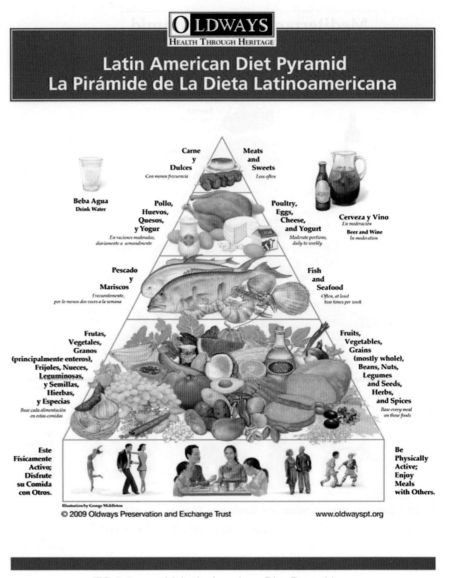

FIG 2-6, cont'd Latin American Diet Pyramid.

Exchange Lists

The food guides refer to eating a number of servings of specific foods daily. But what is a "serving"? A resource for serving sizes is the *Choose Your Foods: Exchange Lists for Meal Planning*, published jointly by the American Diabetes Association (ADA) and the American Dietetic Association (2008), currently known as the Academy of Dietetics and Nutrition. Serving sizes may differ by weight or volume from the portion sizes we receive in restaurants or serve ourselves at home.

Foods are divided into different groups or lists: carbohydrates, meat and meat substitutes, and fats. Each list or exchange contains sizes of servings for foods of that category, and each serving size provides a similar amount of carbohydrate, protein, fat, and kcal. The carbohydrate group is subdivided into lists for starch, fruit, milk, other carbohydrates, and vegetables. The meat and meat substitute group is sorted by fat content (Table 2-1).

The exchange lists were first developed for use by people with diabetes. A dietitian can create an appropriate dietary program that prescribes the number of kcal and units of each exchange category to be consumed daily as well as a plan for when foods should be eaten. By using the exchange lists for carbohydrate counting, an individual can choose favorite foods from each list while controlling the amount and kind of carbohydrates consumed throughout the day.

Guidelines for individuals with diabetes, published by the ADA, deemphasize prescribed calculated kcaloric diets only using the exchange lists (ADA/ADA, 2008). The focus is now on adapting dietary intake to meet individual metabolic nutrition and lifestyle requirements (see Chapter 15).

The exchange lists encourage variety and help to control consumption of kcal and grams of carbohydrates, protein, and fats. As a tool for dietary instruction, these lists have been adapted to meet the needs of weight-reduction programs and nutrition care planning.

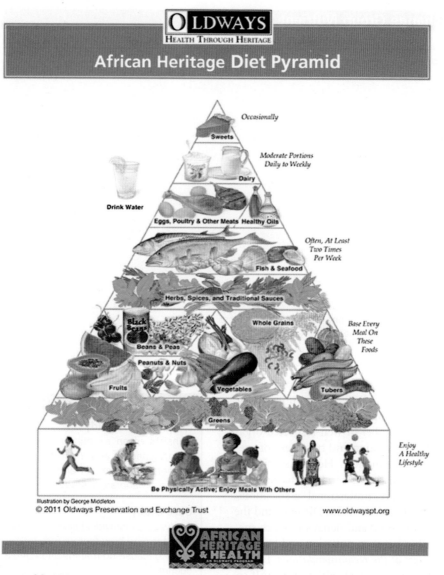

FIG 2-6, cont'd African Heritage Diet Pyramid. (From Oldways Preservation Trust: *Mediterranean Diet Pyramid*, *Latino Diet Pyramid*, *Asian Diet Pyramid*, and *African Heritage Diet Pyramid*, Cambridge, Mass, 2013, Author. Accessed June 15, 2013, from, respectively, http://oldwayspt.org/resources/heritage-pyramids/mediterranean-pyramid/overview/, http://oldwayspt.org/resources/heritage-pyramids/latino-diet-pyramid/overview, and http://oldwayspt.org/resources/heritage-pyramids/african-diet-pyramid/overview/.)

FIG 2-7 Logo for "Fruits & Veggies—More Matters." (Courtesy of Produce for Better Health; retrieved from www.fruitsandveggiesmorematters.org.)

Criteria for Future Recommendations

Although the current recommendations are expected to provide sound advice for a while, other organizations may issue their own guidelines in the future. Which guidelines should we follow? Should we change our eating habits and revise client dietary recommendations for each new study? Or, to avoid confusion, should new recommendations just be ignored?

Following are criteria to use to evaluate future dietary guidelines and recommendations:

Consider the source of the nutrition advice. Are the recommendations from a federal government agency? If so, the work of these agencies is usually reviewed by health and

TABLE 2-1 Exchange Group Nutrient Values

GROUPS/LISTS	CARBOHYDRATE (g)	PROTEIN (g)	FAT (g)	CALORIES
Carbohydrates Group				
Starch	15	3	0-1	80
Fruit	15	—	—	60
Milk:				
Fat-free	12	8	0-3	90
Reduced-fat	12	8	5	120
Whole	12	8	8	150
Other carbohydrates	15	Varies	Varies	Varies
Vegetables	5	2	—	25
Meat and Meat Substitute Group				
Very lean	—	7	0-1	35
Lean	—	7	3	55
Medium-fat	—	7	5	75
High-fat	—	7	8	100
Fat Group	5	45		

This table shows the amount of nutrients in one serving from each list.

From American Diabetes Association/American Dietetic Association: *Choose your foods: Exchange lists for diabetes,* Alexandria, VA/Chicago, 2008, Authors.

nutrition professionals before release to the public. If the advice is from a private nonprofit group, is the group nationally recognized? A number of well-respected organizations are devoted to prevention and treatment of specific diseases, such as the American Heart Association, American Cancer Society, and American Diabetes Association. In addition, there are professional associations, including the Academy of Nutrition and Dietetics and the Society for Nutrition Education and Behavior, which specialize in the relationship between nutrition and health.

Assess the comprehensiveness of the recommendations. Do the recommendations address only one health problem? If so, is that a health problem that affects your clients? Would following these recommendations have any negative effects? Would a category of nutrients be under-consumed if they were followed? Recommendations addressing several health issues are usually more complete and provide a higher level of prevention.

Evaluate the basis of the recommendations. How were the recommendations determined? The current recommendations are based on many research studies on the relationships between diet and diseases. If new recommendations are issued, are they based on the results of new studies? If so, how many and what kinds of studies (Box 2-3)? Collecting this type of information means doing more than just listening to a 2-minute radio announcement or a 5-minute TV report. Some newspaper articles contain in-depth evaluations of research; others just skim the surface. It may be necessary to read the original study in the library or on the Internet, or to discuss the recommendations with other health professionals.

Estimate the ease of application. Can the recommendations be easily adopted? Are they presented in terms of foods

BOX 2-3   Types of Research

Experimental Study

Consists of an experimental group receiving treatment (or dietary change) and a control group receiving no treatment (or dietary change); differences, if any, are then noted; called *clinical* or *laboratory study.*

Case Study

Analyzes an individual case of a disease or health difference to determine how factors may influence health; a naturalistic study because no manipulation of dietary intake or behaviors occurs.

Epidemiologic Study

Studies populations; tracks the occurrence of health or disease processes among populations; may use historical data, surveys, and/or medical records to determine possible factors influencing the health of a group of people.

(easier to apply) or nutrients (harder to apply)? Is a degree in nutrition needed to understand them?

CONSUMER FOOD DECISION MAKING

Community supports can have an impact on the quality of personal nutrition. Most important are the consumer decisions a person makes daily when buying food to be prepared in the home or when eating out.

Food Selection Patterns

Food selection patterns may be estimated by assessing government data gathered through national surveys and programs. One approach is to compare a client's choices with the national recommendations of the online MyPlate SuperTracker. Developed as part of the MyPlate food guidance system, the MyPlate SuperTracker measures the dietary quality of an individual's food intake and physical activity according to the extent to which the intake follows the *Dietary Guidelines* and the Daily Reference Intakes (DRI) recommendations (available at www.supertracker .usda.gov.)

According to research, people with more healthful dietary intakes have higher levels of nutrition knowledge and advanced education levels. Consequently, the data reveal that higher socioeconomic characteristics are related to a greater understanding of nutrition and of the effects of healthy diets in reducing the risks of diet-related disorders (Beydoun and Wang, 2008). This difference may reflect access to resources (e.g., time and financial means) that support preparation and consumption of foods that follow the dietary guidelines.

As a nation we need to improve our nutrient intake. An aspect of doing so must take into account our beliefs about and attitudes toward our dietary intake. A study using national data reveals that only 23% of the surveyed population is interested in improving their intake, whereas 37% are not interested in doing so, and 40% believe their intake does not need to change. Most view healthy eating as too complicated. In addition, the majority views snacking as an unhealthy practice, and as a result, the majority chooses snacks that are also unhealthy (Hartman Group, 2009).

Application to Nursing

When working with clients, we can be aware of their attitudes toward nutrition and dietary change. Although changing dietary intake is a prime strategy to reduce the risk of diet-related chronic disorders, many Americans are not interested in changing their eating behaviors. In addition, the belief that snacking is unhealthy is unfortunate. Snacks do not have to be high fat, high sodium, or calorie laden. Consuming additional fruits, vegetables, and whole-grain foods is often best accomplished through wisely selected additional "mini-meals" or snacks. We may need to educate or remind clients about the nutritional benefits of dietary change as a disease-prevention strategy, and we should definitely emphasize the positive value of snacking on wholesome foods. Providing clients with simple techniques for changing food selection habits is crucial.

Food Consumption Trends

Food consumption trends reflect the food decisions Americans made in the past. Tracking these trends is the responsibility of the USDA. Following changes in consumption trends across the years for specific foods reveals information about food substitutions, including food prices or technologic changes that bring new types of food products to the marketplace. Food consumption trends now show that generally Americans eat more food away from home in larger portions and with additional snacks, resulting in a greater caloric intake than in the past (Guthrie, et al, 2013).

Implications of food consumption trends. Food consumption trends affect the nutritional status of the U.S. population. Consumption can be gauged from grocery purchase data, which show that Americans underspend on fruits, vegetables, and whole grains and overspend on fats, refined grains, sweets, and convenience foods (Guthrie, et al, 2013). Grocery purchase data cover just food purchased for home consumption. They do not show the impact of away-from-home food consumption, which now constitutes one-third of daily caloric intake for the average American. Away-from-home foods tend not be as wholesome as at-home foods (Guthrie, et al, 2013) (Figure 2-8).

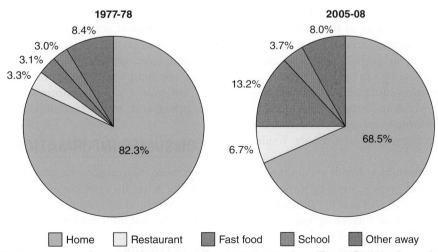

FIG 2-8 Expenditures for away-from-home food are increasing. (From Guthrie J, et al: *Americans' food choices at home and away: How do they compare with recommendations? Amber Waves*, February 21, 2013. Accessed July 5, 2013, from www.ers.usda.gov/amber-waves/2013-february/americans-food-choices-at-home-and-away.aspx#.UdN7InDD8iQ/.)

Factors affecting these trends may include cost, availability, knowledge, and time. Income differences may account for the varying consumption levels. Lower-income households report consuming fewer fruits and vegetables than other households. Costs of fruits and vegetables have been rising because of increased energy and production costs. Because consumers expect seasonal produce to be available year-round, transportation costs rise as produce travels halfway around the world to arrive on our grocer's stands. Although all households are affected, price increases for produce in any form (fresh, frozen, or canned) limits the food-buying power of lower-income households more.

Cost may be tied to availability. If under-consumed foods are in limited supply to be purchased, the price may be higher than if they are easily available. If communities have access to reasonably priced nourishing foods, residents will purchase and eat healthier foods. Improving such access may mean increasing the number of food outlets in both rural and urban areas (Dutko, et al, 2012). A study of locations of supermarkets, super-centers, and large grocery stores finds that there are about 6500 food desert tracts in the United States (Hagan and Rubin, 2013). *Food deserts* are areas where residents do not have adequate access to affordable and quality sources from which to purchase food. There simply are not enough supermarkets or grocery stores to meet the needs of the population. Although poverty is a common factor in both rural and urban communities, other determinants, such as inadequate public and/or personal transportation and communities of color, may increase the likelihood of food deserts (Hagan and Rubin, 2013). Elimination of food deserts will provide access to wholesome foods for residents while strengthening the economic viability of communities through increased food retail employment opportunities.

Does knowledge affect food consumption trends? Everyone knows that fruits and vegetables are healthier options than processed food and snacks, yet highly processed foods and snacks are too often chosen. So what knowledge is needed? Generally, many consumers could learn how to prepare a wider variety of vegetables so they taste and look good and are safe to eat. Consumers need to know that frozen fruits and vegetables can be as nutritious as fresh and are available year round. Teaching how to buy and prepare foods is an adjunct goal of nutrition education. In addition, efforts by the government and private industry to make food labels and point-of-purchase information easier to understand and apply may increase preference for nourishing foodstuff (Guthrie, et al, 2013).

Time as a factor of consumption trends encompasses the limiting of time to shop and prepare meals by work, school, and/or family responsibilities as well as other distractions of contemporary lifestyles (such as increasing use of digital technology). As Michael Pollan, author of *Cooked: A Natural History of Transformation* (2013), remarks:

> Survey research confirms we're cooking less and buying more prepared meals every year. The amount of time spent preparing meals in American households has fallen by half since the mid-sixties, when I was watching my mom fix dinner, to a scant twenty-seven minutes a day. (Americans spend less time cooking than people in any other nation, but the general downward trend is global.) And yet at the same time we're *talking* about cooking more—and watching cooking, and reading about cooking, and going to restaurants designed so that we can watch the work performed live. We live in an age when professional cooks are household names, some of them as famous as athletes or movie stars. The very same activity that many people regard as a form of drudgery has somehow been elevated to a popular spectator sport.

Although these trends reflect per capita consumption patterns based on the total population, it is our individual consumer food decisions that have the greatest influence on our personal level of wellness.

Effective Food-Buying Styles

This chapter is full of information about consumer decisions, but how is it to be applied? How do you and your clients become better shoppers? The first step is to tailor a shopping style to one's particular situation. (See the *Personal Perspectives* box, What's for Dinner?) Consider the following issues to formulate the most effective approach to food shopping:

Food budget: A food budget should take into account the funds needed to keep a moderate amount of food in the home and the money spent on meals away from home.

Consumer diversity: Buying food for a single young adult is different from buying for a family. Lifestyles of household members affect the number and types of meals served and the kinds and amounts of food served.

Dietary preferences: We all have food preferences based on ethnicity, habits, chronic illness, or ethical views such as vegetarianism. Each preference affects food-buying selections.

Shopping frequency: Each household works best with a shopping plan—perhaps weekly, every 2 weeks, or on the way home from school or work when things are needed.

Location and types of food stores: Different types of food stores provide a range of services and products. Conventional supermarkets, superstores, super centers, and super warehouse stores are valuable for fresh produce, perishables, and basic grocery items; wholesale clubs and limited assortment warehouse stores are good for bulk foods at low prices; specialty stores offer unique foods at high prices; and convenience stores "save the day."

CONSUMER INFORMATION AND WELLNESS

The more information consumers have about the food they eat, the better they can choose foods that contribute to wellness. Nutrition education is necessary for consumers to use the additional information appropriately.

Food Labeling

Food labels are the best way for consumers to see how individual foods fit their nutritional needs. The function of food labels is twofold (U.S. Food and Drug Administration [FDA],

What's for Dinner?

LocalHarvest.org, a unique website, is a dynamic nationwide directory of small farms, farmers markets, and other local food sources. The site search engine connects consumers with sources of local sustainably grown food and family farms, some accessible through an online store. In this newsletter issue, Erin Barnett, director of LocalHarvest.org, shares her strategy for "meal planning."

Three years ago this month I started taking a new approach to meal planning. It sounds like an exaggeration, but it really has changed my life. If you're like me, you like to cook, but don't enjoy deciding what's for supper, especially under duress. There is nothing that drains the energy and ratchets up the stress quite like arriving home after work tired and hungry, with no idea what to make. Add a couple of tired and hungry kids to the mix, and it is easy to see why there is often a long line at the drive-through.

My new approach takes about 30 minutes a month, 45 if I get fancy. Around the first of the month—ideally before the new month begins—I sit down with a calendar and jot down a supper menu for every night of the month ahead. Usually I have some idea of which nights are likely to be a little hectic or unusual around the dinner hour, so I can plan simple meals for those nights. ("Tacos and leftover squash.") Similarly, I can plan to do a little extra cooking on the weekends if it is going to be a particularly busy week. ("Quiche and salad; bake a squash for Tuesday.") It really is not that hard, but it has changed how we eat. That far ahead, mood and whim do not factor in—it is easy and neutral. If need or craving arise, I can always change the menu on any given day, but usually I am so glad to have it decided that I just make whatever is on the calendar.

The benefits here are many. Looking at our diet a whole month at a time helps me balance out the protein sources and the kinds of vegetables to make sure we are getting a good variety. It helps me anticipate and create a steady flow of leftovers so we always have something to take for our lunches. I have also found that this method helps eliminate food waste. There are just three people in our family, so it takes us a few meals to get through a roasted chicken or a head of cabbage. By looking ahead, I can shop less often and make a plan to use everything.

Once I was asked to share my calendar, and the friend who looked at it was aghast: "But where's the Pad Thai?" Aha! Lesson learned. We all eat differently, so these calendars are highly individualized and, sadly, not transferable. Nor are they as replicable as I had thought they would be. Initially, I planned to only do this for one full year, thinking that I would just save the calendar and repeat it the following year. My family eats quite seasonally, so I figured that the available produce would be similar to the same month the year before. More or less it is, but our tastes change over time, and some years I have more interest and time for cooking than others. So I look at the past year's calendar for reference, but create an updated version every month. It's time well spent.

How do I know? If I am running a few days behind and planning the whole month starting with tonight, it is that square—tonight—that is invariably the last to be filled in. The rest of the month takes maybe 30 minutes, and I spend another 15 trying to figure out what to make tonight. "What's for supper?" Try this idea, and you'll wrestle with that question only once a month.

As always, eat well and take good care.

From Barnett E: What for dinner? *The LocalHarvest Newsletter*, January 26, 2012. Accessed July 9, 2013, from: www.localharvest.org/newsletter/20120126/.

2000). The first is to help consumers select foods with the most health-providing qualities. The second is to motivate food companies to enhance the nutritional value of food products because labels reveal ingredient and nutrient content.

Food labeling for processed foods in the United States is based on standards established under authority of the 1990 Nutrition Labeling and Education Act. Although nutrition labeling is mandatory for most processed products, it is voluntary for fresh meat, poultry, fish, milk, eggs, and produce. An example of the label for processed foods is shown in Figure 2-9.

The Nutrition Facts panel on the food packaging must list the quantities of energy (kcal), fat, and the following other specific nutrients in a serving:
- Total food energy
- Food energy from fat
- Total fat
- Saturated fat
- *Trans* fat
- Cholesterol
- Sodium
- Total carbohydrates
- Dietary fiber
- Sugars
- Protein
- Vitamins A and C
- Calcium
- Iron

The **Daily Values (DVs)** is a system for food labeling composed of two sets of reference values: reference daily intakes (RDIs) and daily reference values. The percent of Daily Values information (%DV), based on a 2000-kcal diet, is intended to show consumers how much of a day's ideal intake of a particular nutrient they are eating. DVs for selected nutrients and food components based on a 2500-calorie diet are also given at the bottom of the label.

Uses of Percent of Daily Values Information

The %DV is useful to make comparisons between products, to assess nutrient content claims, and to choose a mix of foods to balance nutrient intake. Making comparisons among

FIG 2-9 An example of the food label format that currently is mandatory in the United States. (From U.S. Food and Drug Administration, Center for Food Safety and Applied Nutrition: *How to understand and use the nutrition facts label*, College Park, MD, 2000 [updated November 2004; March 2013], Author. Accessed July 6, 2013, from www.fda.gov/Food/IngredientsPackagingLabeling/LabelingNutrition/ucm274593.htm/.)

%DVs of similar products is possible if the serving sizes are the same. Which brand has the lowest fat content? Which has the highest fiber content? Assessing nutrient content claims is simple when using %DV. By considering the %DVs of fiber in two food products, the consumer can quickly determine the better source of fiber. This can be used for any nutrient content claim. Using %DV to balance nutrient intake is accomplished by combining foods high in %DV of a particular nutrient, such as fat, with foods low in %DV of that nutrient. A person's daily intake of fat can still be less than 100%DV.

Uniform definitions for food descriptors, such as light and low-fat, for nutrient content claims are now clearly established and must be consistently used for all foods (FDA, 2009) (Box 2-4). This information helps consumers who try to control their intakes of specific nutrients and food components.

Manufacturers have increased the proportion of whole-grain ingredients in many products so consumers can more easily achieve the *Dietary Guidelines'* recommendation to consume at least 3 ounces of whole grains daily—and to remain competitive with other products. The Whole Grains Council, an Oldways Program that includes scientists,

manufacturers, and chefs, developed two stamps to appear on packaging that identify the whole-grain content of a product (Figure 2-10). The "100% Whole Grain Stamp" on a product signifies that all of the grain ingredients are whole grains and that each product serving contains a minimum of 16 g of whole grains, which equals one ounce of whole grains. The "Basic Whole Grain Stamp" means that each product serving contains at least 8 g or more of whole grains or half a full serving (equaling 0.5 ounce of whole grains). If the product also contains refined grains, such as extra bran, germ, or refined flour, the Basic Stamp must be used regardless of the total amount of whole grains provided. (Whole-grain content is not the same as dietary fiber content, even though dietary fiber is part of the whole grain.)

Organic Food Standards and Labels

Fresh produce and a variety of foods are labeled "organic." Just what does *organic* mean? The USDA established national standards for food products to be labeled organic, regardless of where they are grown or processed. Farmers who produce organic food focus on the use of renewable resources and soil and water conservation to maintain and/or improve the

BOX 2-4   Food Descriptors

Free

Contains only a tiny or insignificant amount of fat, cholesterol, sodium, sugar, and/or calories. For example, a "fat-free" product contains less than 0.5 g of fat per serving.

Low

"Low" in fat, saturated fat, cholesterol, sodium, and/or calories; can be eaten fairly often without exceeding dietary guidelines. So, "low in fat" means no more than 3 g of fat per serving.

Lean

Contains less than 10 g of fat, 4 g of saturated fat, and 95 mg of cholesterol per serving. "Lean" is not as lean as "low." "Lean" and "extra lean" are US Department of Agriculture terms for use on meat and poultry products.

Extra Lean

Contains less than 5 g of fat, 2 g of saturated fat, and 95 mg of cholesterol per serving. Although "extra lean" is leaner than "lean," it is still not as lean as "low."

Reduced, Less, Fewer

Contains 25% less of a nutrient or calories. For example, hot dogs might be labeled "25% less fat than our regular hot dogs."

Light/Lite

Contains one third fewer calories or one half the fat of the original. "Light in sodium" means a product with one half the usual sodium.

More

Contains at least 10% more of the daily value of a vitamin, mineral, or fiber than the usual single serving.

Good Source of ...

Contains 10% to 19% of the daily value for a particular vitamin, mineral, or fiber in a single serving.

From U.S. Food and Drug Administration, Center for Food Safety and Applied Nutrition: *Guidance for Industry: A food labeling guide: IX. Appendix A: Definitions of nutrient content claims,* College Park, MD, 2009 (October), Author.

Each Stamp also shows a number, telling you how many grams of whole grain ingredients are in a serving of the product.

THE BASIC STAMP	THE 100% STAMP
Product may contain some extra bran, germ, or refined flour.	For products where ALL of the grain is whole grain.
Minimum requirement: 8g (8 grams) whole grain per serving. (one half serving of whole grain)	Minimum requirement: 16g (16 grams) whole grain per serving. (a full serving of whole grain)

FIG 2-10 Whole Grain Stamps. (From The Whole Grains Council, an Oldways Program, Oldways Preservation Trust, Boston, MA. Whole Grain Stamps are a trademark of Oldways Preservation Trust and The Whole Grains Council; www.wholegrainscouncil.org/.)

Consumption of fruits and vegetables may reduce the risk of diet-related disorders. (From thinkstock.com.)

environment for the future. Animal-derived foods such as meat, poultry, eggs, and dairy products are labeled organic if no antibiotics or growth hormones are used in the rearing of the animals. Produce is grown without the use of conventional pesticides, synthetic fertilizers, bioengineering, or radiation. Before a product can be labeled organic, certification by government-approved inspectors is required of farms where foods are grown, as well as of companies that process foods, to ensure that the USDA organic standards are followed (USDA, 2012).

Specific labeling rules exist for foods containing organic ingredients (USDA, 2012). Single-ingredient foods may use the organic seal and the word *organic* on labeling or on display posters. These foods may include fresh fruits, vegetables, cheese, cartons of eggs or milk, meat packages, and other single-ingredient foods. When foods contain more than one ingredient, specific labeling categories are followed (Box 2-5).

The term *natural* may also be used, but it is not the same as organic. *Natural* often signifies that the ingredients of a product are less processed and more wholesome but does not address how the ingredients were grown or the animals

BOX 2-5 Labeling Definitions for Organic Foods

Look for the U.S. Department of Agriculture (USDA) organic seal on raw, fresh products, and processed products that contain organic agricultural ingredients. Or the seal may appear on a sign above an organic produce display.

On multi-ingredient products, the seal is usually placed on the front of the package (principal display panel); however, it may be placed anywhere on the package. When you see this seal, you know the product is at least 95% organic.

The seal may be printed in green and brown (as shown), in black and white, or outlined in black on a transparent background.

From U.S. Department of Agriculture, Agricultural Marketing Service, National Organic Program: *Understanding organic labeling,* Washington, DC, 2010, Author. Accessed July 9, 2013, from http://www.ams.usda.gov/AMSv1.0/ams.fetchTemplateData.do?template=TemplateA&navID=NationalOrganicProgram&leftNav=NationalOrganicProgram&page=NOPUnderstandingOrganicLabeling&description=Understanding%20Organic%20Labeling&acct=nopgeninfo/.

reared. *Organic* means that the food is certified as fulfilling the USDA organic standards for farming and/or rearing of animals, not how the ingredients have been processed during the manufacturing procedures. Organic soda prepared from organically grown sugar and/or high-fructose corn syrup and flavorings is not more nutrient dense or natural than a soda from a national beverage company containing similar ingredients grown under conventional means. Consumers need to be savvy about the nutrient density of the foods chosen regardless of whether the product meets USDA organic standards (see Box 2-5).

Application to nursing. Check the Nutrition Facts panels for products purchased regularly. Ingredients may be changed by manufacturers, and similar products may be created from different formulations. This may result in modifications of ingredients and serving sizes that affect calories and nutrient content. (See the *Teaching Tool* box Just the Facts: Using Labels to Teach Nutrition Literacy for information on how to help clients evaluate food labels.)

✳ TEACHING TOOL

Just the Facts: Using Labels to Teach Nutrition Literacy

Health care providers view nutrition as a basic component of health education and refer patients to nutritionists for nutrition education. Nurses are in the position to reinforce nutrition concepts first presented by dietitian/nutritionists. Although physicians may be viewed as the experts on health, patients who have low literacy skills tend to use their social network of family and friends for health and nutrition information. Consequently, for interventions to be successful, members of social networks should be included. The approach should be visual, interactive, and culturally appropriate. This lesson on label comprehension fits these three criteria.

Clients should be presented with three boxes of cereal or Nutrition Facts labels from three cereal products. Choose three different products. For example, include a heavily presweetened cereal, a lightly sweetened cereal, and one with no added sweeteners. Ask the following questions:

Which has the most kcal per serving? This may be affected by weight, volume of the cereal (popped with air), and the density of added ingredients like raisins.

Which has the largest serving size? Serving sizes are the same by weight for all products in a food category.

Which contains the most dietary fat? Fat is not an issue with cereals, except for granola.

Which contains the most sodium? Some cereals contain about 300 mg, which is high for sodium-sensitive clients.

Which contains the most added sugars? Added sugars can range from none to 13 g per serving.

How many calories come from sugars? Multiply the number of grams of sugars by 4 kcal. By dividing this number by the total kcal per serving and multiplying the decimal by 100, you can determine the percentage of sugar content.

Which contains the most fiber? Fiber content can range from none to about 5 g per serving.

As your study of nutrition continues, you may add other questions and be able to relate client responses to preventive health issues of diet-related diseases or to address specific dietary needs of a patient's nutrition recommendations.

Data from Lee SY et al: Health literacy, social support, and health: a research agenda, *Soc Sci Med* 58(7):1309-1321, 2004.

Health Claims

Health claims relating a nutrient or food component to the risk of a disease or health-related condition now appear on food labels. Only health claims approved by the FDA may be on the label. This information helps consumers select those foods that can keep them healthy and well.

So far, the health claims allowed include relationships between the following:

- Potassium and reduced risk of high blood pressure (hypertension)
- Plant sterol and plant stanol esters and heart disease (Plant sterols and stanols are substances found naturally in certain plant foods that provide health benefits.)
- Whole grains and reduced risk of heart disease and certain cancers
- Soy protein and reduced risk of heart disease
- A diet with enough calcium and a lower risk of osteoporosis
- A diet low in total fat and a reduced risk of some cancers
- A diet low in saturated fat, cholesterol, and *trans* fat and a reduced risk of coronary heart disease
- A diet rich in fiber-containing grain products, fruits, and vegetables and a reduced risk of some cancers
- A diet rich in fiber-containing grain products, fruits, and vegetables and a reduced risk of coronary heart disease
- A diet low in sodium and a reduced risk of high blood pressure
- A diet rich in fruits and vegetables and a reduced risk of some cancers
- Folic acid and a decreased risk of neural tube defect–affected pregnancy
- Dietary sugar alcohols and a reduced risk of dental caries (decay)
- Fluoridated water and reduced risk of dental caries (decay)
- Soluble fiber from certain foods, such as whole oats and psyllium seed husk, as part of a diet low in saturated fat and cholesterol and a reduced risk of heart disease

Food labeling legislation also covers dietary supplements. The Dietary Supplement Health and Education Act of 1994 (DSHEA) requires the FDA to prove that a dietary supplement is unsafe or adulterated or has false or misleading labeling. The act does not allow claims about diagnosis, treatment, or prevention of disease but does allow that claims of certain benefits must be truthful. A standard statement is required on the label by the FDA (FDA, 1995).

TOWARD A POSITIVE NUTRITION LIFESTYLE: *LOCUS OF CONTROL*

Do things just happen to you? Does it seem as if school, family, or society affect what you do without your input? Or do you feel that you have control over what takes place? Do you have a life plan (or weekly plan) that you follow? Locus of control is the perception of one's ability to control life events and experiences. Having an *internal locus of control* means feeling as if you can influence the forces with which you come into contact. You have an inner sense of your ability to guide life events. An *external locus of control* is defined as the perception that you are not able to control what happens to you and that outside forces have power over what you experience.

Let's apply these concepts to your style of making food choices when shopping. In particular, consider the nutritional implications of locus of control. If you have an internal locus of control, you may develop a basic plan of the types of nutritious foods to be purchased during a shopping trip. You may make a few unplanned purchases, but they would be limited. You feel in control of your choices. Having an external locus of control means you might start out with a shopping list, but you are probably easily swayed by in-store promotions, coupons, and even colorful packaging to select products not on your list. You often buy more than needed because so much "looked good."

Awareness of our type of locus of control allows us to develop strategies to improve our food decisions. Individuals with an internal locus of control tend to develop their own approaches for changing food-related behaviors; those with an external locus of control may need a structured program or group support to provide guidance to modify their food behaviors.

SUMMARY

- Personal nutrition is composed of the dietary choices an individual makes that impact health and nutritional status.
  - Food preferences, food choice, and food liking influence selection. These may be altered by biological tendency, availability, media, and marketing.
- Community nutrition is a reflection of the nutritional health of the individuals within the community.
  - Public health programs such as SNAP and WIC focus on the prevention of nutrient deficiencies on the individual and community levels. Other government and/ or private organizations representing specific diet-related disorders such as American Heart Association

and American Diabetes Association develop recommendations to reduce excessive intake of energy and nutrients.

- *Dietary Guidelines, 2010* provides lifestyle and dietary pattern recommendations that ensure nutrient adequacy and primary disease prevention.
  - MyPlate is an interactive food guide to implement the *Dietary Guidelines* recommendations.
- The requirement for consumer information on food product packaging increases the probability that decisions about food choice are based on nutritional value as well as on taste, cost, and availability.

- FDA food labeling regulations require the following:
  - Nutrition Facts panel must list quantity of energy (fat), fat, and other specified nutrients per serving listed as percent of Daily Values.
  - Food descriptors are defined to ensure uniformity of meaning.

- Health claims approved by the FDA may appear on food labels.
- Organic food standards established by USDA determine labeling of products containing multiple ingredients.

◎ THE NURSING APPROACH
MyPlate Teaching Project

Because proper nutrition is an important part of the general health and well-being of all individuals, it is essential that nurses incorporate nutrition into health education. Each learning session should begin with an assessment of the client's learning needs and goals identified by the nurse and client. The overall objective of health education is to change behavior.

Factors that contribute to learning include the person's readiness to learn, ability to exercise and retain information, and motivation. When teaching, it is important to tailor the information to the individual or group. To ensure that the lesson is effective, the teacher should include (1) age-appropriate teaching materials and handouts, (2) relevant and sequential information, (3) feedback and praise when appropriate.

To enhance learning, the nurse can implement a variety of teaching methods, such as explanation, discussion, demonstration, group discussion, and role-playing.

Following is an example of a MyPlate teaching project using the nursing process ADPIE: assessment, diagnosis, planning, implementation, and evaluation.

Assessment
Assess client/learner characteristics:
- Age
- Language and ability to read
- Readiness to learn
- Learning style preference—visual aids, reading, demonstration, hands-on

Diagnosis
Diagnose the knowledge deficit; determine the learning need:
- What does the client/learner already know about MyPlate? About MyPyramid or the traditional food pyramid?
- What does he or she need to know or be able to do?
- What specific aspect of MyPlate is the individual interested in learning?

  Example: Deficient knowledge: types and amounts of food recommended

Planning
Plan the teaching.

Objectives
What measurable behavior changes can result from the learning experience?

  Examples:
  The client/learner will be able to:
- Explain general guidelines for each food group in MyPlate.
- Use MyPlate as a guide for making healthy food choices.
- Seek out the MyPlate website and obtain personalized guidelines.

- Use the SuperTracker to track eating patterns at www.choosemyplate.gov/.
- Set a specific goal for improving food choices, based on MyPlate guidelines.

Content
What information is appropriate for a teaching session 15 to 30 minutes long? Consider how long the individual can focus and how much depth of information will be appropriate for his/her age.

  Examples:
- Purpose of MyPlate (why developed, how it helps the individual)
- MyPlate's general guidelines for activity and healthy eating
- Availability of interactive information and MyPlate SuperTracker at www.choosemyplate.gov/

Teaching Methods
What methods will facilitate change?

  Examples:
- Lecture/discussion.
- Demonstrate use of MyPlate interactive site by sitting at a computer and guiding the client/learner through the program.
- Provide and interpret a visual handout from www.choosemyplate.gov, individualized by age and activity level.

Evaluation Plan
How can learning be measured to determine whether identified goals have been met?

  Examples:
- Administer a short verbal quiz about MyPlate.
- Play a game to sort out different foods and identify best choices to match MyPlate.
- Help the client/learner write a specific measurable goal based on better food choices identified in MyPlate.
- Observe the individual navigating in the MyPlate website and obtaining a personalized plan.

Implementation
Implement the teaching plan:
- Choose a time and place for which there will be no interruptions.
- Revise your plan as needed to match the knowledge and interest of the client/learner.
- Make the process interactive. Check for understanding frequently through an activity or what the individual states regarding the new information.
- Use understandable, age-appropriate terminology.
- Use visual aids and handouts the client/learner can use later.

◎ THE NURSING APPROACH—cont'd

Evaluation
Evaluate.

Client/Learner
- What was the client/learner able to demonstrate at the end of the teaching session?
- Were the behavior change goals met, partially met, or not met?

Nurse/Teacher
- Was the client/learner engaged in the lesson?
- Which teaching method or activity was effective?
- What was ineffective? What could be implemented differently to improve effectiveness next time?
- Was the teaching experience enjoyable? If not, how could the experience be improved?

❓ APPLYING CONTENT KNOWLEDGE

Jennifer and Peter are in their late 40s. Recently Peter was diagnosed with high blood cholesterol levels. His doctor told him to cut down on fats and cholesterol, but he is confused about what to order at the daily business lunches he must attend. Jennifer has noticed that she is starting to put on weight and wonders whether the change has to do with perimenopause or whether she is just eating more than usual. In addition, Jennifer's mother has just moved in with them because she could no longer afford her own home. Jennifer is concerned because her mother seems to eat little during the day. Her mother is alone all day because Jennifer and Peter work. What advice might you give to this family?

■ WEBSITES OF INTEREST

MyPlate Food Guidance System
www.ChooseMyPlate.gov
The official "home" of MyPlate, the interactive food guidance system.

Oldways Preservation Trust
oldwayspt.org
A nonprofit organization promoting good health through heritage.

U.S. Food and Drug Administration (FDA)
www.fda.gov
Gateway website connecting areas serviced and supervised by the FDA.

REFERENCES

American Diabetes Association/American Dietetic Association: *Choose your foods: Exchange lists for diabetes*, Alexandria, VA/ Chicago, 2008, Authors.

Beydoun MA, Wang Y: Do nutrition knowledge and beliefs modify the association of socio-economic factors and diet quality among US adults? *Prev Med* 46(2):145–153, 2008.

Centers for Disease Control and Prevention: State-specific trends in fruit and vegetable consumption among adults—United States, 2000–2009, *MMWR Morbid Mortal Wkly Rep* 59(35):1125–1130, 2010. From: www.cdc.gov/mmwr/preview/ mmwrhtml/mm5935a1.htm?s_cid=mm5935a1_w/. Accessed June 29, 2013.

Centers for Disease Control and Prevention: *State Indicator Report on Fruits and Vegetables*, Atlanta, GA, 2013, Author. From: www.cdc.gov/nutrition/downloads/State-Indicator-Report- Fruits-Vegetables-2013.pdf/. Accessed June 20, 2013.

Dutko P, et al: *Characteristics and influential factors of food deserts (ERR-140)*, Washington, DC, 2012, U.S. Department of Agriculture, Economic Research Service.

Guthrie J, et al: Americans' food choices at home and away: *How do they compare with recommendations? Amber Waves* 2013. From: www.ers.usda.gov/amber-waves/2013-february/americans-food -choices-at-home-and-away.aspx#.UdN7InDD8iQ/. Accessed July 5, 2013.

Hagan E, Rubin V: *Economic and community development outcomes of healthy food retail*, Oakland, CA, 2013, PolicyLink. From: www.policylink.org/publications. Accessed July 6, 2013.

Hartman Group: Healthy eating: Connections to attitudes about aging, *HartBeat* 2009. From: www.hartman-group.com/ hartbeat/healthy-eating-connections-to-attitudes-about-aging/. Accessed July 1, 2013.

Harvard School of Public Health: *The nutrition source: Healthy eating plate*, Cambridge, MA, 2013, Author. From: www.hsph.harvard.edu/nutritionsource/. Accessed June 29, 2013.

Howard AJ, et al: Toddlers' food preferences: The impact of novel food exposure, maternal preferences and food neophobia, *Appetite* 59:818–825, 2012.

Hoyert DL, Xu JQ: Deaths: Preliminary data for 2011, *Natl Vital Stat Report* 61(6), Hyattsville, MD, 2012. National Center for Health Statistics.

Logue AW: *The psychology of eating and drinking: An introduction*, ed 3, New York, 2004, Taylor & Francis Books Inc.

Mennella JA, Beauchamp GK: The early development of human flavor preferences. In Capaldi ED, editor: *Why we eat what we eat: The psychology of eating*, ed 2, Washington, DC, 2001, American Psychological Association.

Moss M: *Salt, sugar, fat: How the food giants hooked us*, New York, 2013, Random House.

Negri R, et al: Taste perception and food choices, *J Pediatr Gastroenterol Nutr* 54(5):624–629, 2012.

Oldways Preservation Trust: *Mediterranean Diet Pyramid, Latino Diet Pyramid, Asian Diet Pyramid, and African Heritage Diet Pyramid*, Cambridge, Mass, 2013, Author. From: www.oldwayspt.org. Accessed June 15, 2013.

Physicians Committee for Responsible Medicine (PCRM): *The Power Plate*, Washington, DC, 2009, Author. From: pcrm.org/. Accessed July 18, 2013.

Pollan M: *Cooked: A natural history of transformation*, New York, 2013, The Penguin Press.

Produce for Better Health Foundation: *Fruits & Veggies—More Matters®*, Hockessin, DE, 2013, Author. From: www.fruitsandveggiesmorematters.org/. Accessed June 29, 2013.

U.S. Department of Agriculture (USDA) and U.S. Department of Health and Human Services (USDHHS): *Dietary guidelines for*

Americans, 2010, ed 7, Washington, DC, 2010, U.S. Government Printing Office. From: www.health.gov/dietaryguidelines/dga2010/DietaryGuidelines2010.pdf/. Accessed July 11, 2013.

U.S. Department of Agriculture (USDA), Agricultural Marketing Service: *National Organic Program: Organic labeling and marketing information*, Washington, DC, 2012, Author. From: www.ams.usda.gov/AMSv1.0/getfile?dDocName=STEL DEV3004446. Accessed May 14, 2014.

U.S. Department of Agriculture, Center for Nutrition Policy and Promotion (USDA/CNPP): *USDA food guidance system (MyPlate)*, Alexandria, VA, 2012, Author. From: www.choosemyplate.gov/. Accessed June 16, 2013.

U.S. Department of Health and Human Services (USDHHS), Office of Disease Prevention and Health Promotion: *Healthy People 2020: Framework: The vision, mission, and goals of Healthy People 2020*, n.d. From: www.healthypeople.gov/2020/Consortium/HP2020Framework.pdf/. Accessed June 14, 2013.

U.S. Food and Drug Administration, Center for Food Safety and Applied Nutrition: *Dietary Supplement Health and Education Act of 1994*, College Park, MD, 1995, (Updated May 2013). Author. From: www.fda.gov/Food/DietarySupplements/default.htm/. Accessed June 23, 2013.

U.S. Food and Drug Administration, Center for Food Safety and Applied Nutrition: *How to understand and use the nutrition facts label*, College Park, MD, 2000, (updated November 2004; March 2013). Author. From: www.fda.gov/Food/IngredientsPackagingLabeling/LabelingNutrition/ucm274593.htm/. Accessed July 6, 2013.

U.S. Food and Drug Administration, Center for Food Safety and Applied Nutrition: *Guidance for industry: A food labeling guide*, College Park, MD, 2009, Author. From: www.fda.gov/FoodLabelingGuide/. Accessed July 6, 2013.

CHAPTER 3

Digestion, Absorption, and Metabolism

The digestive system, which is responsible for processing foods, is itself dependent on the body's nutrient intake for its maintenance.

ⓔ http://evolve.elsevier.com/GRODNER/FOUNDATIONS

LEARNING OBJECTIVES

- List the organs of the gastrointestinal (GI) tract and their functions.
- Identify other supportive structures and organs of the digestion and absorption.
- Describe the three types of muscular actions of the GI tract.
- Discuss the digestive and absorption roles of the small intestine.
- Explain the function of metabolism.

ROLE IN WELLNESS

Gulping down breakfast on the way to class or work, skipping lunch, and then eating dinner late may not seem to affect the health status of adults. However, if this kind of eating becomes routine, it characterizes an individual's lifestyle and may negatively influence health status.

The body's health is based on the nutrients available to support growth, maintenance, and energy needs. Inadequate nutritional intake can affect the body's ability to use the foods consumed. The digestive system, which is responsible for processing foods, depends on nutrient intake for its maintenance. Although the body is resilient, we stress our physical limits when we adopt habits that do not support optimal health. A primary way to decrease the risk of future disease and achieve wellness is to use lifestyle choices that support positive health behaviors.

Physical health begins with the gastrointestinal (GI) tract as the first step to maintain body functioning; unless nutrients in foods are digested and absorbed, life cannot continue. The decision and follow-through to change lifestyle behaviors to positively improve health in relation to digestive disorders is an aspect of *intellectual health*. An individual's emotional state and ability to handle stress may increase the risk of several disorders of the GI tract. Consequently, the *emotional health* effects of lifestyle behaviors may be related to constipation, diarrhea, and heartburn. Reducing the causes of intestinal gas helps guard against socially embarrassing moments.

Our food choices and styles of eating may affect the level of flatus experienced. Negativity associated with body smells is defined by society and thus affects our *social health* dimension. Respecting the sanctity of the human body, thereby acknowledging our *spiritual health* dimension, may include one's willingness to follow dietary and lifestyle changes to enhance the functioning of the GI tract (see the *Cultural Considerations* box Wholeness of Body, Mind, and Self). The *environmental health* dimension considers how we organize our lifestyles to allow adequate time for preparation and consumption of meals.

This chapter presents a brief orientation to the processes of digestion, absorption, and metabolism. These processes work together to provide all body cells with energy and nutrients.

DIGESTION

The main organs of the digestive system form the **gastrointestinal (GI) tract**, or alimentary canal, which creates an open tube that runs from the mouth to the anus (Figure 3-1 and Box 3-1). Everything we eat is processed through the GI tract. The **digestive system** consists of a series of organs that prepare ingested nutrients for **digestion** and absorption and protect against consumed microorganisms and toxic substances. To accomplish these actions, several processes take place. These processes—ingestion, digestion, absorption, and elimination—depend on the motility or movement

⊕ CULTURAL CONSIDERATIONS
Wholeness of Body, Mind, and Self

This text's presentation of digestion and absorption is based on Western perspectives. To most Westerners, body organs tend to be viewed separately from mind and spiritual influences. In contrast, *Ayurveda*, the name of traditional Indian medicine and meaning "the science of life," is based on living a balanced life. Consequently, Ayurveda regards physical disorders as imbalance of the body (organs) or life. Treatment works to bring balance or harmony back to the individual's life. The wholeness of life is represented by body *(shira)*, mind *(manas)*, and self *(atman)*. All three require attention to achieve and maintain health. Because each component is important, Ayurveda is a holistic approach recognizing the interdependent roles of body, mind, and self. A person is viewed as a combination of three forces or humors called *doshas*. Each person is a different combination of these forces, which are *vata, pitta,* and *kapha. Vata* is a force similar to air; *pitta,* a force similar to fire; and *kapha,* a force like mucus and water. Health occurs when these *doshas* are in balance; otherwise disease occurs. If *pitta* is too strong, fever, ulcers, and liver disorders may occur. An individual would need to strengthen the other *doshas* through (1) changes in behaviors and food choices, (2) use of natural medicines, and (3) yoga and meditation to decrease *pitta* and regain balance.

Application to nursing: This concept may assist clients to understand that their health may be affected by other components of their lives. Sometimes health concerns force us to confront factors that may influence our ability to maintain health or to achieve balance in our lives.

Data from Ninivaggi, FJ: *Ayurveda: A comprehensive guide to traditional Indian medicine for the West,* Westport, CT, 2008, Praeger Press.

BOX 3-1 Digestive System Organs

Segments of the Digestive Tract
Mouth
Oropharynx
Esophagus
Stomach
Small intestine
Duodenum
Jejunum
Ileum
Large intestine
Cecum
Colon:
  Ascending colon
  Transverse colon
  Descending colon
  Sigmoid colon
Rectum
Anal canal

Accessory Organs
Salivary glands
Parotid gland
Submandibular gland
Sublingual gland
Tongue
Teeth
Liver
Gallbladder
Pancreas
Vermiform appendix

---

of the GI wall and the secretions of digestive juices and enzymes.

The Mouth

Are you hungry? Are you thinking about your favorite food? Is your mouth watering? Our mouths really do "water" when we think about or begin to eat foods. However, it is not actually water we sense but a thin mucus-like fluid called **saliva**. *Saliva* is the term for the secretions of the three sets of salivary glands of the mouth. As **exocrine glands**, each set of salivary glands produces a different type of secretion that is released into the mouth. The parotid glands create watery saliva that supplies enzymes; the submandibular glands produce mucus and enzyme components; and the sublingual glands, the smallest, create a mucous type of saliva. A reflex mechanism controls these secretions.

Food in the mouth stimulates chemical and mechanical digestion. **Chemical digestion** occurs through the action of saliva that not only moistens the foods we chew but also contains amylase, an enzyme that begins the digestive process of starches.

Another digestive process that occurs in the mouth is **mechanical digestion,** which depends on teeth. Teeth rhythmically tear and pulverize food. The enamel covering teeth is the hardest substance in the body and therefore protects teeth from the harsh effects of chewing. (See the *Personal Perspectives* box, Which came first, the fork and knife or the overbite?) The tongue assists with mechanical digestion by guiding food into chewing positions and then leading the pulverized food into the esophagus. Another function of the tongue is that of taste. More than 2000 taste buds are responsible for our sensations of sweet, bitter, sour, and salty when we taste foods (Figure 3-2).

As toddlers, we have the highest number of taste buds and a higher degree of taste sensitivity, so bland foods are more appealing. The number of taste buds declines as we grow older, explaining why older adults have diminished taste sensitivity. Older adults may need to be encouraged to avoid the use of too much salt, particularly if they have hypertension or cardiac disorders.

Our sense of smell works along with our taste bud sensations. These two combined senses actually account for the perception (and enjoyment) of the flavors of different foods. Our positive or negative response to specific foods based on our sensory perception affects our food choices (Mahan, et al, 2012).

Portions of the pulverized or masticated food are formed into the shape of a ball called a **bolus**. The tongue effortlessly forms the bolus, which is then swallowed and passed by the

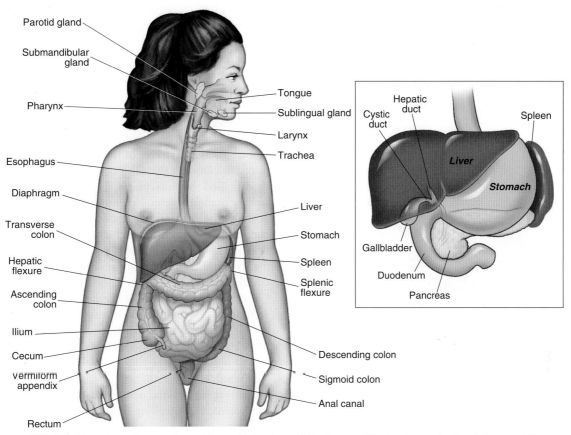

FIG 3-1 The digestive system. (From Thibodeau GA, Patton KT: *Anatomy & physiology,* ed 5, St Louis, 2003, Mosby.)

PERSONAL PERSPECTIVES

Which Came First, the Fork and Knife or the Overbite?

Bee Wilson has written a fascinating account about how we cook around the world and through the centuries in *Consider the Fork: A History of How We Cook and Eat.* Her research reveals the past dangers of cooking throughout history from young children wandering into the flames of families' cooking hearths to the use of young boys and/or dogs to spin roasting meats to prevent charring and uneven cooking while being exposed to searing heat from open flames. Below we consider an example of human physiologic change.

We tend to forget that human physiology changes very slowly over the passage of time. Of course we consider ourselves different than the Neanderthals in our choice of food preparation methods, such as cooked not raw, and how we consume foods based on our cultural customs ranging from using fingers, knives, forks, or chopsticks. According to the historical research of Charles Loring Brace, an anthropology professor, one of the substantial physical changes to human anatomy is as recent as the late eighteenth century: the overbite of the jaw. Previously, an "edge to edge" bite of the top jaw meeting the edge of the lower jaw prevailed and an overbite was not to be found.

The potential cause appears to be not a change in *what* we eat, but *how* we eat our food. In the past, a large quantity of food was put into one's mouth. What could not be contained in the oral cavity was then ripped off by clenching one's teeth. In this circumstance, an edge to edge bite was the efficient way to "cut" the food away from one's mouth. A knife could, carefully, be used to achieve the same purpose, but teeth were safer.

The significant change in physiology may have come about because of how knifes with the assistance of forks to hold the food still, allowed foods to be cut into bite-sized pieces to more easily be chewed. As customs around food evolved, cultures prized the gentile nature of cutting food into smaller and smaller pieces that barely required chewing. Therefore, the overbite—of the top jaw hanging over the lower jaw—emerged as the tearing role of the teeth became obsolete.

Although the knife had been around a very long time, the newer use of the fork to ease the cutting of bite sized pieces of food, allowed the overbite to evolve. We can just wonder what the next physiologic change may be!

Data from: Wilson B: *Consider the fork: A history of how we cook and eat,* New York, 2012, Basic Books.

epiglottis into the esophagus within about 5 to 7 seconds. The epiglottis is a flap of tissue that closes over the trachea to prevent the bolus from entering the lungs.

The Esophagus

The *esophagus* is a muscular tube through which the bolus travels from the mouth to the stomach. The process begins at

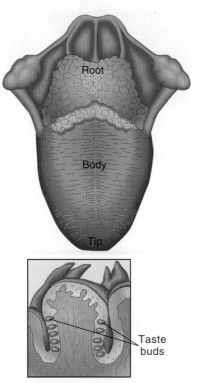

FIG 3-2 Top, Parts of the tongue. **Bottom,** A detailed site of taste buds. (From Thibodeau GA, Patton KT: *Anatomy & physiology,* ed 5, St Louis, 2003, Mosby.)

the top of the esophagus when **peristalsis,** the involuntary movements of circular and longitudinal muscles, begins and draws the bolus farther into the GI tract. This mechanical action further breaks down the size of foodstuff and increases its exposure to digestive secretions. Muscular actions depend on the four layers of tissues that form the tube of the GI tract (Figure 3-3). The **mucosa** is composed of mucous membrane and forms the inside layer. Under the mucosa is the **submucosa,** a layer of connective tissue. Digestion depends on the blood vessels and nerves of the submucosa to regulate digestion. Surrounding the submucosa is a thick layer of muscle tissue called the **muscularis.** The outermost layer of the GI wall is made of serous membrane called **serosa,** which is actually the visceral layer of the peritoneum lining the abdominal pelvic cavity, and covers organs.

The coordination of these layers provides the varied movements required for digestion. Essentially, muscular action controls the movement of the food mass through the GI tract. Churning action within a segment of the GI tract allows secretions to mix with food mass. Circular muscles surround the GI tube. Rhythmic contractions of these muscles cause the wavelike motions of peristalsis, moving food downward. Longitudinal muscles run parallel along the GI tube. The combined effect of the circular and longitudinal muscles causes **segmentation,** a forward-and-backward movement that assists in controlling food mass movement through the GI tract.

Sphincter muscles are stronger, circular muscles that act as valves to control the movement of the food mass in a forward direction. In effect, sphincter muscles prevent reflux by forming an opening when relaxed and closing completely when contracted. At the bottom of the esophagus, the cardiac sphincter controls the movement of the bolus from the esophagus into the stomach. It also prevents the acidic

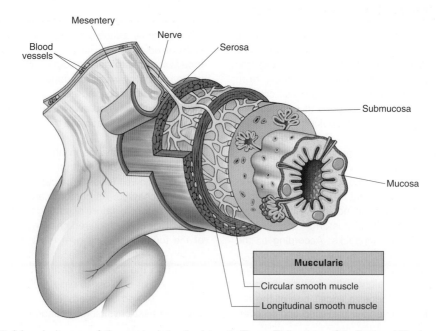

FIG 3-3 Muscle layers of the gastrointestinal tract. (From Thibodeau GA, Patton KT: *Anatomy & physiology,* ed 5, St Louis, 2003, Mosby.)

contents of the stomach from moving upward back through the esophagus.

The Stomach

Functions of the stomach include the following:
- Holding food for partial digestion
- Producing gastric juice
- Providing muscular action that, combined with gastric juice, mixes and tears food into smaller pieces
- Secreting the intrinsic factor for vitamin B_{12} absorption
- Releasing gastrin
- Assisting in the destruction, through its acidity of secretions, of pathogenic bacteria that may have inadvertently been consumed

When the bolus passes through the cardiac sphincter, it enters the fundus, the upper portion of the stomach that connects with the esophagus. The other divisions of the stomach include the body, or center portion, and the pylorus, the lower portion. The stomach wall contains gastric mucosa with gastric pits. At the base of the pits are the gastric glands whose chief cells create gastric juice, a mucous fluid containing digestive enzymes, and parietal cells, which secrete stomach acid called *hydrochloric acid.*

Gastric secretions occur in three phases: cephalic, gastric, and intestinal (Sullivan, et al, 2014). The cephalic phase is called the "psychic phase" because mental factors can stimulate gastrin, a hormone secreted by stomach mucosa. In the gastric phase, gastrin increases the release of gastric juices when the stomach is distended by food. The third phase is the intestinal phase, in which the gastric secretions change as chyme, a semiliquid mixture of food mass, passes through to the duodenum. Gastric secretions are inhibited by exocrine and nervous reflexes of gastric inhibitory peptides, secretin, and cholecystokinin (CCK) (also called pancreozymin), a hormone secreted by intestinal mucosa.

Some gastric juices provide acidity in the stomach to assist the effective function of certain enzymes. As agents of chemical digestion, enzymes are specific in action, working only on individual classes of nutrients and changing substances from one form to a simpler form. Enzymes are "organic catalysts" formed from protein structures. They function at specific pH levels and are continually created and destroyed. Specific enzymes are required for energy release and digestion.

Hormones regulate the release of gastric juices and enzymes, acting as messengers between organs to cause the release of needed secretions. In digestion, hormones affect the secretions from the stomach, intestines, and gallbladder. These secretions may slow or speed digestion and may affect the pH levels of gastric juice. Overall, the mechanical and chemical actions work together to complete the process of digestion.

Gastric *motility,* or movement of food mass through the stomach, requires 2 to 6 hours. The churning and mixing of the food mass with gastric juices create a semiliquid mixture called *chyme.* When chyme enters the pylorus section of the stomach, it causes distention and the release of the hormone gastrin. Gastrin sends a message that hydrochloric acid (HCl)

is needed to continue the breakdown of chyme. As HCl is released from the stomach lining, thick mucus is also secreted to protect the stomach walls from the harsh HCl.

Every 20 seconds chyme is released into the duodenum, the upper portion of the small intestine; this action is controlled by the hormonal and nervous system mechanism of enterogastric reflex. This consists of duodenal receptors in the mucosa that are sensitive to the presence of acid and distention. The impulses over sensory and motor fiber in the vagus nerve cause a reflex restriction of gastric peristalsis. For example, the gastric inhibitory peptide released in response to fats in the duodenum decreases peristalsis of stomach muscles and slows chyme passage. The result is decreased motility, which is why the stomach empties more slowly when a person eats a high-fat diet.

The combined action of mechanical digestion (the strong muscular movements of peristalsis) and chemical digestion (the effects of the gastric juices) works to prepare nutrients for the process of absorption. Chyme is kept in the stomach by the actions of the pyloric sphincter, which slowly releases it into the duodenum.

The Small Intestine

The chyme entering the duodenum soon moves through to the jejunum and ileum of the small intestine. It takes about 5 hours for chyme to pass through the small intestine because of the action of segmentation and peristalsis. Segmentation in the duodenum and upper jejunum mixes chyme with digestive juices from the pancreas, liver, and intestinal mucosa. Peristalsis is controlled by intrinsic stretch reflexes and is initiated by CCK, the hormone secreted by intestinal mucosa.

In the small intestine, the nutrients in chyme are prepared for absorption. The small intestine is the major organ of digestion, and the final stages of the digestive process occur here. Because it is also the site of almost all of the absorption of nutrients, the intestinal lining must be able to accommodate the actions of both digestion and absorption. The intestinal walls are covered with a thin layer of mucus, which protects the walls from digestive juices. The walls are also adapted to enhance the absorption process. Finger like projections called villi greatly increase the amount of mucosal layer available for the absorption of nutrients (Figure 3-4). On the villi are hairlike projections called *microvilli* that also enhance absorption by their structure and movements.

As chyme enters the small intestine, hormones begin sending messages that regulate the release of digestive juices to continue the process of chyme digestion. Some hormones are provided by the small intestine; several are released by other organs into the small intestine. These secretions include enzymes from the small intestines, bile produced in the liver, and digestive juices from the pancreas.

One of the first hormones released by the small intestine is secretin. This hormone causes the pancreas to send bicarbonate to the small intestine to reduce the acidic content of the chyme. As the acidic level decreases, other pancreatic juices enter and begin their work. Another hormone secreted by the small intestine is CCK, which initiates pancreatic

TABLE 3-1	**Digestive Processes**
MECHANISM	**DESCRIPTION**
Ingestion	Process of taking food into the mouth, starting it on its journey through the digestive tract
Digestion	A group of processes that break complex nutrients into simpler ones, thus facilitating their absorption; *mechanical digestion* physically breaks large chunks into small bits; *chemical digestion* breaks molecules apart
Motility	Movement by the muscular components of the digestive tube, including processes of mechanical digestion; examples are *peristalsis* and *segmentation*
Secretion	Release of digestive juices (containing enzymes, acids, bases, mucus, bile, or other products that facilitate digestion); some digestive organs secrete endocrine hormones that regulate digestion or metabolism of nutrients
Absorption	Movement of digested nutrients through the gastrointestinal mucosa and into the internal environment
Elimination	Excretion of the residues of the digestive process (feces) from the rectum, through the anus; defecation

Data from Thibodeau GA, Patton KT: *Anatomy & physiology*, ed 5, St Louis, 2003, Mosby.

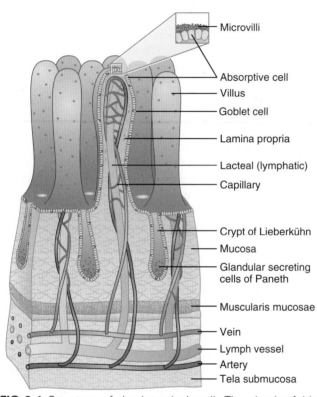

Microvilli
Absorptive cell
Villus
Goblet cell
Lamina propria
Lacteal (lymphatic)
Capillary
Crypt of Lieberkühn
Mucosa
Glandular secreting cells of Paneth
Muscularis mucosae
Vein
Lymph vessel
Artery
Tela submucosa

FIG 3-4 Structure of the intestinal wall. The circular folds, villi, and microvilli multiply the surface area and enhance absorption. (From Mahan LK, et al, editors: *Krause's food & the nutrition care process*, ed 13, Philadelphia, 2012, Saunders.)

exocrine secretions, acts against gastrin by inhibiting gastric HCl secretion, and activates the gallbladder to contract, causing bile to be released into the duodenum.

Bile, which is secreted by the liver and stored in the gallbladder, is released to emulsify fats, aiding in the digestion of lipids. The emulsification creates more surface area, allowing lipid enzymes to digest fats to their component parts. The liver continuously secretes bile, and CCK and secretin spur the gallbladder to release bile for the digestion of fats. In addition, the small intestine produces enzymes to assist in the digestive process. Although much of the chyme is absorbed, the rest—which usually consists of fiber, minerals, and water—passes through the next sphincter (ileocecal valve) and into the large intestine (ascending colon).

The Large Intestine

The large intestine consists of the cecum, colon, and rectum. The cecum is a blind pocket; therefore, the mass bypasses it and enters the ascending colon, which leads into the transverse colon running across the abdomen over the small intestine to the descending colon. The descending colon extends down the left of the abdomen into the sigmoid colon and leads into the descending colon, on to the rectum, and into the anal canal. Finally, any remaining mass passes out through the anus. The journey through the large intestine takes about 9 to 16 hours.

In the large intestine or colon, final absorption of any available nutrients, usually water and some minerals, occurs. Bacteria residing in the large intestine produce several vitamins, which are then absorbed. Water is withdrawn from the fibrous mass, forming solidified feces. Mucous glands in the intestinal wall create mucus that lubricates and covers feces as it forms. Again, peristalsis continues to move substances through the GI tract, resulting in the excretion of feces from the colon through the anus, the last sphincter muscle of the GI tract.

The movement of the food mass through the GI tract is controlled to enhance digestion and absorption. During passage through the GI tract, more than 95% of the carbohydrates, fats, and proteins ingested are absorbed. Some minerals, vitamins, and trace elements may be less absorbed (Sullivan, et al, 2014). Table 3-1 summarizes the primary mechanisms of the digestive system. Details of carbohydrate, protein, and lipid digestion follow in specific chapters.

ABSORPTION

Although the food mass has possibly spent several hours in the tube of the GI tract, it is not yet actually inside the body until its nutrient components are absorbed. **Absorption** is the process by which substances pass through the intestinal mucosa into the blood or lymph. Transport processes provide the means for nutrients to actually pass through the wall of the small intestine. These include passive diffusion and

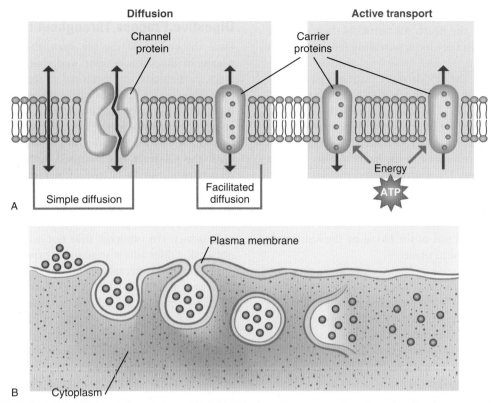

FIG 3-5 A, Methods of absorption. *Simple diffusion,* the movement of molecules from a region of high concentration to low concentration; *facilitated diffusion,* the movement of molecules by a carrier protein across the cell membrane from a region of high to low concentration; *active transport,* the movement of molecules and ions by means of a carrier protein against fluid pressures that require expenditure of cellular energy. **B,** Pinocytosis. (**A** from Mahan LK, et al, editors: *Krause's food & the nutrition care process,* ed 13, Philadelphia, 2012, Saunders; **B** from Nix S: *Williams' basic nutrition & diet therapy,* ed 12, St Louis, 2005, Mosby.)

osmosis, facilitated diffusion, energy-dependent active transport, and engulfing pinocytosis (Figure 3-5).

Passive diffusion occurs when pressure is greater on one side of the membrane and the substance then moves from the area of greater pressure to less pressure, allowing molecules to travel through capillaries. *Facilitated diffusion* takes place when, despite positive pressure flow, molecules may be unable to pass through membrane pores unless aided. Specific integral membrane proteins support the movement by bringing the larger nutrient molecules through the capillary membrane.

Energy-dependent *active transport* happens when fluid pressures work against the passage of nutrients. As an active process, it requires energy. This energy is supplied by the cell and a "pumping" mechanism, which are assisted by a special membrane protein carrier. Engulfing *pinocytosis* takes place when a substance, either a fluid or a nutrient, contacts the villi membrane, which then surrounds the substance and creates a vacuole that encompasses the substance. Passing through the cell cytoplasm, the substance is then released into the circulatory system. The amounts of vitamins and minerals absorbed depend on the body's storage levels and immediate need for these nutrients. Nutrients such as fats, carbohydrates, and protein are easily absorbed regardless of the level of need. The structure of the small intestine, the site

of almost all nutrient absorption, allows for efficient absorption to occur. The microvilli are sensitive to the exact nutrient needs of the body. Their wavelike motions, caused by peristalsis, result in the most exposure of the nutrient-laden chyme to the absorbing cells. This exposure allows needed nutrients to leave the GI tract and pass through the microvilli cells. At this point, the nutrients are truly "inside" the body.

Various factors may affect absorption of nutrients. Combinations of naturally occurring substances such as fiber or binders may move nutrients through the GI tract too quickly for optimum absorption to occur. Individual nutrient absorption and other issues of bioavailability are addressed in other chapters. The relationship between food and drug absorption is also an important issue of medical treatment. Ingesting a medication with food may decrease the absorption rate of the medication and may interfere with the absorption of other nutrients contained in the food consumed. This issue is explored in depth in Chapter 11.

Once "inside" the body, the nutrients enter the circulatory systems of the bloodstream or lymphatic system. The general circulatory or blood system receives absorbed protein, carbohydrates, small parts of broken-down fats, and most vitamins and minerals. This system transports these nutrients throughout the body. The lymphatic system, a secondary circulatory system, receives large lipids and fat-soluble vitamins. The nutrients traveling in the lymphatic system are deposited into the bloodstream near the heart. All nutrients then circulate throughout the body in the blood, providing for the nutrient requirements of cells.

Soon after entering the bloodstream, nutrients pass by the liver. This arrangement allows the liver to have "first choice" of the available nutrients. The liver is a powerhouse organ that provides a wide variety of services and substances; thus, its nutrient needs are a priority. From there, the bloodstream's journey of nutrients continues to the heart to also give it a prime nutrient selection. The journey then continues through the circulatory system to all cells. Some nutrients end up in nutrient storage sites of the body. These sites include the bones, liver, and kidneys. Other nutrients, if not discarded or used by cells, are filtered out of the blood by the kidneys to be reabsorbed or excreted in urine.

Elimination

The expulsion of feces or body waste products is called *defecation*. When the rectum is distended because of waste accumulation, the reflex to defecate occurs. The residue may include substances such as cellulose and other dietary fibers and connective tissue from meat collagen that are unable to be digested by human enzymes. Undigested fats may combine with dietary minerals, such as calcium and magnesium, and form residue. Additional residue may include water, bacteria, pigments, and mucus. Figure 3-6 summarizes the functions of the digestive system, and the *Teaching Tool* box Digesting Food: A Primer for Clients and Patients provides suggestions for client and patient teaching.

Digestive Process Throughout the Life Span

Over the course of the life span, the main and accessory organs of digestion develop and change. The immature GI tract, particularly the intestinal mucosa of a young infant, may allow intact proteins to be absorbed without complete digestion occurring. This incomplete digestion may result in an allergic response by the immune system and is part of the reason to delay the introduction of solid foods (e.g., cereals) until the GI tract has matured sufficiently. Another age-related condition is lactose intolerance, in which the body ceases to produce lactase, the enzyme that breaks down the milk carbohydrate of lactose. For some people, this occurs once the primary growth need for nutrients contained in milk is met. For others, it may not occur until adulthood or not at all. Older adults sometimes experience lactose intolerance when the secretion of enzymes, including lactase, decreases as part of the aging process. Conditions of the middle years include gallbladder disease and peptic ulcers (sores that may occur on the epithelial surfaces of the stomach or small intestine). Older years may be marked by problems of constipation and diverticulosis. These conditions may be associated with age-related reductions in peristalsis and physical activity, and may be worsened by a lifelong history of chronic low dietary fiber consumption. Gastrointestinal disorders are discussed in Chapter 13. Other issues related to aging are discussed in other chapters, particularly Chapter 10.

TEACHING TOOL

Digesting Food: A Primer for Clients and Patients

As health care professionals, we may assume our clients understand the way the body works as easily as we do. More than likely, however, their knowledge is limited, and even if they studied digestion years ago in a health education class, they may have forgotten or replaced facts with misinformation.

When working with clients for health promotion or with patients recovering from GI disorders, the nurse should consider using the summary of digestive organ functions (see Figure 3-6) as a teaching tool. A visual review of the digestive organs and processes can give clients and patients a clearer concept of the purposes of dietary recommendations, and they may therefore find compliance easier.

Overall food transit times for nutrients to move from our plate to our cells are as follows:

Chewing and swallowing	Depends on texture and quantity
Esophagus	5-7 seconds
Stomach	2-6 hours
Small intestine	Approximately 5 hours
Large intestine	9-16 hours
Total	16-27 hours ingestion to elimination

HEALTH DEBATE

Are Specialty Yogurts the Key to "Regularity"?

Yogurts, which contain at least the starter cultures *Lactobacillus bulgaricus* and *Streptococcus thermophilus*, are recognized for their health-promoting value, particularly for the digestive tract. Many yogurt brands contain additional probiotics such as *Lactobacillus rhamnosus*, *Lactobacillus casei*, and *Bifidobacterium animalis DN-173 010* (trademarked by Dannon as *Bifidus regularis* in the United States). These cultures, when listed as "live and active" ingredients of products, are probiotics—beneficial bacteria that reside in the small intestine. Probiotics can replace or push out problematic bacteria, thereby possibly decreasing gas, bloating, and constipation. Some sustain the immune system and may be preventive against antibiotic-related diarrhea.

Marketing campaigns present certain yogurt products, such as *Activia* by Dannon, as able to "naturally regulate your digestive system," because of the added probiotics. Other yogurt brands contain even more probiotics than *Activia* that also influence the digestive and immune systems.

Should we consume probiotics from heavily marketed (expensive and quite sweet) designer food products or from more traditional yogurt products containing similar probiotics? Should probiotics even be a concern, or should they be viewed as a dietary supplement? Do we really need to buy special (and sweetened) products to be "regular"?

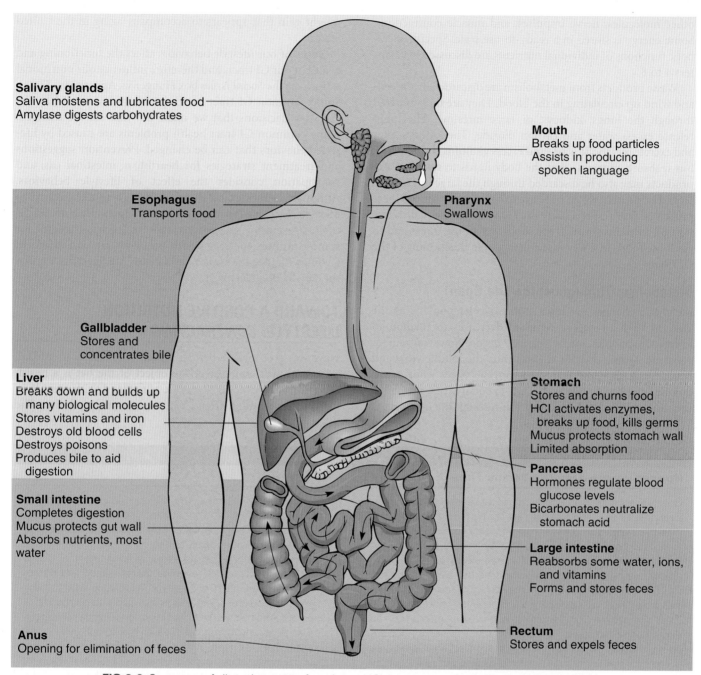

Salivary glands
Saliva moistens and lubricates food
Amylase digests carbohydrates

Mouth
Breaks up food particles
Assists in producing
  spoken language

Esophagus
Transports food

Pharynx
Swallows

Gallbladder
Stores and
concentrates bile

Liver
Breaks down and builds up
  many biological molecules
Stores vitamins and iron
Destroys old blood cells
Destroys poisons
Produces bile to aid
  digestion

Stomach
Stores and churns food
HCl activates enzymes,
  breaks up food, kills germs
Mucus protects stomach wall
Limited absorption

Pancreas
Hormones regulate blood
  glucose levels
Bicarbonates neutralize
  stomach acid

Small intestine
Completes digestion
Mucus protects gut wall
Absorbs nutrients, most
water

Large intestine
Reabsorbs some water, ions,
  and vitamins
Forms and stores feces

Anus
Opening for elimination of feces

Rectum
Stores and expels feces

FIG 3-6 Summary of digestive organ functions. *HCl,* hydrochloric acid. (From Rolin Graphics.)

METABOLISM

It is hard to imagine that a lunch consisting of tuna on rye bread will actually end up being part of the cells of the body. Fortunately, the human body is able to transform the nutrients of the sandwich into substances usable by cells. Metabolism is a set of processes through which absorbed nutrients are used by the body for energy and to form and maintain body structures and functions. The two main processes of metabolism involve catabolism and anabolism. *Catabolism* is the breakdown of food components into smaller molecular particles, which causes the release of energy as heat and chemical energy. *Anabolism* is the process of synthesis

from which substances are formed, such as new bone or muscle tissue. Both processes happen within cells at the same time.

When nutrients finally reach individual cells, they may be chemically changed through anabolism to help form new cell structures or to create new substances such as hormones and enzymes. Some vitamins and minerals assist in the use of other nutrients within the cell. They act as catalysts or coenzymes to initiate and support the transformation and use of carbohydrates, proteins, and lipids. Other nutrients may be used as energy to continue life-supporting processes. These processes include the energy needed to support deoxyribonucleic acid (DNA) reproduction and create proteins and other molecules, nerve impulses, and muscle contractions. Some energy is stored in a ready-to-use state. Specific metabolic functions of individual nutrients are discussed in Chapters 4 to 8.

Waste products from metabolism are discarded by the cells and wind up circulating in the blood. They are then excreted through the lungs, kidneys, or large intestine. The lungs release excess water and carbon dioxide. The kidneys filter and excrete metabolic waste and excess vitamins and minerals but reabsorb nutrients that the body needs to retain. Waste products may also be discarded through the large intestine in feces. Fortunately, we do not have to consciously control these processes. Our responsibility is to provide an adequate selection of nutrients through the foods we choose to eat and to eat those foods in a way that enhances the functioning of the GI tract.

Metabolism Throughout the Life Span

Metabolic changes are most noticeable later in life as the amount of food energy required decreases in relation to lowered metabolic rates. Nutrient needs, however, remain constant. As we (and our clients) enter the middle years and beyond, our challenge is to meet nutrient needs while maintaining or reducing our kcal needs to equal actual metabolic use. Recognition of this change can forestall the unexpected weight gain that appears to accompany aging in the United States.

Some of our lifestyle behaviors affect the functioning and health of our GI tracts and therefore influence our nutritional status (see the *Social Issues* box Hunger vs. Appetite vs. Time). Some common GI tract health problems are caused by the everyday decisions that we make but that can be changed. Some common GI tract health problems are caused by lifestyle behaviors that can be changed. Prevention suggestions and treatment strategies for heartburn, intestinal gas, and constipation consider the effect of lifestyle behaviors. Although vomiting and diarrhea are not usually related to lifestyle, each has an impact on the functioning of the GI tract. Prevention suggestions and treatment strategies for some common GI tract health problems are considered in Chapter 13. (See the *Health Debate* box, Are Specialty Yogurts the Key to "Regularity"?)

TOWARD A POSITIVE NUTRITION LIFESTYLE: *CONTRACTING*

Have you ever made a bet? Contracting is similar to making a bet with a friend, except the object of the bet is a health behavior. A *contract* is a specific agreement with oneself or between you and a friend, spouse, or other relative. The

---

SOCIAL ISSUES

Hunger versus Appetite versus Time

Our daily schedules often determine our responses to hunger. Ever notice how differently you eat during the week compared with the weekend? The weekday mosaic of classes, studying, work, and possibly sports training often makes fitting in time to get to the campus cafeteria a Herculean feat. Or, if you prepare your own meals, time must be set aside for buying and cooking foods. Weekends may be more leisurely without classes or work, or perhaps we find time for socializing.

Yet somehow we manage. Although fewer meals may be eaten during the week, we are not any less hungry nor are energy needs lower. Sometimes, chaotic schedules may be accommodated by telling ourselves we are not really hungry or we just do not have time to eat.

How can we do that? Isn't hunger a physiologic need for energy and nutrients? Can we just think ourselves through the hunger sensation? To understand this process, we need to explore the feeding regulating mechanism of the body.

Our sense of hunger and satiety is governed by the *hypothalamus*, a small portion of the brain. Its purpose is to maintain homeostasis (a state of balance) by regulating food intake through a feeding (hunger) center and a satiety center. The response of the hypothalamus, which initiates the hunger sensation, is thought to be related to either low blood glucose levels or to the lack of chyme in the stomach.

When we eat, blood glucose levels rise and chyme is once again in the stomach. The hypothalamus responds by providing a feeling of satiety or satisfaction, and we stop eating.

When we "feel" hungry, we are recognizing the internal stimuli of hunger. Perhaps our stomach seems to be rumbling or "empty" or we are "starving." These sensations are tied to physical events in our bodies. When we act on these signals, we eat. However, we can also choose to ignore them. This means that we cognitively override the sensation and do not respond. There are physical mechanisms to cope with the lack of new energy sources, but it is still stressful to our bodies.

External stimuli also affect our desire or appetite for eating. Referred to as *environmental cues,* these stimuli include the smell and sight of food, which may artificially increase our hunger. Simply seeing a food commercial on television or talking about food can excite the feeding center even if the stomach is not actually "empty." We also associate eating with specific social settings and time of day, regardless of our physical need for food. How can a birthday be celebrated without a cake? Religious holidays are often associated with special foods or meals. Throughout our elementary school experience, we ate lunch when we were scheduled, not necessarily when we were hungry.

All those years of eating by schedules and events have led us to adapt by overriding our cognitive cues about our real sense of hunger. Now, when personal schedules are more individualized, we may find that the external stimuli supporting our appropriate intake of food are gone; we must develop our own cues to ensure optimal nutritional intakes.

Data from Logue AW: *The psychology of eating and drinking: An introduction,* ed 3, New York, 2004, Freeman; and Mahan LK, et al, editors: *Krause's food & the nutrition care process,* ed 13, Philadelphia, 2012, Saunders.

agreement represents your willingness to attempt to change a health-related behavior. The advantage to contracting is that the goal or behavior change is clearly defined and observable. You also decide on a specific period within which to achieve the goal. As with a bet, you determine a reward or penalty for not completing the contract. (Yes, contracts with oneself are much easier to break.) The expectation is that practicing a new health-related behavior for a specific period makes the change permanent.

A contract with oneself might be to drink eight glasses of water a day for a week to relieve constipation. The change to increase fluid intake is a behavior you can directly control and observe. Although the aim is to alleviate constipation, which may not be a behavior you can consciously change, you can reduce its risk factors. At the end of the week, your reward could be to see a movie with a friend, whereas the penalty might be to clean out your messy bedroom closet.

Perhaps you have noticed that you regularly work through lunch and eat at your desk. The result is that heartburn has become a regular discomfort, and a discussion of remedies is often the topic of work breaks. A co-worker complains that she seems unable to break her habit of buying a high-calorie Danish pastry with her coffee each morning. You could contract with her that for the next 2 weeks you will eat lunch away from your desk, either in the employee cafeteria or at a local restaurant. She contracts with you that she will buy fruit instead of a Danish pastry for her morning snack. If you both complete the contracts, a reward could be to lunch together at a special restaurant. If only one person completes a contract, the penalty could be for the "loser" to pack a brown bag lunch for a week for the "winner." Contracting is applicable to many aspects of contemporary lifestyles and is limited only by our imagination.

■ SUMMARY

- GI tract organs include the mouth, esophagus, stomach, small intestine, and large intestine.
- Other supportive structures and organs are the teeth, tongue, salivary glands, liver, gallbladder, and pancreas.
- The small intestine is the main site of nutrient digestion and absorption.
- Digestion and absorption are achieved through mechanical and chemical digestion.
- Mechanical digestion consists of chewing, peristalsis, segmentation, and the action of sphincter muscles, which regulate the movement of foodstuff through one organ to the next.

- Chemical digestion is the actual breakdown of substances resulting from the production and/or storage of gastric and digestive secretions.
- Nutrients, once absorbed, are transported through the blood circulatory system or the lymphatic system, becoming available to all cells.
- Once nutrients reach the cells, metabolism may occur once. Metabolic changes allow the nutrients to fulfill many cell functions.
- Digestion absorption, and metabolism work together to provide all body cells with energy and nutrients.

◎ THE NURSING APPROACH

Debunking the Myths: Myth or Truth?

The topic of nutrition harbors many myths and misconceptions. People are constantly bombarded with mixed messages from the media, not to mention the various new diets claiming to help you magically and effortlessly lose weight.

You and a few of your classmates decide to volunteer at a local health and wellness event to help screen for diseases and to educate the public on prevention. In your clinical as a nursing student, you noticed that patients often have inaccurate nutrition information. You decide to create a "Myth or Truth" game.

1. *Myth:* Metabolism can't be changed. It's genetic.
   Truth: Metabolism is the process through which the body absorbs nutrients to use them for energy and to form and maintain body structures and functions. Genetics help to determine metabolic rates, but we can increase our metabolism through exercise and by building lean muscle mass. Exercise revs up metabolism, and muscle burns more calories per hour than fat. Muscle mass decreases as we age; therefore, lifting weights may help to improve metabolic rate.

2. *Myth:* Eating late at night leads to weight gain.
   Truth: Little evidence has shown that eating late at night leads to weight gain. Weight gain is more likely caused by mindless eating and poor food choices. The bottom line is that weight gain is caused by consuming too many extra calories.

3. *Myth:* You have to have a bowel movement every day to stay healthy.
   Truth: There is no right number of daily or weekly bowel movements. Normal functioning ranges from once a day to every 3 days. Constipation is difficulty and discomfort due to slow movement of feces through the colon.

4. *Myth:* Spicy foods and stress cause ulcers.
   Truth: An infection caused by the bacteria *Helicobacter pylori* (*H. pylori*) is the most common cause of peptic ulcers. The bacteria attach to stomach cells, causing gastritis, and can stimulate the production of excess hydrochloric acid. Spicy foods and stress do not cause ulcers; however, they can worsen symptoms if an ulcer is present.

5. *Myth:* Heartburn is nothing to worry about.

Continued

◎ THE NURSING APPROACH—cont'd

Truth: Frequent heartburn could be a symptom of a more serious condition called gastroesophageal reflux disease (GERD). If left untreated, it can cause ulcers of the esophagus, strictures (a narrowing of the esophagus), and an increased risk of esophageal cancer.

The event is a great success. However, there are several questions that you are unable to answer. You gather contact information and offer to get back to them with the answers.

The questions are:
1. How long does it take for food to move from our plate into our cells?
2. Where does the majority of absorption occur?

❓ APPLYING CONTENT KNOWLEDGE

James, a senior at the local university, is completing his internship at the rock radio station while continuing to work at his part-time job. Without any time to spare, he has been eating meals whenever he can, often from fast-food restaurants. These meals are usually gobbled quickly in his car. Lately, though, he is feeling stressed and is experiencing heartburn. List three lifestyle behaviors that James could change to possibly reduce heartburn.

■ WEBSITES OF INTEREST

Healthfinder.gov

healthfinder.gov

Provides a wealth of information and tools on health, coordinated by the National Health Information Center, U.S. Department of Health and Human Services.

American Dental Association

www.ada.org

Source of up-to-date news items and search tools related to oral health.

American Medical Association

www.ama-assn.org

The *Patient Education Materials* (under *Resources*) includes the *Atlas of the Human Body*, a good resource for patient education.

REFERENCES

Mahan LK, et al, editors: *Krause's food and the nutrition care process*, ed 13, Philadelphia, 2012, Saunders.

Sullivan S, et al: Nutritional physiology of the alimentary tract. In Ross AC, et al, editors: *Modern nutrition in health and disease*, ed 11, Philadelphia, 2014, Wolters Kluwer/Lippincott Williams & Wilkins.

CHAPTER 4

Carbohydrates

Found primarily in plants, carbohydrates are a convenient and economical source of calories for people throughout the world.

http://evolve.elsevier.com/GRODNER/FOUNDATIONS

LEARNING OBJECTIVES

- Identify the simple carbohydrates and their components.
- Explain the different types of complex carbohydrates.
- List the dietary recommendations (DRI and AMDR) for carbohydrates.
- Discuss the functions of carbohydrates as a source of energy and dietary fiber.

- Describe the differences and health benefits of soluble and insoluble fiber.
- Compare the nutrient content of refined versus unrefined grains.

ROLE IN WELLNESS

Nature has provided us with an excellent source of energy: carbohydrates. Found primarily in plants, **carbohydrates** are a convenient and economical source of calories for people throughout the world. Carbohydrates are organic compounds composed of carbon, hydrogen, and oxygen. These compounds consist of simple carbohydrates, such as glucose and sucrose, and complex carbohydrates, which include starch and dietary fiber. Each type of carbohydrate serves a distinct role in nourishing the body.

In addition to serving as an energy source, some carbohydrates are also used as sweetening agents. When carbohydrate sweeteners are found naturally in foods, such as in fruits, they are accompanied by essential nutrients. The sweetness makes eating nutrient-dense foods even more enjoyable. Some carbohydrates also supply dietary fiber.

The energy value of carbohydrates was discovered in 1844 (Dolan and Adams-Smith, 1978). Recognition that increasing our consumption of carbohydrates from grains, vegetables, and fruits provides preventive health benefits is more recent. Increased levels of complex carbohydrates, particularly dietary fiber, appear to reduce the risk factors associated with chronic diet-related disorders such as heart disease, diabetes, and some cancers. The *Dietary Reference Intake (DRI)* for carbohydrates is 130 g/day for adults between 19 and 30 years of age. The *Acceptable Macronutrient Distribution Range (AMDR)* for carbohydrates is 45% to 65% of kcal intake per day as primarily complex carbohydrates (National Research Council [NRC], 2006). The U.S. Department of Agriculture (USDA) and U.S. Department of Health and Human Services

(USDHHS) *Dietary Guidelines for Americans, 2010,* concurs, recommending that we emphasize a plant-based diet consisting of fruits, vegetables, cooked dried beans and peas, whole grains, and seeds (USDA/USDHHS, 2010). This advice is reflected in the nutrition guide MyPlate. More than three quarters of MyPlate consists of food groups that are excellent sources of carbohydrates: fruits, vegetables, and grains. Although recommendations vary according to individual needs, average suggestions of 2 cups of fruits, 2½ cups of vegetables, and 6 ounces of grains (bread, cereal, rice, and pasta), with at least half being whole grains, provide adequate amounts of complex carbohydrates (Box 4-1).

Considering carbohydrates through the health dimensions provides perspective on their role in wellness. The *physical health* dimension depends on our ability to provide our bodies with enough carbohydrate kcal for energy and enough complex carbohydrates and fiber consumption for optimum body functioning. Issues related to the role of carbohydrates are often in the headlines. Our ability to process research findings and make decisions about our food choices reflects our level of *intellectual*, or reasoning, *health* dimension. For some of us, *emotional health* may depend on the ability to distinguish hypoglycemic (low blood glucose) symptoms. If we are aware of our personal response to normal hypoglycemia, can we then distinguish real emotional issues from those caused by hypoglycemia? The *social health* dimension also may be tested. Social groups can support change or make changes more difficult to achieve. Will you or your client feel comfortable snacking on a banana (a good fiber source) while other people are unwrapping chocolate bars? The *spiritual health* dimension has ties to carbohydrates because several

BOX 4-1 MyPlate: Grains

MyPlate provides a wealth of resources about nutrients, foods, portion sizes, and activity levels related to caloric needs. Highlights of grains food sources are listed here, but the reader should explore the MyPlate site, at ChooseMyPlate.gov, to customize the information to individual needs.

What Foods Are in the Grains Group?

Any food made from wheat, rice, oats, cornmeal, barley, or another cereal grain is a grain product. Bread, pasta, oatmeal, breakfast cereals, tortillas, and grits are examples of grain products.

Grains are divided into two subgroups, whole grains and refined grains.

Whole grains contain the entire grain kernel—the bran, germ, and endosperm.

Examples are:

- Whole-wheat flour
- Bulgur (cracked wheat)
- Oatmeal
- Whole cornmeal
- Brown rice

Refined grains have been milled, a process that removes the bran and germ. Milling is done to give grains a finer texture and improve their shelf life, but it also removes dietary fiber, iron, and many B vitamins.

Some examples of refined grain products are:

- White flour
- De-germed cornmeal
- White bread
- White rice

Most refined grains are *enriched*. This means that certain B vitamins (thiamin, riboflavin, niacin, folic acid) and iron are added back after processing. Fiber is not added back to enriched grains. Check the ingredient list on refined grain products to make sure that the word "enriched" is included in the grain name. Some food products are made from mixtures of whole grains and refined grains.

Key Consumer Message: *Make at least half of your grains whole grains.*

Commonly Eaten Grain Products

Whole Grains

- Amaranth
- Brown rice
- Buckwheat
- Bulgur (cracked wheat)
- Millet
- Oatmeal
- Popcorn
- Rolled oats
- Quinoa
- Sorghum
- Triticale
- Whole-grain barley
- Whole-grain cornmeal
- Whole rye
- Whole-wheat bread
- Whole-wheat crackers
- Whole-wheat pasta
- Whole-wheat sandwich buns and rolls
- Whole-wheat tortillas
- Wild rice
- Ready-to-eat breakfast cereals:
  - Whole-wheat cereal flakes
  - Muesli

Refined Grains

- Cornbread*
- Corn tortillas*
- Couscous*
- Crackers*
- Flour tortillas*
- Grits
- Noodles*
- Pitas*
- Pretzels
- White bread
- White sandwich buns and rolls
- White rice
- Pastas:
  - Spaghetti
  - Macaroni
- Ready-to-eat breakfast cereals:
  - Corn flakes

*Most of these products are made from refined grains. Some are made from whole grains. Check the ingredient list for the words "whole grain" or "whole wheat" to determine whether a food is made from a whole grain. Some foods are made from a mixture of whole and refined grains.

Some grain products contain significant amounts of bran. Bran provides fiber, which is important for health. However, products with added bran or bran alone (e.g., oat bran) are not necessarily whole-grain products.

What Counts as an Ounce Equivalent of Grains?

In general, 1 slice of bread, 1 cup of ready-to-eat cereal, or ½ cup of cooked rice, cooked pasta, or cooked cereal can be considered a 1-ounce equivalent from the Grains Group.

BOX 4-1 MyPlate: Grains—cont'd

The following table lists specific amounts that count as 1-ounce equivalents of grains towards your daily recommended intake. In some cases the number of ounce equivalents for common portions is also shown.

		AMOUNT THAT COUNTS AS 1 OUNCE-EQUIVALENT OF GRAINS	COMMON PORTIONS AND OUNCE-EQUIVALENTS
Bagels	WG: whole wheat RG: plain, egg	1 "mini" bagel	1 large bagel = 4-ounce equivalents
Biscuits	(baking powder/ buttermilk—RG)	1 small (2-in. diameter)	1 large (3-in. diameter) = 2-ounce equivalents
Breads	WG: 100% whole wheat RG: white, wheat, French, sourdough	1 regular slice 1 small slice French 4 snack-size slices rye bread	2 regular slices = 2-ounce equivalents
Bulgur	cracked wheat (WG)	½ cup cooked	
Cornbread	(RG)	1 small piece (2½ in. × 1¼ in. × 1¼ in.)	1 medium piece (2½ in. × 2½ in. × 1¼ in.) = 2-ounce equivalents
Crackers	WG: 100% whole wheat, rye RG: saltines, snack crackers	5 whole-wheat crackers 2 rye crispbreads 7 square or round crackers	
English muffins	WG: whole wheat RG: plain, raisin	Half a muffin	1 muffin = 2-ounce equivalents
Muffins	WG: whole wheat RG: bran, corn, plain	1 small (2½-in. diameter)	1 large (3½-in. diameter) = 3-ounce equivalents
Oatmeal	(WG)	½ cup cooked 1 packet instant 1 ounce (⅓ cup) dry (regular or quick)	
Pancakes	WG: whole wheat, buckwheat RG: buttermilk, plain	1 pancake (4½-in. diameter) 2 small pancakes (3-in. diameter)	3 pancakes (4½-in. diameter) = 3-ounce equivalents
Popcorn	(WG)	3 cups, popped	1 mini microwave bag or 100-calorie bag, popped = 2-ounce equivalents
Ready-to-eat breakfast cereal	WG: toasted oat, whole-wheat flakes RG: corn flakes, puffed rice	1 cup flakes or rounds 1¼ cup puffed	
Rice	WG: brown, wild RG: enriched, white, polished	½ cup cooked 1 ounce dry	1 cup cooked = 2-ounce equivalents
Pasta—spaghetti, macaroni, noodles	WG: whole wheat RG: enriched, durum	½ cup cooked 1 ounce dry	1 cup cooked = 2-ounce equivalents
Tortillas	WG: whole wheat, whole-grain corn RG: flour, corn	1 small flour tortilla (6-in. diameter) 1 corn tortilla (6-in. diameter)	1 large tortilla (12-in. diameter) = 4-ounce equivalents

RG, Refined grains; *WG*, whole grains. This information is shown when products are available both in whole-grain and refined-grain forms.

Modified from U.S. Department of Agriculture, Center for Nutrition Policy and Promotion: *Choose My Plate*, Alexandria, VA, 2011, Author. Accessed July 20, 2013, from www.choosemyplate.gov/.

---

religions view bread, a carbohydrate, as the "staff of life." The *environmental health* dimension may impact our available sources of carbohydrates. Are whole-grain products and snacks accessible and affordable, or are overly refined and/or excessively sweet carbohydrate foods the only options?

FOOD SOURCES

The carbohydrates we consume are primarily from plant sources. As plants grow, they capture energy from the sun and chemically store it as carbohydrates. This process, called *photosynthesis,* depends on water from the earth, carbon dioxide from the atmosphere, and chlorophyll in the plant leaves to form carbohydrates.

All carbohydrates are organic compounds composed of carbon, hydrogen, and oxygen in the form of simple carbohydrates or sugars (Figure 4-1). When linked together, these simple sugars form three sizes of carbohydrates: monosaccharides, disaccharides, and polysaccharides (Figure 4-2).

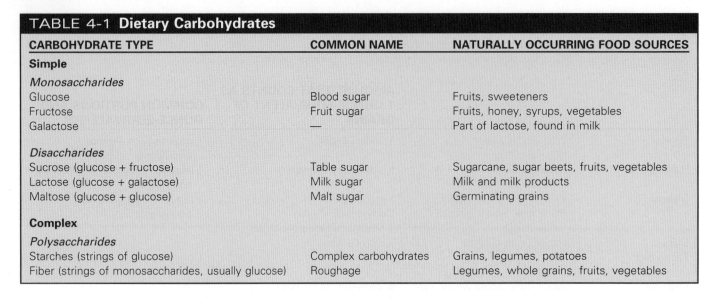

TABLE 4-1 Dietary Carbohydrates

CARBOHYDRATE TYPE	COMMON NAME	NATURALLY OCCURRING FOOD SOURCES
Simple		
Monosaccharides		
Glucose	Blood sugar	Fruits, sweeteners
Fructose	Fruit sugar	Fruits, honey, syrups, vegetables
Galactose	—	Part of lactose, found in milk
Disaccharides		
Sucrose (glucose + fructose)	Table sugar	Sugarcane, sugar beets, fruits, vegetables
Lactose (glucose + galactose)	Milk sugar	Milk and milk products
Maltose (glucose + glucose)	Malt sugar	Germinating grains
Complex		
Polysaccharides		
Starches (strings of glucose)	Complex carbohydrates	Grains, legumes, potatoes
Fiber (strings of monosaccharides, usually glucose)	Roughage	Legumes, whole grains, fruits, vegetables

● = Oxygen
○ = Carbon

FIG 4-1 Structure of a molecule of carbohydrate.

Represents one sugar molecule (or sugar "unit"), such as glucose.

Monosaccharides
Disaccharides
} Sugars or simple carbohydrates

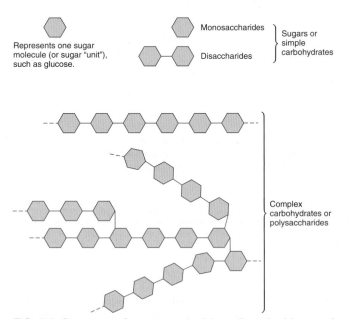

Complex carbohydrates or polysaccharides

FIG 4-2 Structure of monosaccharides, disaccharides, and polysaccharides.

Monosaccharides are composed of single carbohydrate units. Glucose, fructose, and galactose are monosaccharides. **Disaccharides** consist of two single carbohydrates bound together. Sucrose, maltose, and lactose are disaccharides.

Polysaccharides consist of many units of monosaccharides joined together. Starch and fiber are food sources of polysaccharides, whereas glycogen is a polysaccharide stored in the liver and muscles.

The three sizes of carbohydrates are divided into two classifications: *simple carbohydrates* (monosaccharides and disaccharides) and *complex carbohydrates* (polysaccharides) (Table 4-1). Both are valuable sources of carbohydrate energy. There are differences, however, between the health values of simple and complex carbohydrates found in the foods we consume. Although simple carbohydrates primarily provide energy in the form of glucose, fructose, and galactose, complex carbohydrates may provide fiber in addition to glucose.

CARBOHYDRATE AS A NUTRIENT WITHIN THE BODY

Function

Carbohydrates provide energy, fiber, and naturally occurring sweeteners (sucrose and fructose). Energy is the only real nutrient function of carbohydrates; the roles of fiber and carbohydrate sweeteners are discussed later in this chapter. Carbohydrates supply energy in the most efficient form for use by our bodies. If enough carbohydrate is provided to meet the energy needs of the body, protein can be spared or saved to use for specific protein functions. This service of carbohydrates is called the *protein-sparing effect*.

When adequate amounts of carbohydrates are available, both carbohydrates and small amounts of fats are used for energy. When there are not enough carbohydrates available, fat is metabolized, resulting in the formation of ketones, intermediate products of fat metabolism. The body without distress easily disposes of low levels of ketones. If carbohydrate levels continue to be insufficient to meet energy demands, increased levels of ketones overwhelm the physiologic system and ketoacidosis develops; ketoacidosis affects the pH balance of the body, which can be lethal if uncontrolled. Although lipids and proteins can, if necessary, provide energy for most bodily needs, the brain and nerve tissues function best on glucose from carbohydrates.

Digestion and Absorption

Our food sources of carbohydrates tend to be disaccharides (sugars) and polysaccharides (starches). The gastrointestinal (GI) tract has the role of digesting carbohydrates into monosaccharides for easy absorption. The digestive process begins in the mouth. Mechanical digestion breaks food into smaller pieces and mixes the carbohydrate-containing food with saliva, which contains an amylase called *ptyalin*. This begins the hydrolysis of starch into the simpler carbohydrate intermediary forms of dextrin and maltose. In the small intestine, intestinal enzymes and specific pancreatic amylase work on starch intermediary products to continue the breakdown to monosaccharides.

⊕ CULTURAL CONSIDERATIONS

The Missing Enzymes

Approximately 70% of the adult world population is unable to easily digest the lactose found in milk. Among white North Americans, Europeans, and Australians, about 5% to 17% have lactose maldigestion. Those of mixed ethnicity tend to experience a lower prevalence (Lomer, 2008). This condition, lactose intolerance, occurs when the body does not produce enough lactase, a digestive enzyme that breaks lactose into glucose and galactose. When the lactose sits in the large intestine, bacteria begin to ferment the undigested lactose, causing diarrhea, bloating, and increased gas formation.

Lactase deficiency may have a primary or secondary cause. Primary lactose intolerance is caused by a genetic factor that limits the ability to produce lactase. Although small amounts of lactose can often be tolerated, the level of lactose produced cannot be enhanced. The condition is common among Asian/Pacific Islanders (Asian Americans), Africans (African Americans), Hispanics (Hispanic Americans), Latinos, and Native Americans. In the United States the prevalence of lactose intolerance due to maldigestion or low lactose levels is approximately 75% in African Americans and Native Americans, 90% in Asian/Pacific Islanders, 50% in Hispanic Americans, and lowest among whites.

One explanation for primary lactose intolerance is that the ability to digest milk is age related. Consider that the milk of mammals, including humans, was intended for the young to consume during periods of major growth. The ability to digest milk may diminish because the biologic need is lessened as maturity is reached. Older adults may also experience lactose intolerance when the aging process diminishes the production of some digestive enzymes such as lactase. The recent identification of a genetic variation is valuable for future diagnostic testing to determine risk for and severity of lactose intolerance earlier in life.

Sometimes, secondary lactose intolerance occurs when a chronic GI illness affects the intestinal tract, reducing the amount of lactase produced (see Chapter 13). Even a bout of an intestinal virus or flu can cause temporary lactose intolerance. Most individuals in whom this occurs recover and are again able to digest lactose.

Application to nursing: Health professionals can guide clients to determine what amounts of lactose-containing foods can be tolerated despite low lactase levels. Fine-tuning eating styles may require the assistance of a registered dietitian/nutritionist (RDN) to ensure adequate consumption of calcium-containing foods. Depending on the severity of the sensitivity, advice to clients may include additional label reading for lactose-containing foods and medications, especially for clients dealing with conditions such as irritable bowel syndrome.

Data from Lomer MC, et al: Review article: Lactose intolerance in clinical practice—myths and realities, *Aliment Pharmacol Ther,* 27: 93-103, 2008; and National Institutes of Health: *Lactose intolerance: What you need to know* (National Institutes of Health Pub No 11–6187S), Washington, DC, 2011, National Digestive Diseases Information Clearinghouse.

✦ TEACHING TOOL

Lacking Lactose? No Problem!

Lactose intolerance is not an illness and should not undermine a person's sense of wellness. To ensure that clients receive an adequate supply of nutrients usually consumed in lactose-containing dairy products—especially calcium, riboflavin, and vitamin D—without the use of supplements, consider making the following suggestions:

- Experiment with different portion sizes of lactose-containing foods to determine individual levels of tolerance; small amounts up to $\frac{1}{2}$ cup consumed throughout the day can often be tolerated.
- Use over-the-counter lactase-enzyme tablets when consuming dairy products (currently available as Lactaid, Lactrase, Dairy Ease, and others).
- If available, purchase lactose-reduced dairy products such as milk, ice cream, and soft cheeses.
- Try out different milk alternatives such as soy milk and other nondairy beverages. BUT choose only products fortified with calcium, vitamin D, and B_{12} to obtain nutrients similar to those from dairy products.

- Consume foods high in nutrients found in lactose-containing foods; high-calcium foods include broccoli, eggs, kale, spinach, tofu, shrimp, canned salmon, sardines with bones, and calcium-fortified orange juice.
- Consume hard cheeses (in moderate amounts because of fat content) that contain lower lactose levels, such as Swiss, cheddar, Muenster, Parmesan, Monterey, and provolone.
- Avoid softer cheeses (or experiment to learn level of tolerance), such as ricotta, cottage, mozzarella, Neufchatel, and cream.
- Test tolerance of different brands of yogurt; lactose levels may vary according to variations in processing. Generally, lactase bacteria in yogurt culture hydrolyzes some of the lactose.
- Consider supplementation if these dietary modifications are not achieved; consult with a dietitian/nutritionist for an appropriate supplement.

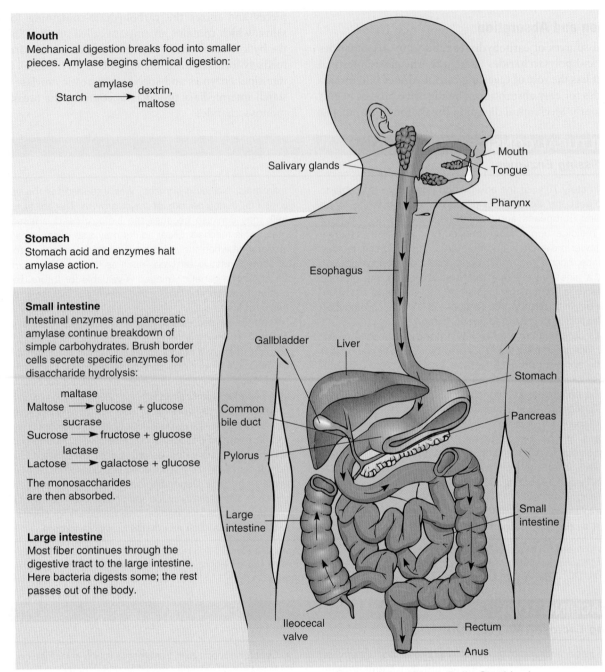

Mouth

Mechanical digestion breaks food into smaller pieces. Amylase begins chemical digestion:

$$\text{Starch} \xrightarrow{\text{amylase}} \text{dextrin, maltose}$$

Stomach

Stomach acid and enzymes halt amylase action.

Small intestine

Intestinal enzymes and pancreatic amylase continue breakdown of simple carbohydrates. Brush border cells secrete specific enzymes for disaccharide hydrolysis:

$$\text{Maltose} \xrightarrow{\text{maltase}} \text{glucose} + \text{glucose}$$
$$\text{Sucrose} \xrightarrow{\text{sucrase}} \text{fructose} + \text{glucose}$$
$$\text{Lactose} \xrightarrow{\text{lactase}} \text{galactose} + \text{glucose}$$

The monosaccharides are then absorbed.

Large intestine

Most fiber continues through the digestive tract to the large intestine. Here bacteria digests some; the rest passes out of the body.

FIG 4-3 Summary of carbohydrate digestion and absorption. (From Rolin Graphics.)

Enzymes specific for disaccharides (lactase for lactose, sucrase for sucrose, maltase for maltose) are secreted by the small intestine's brush-border cells, which then hydrolyze disaccharides into monosaccharides. (For more information, see the *Cultural Considerations* box The Missing Enzyme, and the *Teaching Tool* box Lacking Lactose? No Problem!) After an active absorption process (i.e., one that requires energy input), absorptive cells in the small intestine take up these monosaccharides. Once glucose, fructose, and galactose enter the villi, the portal blood circulatory system transports them to the liver. The liver removes fructose and galactose and converts them to glucose. This glucose may be used immediately for energy or for glycogen formation, a storage form of carbohydrate providing an always-ready source of energy. Figure 4-3 summarizes carbohydrate digestion.

Glycogen: Storing Carbohydrates

Glycogen is carbohydrate energy stored in the liver and in muscles. The amount held in the muscles of an adult is 150 g (600 kcal); 90 g (360 kcal) are stored in the liver. Retrieved as needed for energy, glycogen is quickly broken down by enzymes to produce a surge of energy. The process of converting glucose to glycogen is glycogenesis.

Glycogen levels can be significantly increased through physical training and dietary manipulations (see Chapter 9).

It is still considered a relatively limited source of energy in comparison with the amounts of energy stored in body fat.

Metabolism

A primary aspect of carbohydrate metabolism is the maintenance of blood glucose homeostasis between 70 and 100 mg/dL. Sources of blood glucose, the most common sugar in the blood, may be carbohydrate and noncarbohydrate. Dietary starches and simple carbohydrates provide blood glucose after digestion and absorption; glycogen stored in the liver and muscle tissue is converted back to glucose in a process called glycogenolysis. Intermediate carbohydrate metabolites are also a source of blood glucose. The metabolites include lactic acid and pyruvic acid, which occur when muscle glycogen is used for energy.

Noncarbohydrates can also provide blood glucose. Gluconeogenesis is the process of producing glucose from fat. It is not as efficient as using carbohydrate directly for glucose. As fat is metabolized into fatty acids and glycerol (see Chapter 5), the smaller glycerol portion can be converted by the liver into glycogen, which is then available for glucose needs through glycogenolysis. Protein, which is composed of numerous combinations of amino acids, also may be a source of glucose. Some of these amino acids are glucogenic; if they are not used for protein structures, they can be metabolized to form glucose. Carbohydrate as an energy source is also discussed in Figure 9-2.

Blood glucose is a source of energy to all cells. Glucose may be used immediately as energy or converted to glycogen or fat; both conversions provide energy for the future. Although glycogen can be converted back to glucose, the conversion of glucose to fat is irreversible. Glucose cannot be formed again but is stored as fat and, if needed, is metabolized later as fat, although its original source was carbohydrate.

Glucose is essential for brain function and cell formation, particularly during pregnancy and growth. Because the body can form glucose through gluconeogenesis from protein and fat, glucose technically is not an essential nutrient. Gluconeogenesis can provide some glucose but not enough to meet essential needs if dietary carbohydrate is insufficient. To compensate (as previously discussed), ketone bodies can be used for energy. Ketone bodies are created when fatty acids are broken down for energy when sufficient carbohydrates are unavailable; this process of fat metabolism, however, is incomplete. If dietary carbohydrate continues to be insufficient, a buildup of ketones results, which causes ketosis, possibly leading to acid-base imbalances in the body.

Blood Glucose Regulation

Metabolism of glucose and regulation of blood glucose levels are controlled by a sophisticated hormonal system. Insulin, a hormone produced by the beta cells of the islets of Langerhans, lowers blood glucose levels by enhancing the conversion of excess glucose to glycogen through glycogenesis or to fat stored in adipose tissue. Insulin also eases the absorption of glucose into the cells so the use of glucose as energy is increased.

Whereas insulin lowers blood glucose levels, other hormones raise glucose levels. The pancreas produces two hormones with this function: glucagon and somatostatin. Glucagon stimulates conversion of liver glycogen to glucose, assisting the regulation of glucose levels during the night; somatostatin, secreted from the hypothalamus and pancreas, inhibits the functions of insulin and glucagon. Several adrenal gland hormones also have a role in raising blood glucose levels. Epinephrine enhances the fast conversion of liver glycogen to glucose. Steroid hormones function against insulin and promote glucose formation from protein. Produced by the pituitary gland, growth hormone and adrenocorticotropic hormone (ACTH) function as insulin inhibitors. The thyroid hormone thyroxine affects blood glucose levels by enhancing intestinal absorption of glucose and releasing epinephrine. Hypoglycemia (abnormally low blood glucose level) and diabetes mellitus (DM) (abnormally high blood glucose level) may occur when these systems cannot regulate glucose within normal levels. These conditions are discussed in Chapter 15.

Glycemic Index and Glycemic Load

Although the sophisticated hormonal system controls the metabolism and regulation of blood glucose levels, it is most likely that the composition of foods we consume differ significantly in their effects on blood glucose levels. To account for this, the concepts of glycemic index and glycemic load are used. Glycemic index is the ranking of foods according to the level to which a food raises blood glucose levels compared with a reference food such as a 50-g glucose load or white bread containing 50 g carbohydrate (Keim, et al, 2014). A ranking of 100 is the highest glycemic index level—that is, it raises blood glucose levels the highest. Note the glycemic index rankings of commonly consumed foods listed in Table 4-2.

The glycemic index of a food is affected by the following factors:
- The physical form such as a baked potato compared with a mashed potato
- The fat and protein content in addition to carbohydrate, which slows digestion
- The ripeness, such as in fruits and vegetables, which increases glucose content
- The fiber content, which slows digestion
- The botanic variety of a food, such as the different glycemic indexes of rice species

Because the glycemic index assesses only one food item, another measurement tool is needed because we usually eat several foods at the same time. This is accounted for by the glycemic load, which considers the total glycemic index effect of a mixed meal or dietary plan. It is calculated as the sum of the products of the glycemic index for each of the foods multiplied by the amount of carbohydrate in each food (Keim, et al, 2014). Given that glycemic load accounts for the mixed consumption of foods, it measures the quantity and quality of the effect of carbohydrate on blood glucose and the resulting effect on insulin release (Gallagher, 2012).

TABLE 4-2 Glycemic Index Comparisons of Commonly Consumed Foods

GLYCEMIC INDEX	FOOD
60	Mini-wheat cereal (WG)
60	Raisin bran cereal (WG)
92	Corn flake cereal (RG)
60	Whole-grain bread (WG)
72	White bread (RG)
72	Bagel (RG)
30	Spaghetti/whole wheat (WG)
60	Spaghetti (RG)
50	Brown rice (WG)
60	White rice (RG)
30	Skim milk
40	Apple juice
50	Orange juice
63	Cola
70	Sports drinks
33	Pear
40	Apple
48	Orange
50	Banana
50	Sweet potato
90	Potato (baked, no fat)
14	Peanuts
22	Cashews
30	Legumes (lentils, chickpeas)

GI, Glycemic index; *RG*, refined grains; *WG*, whole grains.
Data from Atkinson FS, et al: International table of glycemic index and glycemic load values: 2008, *Diabetes Care* 31(12):2281-2283, 2008.

Recent epidemiologic work notes associations between glycemic index and glycemic load and the risk of chronic diseases such as type 2 diabetes mellitus (T2DM), cardiovascular disease, and diet-related cancers of the colon and breast. Seemingly, limiting consumption of foods that produce a high glycemic index and overall high glycemic load may reduce risk. Public health recommendations, however, will most likely not be forthcoming until long-term clinical trials demonstrate a clear role for these diet-related effects. Regardless, the concept of glycemic index continues to be explored even though it measures individual foods, not mixed meals within which the carbohydrate effect might vary. These concepts can be helpful for management of diabetes and hypoglycemia (Keim, et al, 2014).

Nonetheless, consider the potential value of the glycemic index in the following situations. The glycemic index of a food may affect a person's blood glucose level, but that same food as part of a meal of several foods (a mix of high and low glycemic indexes) will have a different effect or glycemic load. If a person's dietary goal is to have an even blood glucose level, one could choose foods that provide an even response and, by consuming foods throughout the day, avoid a feasting or fasting experience. Certainly this is what individuals with diabetes (abnormally high blood glucose levels) accomplish through counting carbohydrates and planning nourishment within intentional intervals. For those of us who are prone to hypoglycemia (abnormally low blood glucose level), consuming low glycemic index foods or meals with moderate glycemic loads may maintain adequate blood glucose levels. For the rest of us, having a stable level of blood glucose for energy from the foods we consume provides much-needed stamina. The bottom line to this issue for most of us is that we struggle enough with just preparing and finding time to eat adequate meals. Adding the layer of assessing glycemic index and glycemic loads to foods and meals may fine-tune maintaining stability of blood glucose levels—even within the stressors of our contemporary lifestyles (Box 4-2).

SIMPLE CARBOHYDRATES

Monosaccharides

Glucose, often called *blood sugar,* is the form of carbohydrate most easily used by the body. It is the simple carbohydrate that circulates in the blood and is the main source of energy for the central nervous system and brain. Glucose is rapidly absorbed into the bloodstream from the intestine, but it needs insulin to be taken into the cells, where energy is released.

Fructose is the sweetest of the sugars. Although fruits and honey contain a mixture of sugars, including sucrose, fructose provides the characteristic taste of fruits and honey. After absorption from the small intestine, fructose circulates in the bloodstream. When it passes through to the liver, liver cells rearrange fructose into glucose.

Galactose is rarely found in nature by itself but is part of the disaccharide lactose, the sugar found in milk. Absorbed like fructose, galactose is converted to glucose by the liver.

Disaccharides

Sucrose is formed from the pairing of units of glucose and fructose. We know it as *table sugar.* Sugarcane and sugar beets are two sources of sucrose, which is found naturally in fruits. Because it contains fructose, sucrose is quite sweet. Sucrose has a special place in our history of food consumption and is further explored in the following section.

Maltose is created when two units of glucose are linked. It is available when cereal grains are about to germinate and the plant starch is broken down into maltose. The majority of maltose in human nutrition is created from the breakdown of starch in the small intestine. Maltose is of particular value in the production of beer and other malt beverages. When maltose ferments, alcohol is formed.

Lactose is composed of glucose and galactose. It is sometimes called *milk sugar* because it is the primary carbohydrate in milk.

Sugar—A Special Disaccharide

The term *sugar* is a word with many meanings. Sugar may refer to the simple carbohydrates (monosaccharides and disaccharides). Sucrose, the disaccharide naturally found in many fruits, is also called sugar. White table sugar refers to

BOX 4-2 To Eat, or Not to Eat?

"Carbs" are a part of everyday food talk, much as "fat" used to be. We thought that if only "fat" intake was lower we would be at healthy weights and free of heart disease and other chronic diseases. Not so. As a nation, we gained weight instead. Now, just replace "fat" with "carbs," and the myth continues.

Can Eating Fewer Carbs Lead to Weight Loss?

Yes, it can, but only if total caloric intake is lower. Weight will return, though, if calories and carbohydrate intake are again elevated. Reducing intake to very low levels, such as 20 g a day, is not a long-term weight-loss approach. Our bodies function best when we consume some carbohydrates because daily we must use about 100 g of carbohydrates as glucose for brain function.

Isn't Eliminating Carbs Such as Doughnuts and Sweets a Healthy Approach to Weight Loss?

The answer depends on how carbs are decreased. Replacing carbohydrate calories with saturated fats found in animal proteins is not health promoting. But if nutrient-empty carbohydrate foods are replaced with low-carbohydrate salad greens and vegetables, health benefits may accrue. The key is portion size and calorie control. Moderate intake of all nutrient groups is best. Some of us may feel better with a higher carbohydrate intake, whereas others feel best with a greater proportion of protein (lean, of course) consumption.

What About Eating Lower-Carb Products Such as Breads, Tortillas, and Pasta?

This issue, too, depends on how many calories of carbohydrates a person tends to consume and what kinds of carbohydrates. Whole-grain foods provide more health benefits than refined grain products. Lower-carb products may be labeled as reduced in carbohydrate content because of the addition of dietary fiber to the ingredient formulation of the product. The label statement "reduced carbohydrate content" is based on "net carbs," which are not defined by the U.S. FDA. Manufacturers often present net carbs as equaling total carbohydrates minus dietary fiber and sugar alcohols (which do not quickly raise blood glucose levels). Consuming such products may increase fiber intake, but 100% whole-grain products are the best choice because they most likely contain dietary fiber and less-processed ingredients.

For each of the nutrient categories studied in this book, a "ChooseMyPlate" section is included to emphasize the importance of portion sizes for the MyPlate food categories. For carbohydrates, the focus is on portions of grains.

our clinical use of the term may confuse clients. Concerns about sugar focus on the following three issues: sources in the food supply, consumption levels, and health effects.

Sources in the food supply. Sugar in our food supply may include the following nutritive sweeteners: refined white sugar, brown sugar, dextrose, crystalline fructose, high-fructose corn syrup (HFCS), glucose, corn sweeteners, lactose, concentrated fruit juice, honey, maple syrup, molasses, agave nectar, and reduced energy polyols or sugar alcohols (e.g., sorbitol, mannitol, xylitol) (Fitch and Keim, 2012) (Table 4-3). All forms of sugar are chemically similar; each provides kcal, and most do not contain any other nutrients. Blackstrap molasses does contain iron, but other more nutrient-dense sources of iron are easily available. Honey, which seems less processed than other sweeteners, provides only a trace of minerals and therefore is as nonnutritious as any other sweetener.

The U.S. FDA (2000) categorizes some sweeteners as generally recognized as safe (GRAS) ingredients and others as food additives. For food additives, an acceptable daily intake (ADI) is determined as the amount that a person can safely consume daily over a lifetime without risk. Table 4-3 lists descriptions, regulatory status, and energy amounts provided by sweeteners.

Consumption levels. Our national intake of refined white sugar has declined, whereas consumption of HFCS has greatly increased since the 1970s. In the 1970s, a process was perfected by which HFCS, very sweet-tasting syrup, could be made from corn syrup. HFCS is less expensive to produce than refined sugar and is sweeter. Used extensively in food manufacturing, it has replaced refined white sugar in many products, such as soft drinks.

Health effects. The health concerns regarding sugar consumption include nutrient displacement, dental caries, and the related issues of obesity and diabetes.

Does it matter to our bodies what the source of the sweet taste is? That depends. A major health concern is nutrient displacement. Displacement occurs when whole foods, which are minimally processed, are not eaten and are replaced by foods containing added sugars. If we eat candy, soda, and other sweet snack foods instead of a sandwich and juice for lunch, we lose a number of important nutrients (Figure 4-4).

Foods and drinks with added sugars often contain empty kcal that provide few nutrients. Because all forms of sugar are chemically similar, the sucrose in fruits is actually the same as the sucrose in a cream-filled doughnut. The difference, however, is that naturally occurring vitamins, minerals, and fiber available in the fruit are not available in the doughnut. The doughnut's empty kcal can replace kcal from other foods that might contain a natural sweetener and also provide vitamins, minerals, protein, complex carbohydrates, and fiber. Consumption of excessively sugared food does not support wellness goals because it probably replaces other, more nutrient-dense foods.

Dental caries are related to eating concentrated sweets and sticky carbohydrates. Sugar supports the growth of bacteria, which promotes the formation of plaque. Plaque leads to

sucrose extracted from sugarcane and sugar beets. Sugar may also be an umbrella term used to cover numerous kcal-sweetening agents used in our food production system, although U.S. commercial law defines sugar as "sucrose." There is a distinction between how the term *sugar* is used on a label and how it is used by a biologist, chemist, or nutritionist. Often, blood glucose levels are called *blood sugar levels*. It is important that we, as health professionals, be aware that

TABLE 4-3 Nutritive and Nonnutritive Sweeteners

SWEETENER	kcal/g	REGULATORY STATUS	OTHER NAMES	DESCRIPTION
Sucrose	4	GRAS	Granulated: coarse, regular, fine; powdered; confectioners'; brown; turbinado, Demerara; liquid: molasses	Sweetens; enhances flavor; tenderizes, allows browning, and enhances appearance in baking; adds characteristic flavor with unrefined sugar
Fructose	4	GRAS	High-fructose corn syrups: 42%, 55%, 90% fructose; crystalline fructose: 99% fructose	Sweetens; functions like sucrose in baking Some people experience a laxative response from a load of fructose ≥ 20 g May produce lower glycemic response than sucrose
Monosaccharide Polyols				
Sorbitol	2.6	GRAS (label must warn about a laxative effect)	Same as chemical name	50%-70% as sweet as sucrose Some people may experience a laxative effect from a load of sorbitol ≥ 50 g
Mannitol	1.6	Permitted for use on an interim basis (label must warn about a laxative effect)	Same as chemical name	50%-70% as sweet as sucrose May cause a laxative effect with a load of mannitol ≥ 20 g
Xylitol	2.4	GRAS	Same as chemical name	As sweet as sucrose
Erythritol	0.2	Independent GRAS determination	Same as chemical name	60%-80% as sweet as sucrose
Tagatose	1.5	Independent GRAS determination	Same as chemical name	75%-92% as sweet as sucrose
Nonnutritive				
Saccharin	0	Limited to <12 mg/fl oz in beverages, 20 mg/serving in individual packages, or 30 mg/serving in processed foods ADI: not determined	Sweet'N Low, Sugar Twin	300% sweeter than sucrose Noncariogenic and produces no glycemic response Synergizes the sweetening power of NSs and NNSs Sweetening power is not reduced with heating
Aspartame	4*	Approved as a general-purpose sweetener ADI: 50 mg/kg BW	NutraSweet, Equal	160%-220% sweeter than sucrose Noncariogenic and produces limited glycemic response New forms can increase its sweetening power in cooking and baking
Acesulfame K	0	Approved for use as a tabletop sweetener and as an additive in a variety of desserts, confections, and alcoholic beverages, except not in meat and poultry ADI:15 mg/kg BW	Sunette†	200% sweeter than sucrose Noncariogenic and produces no glycemic response Sweetening power is not reduced with heating Can synergize the sweetening power of other NSs and NNSs
Sucralose	0	Approved for use as a tabletop sweetener and as an additive in a variety of desserts, confections, and nonalcoholic beverages	Splenda‡	600% sweeter than sucrose Noncariogenic and produces no glycemic response Sweetening power is not reduced with heating
Stevia	0	GRAS Approved for use in a variety of food products ADI: 4 mg/kg BW	Truvia, Sun Crystals, Stevia in the Raw	250% sweeter than sucrose

Data from Fitch C, Keim KS: Academy of Nutrition and Dietetics: Position of the Academy of Nutrition and Dietetics: Use of nutritive and nonnutritive sweeteners, *Acad Nutr Diet* 112:739-758, 2012.

ADI, Acceptable daily intake; *BW,* body weight; *GRAS,* generally recognized as safe by the U.S. Food and Drug Administration; *NNS,* nonnutritive sweetener; *NS,* nutritive sweetener.

*Provides limited energy to products because of its sweetening power.

†Hoechst Food Ingredients, Edison, NJ.

‡McNeil Specialty Products Company, New Brunswick, NJ.

FIG 4-4 Consuming products with added sugars *(left)* can displace more nutrient-dense foods *(right)*. (From Joanne Scott/Tracy McCalla.)

tooth decay. Ways to decrease the development of caries are to eat sweets at the end of meals—rather than between meals—and to monitor the quantity and frequency of sugar intake. Sticky, sugary foods are more cariogenic than sweet liquids. Optimal dental hygiene reduces plaque formation and promotes dental health.

A misconception is that obesity is caused by high sugar intake only. In fact, obesity may be caused by an excess intake of kcal from any of the energy nutrients, which is then stored as body fat. Many sugared foods are also high in fat. Because fat is the most energy-dense nutrient, fat intake may be more of a risk factor for obesity than sugar intake.

There is no confirmed relationship between the level of sugar intake and increased risk for development of type 2 diabetes mellitus (NRC, 2006). Once the disorder is confirmed, people with diabetes are counseled to restrict their intake of concentrated sweets to assist the regulation of insulin needs. However, consumption of sweets does not cause the disorder. These issues become complicated because obesity is a risk factor for type 2 diabetes mellitus. Health concerns related to obesity and type 2 diabetes mellitus are explored in Chapters 9 and 15.

A myth that sugar consumption by children produces hyperactivity or attention deficient/hyperactivity disorder (ADHD) continues to be perpetuated. Controlled research studies have consistently failed to support this assertion (Fitch and Keim, 2012). More than likely, excessively active behavior is related to the occasions at which sugared foods such as cake and candy are ingested. If children regularly consume excessive amounts of refined sugar, their overall dietary intake may be nutritionally deficient, possibly resulting in altered behaviors.

So how much sugar is acceptable? Moderate amounts are all right when our diets are low in fat and high in fiber. The *Dietary Guidelines for Americans* suggests consuming sugars in moderation (see Chapter 2). The Dietary Reference Intake (DRI) report on carbohydrates suggests that added sugars be kept to 25% or less of energy intake on a daily basis. Less added sugar intake ensures a dietary intake that is adequate in complex carbohydrates. By following recommendations to

increase consumption of fruits and vegetables to at least five servings or $4\frac{1}{2}$ cups a day and of grains to 6 ounces a day, we can reduce our intake of simple sugars.

Other Sweeteners

Other available sweeteners are sugar alcohols (polyols) and alternative sweeteners. Sugar alcohols, also called *sugar replacers* to avoid confusion with noncarbohydrate alcohol, are nutritive sweeteners because they provide 2 to 3 kcal/g but fewer than the 4 kcal/g of carbohydrates. They occur naturally in fruits and berries. Sorbitol, mannitol, and xylitol are the most commonly used sugar alcohols. Alternative sweeteners are nonnutritive substances produced to be sweet-tasting; however, they provide no nutrients and few, if any, kcal. For food production purposes, sugar alcohols are synthesized rather than derived from natural sources (Fitch and Keim, 2012). Aspartame and saccharin are commonly used alternative sweeteners.

Products containing these sweeteners may be labeled as "sugar free," but this label does not mean "calorie free." Consumers still need to be aware of calories per serving as well as *trans* fat and saturated fat contents. Sometimes when "sugar" is removed, fats are added to improve the taste and texture of the product. This may be problematic for individuals with diabetes who monitor their carbohydrate and dietary fat intake.

Sugar alcohols have several advantages when used to replace sugar. They are less cariogenic than sucrose. In contrast to carbohydrate sugars, sugar alcohols do not encourage the growth of bacteria in the mouth that leads to tooth decay. In fact, xylitol may actually prevent cavity formation and may be protective when used in chewing gum. Although chemically related to carbohydrates, sugar alcohols are absorbed more slowly and incompletely than carbohydrates. The longer absorption time leads to a slower rise in blood glucose levels or reduced glycemic response. People with diabetes may be able to consume moderate amounts of these sweeteners and still control their blood glucose levels.

A disadvantage of sugar alcohols is that if large quantities are consumed, they may ferment in the intestinal tract because of their slower absorption rate. This fermentation may cause gas and diarrhea. The incomplete absorption results in a lower caloric value per gram, and thus less energy is available. Therefore, the sugar alcohols are called *reduced-energy* or *low-energy sweeteners*.

Alternative sweeteners, also called *artificial sweeteners* or *non-nutritive sweeteners* (NNSs), are manufactured to be used as sweetening agents in food products. Their function is to replace naturally sweet substances such as sugar, honey, and other sucrose-containing substances. Alternative sweeteners most commonly used in the United States and approved by the FDA are aspartame, saccharin, acesulfame potassium (K), and sucralose. Often, a combination of alternative sweeteners is used that results in an increased sweetness (Fitch and Keim, 2012).

Aspartame is formed by the bonding of the amino acids phenylalanine and aspartic acid. When consumed, aspartame is digested and absorbed as two separate amino acids. Although aspartame contains the same kcal as sucrose, much less aspartame is needed to get the same sweet taste because it is 160 to 220 times sweeter than sucrose. This provides so few kcal that aspartame can be considered a noncaloric sweetener. Approved in 1981 and used in a wide variety of products such as soft drinks, cereals, chewing gum, frozen snacks, and puddings, aspartame is consumed in more than 100 countries. In 1996, aspartame was approved as a general-purpose sweetener for all foods and beverages.

Several studies have shown aspartame to be safe, yet some individuals have reported side effects thought attributable to its consumption. These included allergic reactions such as rashes; edema of the lips, tongue, and throat; and respiratory difficulties. However, within controlled settings, these reactions were not replicated—meaning that aspartame consumption was not responsible for the allergic reactions (Fitch and Keim, 2012). The Internet has been used by some individuals to spread false information about aspartame, linking its consumption to disorders that range from multiple sclerosis to brain tumors to arthritis. Logically, one substance would not cause such an array of serious disorders. Investigation of the authors of the e-mails revealed sources that were not credible, and therefore the FDA maintains its approval of aspartame.

Individuals with the genetic disorder phenylketonuria (PKU) should not consume aspartame because their bodies cannot break down excess phenylalanine, resulting in a buildup that causes medical problems. All products containing aspartame have a warning label to alert individuals with PKU. This warning should apply to pregnant women as well. Because the fetus would be exposed to excess phenylalanine before the presence of PKU could be determined, the safest approach is to restrict consumption of aspartame during pregnancy.

The general adult population is advised to keep daily aspartame consumption (for a 132-pound person) at or less than 50 mg/kg body weight (the equivalent of 83 packets of Equal, an aspartame product) or 14 12-ounce cans of aspartame-sweetened soda (Fitch and Keim, 2012). Aspartame, when added to products, is often listed by its original brand names, NutraSweet and Equal.

Saccharin has had a stormy history since it was accidentally discovered more than 100 years ago. The storm began when some animal studies indicated an association between excessive saccharin consumption and the development of bladder cancer. In 1977 the FDA proposed a ban on saccharin. Many Americans were upset that the only available noncaloric sweetener was to be banned. The public outcry was so great that Congress, in an unusual move, created a moratorium to prevent the ban. In addition, Congress passed legislation requiring all products containing saccharin to clearly state a warning that the consumption of saccharin may be hazardous to health.

The danger from saccharin is probably minimal. The risk of bladder cancer does not appear to apply to humans because no noticeable increase in rate of bladder cancer has occurred.

In addition, an association between cancers and saccharin is not supported by studies of individuals with diabetes, who tend to consume high amounts of saccharin. Consequently, the moratorium is no longer in effect because the FDA is not pursuing the ban on saccharin. Saccharin is now considered an interim food additive to be used in cosmetics, pharmaceuticals, and foods and beverages (Fitch and Keim, 2012). For food products, the amount of saccharin contained must be identified on the product label. Restrictions include that beverages may contain no more than 12 mg/ounce or less than 30 mg per food serving (FDA, 2000).

Compared with other alternative sweeteners, saccharin has a bitter aftertaste. To mask this flavor, it is often used in combination with other alternative sweeteners. Saccharin is still valuable because it is extremely sweet—300 times sweeter than sucrose. Trade names for saccharin include Sweet'N Low and Sugar Twin.

Acesulfame K received FDA approval in 1988. Synthetically produced, it tastes 200 times sweeter than sucrose, but it is not digestible by the human body and therefore provides no kcal. Acesulfame K is approved for use in a variety of products, from chewing gum to nondairy creamers, but so far its use has been limited. One advantage of this product over aspartame is that it can be used for baking. Heat does not affect its sweetening ability, whereas heat destroys the sweet taste of aspartame. People who must severely limit potassium intake because of nutritional therapy for renal disorders should consult an RD about acceptable levels of acesulfame K intake. The consumer brand name for acesulfame K is Sunette.

Sucralose (trichlorogalactosucrose) was approved by the FDA in April 1998 for use in desserts, candies, and nonalcoholic beverages, and as a tabletop sweetener. Made from chemically altered sucrose, sucralose provides no energy but is 600 times sweeter than sucrose. Because the body poorly absorbs it, sucralose passes through the digestive tract and is excreted in urine. An advantage of sucralose is that it can be used in baking and cooking. Sucralose is currently sold as Splenda.

Another NNS is stevia, which is created from the leaves of a South American shrub. Stevia has been approved as a GRAS food additive by the FDA. Rebiana may be extracted from the stevia leaves and combined with other ingredients to create sweetening products such as Truvia, Sun Crystals, and Stevia in the Raw. Because stevia is used in very small quantities and has no caloric value (depending on other ingredients), individuals with diabetes may use it as another sweetener alternative.

Sweet Decisions

Should you consume foods with real sugar or artificial sugar? Which is the best? Which is the worst? There are no clear answers, but here is a way to decide. A concept used with food safety issues is a benefit-risk analysis. Does the benefit of consuming a substance outweigh the risk? This analysis can be applied to the decision whether to consume artificial sweeteners.

Benefits of consuming artificial sweeteners include experiencing a sweet taste with fewer kcal and a less cariogenic effect than sucrose. Many people believe these sweeteners are an important part of their weight-reduction effort. For most, though, the saved kcal are often replaced by consuming other kcal foods, thereby undermining their weight-loss efforts. Another concern is that recent studies suggest that since non-nutritive sweeteners mimic sweetness, physiologic responses may occur as if a caloric sweetener has been consumed. These responses may promote weight gain. Results have been mixed, so more research is needed. Nonetheless, with the significant consumption of artificially sweetened products, such as diet sodas, beverages, and foods, unforeseen health concerns may surface (Pepino and Bourne, 2011; Shankar, et al, 2013).

As noted, risks associated with the use of alternative sweeteners may involve safety concerns. This is a difficult issue to sort out. Because sucrose in the form of white table sugar has been used for thousands of years, we essentially have a large-scale study of its safety for humans. In contrast, alternative sweeteners have existed only for a century or less. Because alternative sweeteners are not naturally formed in plants or animals, their safety must be determined through research studies.

The research process is difficult. Rather than use humans as test subjects, researchers use animals. The test animals are given extremely large doses of the artificial sweeteners and are followed by researchers for several generations of their species. If the physiology of the animals is affected, particularly in regard to cancerous tumors, the substance may be regarded as too dangerous for consumption by humans. The difficulty is that the extremely large doses given to the animals do not replicate the amounts that would be typically consumed by humans. Concerns raised include whether the substance caused the tumor or whether the excessive quantity interfered with normal cell function. Also, how many animals need to be affected for a substance to be considered dangerous and in what animal generation of the experiment? Attention should also be paid to who funds such studies. If the company manufacturing the substance pays for the research, does that fact affect the interpretation of the results? These are difficult questions with which health scientists and FDA officials grapple.

This is an area, however, in which we can make a personal decision whether to consume products that contain alternative sweeteners. On the basis of our analysis of the benefits and risks, we can decide whether our wellness goals are better met by consuming a moderate amount of sucrose or a reasonable intake of alternative sweetened products.

COMPLEX CARBOHYDRATES: POLYSACCHARIDES

Polysaccharides are many units of monosaccharides held together by different kinds of chemical bonds. These types of bonds affect the ability of the body to digest polysaccharides and therefore account for the classification of polysaccharides as complex carbohydrates.

Starch

All starchy foods are plant foods. Starch is the storage form of plant carbohydrate. The strings of glucose that form starch are broken down by the digestive tract to provide glucose. Food sources of starch include grains, legumes, and some vegetables and fruits. Grains are the best source of starch. Grains provide more carbohydrates than any other food category. Grains are consumed in many forms and include wheat, oats, barley, rice, corn, and rye. The overall health value of processed grain products differs according to their sugar, fat, and fiber content. See the *Personal Perspectives* box, Eat Food, Not Too Much, Mostly Plants.

Breads, bagels, breakfast cereals, pasta, pancakes, grits, oatmeal, and other cooked cereals provide high-quality complex carbohydrates. These grain products may also contain fiber if made with whole grains. Depending on the spreads and toppings served, they may also be low in fat. Main dish items such as pizza, rice casseroles, and pasta mixtures create another category of complex carbohydrate foods. Other foods such as crackers, cakes, pies, cookies, and pastries also provide carbohydrates but often contain considerable amounts of added sugar and fats; they should be eaten in moderation.

Legumes (beans and peas) are another significant source of complex carbohydrates. They are low in fat and are an excellent source of fiber, iron, and protein. Available dried, canned, or frozen, beans can be easily incorporated into commonly eaten foods.

Thai (as above) and other ethnic cuisines can provide a source of complex carbohydrates and variety in the diet.

Multicultural influences have expanded our exposure to inexpensive and versatile legumes. Mexican foods feature kidney beans as an ingredient of taco fillings and chili. Puerto Rican and Caribbean meals highlight rice and beans in savory sauces. Hearty Italian-style soups often depend on white and kidney beans combined with pasta. An African influence is reflected in dishes that combine black-eyed peas with meats or green vegetables. Hummus, a chickpea paste dip of Middle

PERSONAL PERSPECTIVES
"Eat Food, Not Too Much, Mostly Plants"

"Eat food. Not too much. Mostly plants" is the succinct nutrition/food consumption advice of author Michael Pollan for eating wisely. These seven words sum up his many years of extensive journalistic research about "What should I eat?" His results are presented in two of his best sellers: *The Omnivore's Dilemma* and *In Defense of Food: An Eater's Manifesto.* Mark Bittman, a journalist, a researcher, and a food lover, also influences attitudes about what to eat and how to prepare foods through his numerous best-selling cookbooks and writings. His latest book, *Food Matters: A Guide to Conscious Eating,* provides "doable" strategies for consuming "more plants, fewer animals, and as little highly processed food as possible." Here are simple suggestions based on his writings that pertain to ecologically, mindful, healthful, and satisfying consumption of carbohydrates and plants.

Eat Fewer Animal-Derived Foods. Eat More Plant Foods
Why
Production of animal-derived foods substantially affects the global environment, particularly climate change. For example, livestock production releases greenhouse gases into the atmosphere. The amount created accounts for 20% of all greenhouse gases produced. Animal-derived foods tend to be energy intensive. More energy is used to create these foods from animals than their actual food energy value. And finally, animal-derived foods tend to provide more saturated fats, dietary cholesterol, and energy than plant-based foods; these substances are potential risk factors for diet-related chronic disorders.

How
If less meat is eaten, more plant food easily takes its place. Smaller portion sizes are a good way to start. Rather than filling half the dinner plate with meat (beef, pork, chicken, fish, cheese, or eggs), restructure proportions to one part meat (a quarter of the plate); two parts vegetables (half of the plate); and one part grains (a quarter of the plate). Legumes (such as chickpeas, kidney beans, and black beans) can be used to replace some or all of the meat or added to the vegetables or grains.

Eat Real Food
Why
Real food is closest to the form found in nature. Foodstuff may be cleaned of outer inedible parts, eaten raw or cooked, eaten alone or with other ingredients. But the plant or animal source is whole, not taken apart and put back together again with some parts containing nutrients removed (and not returned).

Avoid heavily processed foods. Why? The energy cost to create and package processed foods is substantial. Nutrients are lost during manufacturing. Often, these nutrients are not returned to the product. Preservatives are added to maintain "freshness" so products can have a long shelf life, allowing processed foods to be shipped worldwide. The energy used for transportation adds to the actual cost of processed foods. Real food products, though, should not last forever!

How
We have lost the connection between the means of producing our food and our level of health. That a food product exists does not mean that it is worth consuming or is sufficiently valuable to expend our planet's limited energy and resources for its production.

We can take responsibility for our food intake. Michael Pollan, as described in *The Omnivore's Dilemma,* set out to procure all the ingredients for a meal, including participating in a hunt for a wild pig that he then helped eviscerate and cook as well as foraging for wild mushrooms in secretive forest areas in California. His intent was to realize the effect of his consumption on the earth in a very concrete manner.

Although we don't need to repeat his experience, we can take action by learning how to cook simple meals from scratch. We can return to our kitchens (and to simple cookbooks or Internet recipes) and begin planning and preparing real food. Bittman's advice is that with a little planning, we can alter our lifestyles to nourish our bodies while reducing our impact on the environment.

Data from: Bittman M: *Food matters: A guide to conscious eating,* New York, 2009, Simon & Schuster; Pollan M: *The omnivore's dilemma: A natural history of four meals,* New York, 2007, Penguin Group (USA) Inc.; and Pollan M: *in defense of food: An eater's manifesto,* New York, 2008, Penguin Group (USA) Inc.

Eastern heritage, is often served with pita bread or vegetables.

Among vegetable sources of starch, potatoes lead the way. We consume potatoes in so many ways that we sometimes forget their humble "roots." As a root vegetable, the potato is a powerhouse of complex carbohydrates, fiber, vitamins, and even some protein. Unfortunately, some of the ways we prepare potatoes undo their positive health benefits. Most potatoes are processed into products loaded with fat and sodium. Nutritionally, potato chips have little in common with baked potatoes. The best health value is to eat potatoes in the least-processed form. Instead of French fries, choose a baked potato, or prepare mashed potatoes with skim milk and a small amount of margarine.

Other starchy root vegetables are parsnips, sweet potatoes, and yams. Sweet potatoes and yams provide the same nutrients as white potatoes plus significant amounts of beta carotene. Carrots and some varieties of squash, such as acorn and butternut, also provide starch and beta carotene. Beta carotene, a substance the body can convert into vitamin A, may have a protective effect against some forms of cancer.

Fiber

Fiber, like starch, consists of strings of simple sugars. Unlike starch, however, fiber cannot be broken down by human digestive enzymes. Dietary fiber consists of substances in plant foods, including carbohydrates and lignin, that for the most part cannot be digested by humans. We do not produce

TABLE 4-4   Types, Composition, Sources, and Functions of Fibers

TYPE OF FIBER	MAJOR CHEMICAL COMPONENT(S)	SOURCES	MAJOR FUNCTION(S)
Less Soluble Fiber			
Cellulose	Glucose (β1-4 linkages)	Whole wheat, bran, vegetables	Increase water-holding capacity, thus increasing fecal volume and decreasing gut transit time
Hemicellulose	Xylose, mannose, galactose	Bran, whole grains	
Lignin	Phenols	Fruits and edible seeds, mature vegetables	Fermentation produces short-chain fatty acids associated with decreased risk of tumor formation
More Soluble Fibers			
Gums	Galactose and glucuronic acid	Oats, legumes, guar, barley	Cause gel formation, thus decrease gastric emptying, and slow digestion, gut transit time, and glucose absorption
Pectins	Polygalacturonic acid	Apples, strawberries, carrots, citrus	Also bind minerals, lipids, and bile acids, increasing excretion of each, thus decreasing serum cholesterol
Functional Fibers*			
Chitin	Glucopyranose	Supplement from crab or lobster shells	Reduces serum cholesterol
Fructans (including inulin)	Fructose polymers	Extracted from natural sources: chicory, onions, etc.	Prebiotics that stimulate growth of beneficial bacteria in gut; used as fat replacers
β-Glucans	Glucopyranose	Oat and barley bran	Reduces serum cholesterol
Algal polysaccharides (carrageenan)		Isolated from algae and seaweed	Gel forming—used as thickeners, stabilizers (can be toxic)
Polydextrose, polyols	Glucose and sorbitol, etc.	Synthesized	Used as a bulking agents or sugar substitutes
Psyllium		Extracted from psyllium seeds	Has a high water-binding capacity (choking hazard)

*Isolated or extracted.

Modified from Gallagher ML: The nutrients and their metabolism. In Mahan K, et al, editors: *Krause's food & the nutrition care process,* ed 13, St. Louis, 2012, Saunders/Elsevier.

digestive juices strong enough to break down the bonds that hold the simple carbohydrates of most plant fibers, so fiber "passes through" our bodies without providing kcal or nutrients. Its texture provides bulk that thickens chyme and eases the work of the GI muscles that regulate movement of the food mass (Table 4-4).

Although human digestive juices cannot digest fiber, microflora that normally reside in the colon use fiber as a medium for microbial fermentation, resulting in the synthesis of vitamins and the formation of short-chain fatty acids (SCFAs). The bacteria that reside in the colon synthesize several vitamins, including vitamin K, biotin, B_{12}, folate, and thiamin. Only vitamin K and biotin can be absorbed in sufficient amounts from the colon to be significant; the other vitamins are absorbed from the small intestine so that the synthesized vitamins are not bioavailable. The SCFAs that are produced can be absorbed and used for energy by the mucosa of the colon, thereby maintaining the health of the colon epithelial cells (Sullivan, et al, 2014). The effects of SCFAs also increase fecal matter bulk.

Dietary fiber actually refers to several kinds of carbohydrate substances from different plant sources; all serve similar functions in the human body. Dietary fibers are divided into two categories based on their solubility in fluids. Soluble dietary fibers dissolve in fluids, include pectin, mucilage, psyllium seed husk, guar gum, and other related gums. Soluble fiber thickens substances. Insoluble dietary fibers do not dissolve in fluids and therefore provide structure and protection for plants. Some insoluble dietary fibers are cellulose and hemicellulose. Lignin, considered a dietary fiber, is composed of chains of alcohol rather than carbohydrate.

Foods are sometimes classified according to the predominant type of fiber they contain. Oatmeal is a good source of soluble fiber because oat bran, part of the whole oatmeal grain, is particularly high in soluble fiber. But the whole grain is a good source of insoluble fiber as well. Although Table 4-5 specifically lists foods containing soluble and insoluble dietary fiber, many fiber-rich foods contain some of each kind of fiber. For example, an apple is a source of the soluble dietary fiber pectin, which is part of the inside "stuff" of the apple. An apple also provides cellulose, an insoluble dietary fiber that forms the structure of the apple and gives it its characteristic shape (Figure 4-5). Popcorn is another source of insoluble dietary fiber that has been with us for a long time (see the *Cultural Considerations* box The "Pop" Heard through the Centuries).

⊕ CULTURAL CONSIDERATIONS
The "Pop" Heard through the Centuries

The next time you're at the movies digging into a giant tub of popcorn, be sure to appreciate one of the tastier contributions of Native Americans to our food supply: popping corn, first created over an open fire 5000 years ago. The delectable popcorn added variety to ways to prepare corn, a mainstay of the Native American diet. Gifts of popcorn necklaces and popcorn beer were made by the Indians of the Caribbean in the 1500s, and the Aztecs used popcorn in religious ceremonies. And what would Thanksgiving have been without some popped corn—compliments of the Wampanoag tribe?

Popcorn most likely originated in Mexico, but it was also grown in India, Sumatra, and China years before Columbus "discovered" America. Biblical stories of "corn" in Egypt were not entirely true. The term *corn* meant the most commonly used grain of a region. In Scotland and Ireland, *corn* referred to oats; in England, *corn* was wheat. In the Americas, the common grain was maize, and the two terms, *corn* and *maize*, became synonymous.

Today special varieties of corn have been developed for their "popping" characteristics. When a corn kernel is heated, water in it creates steam. This steam, unable to escape through the heavy skin of the kernel, causes an explosion that exposes the white starchy center. Fortunately, the skin remains attached to the starch, making popcorn an excellent source of dietary fiber.

Although all popcorn provides dietary fiber, some of the ways it is prepared negate this health benefit. Popcorn laden with butter and covered with salt is not a healthful snack nor is a batch popped with the aid of oil, even if vegetable oil is used. Microwaveable packets of popcorn are equally deceiving because they contain oil and other additives. We also may easily be misled into eating more than we should because each bag contains four servings, which most of us devour singlehandedly.

Instead, return to the native style—fresh air-popped corn. Air-popping appliances and microwave containers eliminate the need for oil. Better toppings include sodium-reduced salt, garlic powder, and Cajun spices. While devouring your wholesome snack, remember to acknowledge the inventiveness of Native Americans.

Data from Popcorn Institute: *Early popcorn history,* Chicago, 1996, Author; and National Agricultural Library, Special Collections: *Popcorn: Ingrained in America's agricultural history,* 2002 (updated July 25, 2013). Accessed July 27, 2013, from www.nal.usda.gov/speccoll/images1/popcorn.html/.

Health Effects

All the health benefits of fiber improve the physical functioning of the human body. The benefits are not directly nutritional but instead allow the body to function at a more efficient level. Each of the following disorders listed may develop because of genetic predisposition, environmental factors, or lifestyle behaviors. However, the risk of developing these disorders seems to increase when consumption of dietary fiber is low. Because eating sufficient fiber appears to

TABLE 4-5 Dietary Fibers and Food Sources

FIBERS	FOOD SOURCES
Insoluble	
Cellulose	Whole grains, brown rice, buckwheat
Hemicellulose	groats, whole-wheat flour, whole-wheat
Lignin	pasta, oatmeal, unrefined cereals, vegetables, wheat bran, seeds, popcorn, nuts, peanut butter, leafy green vegetables such as broccoli
Soluble	
Pectin	Kidney beans, split peas, lentils,
Mucilage	chickpeas (garbanzo beans), navy beans,
Guar and other gums	soybeans, apples, pears, bananas, grapes, citrus fruits (oranges and grapefruits), oat bran, oatmeal, barley, corn, carrots, white potatoes

Pectin: soluble fiber

Cellulose: structural insoluble fiber

FIG 4-5 In an apple, insoluble fiber (cellulose) inside and in the skin provides structure, and soluble fiber (pectin) inside adds substance.

be a preventive factor, we consider the benefits of fiber for primary disease prevention. Primary prevention aims to avert the initial development of a disorder or health problem. The risk for development of obesity, constipation, hemorrhoids, diverticular disease, and colon cancer may be decreased by regular consumption of sufficient amounts of fiber. Each of these topics is discussed in Part IV of this book, Overview of Nutrition Therapy. A brief introduction to the relationship between fiber consumption and reduced risk of these disorders is given here.

Obesity. Eating high-fiber foods seems to make weight control easier. The volume of such foods makes us feel fuller, so we consume less food. Often, high-fiber foods replace those that are higher in fat and kcal. Regularly eating foods high in fiber and low in fat may reduce or prevent obesity.

Constipation. Fiber, particularly insoluble fiber such as wheat bran and whole grains, prevents the dry, hard stools of constipation (see Chapter 13). A sufficient fiber intake plus adequate fluid intake ensures larger, softer stools that are easier to eliminate. Less straining during elimination also reduces the risk of hemorrhoids (enlarged veins in the anus) and diverticular disease.

Diverticular disease. Diverticular disease affects the large intestine. Pockets (diverticula) develop on the outside walls of the intestine. Low-fiber diets may create increased internal pressure from segmentation muscles attempting to move the food mass because the bulk of fiber is not available, which may then weaken intestinal muscles. Weakened muscles are more at risk for the formation of diverticula. If feces get caught in the pockets, bacteria may develop, multiply, and cause serious and painful inflammation (diverticulitis). Medical treatment and nutritional recommendations are necessary and are discussed in Chapter 13.

Cancer. Eating enough dietary fiber may also reduce the risk of colon cancer. Two potential risk factors for colon cancer related to fiber intake are a high dietary fat intake and exposure to carcinogenic substances in the GI tract (Keim, et al, 2014). If we eat more fiber, we tend to eat less fat. High-fiber foods tend to replace foods that are high in fat. Because foods containing fiber are bulkier, they seem to fill the stomach quicker, providing satiety sooner and with fewer kcal than foods containing fat. Fiber-containing foods such as fruits and vegetables may contain other substances that may be protective for the colon.

Heart disease. Two heart disease risk factors are high blood cholesterol and increased lipid levels (see Chapter 17 for recommended levels). Increasing dietary fiber consumption can lower blood cholesterol and lipid levels in two ways: (1) high-fiber foods replace higher-fat foods, particularly those containing dietary cholesterol and saturated fats; (2) soluble fiber such as pectin (citrus fruits and apples), guar gum (legumes), and oat gum (oat bran) binds lipids and cholesterol as they move through the intestinal tract and are then excreted with the fiber (Willis and Slavin, 2014).

Diabetes control. Dietary fiber intake may help people with diabetes to stabilize blood glucose levels. Diabetes mellitus affects the body's ability to regulate blood glucose levels. When fiber is consumed, particularly soluble fiber, glucose may be absorbed more slowly. The slower absorption rate of glucose may keep blood glucose within acceptable levels.

Potential Health Risks of Dietary Fiber

When the recommended increase of dietary fiber intake is fulfilled by fiber-containing foods, there tend to be few health risks. Problems may develop when fiber supplements or other forms of processed or purified fiber, such as oat or wheat bran, are consumed in large quantities. When used as a supplement, excessive quantities of purified fiber can overwhelm the GI tract and lead to blockages in the small intestine and colon (Willis and Slavin, 2014). This is a serious medical condition that fortunately is rare.

Bioavailability of minerals may be lowered by the presence of fiber-containing foods. Some fibers and substances in whole grains, such as phytates and oxalates, may bind minerals, making them unable to be absorbed. However, higher-fiber dietary patterns tend also to be higher in mineral content; therefore, absorption of minerals remains adequate.

As fiber passes through the GI tract, it provides several health-promoting services that are still being analyzed. Some foods that contain fiber also contain an assortment of essential nutrients. That is why it is best to get fiber from real foods rather than from supplements.

Because some benefits do vary between soluble and insoluble fibers, should daily intakes of each kind of fiber be calculated? Not at all. Increase total dietary fiber to recommended levels slowly by gradually substituting whole-grain foods, fresh fruits, and vegetables for some lower-fiber foods (see the *Teaching Tool* box, What's Your Fiber Score Today?). This allows the body to adjust to the additional fiber, reducing the possible formation of intestinal gas.

✳ TEACHING TOOL

What's Your Fiber Score Today?

Although the following foods are particularly good sources of dietary fiber, many other foods—all fruits and vegetables—contain smaller amounts that add up by the day's end. Does your typical intake meet the recommended levels of about 25 to 38 g per day?

Approximately 2 g per Serving

Apricot	Grapefruit
Banana	Oatmeal
Blueberries	Peach
Broccoli	Pineapple
Cantaloupe	Rye crackers
Carrot	Whole-wheat bread
Cauliflower	Whole-wheat cereals

Approximately 3 g per Serving

Apple with skin	Potato with skin
Corn	Raisins
Orange	Shredded wheat cereal
Pear	Strawberries
Peas	

Approximately 4 g or More per Serving

Baked beans	Lentils
Bran cereals	Navy beans
Kidney beans	Whole-wheat spaghetti

Data from U.S. Department of Agriculture, Agricultural Research Service: *USDA national nutrient database for standard reference* (Release 26). 2012, Nutrient Data Laboratory. Accessed from www.ars.usda.gov/ba/bhnrc/ndl/.

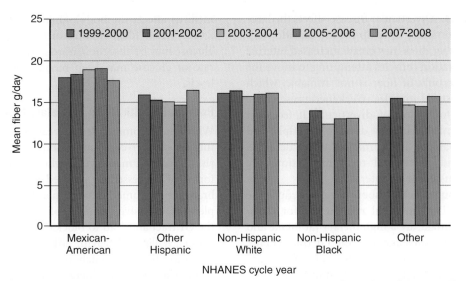

FIG 4-6 Dietary fiber intake of Americans by race/ethnicity and year. (From King DE, et al: Trends in dietary fiber intake in the United States, 1999-2008, *J Acad Nutr Diet*, 112:642-648, 2012.)

FOOD SOURCES AND ISSUES

Although dietary fiber is not absorbed and does not serve a nutrient function in the body, the effects of fiber are important for optimum health. An Adequate Intake (AI) of dietary fiber is about 25 to 38 g per day, depending on age and gender (NRC, 2006). Most Americans consume much lower levels of fiber; adults often average less than 16 g of fiber per day, whereas children and young adults average 12 g (King, et al, 2012).

This situation arises from several factors. First, many Americans do not consume enough fruits and vegetables on a daily basis. Somehow, high protein and fat dietary intakes have pushed fruits and vegetables out of our meal patterns. This is most likely due to the increased consumption of meals away from home tied with the fact that sugared beverages account for a significant percentage of daily caloric intake for many people.

Also, and possibly the most significant factor, is that many Americans regularly eat foods made with refined grains from which dietary fiber has been removed. Consumption of legumes and high-fiber cereal foods provides considerably more fiber. Fiber intake also differs by race/ethnicity (Figure 4-6). Some of the difference is probably due to the fiber levels of traditional foods consumed. For example, Mexican-American consumption of fiber is the highest, whereas African American consumption of fiber is the lowest.

Unrefined versus Refined Grains

Unrefined grains are prepared for consumption while they contain their original components. These grains are really seeds or kernels that include all the nutrients necessary to support plant growth and are segmented inside the kernel to be used when needed. Whole-grain products refer to food items made using all the edible portions of kernels.

In contrast, refined grains have been taken apart. Only portions of the edible kernel are included in refined grain

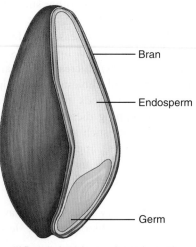

FIG 4-7 Inside a wheat kernel.

products. Although both unrefined and refined grain products are good sources of complex carbohydrates, other nutritional qualities of the whole grain are lost when grains are refined. Grains most often refined are wheat, rice, oats, corn, and rye.

To better understand how the nutrients are lost, consider the wheat kernel shown in Figure 4-7. The kernel consists of three nutrient-containing components. The outer layer, bran, is an excellent source of cellulose dietary fiber and contains magnesium, riboflavin, niacin, thiamin, vitamin B_6, and some protein.

The germ found in the base of the kernel contains a wealth of nutrients to support the sprouting of the plant. Some of these are thiamin, riboflavin, vitamin B_6, vitamin E, zinc, protein, and wheat oil (polyunsaturated vegetable oil). The endosperm, the largest component of the kernel, contains starch, the prime energy source for the sprouting plant. It also contains protein and riboflavin but much smaller amounts of niacin, thiamin, and B_6.

When flour is refined, the bran and germ are removed; the bran affects the physical lightness of the flour, and the oil in the germ may become rancid, reducing the shelf life of the flour. Only the starchy endosperm is used to mill refined flour. Because flour is the mainstay of grain products, the loss of nutrients for the population is significant. In the 1940s it was determined that deficiencies of thiamin, riboflavin, niacin, and iron occurred because of the refining process. To counteract this loss, those four nutrients were added back to flour. Now, flour with these specific nutrient additives is called *enriched flour.*

Enrichment is the replacement of nutrients to the level that was present before processing. Although the four lost nutrients are replaced in enriched flour, other vitamins, minerals, and fiber originally in whole wheat are not. Zinc, magnesium, vitamin E, and dietary fiber are not returned to the refined white flour. Consequently, any product made with enriched white flour is still nutritionally inferior to one made with whole-wheat flour (see the *Health Debate* box, If Dietary Fiber Is So Important, Should Grain Products Be Allowed to Be Refined?)

HEALTH DEBATE

If Dietary Fiber Is So Important, Should Grain Products Be Allowed to Be Refined?

This chapter highlights the health benefits of eating the recommended levels of fiber. Also emphasized are nutrition losses that occur when fruits, vegetables, and grains are processed or refined. The process of refining can lead to the extensive loss of fiber and various nutrients. Although some nutrients are replaced, some, such as dietary fiber, are not.

If health benefits of dietary fiber and nutrients are so valuable, should there be government regulations to restrict or prohibit the removal of valuable nutrients and dietary fiber? Several of the diseases associated with low fiber intake are chronic. Treating these long-term diseases places a burden on the entire U.S. health care system.

Is it fair for all of us to bear the financial burden for those not consuming the most healthful form of foods available? Should there be a law against the processing of whole grains? Should white flour production be restricted? Or is the availability of white (or wheat) and whole-wheat products sufficient? Is it our "freedom of choice" to be able to select among different food products even though some are more beneficial to health than others?

What do you think?

The preference for refined complex carbohydrates may be changing. The health benefits of dietary fiber have been so newsworthy and the focus of such intensive advertising that consumer perception of fiber has evolved from a negative selling point to a positive one. Twenty years ago, if products claimed to be high in fiber or made from whole grains, sales would decline. Today, high-fiber food items are among the better sellers in categories such as cereals and breads (see the *Cultural Considerations* box, Cereals around the World).

CULTURAL CONSIDERATIONS

Cereals Around the World

Hot cereals have been the mainstay of carbohydrate breakfast calories among cultures in colder climates. The adage "sticking to the ribs" foods refers to the warming and filling effects of freshly cooked cereals such as oatmeal, cream of wheat, and oat bran. Just as the Inuit have many words for snow to reflect its many variations in a climate often characterized by snow, Norway, another cold country, has many kinds of porridge or hot cereal. In Norway, porridges may include oats, wheat, barley, rye, and rice. Porridge is often eaten as a winter dinner and can be served cold as dessert pudding topped with fruit sauce. Porridge also has social significance. Extra-creamy porridge is served to women who just gave birth as a way to boost their nutrition. A lucky individual may refer to good luck as being "in the middle of a butter island," meaning the kind of melting butter found in a bowl of steaming porridge.

Consider your own cultural background. Is there a grain or carbohydrate food that has special significance to your family because of its ethnic or regional influence?

Data from The Norwegian Table: *Some like it hot,* Norway, 2001. Accessed July 27, 2013, www.fromnorway.net/norwegian_food/199910/foodcultureone.htm.

TOWARD A POSITIVE NUTRITION LIFESTYLE: *TAILORING*

Consider what a tailor does. A tailor takes a bolt of cloth and by cutting, shaping, and sewing, fits a garment to a person's exact measurements. Tailoring as a behavior-change technique takes a health recommendation and by "cutting," "shaping," and "sewing," fits the recommendation to the limitations or requirements of our individual lifestyles.

Strong recommendations to increase our fiber intake are made in this chapter. Ideally, fiber intake should be about 25 to 38 g a day. The most efficient means of intake would be to replace all refined grain products with whole-grain products. But is that possible if one considers contemporary lifestyles? Often we are not able to control available food choices, and thus we have difficulty changing our behavior to implement this type of recommendation. By tailoring the recommendation or goal to our individual lifestyles, we can succeed. Following are some recommendations for "tailoring" in practice:

- Overwhelmed by the thought of eating only whole-grain foods? Decide to eat more whole-grain products for breakfast and dinner, which are eaten at home, where control is easier.
- No time to cook vegetables? Prepare or order salads and keep fresh fruits of any kind handy.
- Need to add fiber to your diet? When possible, choose fiber-rich foods for lunch. Be realistic, however, because foods available at the cafeteria or coffee shop are limited.

- Attending a family holiday dinner or special event or going on vacation? Enjoy what's served. Then resume a regular fiber-rich dietary pattern when back at work or school.

Although the goal is to increase fiber intake, the objective is to fit positive dietary choices and habits to the shapes of our nutrition lifestyles.

SUMMARY

- Carbohydrates are organic compounds composed of carbon, hydrogen, and oxygen in the form of simple carbohydrates.
  - There are three sizes of carbohydrates: monosaccharides (glucose, fructose, and galactose); disaccharides (sucrose, maltose, and lactose); and polysaccharides (starch, fiber, and glycogen).
  - Food carbohydrates are divided into two categories: simple carbohydrates (monosaccharides and disaccharides) and complex carbohydrates (polysaccharides, excluding glycogen).
  - Dietary recommendations for carbohydrates are:
    - *Dietary Reference Intake (DRI)* for carbohydrates is 130 g/day for adults between 19and 30 years of age.
    - *Acceptable Macronutrient Distribution Range (AMDR)* is 45% to 65% of kcal intake per day as primarily complex carbohydrates.
    - *Dietary Guidelines* recommends emphasizing a plant-based diet including fruits, vegetables, cooked dried beans and peas, whole grains, and seeds.
- Carbohydrates are an abundant food source of energy and dietary fiber.
  - Energy circulates in the bloodstream as glucose.
    - Blood glucose levels are regulated and balanced through hormonal systems.
- Hypoglycemia and diabetes mellitus may occur when these systems cannot regulate glucose within normal levels.
- Dietary fiber does not provide energy; it is not digestible by humans.
  - Consuming adequate quantities of soluble and insoluble fiber has significant health benefits.
  - The DRI for dietary fiber is 25 to 38 g for adult women and men, respectively.
- Best carbohydrate food energy sources: grains, legumes, and starchy root vegetables.
- Best dietary fiber sources: fruits, vegetables, and whole-grain products.
- Nutrients are lost when unrefined (whole) grains are refined.
- *Dietary Guidelines* recommends increased consumption of complex carbohydrates:
  - MyPlate proposes 6 ounces of grains (with at least 3 ounces whole grains), 4½ cups of vegetables, and 2 cups of fruits.

◎ THE NURSING APPROACH

Case Study: Fiber (Constipation)

Mary, age 62, is in the nurse practitioner's (NP's) office for a routine annual physical examination. When collecting the health history, the NP finds that Mary frequently has had abdominal discomfort and constipation. Past medical history indicates a medical diagnosis of diverticulosis. The NP interviews Mary and performs an abdominal examination.

Assessment
Subjective (from Patient Statements)
- Small, hard, pebble-like stools, usually two times a day
- Uncomfortable straining with bowel movements
- Bloating and gas
- Drinks 4 to 6 glasses of water per day
- Prefers white bread and refined grains
- Eats few fruits and vegetables and peels those she does eat
- Does not exercise regularly

Objective (from Physical Examination)
- Abdomen distended, nontender
- Bowel sounds hypoactive

Diagnosis (Nursing)
Constipation related to low fiber and fluid intake, and lack of exercise as evidenced by hypoactive bowel sounds and patient statements about small, hard stools and uncomfortable straining with bowel movements

Planning
Patient Outcomes
Short term (at the end of this visit):
- Mary will identify foods high in fiber and develop plans to gradually include them in her diet.
- Mary will verbalize intention to drink at least 8 glasses of water and walk at least 15 minutes per day.
Long term (at the follow-up visit in 1 month):
- Mary will report she was able to follow her plan.
- Mary will report regular soft bowel movements with no discomfort or straining.

Nursing Interventions
1. Teach Mary about the causes of constipation and diverticulosis.

◎ THE NURSING APPROACH—cont'd

2. Teach Mary about lifestyle changes that will prevent constipation.

Implementation

1. Explained causes of constipation and how constipation can lead to diverticulosis and diverticulitis.
   Common causes of constipation are insufficient fiber, fluids, and activity. Strained defecation increases intracolonic pressure and can weaken the muscles in the bowel, allowing outpouching of the intestinal wall (diverticulosis). If fecal matter gets caught in the diverticula, infection can result (diverticulitis). For diverticulosis, a high-fiber diet is prescribed. For diverticulitis, the patient may receive nothing by mouth temporarily or may consume only low-fiber foods and fluids, in order to allow healing of the irritated bowel.
2. Encouraged Mary to add fiber gradually until she is eating at least six servings of whole-grain breads and cereals and five servings of fruits, vegetables, and legumes per day.
   Fiber adds bulk to stools and stimulates peristalsis. Increasing fiber intake too quickly can lead to bloating, gas, cramps, abdominal discomfort, and diarrhea. Generally, one high-fiber food can be added every 2 weeks, until the client is eating 25 to 38 g of fiber per day.
3. Provided written information on types and sources of fiber and explored food likes and preferences to determine high-fiber foods acceptable to Mary.
   Substituting high-fiber foods for low-fiber foods can prevent constipation, but the diet needs to be individualized. Examples of high-fiber foods are whole-wheat bread, bran cereal, kidney beans, prunes and other fruits with peelings, and broccoli.
4. Encouraged Mary to drink 8 to 12 glasses of fluid per day, especially water and fruit juices.
   Fluid softens stools and increases bulk, promoting peristalsis. As fiber is increased, fluids must be increased to prevent further constipation, intestinal blockage, and abdominal pain.
5. Encouraged Mary to exercise regularly—for example, start by walking for at least 15 minutes five times a week.
   Activity promotes peristalsis. It is recommended that adults get 2 hours 30 minutes of moderate-intensity aerobic activity every week and participate in muscle-strengthening activities 2 or more days per week.

Evaluation

Short term (at the end of the visit):
  Mary wrote down specific goals for lifestyle changes to correct constipation.
- Changes to make right away:
  - Substitute whole-wheat bread for white bread.
  - Eat 3 servings of fruits and vegetables per day.
  - Drink 8 glasses of water per day.
  - Walk for 15 minutes three times a week.
- Changes to make gradually, starting in 2 weeks:
  - Replace one low-fiber food with one new high-fiber food every 2 weeks.
  - Increase walking to 20 minutes five times a week.
- Changes not willing to make: drinking prune juice
Short-term outcomes achieved.
Mary set up an appointment for follow-up in 1 month.

Discussion Questions

At her follow-up appointment, Mary said her stools had been softer, better formed, and more comfortable to eliminate. She said she had eaten whole-wheat bread 3 days per week, had eaten 3 fruits per day, had drunk about 5 glasses of water per day, and had walked for 15 minutes twice a week. Last week she began eating raisin bran cereal 4 days per week.

1. How would you judge Mary's goal achievement—met, partially met, or not met at all? What was the basis for your answer?
2. If you were the nurse, what would you say to Mary about her report? What questions would you ask?
3. What other high-fiber foods could you recommend?

❓ APPLYING CONTENT KNOWLEDGE

You are at a restaurant having lunch with friends. After hearing you order a sandwich on whole-wheat bread, the friend comments, "Whole-wheat bread, white bread, what's the big deal? They're all complex carbohydrates." How would you respond?

▮ WEBSITES OF INTEREST

American Public Health Association
  www.apha.org
  Promotes and protects the public's health to achieve a healthy global society.

Wheat Foods Council
  www.wheatfoods.org
  Provides nutrition and food preparation resources for incorporating more grains into the American diet.

USA Rice Federation
  www.usarice.com
  Offers information about rice production, preparation, research, and environmental issues.

REFERENCES

Dolan JP, Adams-Smith WN: *Health and society: A documentary history of medicine*, New York, 1978, The Seabury Press.

Fitch C, Keim KS, Academy of Nutrition and Dietetics: Position of the Academy of Nutrition and Dietetics: Use of nutritive and nonnutritive sweeteners, *J Acad Nutr Diet* 112:739–758, 2012.

Gallagher ML: The nutrients and their metabolism. In Mahan K, et al, editors: *Krause's food & the nutrition care process*, ed 13, St. Louis, 2012, Saunders/Elsevier.

Keim NL, et al: Carbohydrates. In Ross AC, et al, editors: *Modern nutrition in health and disease*, ed 11, Philadelphia, 2014, Wolters Kluwer/Lippincott Williams & Wilkins.

King DE, et al: Trends in diet fiber intake in the United States, 1999-2008, *J Acad Nutr Diet* 112:642–648, 2012.

National Research Council: *Dietary reference intakes: The essential guide to nutrient requirements*, Washington, DC, 2006, The National Academies Press.

Pepino MY, Bourne C: Non-nutritive sweeteners, energy balance, and glucose homeostasis, *Curr Opin Clin Nutr Metab Care* 14(4):391–395, 2011.

Shankar P, et al: Non-nutritive sweeteners: Review and update, *Nutrition* 29:1293–1299, 2013.

Sullivan S, et al: Nutritional physiology of the alimentary tract. In Ross AC, et al, editors: *Modern nutrition in health and disease*, ed 11, Philadelphia, 2014, Wolters Kluver/Lippincott Williams & Wilkins.

U.S. Department of Agriculture and U.S. Department of Health and Human Services: *Dietary Guidelines for Americans, 2010*, ed 7, Washington, DC, 2010, U.S. Government Printing Office. From: www.health.gov/dietaryguidelines/dga2010/DietaryGuidelines2010.pdf/. Accessed July 11, 2013.

U.S. Food and Drug Administration (FDA): *Code of federal regulations: Food and drugs*, Parts 1 to 99. Washington, DC, 2000, The Office of the Federal Register. From: www.gpo.gov/fdsys/pkg/CFR-2000-title21-vol1/pdf/CFR-2000-title21-vol1.pdf. Accessed May 14, 2014.

Willis HJ, Slavin JL: Dietary fiber. In Ross AC, et al, editors: *Modern nutrition in health and disease*, ed 11, Philadelphia, 2014, Wolters Kluver/Lippincott Williams & Wilkins.

CHAPTER 5

Fats

Fat is the densest form of stored energy in food and our bodies. This means that gram for gram, food fat—in the form of triglycerides—can produce more than twice the energy in kcal as that provided by carbohydrate or protein.

ⓔ http://evolve.elsevier.com/GRODNER/FOUNDATIONS

LEARNING OBJECTIVES

- List the major functions of triglyceride in food and physiologically in the body.
- State the functions of phospholipids and cholesterol.
- Summarize the structures and sources of the three types of lipids.
- Discuss the function and sources of the linolenic and linoleic essential fatty acids.

- Explain the digestion, absorption, and transportation of lipids in the body.
- Identify the three different types of lipoproteins and their functions.
- Describe the potential health concerns related to dietary fat intake.

ROLE IN WELLNESS

It may be time for a truce about the consumption of dietary fat. Since the 1970s, consumption of fats gained a negative reputation as a possible source of diet-related disorders and a factor in the increasing waistlines of Americans. We are now recognizing that the types and amount of fats being consumed determine the impact on our bodies. Some dietary fats are essential, and others are not. Some actually confer additional health benefits, and a few, when eaten in large amounts, may increase the risk of certain diseases. This chapter explores these issues.

Fat is valuable and necessary to health. It is important to learn about fat in food, what the fat we eat does in our bodies, and how it can be both helpful and harmful to our health. Individual preference for fat is developed in either infancy or early childhood; innate preferences for sweet taste are observed at birth (Drewnowski, 2000). Thus children learn to prefer tastes, flavors, and textures that are associated with foods that are rich in fat, sweet, or both. Aging may be associated with increasing acceptance of bitter tastes and consumption of more fruits, vegetables, and whole grains (Drewnowski, 2000). Nonetheless, reducing fat consumption takes time and effort, perhaps because of food selection habits, symbolic meaning associated with certain foods, and sensory values of fats in foods.

The six dimensions of health provide ways to think about the effects of changing dietary fat consumption. *Physical health* is maintained by consuming dietary fats that are necessary for essential fatty acids (EFAs), for energy, and for fat-soluble vitamins. Excessive intake of fats, though, may increase the risk of obesity and diet-related diseases. The *intellectual health* dimension encompasses the skills necessary to assess the type of dietary fat modification most appropriate for our clients' and our own health needs. How we emotionally approach nutritional lifestyle changes for our clients and ourselves affects success, which reflects the *emotional health* dimension. Can these emotions be expressed, or are changes simply disregarded because they make us feel uncomfortable? The *social dimension* is tested as change is initiated. Are relationships of family and friends based on sharing high-fat meals? Can you or your clients refuse to take part in social situations without jeopardizing relationships or making others feel defensive? Can you or your clients make food preparation suggestions to lower the fat content without seeming overly critical? Some religions maintain that taking care of one's body is necessary to achieve spiritual goals. Adopting a healthier fat intake supports these *spiritual health* dimension goals. The *environmental health* dimension may require seeking or making available foods that contain healthier fats. Some food stores and restaurants may better support one's dietary fat intake goals.

Fat actually refers to the chemical group called *lipids.* Lipids are divided into three classifications: fats (or triglycerides), and the fat-related substances phospholipids and sterols. Triglycerides, the largest class of lipids, may be in the form of fats (somewhat solid) or oils (liquids). Approximately 95% of the lipids in foods and in our bodies are in the triglyceride form of fat. Of the other two lipid classifications, lecithin is the best-known phospholipid, and cholesterol is the best-known sterol. All are organic—composed of carbon, hydrogen, and oxygen—and cannot dissolve in water.

FUNCTIONS

The functions of lipids may be divided into two categories: (1) specific characteristics of foods that arise from lipids and (2) maintenance of the physiologic health of our bodies.

Food Functions

Source of Energy

Fat is the densest form of stored energy in food and our bodies. This means that gram for gram, food fat—in the form of triglycerides—can produce more than twice the energy in kcal that carbohydrate or protein can. For example, a gram of nearly pure fat (9 kcal), such as butter, provides more than twice the kcal provided by a gram of nearly pure carbohydrate (4 kcal), such as sugar, or a gram of nearly pure protein (4 kcal), such as dried, lean fish.

Palatability

Fat makes food smell and taste good. Deep-fat fried potatoes outrank all other vegetable choices among North Americans. Whether it's bread with butter (or margarine), salad with dressing, or desserts with cream, fat makes foods taste pleasant for many people. For patients who are anorexic because of illness, strategically adding small amounts of fats to meals may increase nutrient intake.

Satiety and Satiation

Fat helps prevent hunger between meals. Fat slows down digestion because of the hormones released in response to its presence in the gastrointestinal (GI) tract, causing us to feel full and satisfied; we call this feeling *satiety. Satiation* is another, different aspect of fat consumption that occurs during, not after, eating. In contrast to satiety, satiation tends to increase our desire to eat more fatty food, not less. The effect of fat on satiation is likely to be more important than its effect on satiety and may lead to overeating (Tso and Liu, 2004). A satiation that often occurs with the last slice of pizza provides a good example: You want it, you eat it, and half an hour later, you feel too full.

Food Processing

Certain qualities of lipids, besides their nutritional purposes, make them a valuable resource for the processing of foods. The use of processed hydrogenated fats helps keep the fat in food products from turning rancid. Lecithin, a phospholipid, has an extensive role as an emulsifier—a substance that works by being soluble in water and fat at the same time. These functions, which are described in more detail, also increase our overall intake of lipids by allowing their use in numerous processed foods.

Nutrient Source

Some fats contain or transport the fat-soluble nutrients of vitamins A, D, E, and K and the EFAs of linoleic and linolenic fatty acids.

These essential fatty acids (EFAs), components of fat triglycerides, are polyunsaturated fatty acids (PUFAs) that

FIG 5-1 Essential fatty acid deficiency. **A,** Biochemical abnormalities and skin lesions have developed in a patient receiving fat-free parenteral nutrition. **B,** Resolution in same patient after 2 weeks of treatment. (Courtesy Dr. M.C. Riella. From McLaren DS: *A colour atlas and text of diet-related disorders,* ed 2, London, 1992, Mosby.)

cannot be made in the body and must be consumed in the diet. EFAs are necessary materials for making compounds, such as prostaglandins, that regulate many body functions, including blood pressure, blood clotting through platelet aggregation, gastric acid secretions, and muscle secretions. The overall strength of cell membranes depends on EFAs.

Overt symptoms of EFA deficiency include skin lesions and scaliness (eczema) caused by increased permeability, which leads to membrane breakdown throughout the body (Figure 5-1). Inflammation of epithelial tissue and increased susceptibility to infections throughout the body are also possible. Because the minimum amount of EFA required is contained in only about 2 teaspoons of polyunsaturated vegetable oil, deficiencies of EFAs were thought to be rare. However, deficiencies have been noted in (1) older patients with peripheral vascular disease (a potential complication of diabetes mellitus), (2) patients with fat malabsorption, such as cystic fibrosis, and (3) patients receiving treatment for protein malnutrition with low-fat, high-protein diets. Individuals recovering from serious accidents and burns are also at risk. It is possible that individuals who strive to achieve extremely low dietary fat intake for perceived health reasons or from disordered eating could experience EFA deficiencies.

Physiologic Functions

Stored Energy

Body fat cells contain nearly pure fat, also in the form of triglycerides. This means that a pound of adipose tissue, the storage depot of body fat, could produce about 3500 kcal as energy. Because glucose stored in our bodies as glycogen is stored with water, carbohydrate is a bulkier form of stored energy than body fat. Adipose tissue provides important fuel during illness or times of food restriction and is a major energy source for muscle work.

Organ Protection

Stored fat safely cushions and protects body organs during bumpy activities, such as participating in impact aerobics and snowboarding.

Temperature Regulation

The fat layer just under our skin serves as insulation to regulate body temperature by minimizing the loss of heat.

Insulation

A substance composed largely of fatty tissue, called *myelin*, covers nerve cells. This covering provides electrical insulation that allows for transmission of nerve impulses.

Functions of Phospholipids and Sterols

So far, we have discussed the major roles of triglycerides. Phospholipids are also important because they form part of all cell membrane structure and serve as emulsifiers to keep fats dispersed in body fluids.

Lecithin is the main phospholipid. Lecithin is a constituent of lipoproteins—carriers or transporters of lipids—including fats and cholesterol in the body. This characteristic has earned lecithin a reputation for carrying fat and cholesterol away from plaque deposits in the arteries. Although lecithin does play a role in transporting fat and cholesterol, supplementary lecithin from sources outside the body does not help make the body's transportation system more efficient. Instead, dietary lecithin is simply digested and used by the body as any other lipid.

As a lipid group, sterols are critical components of complex regulatory compounds in our bodies and provide basic material to make bile, vitamin D, sex hormones, and cells in brain and nerve tissue. Cholesterol in particular is a vital part of all cell membranes and nerve tissues and serves as a building block for hormones. When exposed to ultraviolet light, a cholesterol substance in our skin can be converted to vitamin D by the kidneys and liver. The liver synthesizes cholesterol to make bile, the emulsifying substance necessary to absorb dietary lipids.

STRUCTURE AND SOURCES OF LIPIDS

Fats: Saturated and Unsaturated

Triglycerides are the largest class of lipids found in food and body fat. A **triglyceride** is a compound consisting of three fatty acids and one glycerol molecule (Figure 5-2). The glycerol portion is derived from carbohydrate, but it is a small part compared with the fatty acids, which may be alike or different from each other. Fatty acids can be made of long or short chains of carbon atoms. Each carbon atom has four bonding sites or imaginary arms where it can attach to other atoms. To form a carbon chain, one site on each side of the carbon bonds to a neighboring carbon, as if one arm on each side were outstretched to form a chain. Because these atoms have four arms, the two extra arms each attach to a hydrogen atom, making the chain saturated with hydrogen.

If a hydrogen atom is removed from two neighboring carbons, freeing the extra arm on each, the carbons are bonded to each other at two sites. The two arms on the same side both clasp the two arms of the neighboring carbon, forming a double bond. We call this an *unsaturated carbon chain,* because there is a possibility that hydrogen could come along and saturate the chain by breaking one set of clasped arms and attaching to them. In foods, this is sometimes done artificially through the process of **hydrogenation**, which

Three fatty acids join to glycerol in a condensation reaction to form a triglyceride.

Glycerol + 3 fatty acids → Triglyceride + 3 water molecules

A bond is formed with the O of the glycerol and the C of the last acid of the fatty acid because of the removal of water from the glycerol and fatty acids.

Three fatty acids attached to a glycerol form a triglyceride. Water is released. Triglycerides often contain different kinds of fatty acids.

FIG 5-2 Formation and structure of a triglyceride.

forces hydrogen atoms to break a double bond and attach to the carbons, creating a saturated fat (Figure 5-3). Hydrogenation is discussed in the section on processed fats.

All natural fats are mixtures of different types of fatty acids. Plants contain mostly polyunsaturated fats, but most plant oils contain some saturated fatty acids (Figure 5-4). Animal fats, although high in saturated fats, contain amounts of polyunsaturated fats. The predominant type of fat in a food determines its category.

A **saturated fatty acid** has a single-bonded carbon chain that is fully saturated because hydrogen atoms are attached to all available bonding sites. Palmitic acid (16 carbon atoms) (Figure 5-5A), a saturated fatty acid, is contained in meats, butterfat, shortening, and vegetable oils. Other saturated fatty acids are stearic acid (18 carbon atoms), myristic acid (14 carbon atoms), and lauric acid (12 carbon atoms). Additional food sources of saturated fatty acids are primarily animal, including beef, poultry, pork, lamb, luncheon meats, egg yolks, and dairy products (milk, butter, and cheeses); the only major plant sources are palm and coconut oils (often called *tropical oils)* and cocoa butter.

FIG 5-3 Process of hydrogenation.

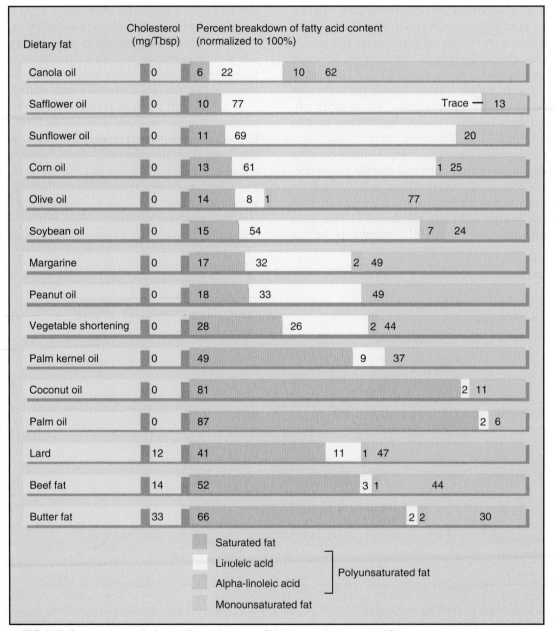

Dietary fat	Cholesterol (mg/Tbsp)	Percent breakdown of fatty acid content (normalized to 100%)				
Canola oil	0	6	22		10	62
Safflower oil	0	10	77			Trace — 13
Sunflower oil	0	11	69			20
Corn oil	0	13	61			1 25
Olive oil	0	14	8 1			77
Soybean oil	0	15	54		7	24
Margarine	0	17	32		2	49
Peanut oil	0	18	33			49
Vegetable shortening	0	28	26		2	44
Palm kernel oil	0	49			9	37
Coconut oil	0	81				2 11
Palm oil	0	87				2 6
Lard	12	41		11	1	47
Beef fat	14	52		3 1		44
Butter fat	33	66		2 2		30

- ▮ Saturated fat
- ▯ Linoleic acid
- ▯ Alpha-linoleic acid } Polyunsaturated fat
- ▯ Monounsaturated fat

FIG 5-4 Comparison of dietary fats in terms of cholesterol, saturated fat, and the most common unsaturated fats.

FIG 5-5 Examples of Fatty Acids Found in Foods. Foods with these fatty acids include: **A,** animal-derived foods (beef, poultry, lamb, pork, eggs, dairy, tropical oils); **B,** olive oil, peanuts (butter and oil), canola oil; **C,** vegetable oils (margarine and salad dressings), some animal fats, prepared foods; and **D,** fatter fish (bluefish, tuna, salmon, etc.), fish, canola oil.

TABLE 5-1 **Food Sources of Omega-3 Fatty Acids**	
Fish sources	Salmon
	Mackerel
	Herring
	Tuna
	Rainbow trout
	Sardines
Plant sources	Canola oil
	Walnuts and walnut oil
	Soybean and soybean oil
	Flaxseed ground and oil
	Wheat germ and oat germ
	Green leafy vegetables

Each unsaturated fatty acid has one or more unsaturated double bonds along the carbon chain. If a carbon chain has only one unsaturated double bond, it is a monounsaturated fatty acid (MUFA), Oleic acid (see Figure 5-5B) is the main MUFA in foods. Dietary sources include olive oil, peanuts (peanut butter and peanut oil), and canola oil.

If a carbon chain has two or more unsaturated double bonds, it is a polyunsaturated fatty acid (PUFA). Food sources include vegetable oils (corn, safflower, wheat germ, canola, sesame, and sunflower), fish, and margarine.

PUFAs are categorized by the location of the unsaturation in the molecular structure of the fatty acid. Two categories of PUFAs, omega-6 and omega-3, contain two fatty acids (linoleic and linolenic) that our bodies cannot manufacture; these acids are EFAs and must be provided by dietary intake. The characteristic that distinguishes them from other PUFAs is the position of the final double bond in relation to the end of the carbon chain. The final double bond is at the sixth carbon from the omega end of the chain in linoleic acid (see Figure 5-5C), the main member of the omega-6 family. The first double bond is at the third carbon atom from the omega end in linolenic acid (see Figure 5-5D), the main member of the omega-3 family.

Americans consume an abundance of linoleic acid from consumption of large amounts of vegetable oils, such as margarine and salad dressing, and large amounts of prepared foods. Another source of linoleic acid may be animal foods; for example, although poultry fat is predominantly saturated, it also contains some PUFAs, including linoleic acid.

In contrast, American consumption of linolenic acid is not abundant at all. Linolenic acid is associated with fish consumption because that is how it was first recognized as important in health. A low incidence of heart disease among the native people of Greenland and Alaska, in spite of a very high-fat diet, was traced to the oils in deep-water fish, the staple in their diet (Harris, 1989). One of the main omega-3 fatty acids in fish is eicosapentaenoic acid (EPA), which is derived from linolenic acid. Fish are more efficient in this conversion of fatty acids than humans. Omega-3 fatty acids appear to lower the risk of heart disease by reducing the blood clotting process; clots can cause blockages in the arteries in the presence of plaques. Although consuming extra omega-3 fatty acids is likely to have little effect on blood cholesterol levels, it may reduce the risk of clots that may cause a myocardial infarction (heart attack) and appears to reduce risk of sudden death, such as from arrhythmias. According to prospective studies, reduced risk of *cardiovascular disease (CVD)* because of higher consumption of fish or omega-3 fatty acids appears applicable to men and women (Jones and Rideout, 2014).

Certain fish provide more omega-3 fatty acids than others. Good sources are tuna, salmon, bluefish, halibut, sardines, and rainbow trout. Table 5-1 lists additional sources. Eating fish twice a week or using canola oil, another source of linolenic acid, should provide an adequate balance between sources of omega-6 and omega-3 fatty acids, although the best balance is still unknown.

Inuits consume 4 to 5 g of EPAs daily, about the amount in 1.5 to 3 pounds of certain deep-water fish (Harper and Jacobson, 2005). Because it is unlikely that most Americans will consume this quantity of fish, fish oil supplements of these fatty acids are manufactured. However, questions about proper dosages, safety, and side effects are still being researched. Large doses can decrease immunity. Therefore, supplements should be taken only when prescribed by a health care provider.

Phospholipids

Phospholipids are lipid compounds that form parts of cell walls and act as fat emulsifiers. Similar to triglycerides,

FIG 5-6 A phospholipid: lecithin.

Cholesterol

FIG 5-7 A sterol: cholesterol. Foods containing cholesterol include animal-derived foods such as beef, pork, chicken, bacon, luncheon meats, eggs, fish, and dairy products.

phospholipids contain fatty acids, but they have only two fatty acids; the third spot contains a phosphate group. The body manufactures phospholipids, which are found in every cell; therefore, they are not essential nutrients. Lecithin, the main phospholipid, contains two fatty acids, with the third spot filled by a molecule of choline plus phosphorus (Figure 5-6). In the body, lecithin's function as an emulsifier is to work by being soluble in water and fat at the same time.

Lecithin from soybeans is used in food processing to perform an emulsification role. Naturally found in egg yolks, lecithin is the versatile ingredient in mayonnaise that prevents separation of vinegar and oil. Lecithin is also used in manufacturing chocolates to keep the cocoa butter and other ingredients combined and in cakes and other bakery products to maintain freshness.

Sterols

Sterols, a fatlike class of lipids, serve vital functions in the body. Sterol structures, including cholesterol, are carbon rings intermeshed with side chains of carbon, hydrogen, and oxygen, making them more complex than triglycerides (Figure 5-7). Like phospholipids, sterols are synthesized by the body and are not essential nutrients. For example, if dietary cholesterol is not consumed, the liver will produce the amount required for body functions.

Generally, dietary cholesterol accounts for about 25% of the cholesterol in the body. The rest, which is made in the liver, seems to be produced in relation to how much is needed.

The only food sources of cholesterol are animal and include beef, pork (bacon), chicken, luncheon meats, eggs, fish, and dairy products (milk, butter, and cheeses); plant foods do not contain cholesterol.

FATS AS A NUTRIENT IN THE BODY

Digestion

Mouth

The mouth's primary fat-digestive process is mechanical, as teeth masticate fatty foods. The glands of the tongue produce a fat-splitting enzyme (lingual lipase) released with saliva that begins digestion of long-chain fatty acids such as those found in milk.

Stomach

Mechanical digestion continues through the strong actions of peristalsis. Fat-splitting enzymes such as gastric lipase hydrolyze some fatty acids from triglycerides.

Small Intestine

Fats entering the duodenum initiate the release of cholecystokinin (CCK) hormone from the duodenum walls. CCK, as described in Chapter 3, then sparks the gallbladder to release bile into the small intestine. The bile emulsifies fats to facilitate digestion. Mechanical digestion through muscular action allows for increased exposure of the emulsified fat globules to pancreatic lipase. This enzyme is the primary digestive enzyme that breaks triglycerides into fatty acids, monoglycerides, and glycerol molecules. Note that fats may not be completely broken down. Some may also pass through without being digested or absorbed. Figure 5-8 summarizes digestion of triglycerides.

Use of Medium-Chain Triglycerides

Triglycerides are composed of long chains of fatty acids. To aid fat digestion in those patients with malabsorption, synthetically manufactured medium-chain triglycerides (MCTs) may be incorporated into a patient's dietary intake. MCTs should not be used to completely replace dietary fats because they do not contain EFAs.

Absorption

Bile salts help fatty acids, monoglycerides, and cholesterol move from the lumen to the villi for absorption. Micelles, created by bile salts encircling lipids, aid diffusion through the membrane wall. Once through the membrane wall, fatty acids and glycerol combine back into triglycerides. These triglycerides are incorporated into **chylomicrons**, which are the first lipoproteins formed after absorption of lipids from food. They contain fats and cholesterol and are coated with protein. The protein coating allows them to travel through the lymph system to the blood circulatory system and then toward the hepatic portal system and the liver. Some glycerol and any short- and medium-chain fatty acids are absorbed directly into the blood capillaries leading to the portal vein and liver.

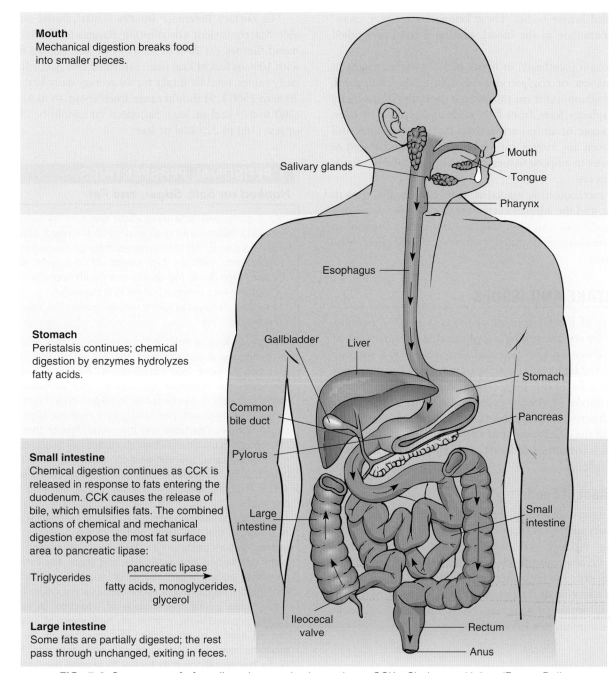

Mouth
Mechanical digestion breaks food into smaller pieces.

Stomach
Peristalsis continues; chemical digestion by enzymes hydrolyzes fatty acids.

Small intestine
Chemical digestion continues as CCK is released in response to fats entering the duodenum. CCK causes the release of bile, which emulsifies fats. The combined actions of chemical and mechanical digestion expose the most fat surface area to pancreatic lipase:

Triglycerides $\xrightarrow{\text{pancreatic lipase}}$ fatty acids, monoglycerides, glycerol

Large intestine
Some fats are partially digested; the rest pass through unchanged, exiting in feces.

Salivary glands — Mouth — Tongue — Pharynx — Esophagus — Gallbladder — Liver — Stomach — Common bile duct — Pancreas — Pylorus — Small intestine — Large intestine — Ileocecal valve — Rectum — Anus

FIG 5-8 Summary of fat digestion and absorption. *CCK,* Cholecystokinin. (From Rolin Graphics.)

At the cell membranes, the triglycerides in the chylomicrons are broken down into fatty acids and glycerol with assistance from an enzyme called *lipoprotein lipase.* Muscle cells, adipose cells, and other cells in the vicinity take up most of the fatty acids released by the breakdown of chylomicrons. Cells can either use the absorbed fatty acids immediately as fuel or reform them into triglycerides to be stored as reserve energy supplies.

Metabolism

Lipid metabolism consists of several processes. Catabolism (breakdown) of lipids for energy involves the hydrolysis of triglycerides into two-carbon units that become part of **acetyl coenzyme A (acetyl CoA).** Acetyl CoA is an important intermediate byproduct in metabolism formed from the breakdown of glucose, fatty acids, and certain amino acids. The acetyl CoA then enters the series of reactions called the **TCA (tricarboxylic acid) cycle,** eventually leading to the oxidation of the carbon and hydrogen atoms derived from fatty acids (or carbohydrates or amino acids) to carbon dioxide and water with the release of energy as adenosine triphosphate (ATP) (see Figure 9-2). If fat catabolizes quickly because of a lack of carbohydrate (glucose) for energy, the liver cells form intermediate products from the partial oxidation of fatty acids called *ketone bodies.* These ketone bodies may excessively accumulate in the blood, causing a condition called ketosis.

Anabolism (synthesis) of lipids, or lipogenesis, results in the formation of triglycerides, phospholipids, cholesterol, and prostaglandins for use throughout the body. Triglycerides and phosphates form from fatty acids and glycerol or from excess glucose or amino acids. Extra carbon, hydrogen, and oxygen from any source can be converted to and stored as triglycerides in adipose tissues, so we can gain fat from foods other than fat.

Lipid metabolism is regulated mainly by insulin, growth hormone, and the adrenal cortex hormones; adrenocorticotropic hormone (ACTH), which stimulates secretion of more hormones; and glucocorticoids, which affect food metabolism.

FAT INTAKE AND ISSUES

Awareness of the fat content of foods is steadily growing. Whether we are consuming a sophisticated gourmet feast or chowing down on hot dogs and hamburgers at a summer barbecue, the fat levels of our meals may be of interest. Concerns about fat in our diets center on health issues such as excessive intake of energy, excessive fat intake that replaces other nutrients, and the relationship between dietary fat intake and the development of chronic diet-related diseases. Some lipids consumed in foods are essential to our bodies to achieve wellness.

Fat Content of Foods

High-fat foods are almost always high-calorie foods. This is because fats are the most concentrated source of food energy, supplying 9 kcal/g; carbohydrates and proteins supply 4 kcal/g. Because most foods contain a mixture of nutrients, we can identify the fat content of food by the number of fat grams in a serving or the percentage of daily value of recommended fat intake in a serving. Nutritional labels on packaged food contain this information.

To reduce fat intake, trim meat before cooking. (From Thinkstockphotos.com.)

The Dietary Reference Intakes (DRIs), based on Acceptable Macronutrient Distribution Ranges (AMDRs), recommend that we eat 20% to 35% of our kcal intakes from fats, with 10% or less of kcal from saturated fats. According to the daily values, total fat intake for an average daily kcal intake of 2000 to 2500 kcal should range from about 40 to 97 g or less (400 to 875 kcal or less). Saturated fat should be 20 to 25 g or less (180 to 225 kcal or less).

Most Americans consume 35% to 40% of total energy intake as fat (Jones and Rideout, 2014), even though many believe they are avoiding or limiting high-fat foods. One reason may be that high-fat foods have both potent sensory qualities and high-energy density; overeating is then often more passive than active. Another reason is that people who eat a lot of high-fat foods are unsure whether their diets are high in fat because the rate of home cooking has fallen sharply; the cook no longer knows exactly what goes into each dish. Also, portion sizes at restaurants are often twice the size of those recommended for good health by MyPlate. Then there is the "less fat, more carbs" message that has been incorrectly translated into sweet, kcal-dense, low-fiber carbohydrate foods, so the low-fat diet has become a high-calorie, processed-carbohydrate diet. It is also likely that people are misled by labels on "reduced fat" foods and thus actually *increase* the total intake of such foods. The individual foods we eat daily may have a higher or lower fat content, but overall we should generally average 25% to 30% of kcal fat intake from all the foods we eat each day (see the *Teaching Tool* box Calculating Your Daily Fat Intake).

✳ TEACHING TOOL

Calculating Your Daily Fat Intake

Use the following steps to calculate your daily grams of fat:
1. Use the Recommended Energy Intake chart in Chapter 9 to determine your appropriate energy needs for the day. Multiply that number of kcal by 0.25 for 25% fat intake or by 0.30 for 30% fat intake.
2. Divide that number by 9, because each gram of fat has 9 kcal. For example, if you consume 1800 kcal a day and want to get 25% of those kcal from fat: $0.25 \times 1800 = 450$. Then divide 450 by 9 to get 50 g of fat. Energy needs for the day kcal $\times$ 0.30 = kcal fat intake/day. Kcal fat intake/day $\div$ 9 kcal = g of fat/day.
3. Next, check food labels and/or use food composition tables (available at Evolve website) for the grams of fat per food serving. Then compare the sum of the fat grams consumed with the recommended levels for your particular energy needs.

How do we measure the fat in foods without labels, such as fresh foods, home-cooked recipes, and restaurant items? One way is to classify foods into groups according to fat content. The Exchange List uses this system by listing protein foods on the basis of their "leanness" (see Chapter 2). In contrast, MyPlate devotes a section to oils (fats that are liquid at room temperature) and provides information on the dietary fat content of foods in the oil category as well as foods in fruit, meats, and bean categories that contain oils. Oils are not considered a food group but *are* recognized as needed for good health. MyPlate emphasizes the health-promoting oils from plants and fish, rather than the solid, more saturated fats from palm kernel oil and coconut oil and many animal foods and from hydrogenation of vegetable oils. As shown in Box 5-1, frequently consumed oils are canola, corn, olive, cottonseed, safflower, and soybean. Foods listed as good sources of oils are nuts, certain fish, avocado, and olives. Table 5-2 provides examples of fat in servings from different foods. Common solid fats include butter, lard (pork fat), shortening, beef fat (suet, tallow), stick margarine, and chicken fat.

Detecting Dietary Fat

Some fats are visible; others are invisible. Visible fat is fairly easy to find and control; just cut off the white fat on the outside of a steak and measure the butter or sour cream on the baked potato. Invisible fat is harder to measure. Fat in milk, cheese, and yogurt is nearly impossible to see, but many people learn to taste the difference between whole- and

TABLE 5-2 Fat in Food Servings

FOOD	SERVING SIZE	FAT CONTENT
Butter/margarine	1 Tbsp	11 g
Salad dressing	1 Tbsp	7 g
Mayonnaise	1 Tbsp	11 g
Cream cheese	1 Tbsp	10 g
Carrots	½ cup	Trace
Broccoli	½ cup	Trace
Potato, baked	1	Trace
French fries	1 cup	8 g
Apple	1	Trace
Orange	1	Trace
Banana	1	Trace
Fruit juice	1 cup	Trace
Rice or pasta	½ cup	Trace
Bagel	1	Trace
Muffin	1 medium	6 g
Danish pastry	1 medium	13 g
Skim milk	1 cup	Trace
Low-fat milk	1 cup	5 g
Whole milk	1 cup	8 g
American cheese	2 oz	18 g
Cheddar cheese	1½ oz	14 g
Frozen yogurt	½ cup	2 g
Ice milk	⅓ cup	3 g
Ice cream	⅓ cup	7 g
Lean beef	3 oz	6 g
Poultry	3 oz	6 g
Fish	3 oz	6 g
Ground beef	3 oz	16 g
Bologna (2 slices)	1 oz	16 g
Egg	1	5 g
Nuts (⅓ cup)	1 oz	22 g

low-fat dairy products. In addition, dairy foods are all labeled so fat content is known. Some foods give other clues that they contain fat. Press a napkin on a slice of pizza, a Danish pastry, or an egg roll. Look for oil around the edge of stir-fried Chinese food.

Be aware of general characteristics that signal the level of fat in foods. Some cooking methods, such as deep-frying, add fat. The way a prepared food is usually eaten may also increase fat intake, such as spreading butter or oil on bread rather than just dipping it in soup. Whether you are eating in or dining out, the amount of food regularly selected from high-fat animal sources such as meat and cheese compared with the amount of food consumed from low-fat grains, vegetables, and fruit affects total dietary fat consumption levels.

Government and consumer groups have encouraged restaurants and institutional food service operations to offer identifiable low-fat, low-calorie food choices. These choices allow clients to meet health promotion goals while maintaining social interactions. Encourage clients to identify healthy menu choices when eating away from home.

The cuisines of China and Italy are based on rice, pasta, and bread. When prepared with small amounts of fat and eaten with little fatty meat and plenty of vegetables, these cultural food patterns are excellent examples of healthful

BOX 5-1 MyPlate: Oils

What Are "Oils"?

Oils are fats that are liquid at room temperature, like the vegetable oils used in cooking. Oils come from many different plants and from fish. Oils are NOT a food group, but they provide essential nutrients. Therefore, oils are included in U.S. Department of Agriculture food patterns.

Some commonly eaten oils include:

- Canola oil
- Corn oil
- Cottonseed oil
- Olive oil
- Safflower oil
- Soybean oil
- Sunflower oil

Some oils are used mainly as flavorings, such as walnut oil and sesame oil. A number of foods are naturally high in oils, like: nuts, olives, some fish, and avocados.

Foods that are mainly oil include mayonnaise, certain salad dressings, and soft (tub or squeeze) margarine with no *trans* fats. Check the Nutrition Facts Label to find margarines with 0 grams of *trans* fat. Amounts of *trans* fat are required to be listed on labels.

Most oils are high in monounsaturated or polyunsaturated fats, and low in saturated fats. Oils from plant sources (vegetable and nut oils) do not contain any cholesterol. In fact, no plant foods contain cholesterol.

A few plant oils, however, including coconut oil, palm oil, and palm kernel oil, are high in saturated fats and for nutritional purposes should be considered to be solid fats.

Solid fats are fats that are solid at room temperature, like butter and shortening. Solid fats come from many animal foods and can be made from vegetable oils through a process called hydrogenation. Some common fats are:

- Butter
- Milk fat
- Beef fat (tallow, suet)
- Chicken fat
- Pork fat (lard)
- Stick margarine
- Shortening
- Partially hydrogenated oil

How Are Oils Different from Solid Fats?

All fats and oils are a mixture of saturated fatty acids and unsaturated fatty acids. Solid fats contain more **saturated fats** and/or *trans* fats than oils. Oils contain more MUFAs and PUFAs. Saturated fats, *trans* fats, and cholesterol tend to raise "bad" (low-density lipoprotein [LDL]) cholesterol levels in the blood, which in turn increase the risk for heart disease. To lower risk for heart disease, cut back on foods containing saturated fats, *trans* fats, and cholesterol.

How Do I Count the Oils I Eat?

The following table gives a quick guide to the amount of oils in some common foods:

	AMOUNT OF FOOD	AMOUNT OF OIL (tsp/g)	CALORIES FROM OIL (APPROXIMATE CALORIES)	TOTAL CALORIES (APPROXIMATE CALORIES)
Oils: Vegetable oils (such as canola, corn, cottonseed, olive, peanut, safflower, soybean, and sunflower)	1 Tbsp	3 tsp/14 g	120	120
Foods rich in oils:				
Margarine, soft (*trans* fat free)	1 Tbsp	2½ tsp/11 g	100	100
Mayonnaise	1 Tbsp	2½ tsp/11 g	100	100
Mayonnaise-type salad dressing	1 Tbsp	1 tsp/5 g	45	55
Italian dressing	2 Tbsp	2 tsp/8 g	75	85
Thousand Island dressing	2 Tbsp	2½ tsp/11 g	100	120
Olives, ripe, canned*	4 large	½ tsp/ 2 g	15	20
Avocado*	½ med	3 tsp/15 g	130	160
Peanut butter*	2 T	4 tsp/ 16 g	140	190
Peanuts, dry roasted*	1 oz	3 tsp/14 g	120	165
Mixed nuts, dry roasted*	1 oz	3 tsp/15 g	130	170
Cashews, dry roasted*	1 oz	3 tsp/13 g	115	165
Almonds, dry roasted*	1 oz	3 tsp/15 g	130	170
Hazelnuts*	1 oz	4 tsp/18 g	160	185
Sunflower seeds*	1 oz	3 tsp/14 g	120	165

g, Gram; *Tbsp*, tablespoon; *tsp*, teaspoon.

*Avocados and olives are part of the Vegetable Group; nuts and seeds are part of the Protein Foods Group. These foods are also high in oils. Soft margarine, mayonnaise, and salad dressings are mainly oil and are not considered to be part of any food group.

Modified from U.S. Department of Agriculture, Center for Nutrition Policy and Promotion: *Oils: What are oils?* From www.choosemyplate.gov/food-groups/oils.html; U.S. Department of Agriculture, Center for Nutrition Policy and Promotion: *Oils: How are oils different from solid fats?* www.choosemyplate.gov/food-groups/oils-how.html; and U.S. Department of Agriculture, Center for Nutrition Policy and Promotion: *Oils: How do I count the oils I eat?* From www.choosemyplate.gov/printpages/MyPlateFoodGroups/Oils/food-groups.oils-count.pdf. Accessed January 22, 2014.

diets. Yet, when Chinese and Italian foods are prepared to please the American palate, large amounts of fat are used in cooking the food, and portion sizes are larger than usual for specific ethnic tradition (see the *Cultural Considerations* box Choosing Lower-Fat Ethnic Dishes).

🌐 CULTURAL CONSIDERATIONS

Choosing Lower-Fat Ethnic Dishes

Perhaps you've grown up eating rice and beans, homemade gravy on lasagna, or Chinese takeout. Regardless of who prepares the food, Americans are consuming more international foods than ever before. We have a smorgasbord of ethnic food from which to choose. Chinese, Indian, Mexican, and Greek dishes have become commonplace.

We may assume, however, that because these foods are different and exotic, they are healthier for us. After all, aren't hamburgers and hot dogs—all-American favorites—the worst offenders for our health? However, although some ethnic dishes are lower in fat and higher in dietary fibers, others aren't much better than traditional American favorites.

The Chinese foods eaten in America would be considered far too rich (and high in fat) by the Chinese; they are reserved for banquets and even then are eaten in moderation. To enhance the healthfulness of prepared Chinese foods, avoid fried dishes, especially egg rolls and deep-fried breaded meats or poultry. Top the rice with moderate portions of entrees of chicken or seafood mixed with vegetables.

Italian dishes of pasta and "gravy" (i.e., tomato sauce) are healthful but become problematic when teamed with sausage, meatballs, fried breaded meats, and layers of cheeses or when tomato sauce is replaced by a cream Alfredo sauce. Each adds substantial amounts of saturated fats. Be aware of portion sizes, and focus on large portions of pasta served with smaller servings of the high-fat foods.

Mexican and Latino foods are sometimes made with lard, a heavily saturated animal fat, and with fatty portions of pork. These negatives, however, are somewhat offset by the generous (and delicious) use of beans, rice, and soft tortillas made from corn or wheat. When possible, avoid or reduce the use of lard; vegetable oils are a good substitute. Generally the less fat used, the healthier the entrée. For example, a taco made with a soft tortilla contains less fat than one made with a hard-fried tortilla. And be sure to pile on lots of lettuce, tomatoes, and salsa!

Application to nursing: Become familiar with the exotic tastes of international cuisines. By doing so, you'll be able to help clients understand the fat content of their ethnic favorites. Guide them to resources such as a dietitian to suggest strategies to prepare their meals with less dietary fat. Just remember that the palatability of fat is a worldwide phenomenon, so choose wisely.

Fast but High-Fat Foods

Contemporary lifestyles sometimes leave little room for meal planning and preparation. Often we may find ourselves heading for the nearest fast-food restaurant or snack bar as we dash off to school or work. What impact do these meals have on our nutritional status? A positive trend among fast-food chains is the use of less saturated fat in fried potatoes and the addition of items such as salads and skim milk to the menu. On the negative side, between 40% and 50% of fast-food kcal comes from fat—far higher than the recommended 30%.

When we study the major food contributors of fat in the American diet, hamburgers, cheeseburgers, meat loaf, and hot dogs top the list. Whole-milk beverages, including shakes, are next, followed by cheese and salad dressings. Doughnuts, cookies, and cake tie with fried potatoes (Cotton, et al, 2004). It is no surprise that the majority of fat in the American diet happens to appear in menu favorites served in fast-food restaurants and at sporting events. In addition, the majority of fat in these foods tends to be saturated, with hamburgers and cheeseburgers leading the pack.

One may wonder why some foods that are fast to fix, such as apples, oranges, and bananas, are not considered fast foods, nor are they sold in fast-food restaurants. The answer probably has to do with the fact that fat lends a seductive flavor to fast-food favorites (see the *Teaching Tool* box But Fast Foods Are So Convenient!).

✳️ TEACHING TOOL

But Fast Foods Are So Convenient!

Our advice to clients needs to be realistic, which means accepting the fact that most people occasionally eat at fast-food restaurants. Rather than attempting to dissuade them from going at all, we should give clients the following tools for helping to make lower-fat selections:

Most menus now include healthier options. For restaurant chains, visit Internet sites to determine nutrition information and newer specialty items that are more nutrient dense and lower in overall calories and fat content.

- Avoid breaded fried chicken and fish sandwiches. Chicken and fish, if grilled, can be lower in fat and cholesterol than beef, but a breaded and fried chicken or fish sandwich may provide more fat (and calories) than a hamburger.
- Choose grilled chicken sandwiches and leave off the high-fat sauces.
- Order a hamburger, plain, and add your own serving of ketchup or mustard.
- If French fries are a necessity, order a small size. Today's small sizes were considered the large size in the past!
- Realize that soda and sweetened ice tea contain empty calories. Therefore, the larger the container size, the more calories consumed. Better to enjoy the calories as filling food items than to guzzle sugary beverages.
- Always order a side salad or add lettuce and tomatoes to sandwiches, when possible.
- Salad bars can be deceiving. Salad greens are fine, but mayonnaise-based cole slaw and potato salad can pile on calories, especially when topped with creamy salad dressings. Selecting carrots, greens, other sliced vegetables, beans, and unprocessed fruits and consuming them with a small amount of dressing, provides a filling side or main dish. Keep dressing use to a minimum by dipping a fork into dressing and then into the salad—same taste with less fat.

How can fat intake be lowered? First, start early to include children and the whole family in buying food, preparing it, and having low-fat foods on hand. Many people prefer fast food because they don't have fresh or partly prepared foods ready to cook. Teaching children cooking skills from simple recipes, from videos, and through friends establishes low-fat food preferences early. Individuals are more likely to adopt low-fat diets if eating partners or families do the same by modeling healthy eating patterns.

Second, most major secondary and tertiary health care settings have an active dietetic department, often geared to pediatrics and family practice. Programs offered may include healthy cooking classes for children and their parents or nutrition and wellness classes. Providing lists of such programs is a valuable resource for clients.

Third, never say never. It is okay to include some high-fat foods in food plans because they taste good. If a mixture of low-fat and high-fat foods is eaten, preferences for both are developed; this practice automatically controls overdoing the fatty foods. The *Teaching Tool* that discusses fast foods is packed with other strategies for fast-food, low-fat eating patterns.

Preserving Fats in Food

Processed Fats and Oils: Hydrogenated and Emulsified

A problem with unsaturated fats in foods is that oxygen attacks the unsaturated double bonds (oxidation), causing damage that makes them rancid; rancid fats have an odor and bad flavor and may cause illness. One way to reduce vulnerability to oxidation is to artificially saturate the fatty acids by adding hydrogen at the double bonds. This process of *hydrogenation* makes the fat solid and more stable, which provides cooking benefits. When vegetable oil, which is polyunsaturated, is completely hydrogenated, it becomes a white, waxy, or plastic-like substance called *vegetable shortening.* Because it is saturated with hydrogens, the body processes it as if it were a saturated fat.

The ingredient list on a product label can truthfully state that the product contains more unsaturated liquid oil, although it is mixed with the partially hydrogenated fat. Partially hydrogenated fats are used in a variety of food products.

Sometimes the solution to one problem causes another problem. Although it stabilizes fat, hydrogenation changes the structure of some of the fatty acids, from *cis* fatty acids to *trans* fatty acids (Figure 5-9). Most fatty acid double bonds in natural foods are in the *cis* form, but margarine and vegetable shortening may contain high concentrations of *trans* fatty acids (*trans* fats). *Trans* fatty acids have unusual double-bond structures caused by hydrogenated unsaturated oils. Most margarines are now processed to contain no *trans* fatty acids. Often manufacturers will note whether their margarine products are free of *trans* fatty acids. Controversy over the effect of *trans* fats in relation to cancer vulnerability and elevated blood cholesterol values has confused the public.

Many commercially produced foods, such as French fries, potato chips, and bakery products, are made from partially

FIG 5-9 *Cis* bond to *trans* bonds.

hydrogenated vegetable oils. Many margarines and other products are now offered as "*trans* free." On the other hand, of the average 35% of kcal consumed as fat by Americans, only about 2% to 7% of total kcal comes from *trans* fats (Jones and Rideout, 2014).

Nonetheless, *trans* fat consumption appears to increase risk for CVD. Risk is increased because the *trans* fat raises the blood cholesterol component LDLs that delivers cholesterol throughout the body and, while doing so, may contribute to plaque formation in arteries. *Trans* fat also decreases the blood cholesterol component (high-density lipoproteins [HDLs]) that removes excess and used cholesterol from the body. Maintaining higher levels of this component decreases risk of CVD. Considering these effects on blood cholesterol, total consumption of *trans* fatty acids formed from partially hydrogenated oils or naturally occurring in ruminant animal foods should be limited (Evidence Analysis Library, 2013).

Since January 2006, listing *trans* fatty acid content on nutrition labels has been mandatory. This requirement led manufacturers to reformulate products without *trans* fats. "Partially hydrogenated fat or oil" as an ingredient is another clue that *trans* fat is present in a product. When possible, *trans* fat should be replaced by a monounsaturated fat such as canola oil. Guidelines currently suggest as a priority to reduce overall food fat to 30% of total kcal; less fat means less *trans* fat as well. Depending on product formulation, this may mean eating less margarine, French fries, potato chips, cakes, and cookies, as well as less fried chicken, fried fish, fatty meat, and ice cream.

Ordinances banning the use of artificial *trans* fats in the preparation of foods for direct consumption by consumers in restaurants and other food outlets have been implemented in several cities in the United States. The U.S. Food and Drug

Administration (FDA) recently proposed removing artificial *trans* fat from the Generally Recognized As Safe (GRAS) list of ingredients because of its effect on blood cholesterol levels. The use of *trans* fat would be as a food additive requiring specific regulations to allow for its use.

Antioxidants

Another way to preserve polyunsaturated fats without hydrogenation is through the use of antioxidant additives. These substances block oxidation, or the breakdown of double bonds by oxygen. Food manufacturers can use either natural or synthetic forms of antioxidants. Natural sources include vitamin E (tocopherol) and vitamin C (ascorbic acid). Their use not only helps to preserve foods but also adds essential vitamins. Synthetic forms consist of the food additives butylated hydroxyanisole (BHA) and butylated hydroxytoluene (BHT). These forms are used in packaging as well to help prevent oxidation of the foods.

Food Cholesterol versus Blood Cholesterol

Cholesterol is a waxy substance found in all tissues in humans and other animals; thus all foods from animal sources, such as meat, eggs, fish, poultry, and dairy products, contain cholesterol. The highest sources of cholesterol are egg yolks and organ meats (liver and kidney). No plant-derived food contains cholesterol, not even avocado or peanut butter, both of which are very high in fat. People often misunderstand this issue because they confuse food (dietary) cholesterol with blood cholesterol.

A high level of cholesterol in the blood is a risk factor for CVD. For an understanding of blood cholesterol levels, the role of lipoproteins—specialized transporting compounds—needs clarification. Lipoproteins are compounds that contain a mix of lipids—including triglycerides, fatty acids, phospholipids, cholesterol, and small amounts of other steroids and fat-soluble vitamins—that are covered with a protein outer layer (Figure 5-10). The outer layer of protein allows the compound to move through a watery substance, such as blood. Lipoproteins transport fats in the circulatory system.

The amounts of fat and protein determine the density or weight of the lipoprotein. The more fat and lipid substances present, the lower the density of (or the lighter) the

compound. Four forms of these compounds are most important for understanding the route of cholesterol in the body; they are chylomicrons, very low-density lipoproteins, LDLs, and HDLs.

Chylomicrons transport absorbed fats from the intestinal wall to the liver cells. Fats are then used for synthesis of lipoproteins. Very low-density lipoprotein (VLDL) leaves the liver cells full of fats and lipid components to transfer newly made (endogenous) triglycerides to the cells. Low-density lipoprotein (LDL) forms from VLDL because density is reduced as fats and lipids are released on their journey through the body. LDL carries cholesterol throughout the body to tissue cells for various functions.

In contrast to the delivery functions of the first three lipoproteins, high-density lipoprotein (HDL) is formed within cells to remove cholesterol from the cell, bringing it to the liver for disposal.

A total blood cholesterol reading reflects the level of cholesterol contained in LDL and HDL. To get a clearer assessment of cholesterol activity in the body, the individual levels of LDL and HDL are valuable. The risk of CVD associated with blood cholesterol levels is presented in Table 17-1. LDL levels reflect the amount of cholesterol brought to cells that has the potential to be dropped off along the way to clog vessels and arteries, contributing to plaque formation. Plaques are deposits of fatty substances, including cholesterol, that attach to arterial walls. As this happens, HDLs remove cholesterol from the circulatory system. Removal of cholesterol is a positive action that reduces CVD risk.

Health guidelines generally recommend a dietary cholesterol intake of 300 mg or less per day. Table 5-3 lists the cholesterol content of selected foods. However, the major culprit that raises blood cholesterol is not dietary food cholesterol but too much *food fat* (dietary triglycerides),

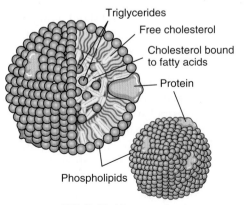

FIG 5-10 Lipoprotein.

Triglycerides
Free cholesterol
Cholesterol bound to fatty acids
Protein
Phospholipids

TABLE 5-3 Cholesterol Content of Selected Foods*

FOOD	AMOUNT	CHOLESTEROL (mg)
Milk, nonfat/skim	1 cup	4
Mayonnaise	1 Tbsp	8
Cottage cheese, low-fat 2%	½ cup	10
Milk, low-fat/2%	1 cup	18
Cream cheese	1 oz	28
Hot dog†	1	29
Ice cream, 10% fat	½ cup	30
Cheddar cheese	1 oz	30
Butter	1 Tbsp	31
Milk, whole	1 cup	33
Clams, fish fillets, oysters	3 oz	50-60
Beef,† pork,† poultry	3 oz	70-85
Shrimp	3 oz	166
Egg yolk†	1	213
Beef liver	3 oz	410

*In ascending order.
†Leading contributors of cholesterol to U.S. diet.

particularly saturated fats; food cholesterol alone makes a minor difference for most people. Too much food cholesterol becomes a problem when it is eaten in conjunction with very high-fat diets. Sometimes, this extra cholesterol in the blood may be dropped off, staying in the vessels and arteries. It may be a factor involved in the development of lesions that may block arteries, leading to CVD. This topic is discussed in detail in Chapter 17.

One reason for the confusion is the way food is cooked and eaten. Eggs, for example, are high in cholesterol and are often cooked and served with high-fat bacon or sausage. The combined meal of eggs and bacon then gets a bad reputation for raising blood cholesterol. The fact is that the large amount of fat in bacon and sausage is more likely to raise blood cholesterol than the food cholesterol in eggs. Shrimp are high in cholesterol but low in fat—that is, low in fat if the shrimp are steamed or broiled, not encased in a deep fat–fried coating. Of course, moderation is recommended for eating eggs and shrimp.

Another source of confusion is that cooking oils made from corn, safflower, and soybeans are often labeled as cholesterol free. Of course, they are cholesterol free; only foods from animals contain cholesterol. Yet vegetable oils are virtually 100% food fat, and large amounts of dietary fat can also raise blood cholesterol.

To be a savvy consumer (and teach your clients), read ingredient labels and be aware of some finer points of fat education:

- Hydrogenated vegetable oils—corn, soybean, and cottonseed—contain *trans* fatty acids, and these cholesterol-forming saturated fats are often used to prepare potato and corn chips.
- Tropical oils of palm, palm kernel, and coconut are the only plant sources of naturally saturated fat. Found in many food products, they should be consumed only occasionally. (Popcorn popped in tropical oils came under fire; many movie theater chains now offer air-popped popcorn in addition to traditionally prepared popcorn.)
- Margarines are cholesterol free if made from vegetable oils but still contain the same number of calories as butter; both are about 100% lipid. Margarines, however, contain unsaturated fatty acids. Note that the level of hydrogenation used to form the margarine affects the amounts of *trans* and saturated fatty acids contained. Use label information to select the least saturated product.
- Advise clients to check the labels of foods they eat regularly; a cholesterol-free product might not be as healthy as it seems.

In addition to the amount of fat, another characteristic of food fat that causes it to affect blood cholesterol differently is whether the fat is saturated or unsaturated—that is, whether the fat contains mostly saturated or unsaturated fatty acids. Saturated fatty acids generally raise blood cholesterol by providing the liver with the best building blocks for making cholesterol.

A simple guideline followed by many people is that blood cholesterol is *raised* by eating solid saturated fats and *lowered* by eating unsaturated and monounsaturated liquid fats. However, this rule is oversimplified for two reasons. First, food fats are a mixture of the three types. Second, although saturated fatty acids as a group raise cholesterol, some individual ones do not. Therefore, although we classify food fats as cholesterol-raising (butter/saturated) and cholesterol-lowering (corn oil/PUFA and olive oil/monounsaturated), these guidelines are based on the proportion of specific fatty acids in each food and how much each fatty acid affects blood cholesterol. Total fat intake can also influence blood cholesterol levels regardless of the source. Table 5-2 and Figure 5-5 clear up some confusion over the finer points of fat.

Synthetic Fats and Fat Replacers

Many people dream about eating brownies and ice cream that are magically stripped of fat but still richly satisfying in taste and texture. Although surveys show that sugar substitutes have not reduced the amount of sugar we consume, optimists hope fat substitutes will reduce fat in our diets. Scientists are working to develop reduced-fat or fat-free substances that replace fat yet retain the taste and mouth-feel of fat in foods.

Fat replacers, as they are called, are generally classified two ways: already existing in nature or synthesized in the laboratory. The naturally occurring ones do not change chemically and thus require less rigorous testing before the U.S. FDA allows them to be used in foods. Heating and then blending protein from milk or eggs in a process called *microparticulation* produces one type of fat replacer. Simplesse is an example. Food applications include ice cream, frozen yogurt, and salad dressings—but not baked or deep-fried foods.

Carrageenan, a carbohydrate extracted from seaweed, has been used for centuries to thicken foods. Added to lean ground beef, carrageenan yields moist, juicy cooked meat with the texture of higher-fat beef. Similar gumlike products from oats, corn, and potatoes are under development and would provide lower kcal fatlike properties in food.

Salatrim, which stands for *short- and long-chain triglyceride molecules,* is made in the laboratory and provides sensory qualities with reduced energy content (5 kcal/g vs. 9 kcal/g). Olestra is a fat replacer made in the laboratory that binds fatty acids to sugar in a nontraditional way so that enzymes in the digestive tract are not able to break away the fatty acids. Olestra resembles standard fats and oils in many ways, including the ability to withstand frying and baking at high temperatures. Several characteristics of olestra are attractive to manufacturers and consumers, including the sensory properties of taste and texture, the no-kcal value because of the body's inability to digest it, and the reduced absorption of fat and cholesterol from the intestine. Potato chips cooked in olestra have 75 kcal/oz—half that of regular chips. A disadvantage is that olestra passes through the gut swiftly, possibly causing abdominal cramping and loose stools and loss of fat-soluble nutrients such as vitamins and carotenoids.

As the story of fat replacers continues to unfold, we need to study their effect on people's food choices. Will we be misled into thinking that low- or no-fat foods automatically are low in kcal? Many fat-reduced foods have increased amounts of other ingredients, such as carbohydrates, and are not low-kcal items.

To what degree will products containing fat replacers stimulate mechanisms to compensate for reduction in fat? Some studies suggest that incorporating reduced-fat products into the diet results in total fat reduction. Yet diets reduced in fat may not result in a reduction of total kcal. Thus, fat-free foods help some people consume fewer kcal overall; other times people eat a fat-free food at one meal and then make up the kcal by eating more at the next. What about appetite guiding what we eat? If mouth-feel is maintained in reduced-fat foods, we may not distinguish between high- and reduced-fat foods. Then there is the "bargain" appeal. In studies in which people did not know which chips were regular and which were made with olestra, they ate similar amounts of each. When they did know, they ate significantly more olestra chips, thus mistakenly thinking they got two for the "fat price" of one.

Although fat replacers are widely available, the most prudent and health-promoting approach is for products to be reformulated or developed without the use of fat replacers so products contain lower-fat ingredients without added sugars and still taste good. Consistently consuming a low-fat diet can lead to a decrease in the preference for fat. Is it possible that fat replacers could undermine this healthful change? Nutritionists and scientists undoubtedly will continue to seek answers to make our fat-free brownie and ice cream dreams come true—without side effects.

Energy Intake

Foods containing significant amounts of dietary fat will naturally provide more kcal than other lower-fat foods. Although high-fat treats are fine occasionally, indulging too often or not even realizing which foods are fat laden can result in consumption of too many kcal that may end up stored as body fat in adipose tissues.

Fat is even more efficient at being stored than carbohydrate and protein, which means that we may gain more body fat from eating fat kcal than eating the same number of carbohydrate kcal (see Figure 9-2). The evidence for this effect comes from studying people who eat low-fat, high-calorie diets, as discussed earlier. A likely explanation is that the energy cost to convert dietary fat to body fat requires only 3% of the kcal consumed, whereas carbohydrate requires 23% of the energy consumed to be converted to body fat. Both storage and oxidation of fats differ from those of carbohydrates and protein.

Diets high in fat are not the primary cause for the high prevalence of excess body fat in our society. We have an "all-food-all-the-time" lifestyle coupled with an aversion to physical activity. Overeating and underactivity are likely reasons for the steady increase in overweight and obese Americans (see the *Personal Perspectives* box Hooked on Salt, Sugar, Fat). Another reason may be the ability to be aware of internal cues of hunger. Consider whether we mistake fatigue as a cue of hunger. Consumption of food becomes a way to relieve tiredness, which of course does not work. Still, for many individuals struggling with moderate or even excessive weight, awareness of their dietary fat intake sources can make a difference. If we gradually reduce fat intake—without increasing carbohydrate intake—energy intake decreases and weight maintenance becomes easier.

Reduced Intake of Other Nutrients

Even if dietary fat consumption does not result in weight gain, foods high in fat tend not to contain much dietary fiber and may be low in other nutrients. Not consuming enough dietary fiber, as noted in Chapter 4 (and in Chapters 13 and 17), is a risk factor for several chronic conditions. The seductive nature of foods containing fats may lead us to crave these foods and neglect others (see the *Personal Perspectives* box Hooked on Salt, Sugar, and Fat). The best guarantee for achieving the goal of nutritional wellness is to consume a balanced intake of nutrients, based on recommended guidelines, through consumption of at least five to seven servings of naturally low-fat fruits and vegetables per day.

Dietary Fat Intake and Diet-Related Diseases

The presence in the American diet of too much fat is directly related to several chronic diseases, such as CVD and certain types of cancer. High-fat diets are indirectly related to type 2 diabetes mellitus and hypertension. Health guidelines to prevent and treat these diseases call for less dietary fat than the average American eats. The DRI daily recommendations are to eat a total fat intake of 30% or less of kcal, and intake of saturated fatty acid less than 10% of kcal, and less than 300 mg of cholesterol. The average intakes of Americans are actually above those levels. Considerations of how this intake affects the risk for these diet-related disorders are presented in Chapters 14, 15, 17, and 20.

TOWARD A POSITIVE NUTRITION LIFESTYLE: GRADUAL REDUCTION

It's the subject of TV situation comedies. One member of the family becomes a health food fanatic, serving blades of grass, sprouts, and weird mixtures of soybeans, nuts, and who knows what. And what is the immediate response of the sitcom family? Disgust and rebellion, of course.

As we make recommendations to our clients (and perhaps decide for ourselves and our families) to reduce or modify the type of fat consumed , we should consider that often the most effective way to achieve permanent change is through gradual reduction. That's the mistake made by the TV character: too many changes made too quickly. An action plan for gradual reduction of dietary fat intake could consist of the following steps:

1. For 1 week, record all food and beverages consumed.
2. On the basis of reading this chapter, assess which foods are likely to be high in fat. Particularly note whether one high-fat food item, such as whole milk, is consumed often or whether a certain meal or snack regularly includes fatty

foods. Perhaps scrambled eggs and bacon are eaten almost every morning for breakfast, and an afternoon coffee break always includes either a sweet Danish pastry or a huge, buttery muffin.

3. The next week, choose one item and either reduce its consumption or replace it with a lower-fat substitute. Instead of whole milk, use 2% or 1% fat milk, or replace the coffee break treat with an English muffin with a bit of butter or margarine and jelly.

4. The following week, select another food item or meal and make a simple substitution.

This process can continue with small changes—gradual reductions—resulting in major reductions in dietary fat intake.

SUMMARY

- Functions of lipids include specific characteristics of foods that arise from lipids and maintenance of the physiologic health of the body.
  - Triglycerides provide food functions of energy, palatability, satiety, food processing, and source of nutrients. Physiologic functions include form of stored energy; organ protection; temperature regulation; and insulation.
  - Phospholipids are a component of all cell membrane structures; emulsifiers of fluids within of the body; and part of the transport of lipids throughout the body.
  - Sterols are part of complex regulatory compounds within the body; a basic material to make bile; vitamin D; sex hormones; and cells in brain and nerve tissues. Cholesterol, a sterol, is a vital part of all cell membrane and nerve tissues; and of building blocks for hormones.
- Lipids are organic, composed of carbon, hydrogen, and oxygen.
  - Triglycerides are composed of one glycerol molecule and three fatty acids.
    - Fatty acids may be saturated, monounsaturated, or polyunsaturated, depending on the number of double bonds.

- Phospholipids are composed of one glycerol molecule with only two fatty acids; the third spot contains a phosphate group.
- Sterol structures, including cholesterol, are carbon rings intermeshed with side chains of carbon, hydrogen, and oxygen.
- All three types of lipids can be manufactured by the body, except for linolenic and linoleic fatty acids (found in triglycerides), which therefore are essential nutrients.
- Digestion of lipids occurs mainly in the small intestine; absorption depends on the transportation of lipids through the lymph and blood circulatory systems.
  - Lipids travel through the body in lipoprotein packages containing triglycerides, protein, phospholipids, and cholesterol.
  - Lipoproteins differ according to the proportions or ratio of these ingredients. Very low-density lipoprotein (VLDL), low-density lipoprotein (LDL), and high-density lipoprotein (HDL) are found in the blood.
- Health concerns about dietary fat intake fall into several categories: appropriate energy intake, reduced intake of other nutrients because of excessive dietary fat consumption, and the relationship between dietary fat intake and diet-related disorders.

◎ THE NURSING APPROACH

Low-Fat Project

In preparation for the opening of a new wellness and fitness center on the college campus, the new director surveyed students, faculty, and staff about their needs and interests. Results revealed great interest in nutrition. The director met with a committee of students, faculty, and staff to share ideas and plan for possible nutrition education. Ideas included offering nutrition courses, providing guest lecturers for short education sessions, arranging for consulting dietitians, posting nutrition information near the cafeteria menu, disseminating nutrition handouts, and creating a health and wellness website or blog.

The first nutrition topic selected by the committee was reducing fat intake by choosing lower-fat foods. Nursing students were assigned to create posters and contribute articles and recipes for the website. Their task was to identify the following important questions for discussion:

1. Why is it beneficial to limit total fat intake to about 30% of the daily kcal? How many kcal are produced by 1 g of fat? How many grams of fat are in food commonly consumed, such as a glass of 2% milk, a serving of potato chips, or a 4-oz. steak?

2. Why should saturated fats be limited to 10% or less of daily kcal? What are the potential harmful effects of saturated fats and cholesterol? Which foods contain saturated fats? Which animal products should be limited?

3. What are *trans* fats, and what are the disadvantages of consuming them? How can they be avoided? Is butter or margarine healthier?

◎ THE NURSING APPROACH—cont'd

4. What are common food sources of monounsaturated and polyunsaturated fats? What is the best salad oil? What is the best cooking oil?
5. Why are omega-3 fatty acids health promoting? What are food sources of omega-3 fatty acids? Is it more beneficial to eat fish or to take fish oil supplements?
6. How can a consumer purchase healthy low-fat products? How can one interpret the nutrition label?
7. What lower-fat snacks and desserts can be substituted for high-kcal, high-fat, and high-sugar snacks and desserts?
8. Which fast foods and restaurant meals are lower in fat?
9. What are the benefits and drawbacks of artificial fat substitutes such as Simplesse, Carrageenan, Saltrim, and Olestra?

10. What food preparation techniques are best for low-fat eating? How can recipes be modified to make them lower in fat?
11. What proportions of each food group are on MyPlate? How can this tool help with portion control?
12. What websites have good information about lowering fat in the diet?

After identifying these questions, the students organized into groups. Questions were divided and assigned to individual groups. Students researched the answers to the questions and then each group created an educational program for the center. The resulting programs were reviewed by a subcommittee that then compiled all the programs into a coherent project.

❓ APPLYING CONTENT KNOWLEDGE

Disease prevention for chronic diet-related diseases depends on changes in lifestyle behaviors. Consider the lifestyle behaviors John Mason could adopt on the basis of his personal history. John Mason is a 20-year-old white male; his mother and father both have high cholesterol levels and family history of CVD. Although John's cholesterol level is average for his age, what three disease prevention strategies could he pursue? Would these strategies be primary, secondary, or tertiary?

▌ WEBSITES OF INTEREST

USDA Nutrient Database Laboratory (Food Composition Tables)
www.ars.usda.gov/Services/docs.htm?docid=8964
Creates and supports nutrient databases through the most advanced procedures to obtain, assess, collect, and distribute composition data on foods accessible in the United States.

Center for Science in the Public Interest (CSPI)
www.cspinet.org
Improving the American food supply through educative, legislative, regulatory, and judicial advocacy and by publication of the monthly *Nutrition Action Healthletter*.

Eating Well On-Line
www.eatingwell.com
Online version of the magazine *Eating Well: Where Good Taste Meets Good Health*; has information on nutrition, food, and low-fat cooking.

REFERENCES

Cotton PA, et al: Dietary sources of nutrients among U.S. adults, 1994 to 1996, *J Am Diet Assoc* 104(6):921–930, 2004.

Drewnowski A: Sensory control of energy density at different life stages, *Proc Nutr Soc* 59(2):239–244, 2000.

Evidence Analysis Library: *What effect does consuming natural (ruminant) vs. synthetic (industrially hydrogenated) trans fatty acids have on LDL-, HDL- and Non-HDL cholesterol?* 2013, Academy of Nutrition and Dietetics. From: www.adaevidencelibrary.com/. Accessed October 5.

Harper CR, Jacobson TA: Usefulness of omega-3 fatty acids and the prevention of coronary heart disease, *Am J Cardiol* 96(11):1521–1529, 2005.

Harris WS: Fish oils and plasma lipid and lipoprotein metabolism in humans: A critical review, *J Lipid Res* 30:785–807, 1989.

Jones PJH, Rideout T: Lipids, sterols, and their metabolites. In Ross AC, et al, editors: *Modern nutrition in health and disease*, ed 11, Philadelphia, 2014, Lippincott Williams & Wilkins.

Tso P, Liu M: Ingested fat and satiety, *Physiol Behav* 81(2):275–287, 2004.

Protein

Protein in food is our only source of amino acids, which are absolutely necessary to make the thousands of proteins that form every aspect of the human body.

ⓔ http://evolve.elsevier.com/GRODNER/FOUNDATIONS

LEARNING OBJECTIVES

- Define the composition of protein.
- Describe how the composition of protein differs from carbohydrate and lipid.
- Define essential and nonessential amino acids.
- Distinguish between complete proteins and incomplete proteins.

- Discuss how protein is digested, absorbed as amino acids and becomes available to cells.
- List the functions of protein.

ROLE IN WELLNESS

In 1928 a political slogan promised "a chicken in every pot!" At that time, being able to afford animal protein on a daily basis was the mark of a high standard of living and an assurance of good health. Today the phrase might be "rice and beans for all of us!" We now know that there are many sources of protein available in our food supply. Some offer advantages over others by being lower in fat and higher in other nutrients such as complex carbohydrates and fiber.

Protein in food is our only source of amino acids, which are absolutely necessary to make the thousands of proteins that form every aspect of the human body. It is no wonder that protein, which is plentiful in our food supply, has gained the status of a super-nutrient for Americans. A common but inaccurate belief is that we expect that the more protein we eat, the stronger our immune system will be, the less we will weigh, and the more muscles we will develop.

Although proteins formed by our bodies do have a role in those functions, the amounts we consume are often greater than we need. Awareness of protein sources and portion sizes is important as we work toward achieving health promotion goals to decrease our risk of diet-related diseases (Box 6-1).

The six dimensions of health provide ways to think about the effects of protein consumption. Our overall *physical health* and well-being depend on our eating enough essential amino acids for body protein synthesis. The ability to comprehend and apply new approaches to protein consumption by adapting to different protein sources (e.g., legumes and grains) and reducing portion sizes depends on our *intellectual health* capacity to implement change. Protein is a super-status

food for some Americans; favorite sources may provide *emotional health* security. Clients needing to make dietary changes, such as changing to lower-fat sources of protein (e.g., cutting back on sausages), may need our advice on coping strategies. Because we and our clients follow different eating patterns, such as practicing vegetarianism or reducing consumption of animal protein, family and social dynamics may be affected when one member changes and thereby tests our level of *social health*. Religious and *spiritual health* beliefs lead individuals to nourish their bodies through a harmless philosophy that views humans as civilized enough to nourish their bodies without taking life. *Environmental health* concerns are being raised because of the ecological impact of byproducts of production of animal sources, such as manure polluting farmlands.

STRUCTURE OF PROTEIN

Proteins are organic compounds formed by the linking of many smaller molecules of amino acids. Amino acids, like glucose, are organic compounds made of carbon, hydrogen, and oxygen. However, amino acids also contain nitrogen, which clearly distinguishes protein from other nutrients.

There are 20 amino acids from which all the proteins that are required by plants and animals are made. The human body is able to manufacture some of the amino acids for its own protein-building function; however, 9 amino acids cannot be made by the cells of the body. Therefore, these essential amino acids (EAAs) must be eaten in food, digested, absorbed, and then brought to cells by circulating blood. The remaining 11 are nonessential amino acids (NEAAs)

BOX 6-1 MyPlate: Protein Foods

The meat and beans group includes not only meat and dry beans or peas but also poultry, fish, eggs, nuts, and seeds, all of which provide protein. Choose lean or low-fat cuts of meat and poultry, trimming fat and removing skin. Some fish (such as tuna, salmon, and trout), nuts, and seeds (walnuts and flax) contain healthy oils and are good sources of omega-3 fatty acids, which may reduce the risk for CVD. Other nuts and seeds (almonds, hazelnuts, and sunflower seeds) provide vitamin E. Eating an assortment of protein sources means consuming other valuable nutrients as well.

What Counts as an Ounce?

In general, 1 ounce of meat, poultry, or fish; $\frac{1}{4}$ cup of cooked dry beans; 1 egg; 1 Tbsp of peanut butter; or $\frac{1}{2}$ ounce of nuts or seeds can be considered a 1 ounce-equivalent from the meat and beans group.

PROTEIN SOURCE	AMOUNT THAT COUNTS AS 1 OUNCE-EQUIVALENT IN THE MEAT AND BEANS GROUP	COMMON PORTIONS AND OUNCE-EQUIVALENTS
Meats	1 ounce cooked lean beef 1 ounce cooked lean pork or ham	1 small steak (eye of round, filet) = $3\frac{1}{2}$ to 4 ounce-equivalents 1 small lean hamburger = 2 to 3 ounce-equivalents
Poultry	1 ounce cooked chicken or turkey, without skin 1 sandwich slice of turkey ($4\frac{1}{2} \times 2\frac{1}{2} \times \frac{1}{8}$ inches)	1 small chicken breast half = 3 ounce-equivalents $\frac{1}{2}$ Cornish game hen = 4 ounce-equivalents
Fish	1 ounce cooked fish or shellfish	1 can of tuna, drained = 3 to 4 ounce-equivalents 1 salmon steak = 4 to 6 ounce-equivalents 1 small trout = 3 ounce-equivalents
Eggs	1 egg	
Nuts and seeds	$\frac{1}{2}$ ounce of nuts (12 almonds, 24 pistachios, 7 walnut halves) $\frac{1}{2}$ ounce of seeds (pumpkin, sunflower, or squash seeds, hulled, roasted) 1 Tbsp of peanut butter or almond butter	1 ounce of nuts or seeds = 2 ounce-equivalents
Dry beans and peas	$\frac{1}{4}$ cup of cooked dry beans (such as black, kidney, pinto, or white beans) $\frac{1}{4}$ cup of cooked dry peas (such as chickpeas, cowpeas, lentils, or split peas) $\frac{1}{4}$ cup of baked beans, refried beans $\frac{1}{4}$ cup ($\approx$ 2 ounces) of tofu 1 ounce tempeh, cooked $\frac{1}{4}$ cup of roasted soybeans 1 falafel patty ($2\frac{1}{4}$ inches, 4 ounces) 2 Tbsp hummus	1 cup split pea soup = 2 ounce-equivalents 1 cup lentil soup = 2 ounce-equivalents 1 cup bean soup = 2 ounce-equivalents 1 soy or bean burger patty = 2 ounce-equivalents

From U.S. Department of Agriculture, Center for Nutrition and Promotion: *MyPlate protein foods*, 2011. Accessed November 3, 2013, from www.choosemyplate.gov/food-groups/protein-foods-counts.html.

(Box 6-2). The liver can create NEAAs as long as structural components, including nitrogen, from other amino acids are available.

Each cell constructs or synthesizes the proteins it needs. To build proteins, the cell must have access to all 20 amino acids. This available supply of amino acids is in the metabolic amino acid pool. The amino acid pool is a collection of amino acids that is constantly resupplied with EAAs (from dietary intake) and NEAAs (synthesized in the liver). The pool allows the cell to build proteins easily.

Protein Composition

The functions of proteins are closely related to their structures. The complex composition of proteins is best understood through four structural levels: primary, secondary, tertiary, and quaternary (Figure 6-1).

BOX 6-2 Amino Acids

Essential Amino Acids	Nonessential Amino Acids
Histidine	Alanine
Isoleucine	Arginine
Leucine	Aspartic acid
Lysine	Cysteine
Methionine	Cystine
Phenylalanine	Glutamic acid
Threonine	Glutamine
Tryptophan	Glycine
Valine	Proline
	Serine
	Tyrosine

FIG 6-1 Structural levels of protein. **A,** Primary structure: determined by number, kind, and sequence of amino acids in the chain. **B,** Secondary structure: hydrogen bonds stabilize folds of helical spirals. **C,** Tertiary structure: globular shape maintained by strong intramolecular bonding and by stabilizing hydrogen bonds. **D,** Quaternary structure: results from bonding between more than one polypeptide unit. (Courtesy Bill Ober. In Thibodeau GA, Patton KT: *Anatomy & physiology,* ed 4, St Louis, 1999, Mosby.)

The *primary* structure of protein composition is determined by the number, assortment, and sequence of amino acids in polypeptide chains. Amino acids are linked together by peptide bonds to form a practically unlimited number of proteins. The peptide bond occurs at the point at which the carboxyl group of one amino acid is bound to the amino group of another amino acid (Figure 6-2).

The 20 amino acids form chains that may contain any combination or assortment of amino acids, allowing for thousands of different proteins to be formed. Two proteins

FIG 6-2 Peptide bonds.

may contain the same assortment and number of amino acids yet still have different functions because of the sequencing or order of the amino acids.

The *secondary* structure level of proteins affects the shape of the chain of amino acids; they may be straight, folded, or coiled. The *tertiary* structure results when the polypeptide chain is so coiled that the loops of the coil touch, forming strong bonds within the chain itself. At the *quaternary* structural level, proteins contain more than one polypeptide chain.

A protein may not be able to perform its original function if its structure or shape changes. The shape may be changed by heat (cooking), ultraviolet light (exposure to sunlight), acids (vinegar), alcohol, or mechanical action. A protein has been **denatured** and physically changed when the shape of a protein is affected (e.g., a folded chain unfolding).

An example of denaturing a food protein is the change that occurs when the white of an uncooked egg (a clear liquid) is beaten. The clear liquid turns white, foamy, and stiff. Although the protein in the egg has been denatured, it is still a valuable source of amino acids. The amino acids are not affected; only the shape of the chain has been changed.

Inside the body, denaturing of proteins is controlled by mechanisms that keep the internal body environment from getting too basic or too acidic. Either extreme can lead to the denaturation of vital proteins within the body. Body temperature also affects the protein structure of the body. High fevers can become lethal when protein structures within the body become denatured. When body proteins are denatured, they cannot perform their original functions.

Although uncontrolled denaturation can be dangerous, it is helpful for digestion. Denaturing changes the three-dimensional structure of a protein, providing more surface area on which digestive juices act to release the amino acids of the food proteins.

PROTEIN AS A NUTRIENT IN THE BODY

The proteins we consume in foods are not the same proteins used by our bodies. Actually, the only nutrient role protein in foods serves is to provide amino acids, the building blocks of all proteins.

Digestion and Absorption

Because of the complex structure of proteins, a number of protein enzymes, or proteases, produced by the stomach and pancreas are required to hydrolyze proteins into smaller and smaller peptides until individual amino acids are ready for absorption (Figure 6-3).

Mouth

Only mechanical digestion of protein occurs in the mouth. Mastication breaks protein-containing food into smaller pieces that mix with saliva passing through to the stomach.

Stomach

Pepsinogen, an inactive form of the gastric protease pepsin, is secreted by the stomach mucosa. Pepsin becomes activated when it mixes with hydrochloric acid (HCl), also produced by stomach secretions. Pepsin then begins the process of protein hydrolysis, breaking the bonds linking the amino acids of the protein peptide. The result is smaller polypeptides rather than single amino acids or dipeptides. The polypeptides pass through to the small intestine for further hydrolysis.

Rennin, an important gastric protease, is produced only during infancy. It functions with calcium to thicken or

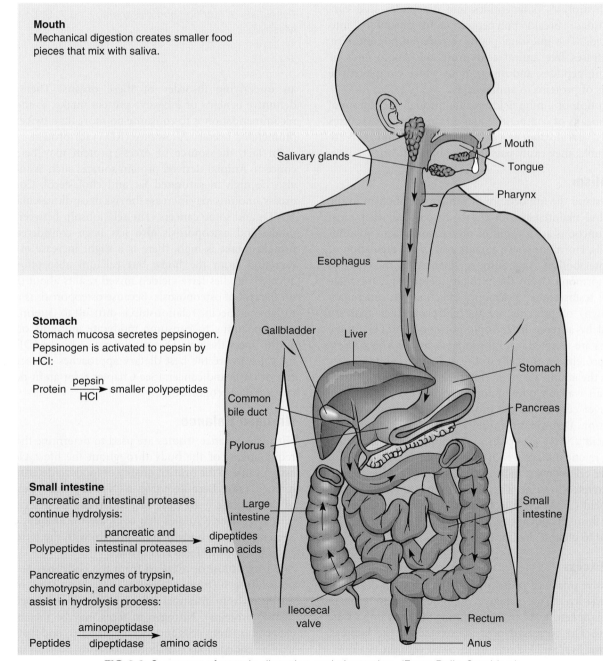

Mouth
Mechanical digestion creates smaller food pieces that mix with saliva.

Stomach
Stomach mucosa secretes pepsinogen. Pepsinogen is activated to pepsin by HCl:

$$\text{Protein} \xrightarrow[\text{HCl}]{\text{pepsin}} \text{smaller polypeptides}$$

Small intestine
Pancreatic and intestinal proteases continue hydrolysis:

$$\text{Polypeptides} \xrightarrow[\text{intestinal proteases}]{\text{pancreatic and}} \begin{array}{l} \text{dipeptides} \\ \text{amino acids} \end{array}$$

Pancreatic enzymes of trypsin, chymotrypsin, and carboxypeptidase assist in hydrolysis process:

$$\text{Peptides} \xrightarrow[\text{dipeptidase}]{\text{aminopeptidase}} \text{amino acids}$$

Labels: Salivary glands, Mouth, Tongue, Pharynx, Esophagus, Gallbladder, Liver, Stomach, Common bile duct, Pancreas, Pylorus, Large intestine, Small intestine, Ileocecal valve, Rectum, Anus

FIG 6-3 Summary of protein digestion and absorption. (From Rolin Graphics.)

coagulate the milk protein casein; thickening slows the movement of milk nutrients from the stomach, allowing additional digestion time.

Small Intestine

In the small intestine, pancreatic and intestinal proteases continue the hydrolysis of polypeptides. As these smaller peptides touch the intestinal walls, peptidases are released that complete the hydrolysis of protein into absorbable units of individual amino acids and dipeptides.

The primary pancreatic enzyme is trypsin. It is first secreted as trypsinogen, an inactive form. The intestinal hormone enteropeptidase activates trypsinogen into trypsin, which continues the hydrolysis of polypeptides. Two other pancreatic enzymes assist in the hydrolysis process: chymotrypsin hydrolyzes polypeptides into dipeptides, and carboxypeptidase breaks polypeptides and dipeptides into amino acids. Two intestinal peptidases are aminopeptidase, which releases free amino acids from the amino ends of short-chain peptides, and dipeptidase, which completes the hydrolysis of proteins to amino acids.

Absorption of amino acids occurs through the intestinal walls by means of competitive active transport that requires vitamin B_6 (pyridoxine) as a carrier. Because amino acids are water soluble, they easily pass into the bloodstream.

Metabolism

To understand the importance of protein metabolism in the growth and maintenance of the body, consider that most protein functions are a result of protein anabolism (synthesis) in cells. Hormones have a major role in the regulation of protein metabolism. Anabolism is enhanced by the effect of growth hormone (from the pituitary gland) and the male hormone testosterone. Hormones affecting the catabolism (breakdown) of proteins are the glucocorticoids that are enhanced by adrenocorticotropic hormone (ACTH); these hormones are secreted from the adrenal cortex. This process releases proteins in the cells to break down to amino acids, and then the amino acids travel in the bloodstream, contributing to an available pool of amino acids (Figure 6-4).

The liver cells begin the process of catabolism through deamination. Deamination results in the breaking off of an amino acid (NH_2) group from an amino acid molecule, resulting in one molecule each of ammonia (NH_3) and a keto acid. Liver cells convert most of the ammonia to urea, which is later excreted in urine. The keto acid may enter the tricarboxylic acid (TCA) cycle to be used for energy (see Figure 9-2) or, through gluconeogenesis and lipogenesis, may be converted to glucose and fat (see Figure 6-4).

Protein Excess

An excessive intake of protein results in increased deamination by the liver. The increased deamination may result in high levels of keto acids, possibly putting the body into a state of ketosis. The increased urea is excreted by the kidneys. Because the liver and kidneys are involved with the deamination process, the increased stress on the organs could initiate

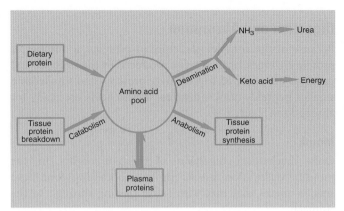

FIG 6-4 The body's equilibrium depends on a balance between the rates of protein breakdown (catabolism) and protein synthesis (anabolism). (Modified from Williams SR: *Essentials of nutrition and diet therapy,* ed 7, St Louis, 1999, Mosby.)

an underlying disorder of these organs. There are no definitive benefits of excessive protein intake, so the general recommendation is to consume no more than twice the Recommended Dietary Allowance (RDA) for protein.

In fact, the source of excess protein may be a health concern. Animal-derived protein sources such as meats may also be high in saturated fat and cholesterol. Consuming excess amounts may increase the risk of cardiovascular disease (CVD) and some cancers. The relationship between protein intake and osteoporosis also has been considered. When protein intake is high, there is a slight increase of calcium excretion from the body, but calcium absorption is not affected. Studies have yielded mixed results about this effect on the risk of osteoporosis. Because osteoporosis is multifactorial, this specific relationship is difficult to determine. Recommendations to consume moderate amounts of protein and to meet the new Dietary Reference Intake (DRI) levels for calcium are the best dietary approaches to decrease the risk of CVD and cancer. (See Chapter 8 for an in-depth discussion of osteoporosis.)

Nitrogen Balance

Nitrogen-balance studies are used to determine the protein requirements of the body throughout the life cycle and to assign value to the protein quality of foods to determine their biologic value. Because nitrogen (N) is a primary component of protein, the body's use of protein can be determined by nitrogen-balance studies that compare the amount of nitrogen entering the body in food protein with the nitrogen lost from the body in feces and urine.

Nitrogen lost or excreted from the body may be endogenous nitrogen (from catabolism of body protein), metabolic nitrogen (from intestinal cells), or exogenous nitrogen (from dietary proteins). Nitrogen in feces may be metabolic and exogenous (from cells and dietary proteins) and that in urine may be endogenous (catabolism of body protein) and exogenous (from dietary proteins).

An individual is in nitrogen equilibrium or zero nitrogen balance if the amount of nitrogen consumed in foods equals the amount excreted. This state occurs in normal, healthy adults when nitrogen in food protein entering (input) the body equals the nitrogen leaving the body (output). Because adults are no longer growing, the nitrogen that enters the body is not needed to build new tissue but is used simply to maintain the body.

Positive nitrogen balance occurs when more nitrogen is retained in the body than excreted. The nitrogen is used to form new cells for growth or healing. This state occurs in growing children and in pregnant women who require additional nitrogen (and protein) for the growth of the fetus. Individuals recovering from illness or injury may be in positive nitrogen balance as the body heals. Negative nitrogen balance happens when more nitrogen is excreted from the body than is retained from dietary protein sources. It occurs when there is a breakdown of proteins within the body, such as in muscles and organs. Negative nitrogen balance may be caused by aging, physical illness, extreme stress, starvation, surgery, or eating disorders.

FUNCTIONS

Proteins created in our bodies perform numerous functions, including the following:
- Growth and maintenance
- Creation of communicators and catalysts
- Immune system response
- Fluid and electrolyte regulation
- Acid-base balance
- Transportation

Growth and Maintenance

Each body cell contains proteins. All growth depends on a sufficient supply of amino acids. The amino acids are needed to make the proteins required to support muscle, tissue, bone formation, and the cells themselves.

Maintaining our bodies also requires a constant supply of amino acids. There is a continual turnover of body cells, which are composed of protein. The cells break down and must immediately be replaced. Each replacement cell requires the formation of additional protein.

Also needed for growth and maintenance is the protein collagen, found throughout the body. Collagen forms connective tissues such as ligaments and tendons and acts as a glue to keep the walls of the arteries intact. In addition, collagen has a role in bone and tooth formation by forming the framework structure, which is then filled with minerals such as calcium and phosphorus. Synthesis of scar tissue also depends on collagen. Wound healing depends on an adequate intake of protein. Other structures, such as hair, nails, and skin, are composed of similar protein substances.

Creation of Communicators and Catalysts

Many vital substances produced by our bodies are formed of protein. Some hormones are proteins. Hormones act as communicators to alert different parts of the body to changes or to regulate functions of organs. Insulin, a hormone that directs cells to take in glucose, is a protein. Enzymes are also proteins. Enzymes are catalysts that enable chemical reactions or biologic changes to occur within the body. Each enzyme has a specific target; consequently, numerous enzymes are continually formed.

Blood clotting depends on protein substances as well. Twelve blood clotting factors must be in place for blood to clot when injury has occurred; several of the factors, such as fibrogen, are composed of protein.

Immune System Response

The defense system of our bodies depends on proteins produced in response to foreign viruses and bacteria that invade our bodies. The proteins, or antibodies, are specific to each intruder. If sufficient levels of amino acids are not available to form these antibodies, we may have difficulties maintaining our health. Our overall immunologic response—our resistance to disease—depends on proteins formed within our bodies.

Fluid and Electrolyte Regulation

Water is balanced among three compartments in the body: intravascular (within veins and arteries), intracellular (inside cells), and interstitial (between cells). Proteins and minerals attract water, creating osmotic pressure. As proteins circulate through our bodies, they maintain body fluid and electrolyte balance by keeping water appropriately divided among the three compartments.

Acid-Base Balance

Some reactions occurring within the body lead to the release of acidic substances; others cause basic matter to enter the fluids of the body. Blood proteins can buffer the effects of fluids to maintain a safe acidic level in body fluids. The ability of protein to regulate the balance between the acidic and base characteristics of fluids is called the *buffering effect* of protein. Because the chemical structure of amino acids combines an acid (the carboxyl group [COOH]) and base (amine), an amino acid can function as either an acid or a base, depending on the pH of its medium. This is why the buffering effect of blood proteins is possible. This function is crucial to protect all proteins in the body. If fluids become either too acidic or too basic, the shapes of proteins are altered or denatured. Denatured proteins are not able to perform their usual functions.

Many of the constituents of blood are protein based, and if protein functions are affected, the result can be lethal. Therefore, proteins maintain a delicate pH level to ensure the proper functioning of all body systems (Box 6-3).

Transportation

Throughout our bodies, proteins are able to transport nutrients and other vital substances. For individual cells, proteins act as pumps, assisting the movement of nutrients in and out of cells. Many nutrients, including lipids, minerals, vitamins,

---

BOX 6-3   Genetic Disorders

Phenylketonuria (PKU) is a genetic disorder with a protein link. This disorder is characterized by the inability to use or break down excess phenylalanine, an essential amino acid. The excess phenylalanine circulating inside the body can cause various health problems. Infants with this disorder consume low-phenylalanine formulas, whereas children and adults with PKU follow a limited-protein diet to control the intake of phenylalanine.

Another genetic protein disorder is sickle cell disease, which affects the shape of red blood cells. Because of abnormalities of the hemoglobin molecule, the red blood cell is curved or sickle shaped rather than round. The sickle shape can cause these blood cells to clog small blood vessels. This clogging can be painful, may cause damage to internal organs such as the kidneys and heart, and may lead to frequent infections throughout the body. Early screening followed by long-term penicillin treatment can prevent secondary infections.

Having the sickle cell disease trait is not the same as having the disease itself. Both parents have to have the trait for a child to be at risk. Even then, there is only a 25% chance of development of the disorder. Sickle cell disease may occur in any ethnic group, but it is more common among Africans and African Americans; some states screen all infants to determine susceptibility.

BOX 6-4   Sources of Complete and Incomplete Proteins

Foods Containing Complete Proteins	Foods Containing Incomplete Proteins
Fish	Cereals:
Shellfish	Ready-to-eat
Chicken	Oatmeal
Turkey	Wheatena
Duck*	Grains:
Beef*	Wheat
Lamb*	Rice
Pork*	Corn
Eggs*	Oats/oatmeal
Soybeans (tofu)	Barley
Cheese:	Spaghetti/pasta
Hard cheeses:	Bagels
Cheddar	Bread
Muenster	Legumes:
Swiss	Black-eyed peas
Soft cheeses:	Lentils
Cottage cheese†	Beans
Ricotta†	Peanuts/peanut butter
Milk†	Chickpeas
Ice milk/reduced-fat ice	Split peas
cream	Broccoli
Yogurt†	Potatoes
Frozen yogurt	Green peas
	Leafy green vegetables

*Possible high-fat source of protein.
†Protein in skim, 2%, and whole milk products.

---

and electrolytes, are carried in the blood by proteins such as lipoproteins. This allows the nutrients to be available to all parts of the body. Hemoglobin, a special carrier composed of protein, transports oxygen in the blood. Oxygen is stored in our muscles in another protein carrier, myoglobin. These protein carriers, hemoglobin and myoglobin, are essential for a well-functioning body.

FOOD SOURCES

Quality of Protein Foods

The proteins in foods are categorized by the EAAs they contain. Complete protein contains all nine EAAs in sufficient quantities that best support growth and maintenance of our bodies. Animal-derived foods, including meat, poultry, fish, eggs, and most dairy products, contain complete protein. (A notable exception is gelatin, which is incomplete.) Soybeans are the only plant source that provide all nine essential amino acids. Foods that contribute the best balance of EAAs and the best assortment of NEAAs for protein synthesis and are easily digestible are high-quality protein foods. The two highest-quality protein foods are eggs and human milk. The egg is of high quality because it contains all the necessary nutrients to support life. Human breast milk is the perfect food; its nutrient profile is ideal for human growth.

Incomplete protein lacks one or more of the nine essential amino acids. Incomplete proteins will not provide a sufficient supply of amino acids and will not support life (Box 6-4). Many plant foods contain considerable amounts of incomplete proteins. Some of the better sources are grains and legumes.

The EAAs that those incomplete proteins lack are called limiting amino acids. The limiting amino acid reduces the value of the protein contained in the food. Unless the limiting amino acid is consumed in other foods, the amino acid pools inside the cells would be missing some of the EAAs. Protein production within the cell would be affected, and fewer proteins could be formed. Consequently, limiting amino acids reduces the number of proteins our bodies can make. Generally, we consume a sufficient mix of complete and incomplete proteins; therefore, this is not a health problem. Only those who adopt a dietary pattern restricting certain types of protein foods are at risk for an imbalanced intake.

Complementary Proteins

If different kinds of plant foods are eaten throughout the day, the total protein intake will equal that of complete proteins found in animal-related products. The advantages to complementary proteins are that plant foods cost less and tend to contain less fat; consuming less dietary fat is a prevention strategy for several chronic diet-related diseases.

A balance of amino acids is required throughout the day for protein synthesis. A sufficient assortment of EAAs is provided without planning if both animal and plant protein foods are eaten. If animal foods are not eaten, more care is

BOX 6-5 Food Combinations That Provide Complete Proteins

Grains + Legumes = Complete Protein
Peanut butter sandwich
Tacos with refried beans
Rice and beans
Split pea soup with croutons
Falafel (chickpea balls) on pita bread
Lentil soup with rye bread
Baked beans with bread

Grains or Legumes + Animal Protein (Small Amount) = Complete Protein
Chili with beans and cornbread
Ready-to-eat cereal with skim milk
Cheese sandwich
Pasta with cheese
Rice pudding
French toast
Pancakes (made with milk and/or eggs)
Tuna casserole

required to ensure that limiting amino acids are consumed. Combinations of plant foods that provide all the EAAs are grains (e.g., wheat or rice) with legumes (e.g., kidney beans or chickpeas) and grains or legumes with small amounts of animal protein from dairy, meat, poultry, or fish (Box 6-5).

Measures of Food Protein Quality

Many foods contain protein, but the value of specific foods as protein sources varies. Perhaps the protein contained is incomplete or is difficult to digest (bound tightly to fiber). If food proteins are not digested, the amino acids can't be absorbed to nourish our bodies.

Several methods are used to analyze the quality of proteins in food, including biologic value, amino acid score, and protein efficiency ratio. Biologic value measures how much nitrogen from a protein food is retained by the body after digestion, absorption, and excretion. This measurement of nitrogen balance reveals how available the protein of that food is to the human body. An egg has the highest reference protein score, 100; all of the egg protein can be used. It has become a standard against which all other food proteins are judged. Fish has a score of 75 to 90, and corn, which contains protein but also has lower amino acid ratios, has a score of 40 (Matthews, 2014).

The amino acid score is a simple measure of the amino acid composition of a food in comparison with a reference protein. The score is based on the limiting amino acid(s) of the food. Digestibility of the protein is not considered.

A third method for assessing protein quality is protein efficiency ratio (PER). With this this method, rats are fed a set amount of protein, and then, on the basis of weight gain, the physiologic value of the food protein consumed is determined as follows (Matthews, 2014):

$$PER = \frac{Weight\ gain}{Protein\ intake}$$

Protein RDA

The RDA for protein provides for sufficient intake of the EAAs and enough total protein to provide the amino groups needed to build new NEAAs. Other factors that affect the RDA for protein are age, gender, physiologic state, and sources of protein.

Age affects protein requirements because when growth occurs, such as during childhood, a greater percentage of dietary intake of protein is needed than in adulthood. Growth results in additional muscle and tissues, all of which require the amino acids contained in dietary protein. Theoretically, older adults may require lower levels of protein because muscle mass is reduced as we age; protein use may also be affected by variables such as decreased physical activity, illness, and long-term use of medications. However, few studies exist to confirm a lower requirement, so the protein RDA for adults 50 years and older is the same as for younger adults (National Research Council [NRC], 2006). Gender differences also affect protein needs. Men tend to have more lean body mass or muscle than women. Lean body mass requires more protein for maintenance.

Certain physiologic states, such as pregnancy and lactation, require different amounts of nutrients. A pregnant woman should consume additional protein to meet the needs of the growing fetus as well as those of her own body. RDA recommendations for protein are 25 g protein/day higher for pregnant women (71 g). Lactation, the production of breast milk, also requires consumption of additional protein. Breast milk contains high-quality protein that is formed from amino acids provided by the woman. The protein RDA for lactation is the same as for pregnancy (71 g). Special circumstances—serious physical illness, wound healing, fevers (increased metabolic rate), and unusual stress—may also increase protein needs.

The type of food source also affects the amount of protein needed. In the United States, most of the protein eaten is complete protein from animal sources. These sources are considered when the RDA for protein is set. Other countries rely on more plant sources of incomplete proteins, so worldwide recommendations, such as those of the World Health Organization, differ from the U.S. guidelines.

The RDA for protein is 0.8 g/kg (or 2.2 pounds) (NRC, 2006). For an average adult man, the RDA is 56 to 63 g; for an average adult woman, the RDA is 46 to 50 g. Research suggests that recommended levels for athletes are 1.2 to 1.7 g protein/kg body weight, depending on whether a sport requires endurance or strength (Rodriguez, et al, 2009). Because most Americans eat more protein than recommended, even athletes tend to easily meet protein recommendations. Determine your recommended protein intake using the formula in the *Teaching Tool* box Calculating Your Recommended Protein Intake.

The Acceptable Macronutrient Distribution Ranges (AMDRs) suggest that protein consumption account for

Calculating Your Recommended Protein Intake

To determine your personal protein recommendation, compute the following:

1. Divide your body weight by 2.2 to determine your weight in kilograms (kg):

   Weight in lb ÷ 2.2 = Weight in kg

   Example:

   140 ÷ 2.2 = 63.63 kg

2. Multiply the kilogram weight by 0.8 g/kg to determine your protein RDA (i.e., weight in kg × 0.8 g/kg = g of protein/RDA).

   Example:

   63.5 kg × 0.8 g/kg = 50.9 g protein/RDA

between 10% and 35% of energy intake. Depending on the percentage of protein energy consumed, consumption of energy from carbohydrates and lipids should be adjusted accordingly.

VEGETARIANISM

Vegetarianism, particularly veganism, has recently gained more acceptance as awareness grows of the values resulting from plant-based food plans. Advantages include health benefits such as reduced risk of diet-related disorders, protection of environmental resources, and recognition for the ethical treatment of animals, including avoiding the use of hormones and antibiotics to enhance animal food production. Instead of animal protein sources, vegetarian dietary categories focus on plant proteins to provide EAAs (Table 6-1). The vegan dietary pattern consists of only plant foods, including grains, legumes, fruits, vegetables, seeds, and nuts; no animal-derived products are eaten. The lacto-vegetarian dietary pattern is a food plan composed of only plant foods plus dairy products. It contains all the vegan foods plus dairy products such as milk, cheese, yogurt, and butter. The ovo-lacto-vegetarian dietary pattern or food plan consist of plant foods plus dairy products and eggs. It incorporates eggs into the lacto-vegetarian assortment of foods.

The Benefits of Vegetarianism

Vegetarian dietary patterns may be followed to achieve health, spiritual, economic, and/or environmental benefits. When well planned, vegetarian dietary patterns result in health benefits that are similar to those of a low-fat, high-fiber diet and

consist of reduced risks for obesity, CVD, type 2 diabetes mellitus, hypertension, gastrointestinal disorders, and certain cancers such as lung and colorectal cancers (Craig, et al, 2009).

Because animal foods are our primary source of saturated fat and our only source of cholesterol, plant-based vegetarian dietary patterns tend to be lower in total fat and cholesterol. This reduced intake, combined with the high fiber content of plant foods, often results in lower blood cholesterol levels. Other nutrients that are usually higher in vegan diets are magnesium, folic acid, vitamins C and E iron, and phytochemicals (Craig and Mangels, 2009). In addition, the body weights of individuals following vegetarian dietary patterns are generally lower. This effect also reduces the risk for development of hypertension and diabetes.

The spiritual rationale for some individuals who are vegetarians is based on the belief in nonharming. Several religions, including Hinduism and Seventh-Day Adventists, see the consumption of animal flesh as being unhealthy or polluting to the body. Other vegetarians do not follow a formal religion but believe strongly in the protection of animal rights and are opposed to the slaughter of animals for human consumption. Information about the treatment of animals before and during the slaughtering process is now more available to the public because of increased exposure through Internet videos and websites.

The economic approach addresses the belief that animal-related products cost more than plant protein foods, not only financially but in terms of costs to our natural environment as well. Livestock and other domesticated animals are inefficient producers of protein. Although protein foods from cattle and chicken are of high quality, many pounds of grains are used by these animals to produce one pound of edible food. Some people maintain that eating from lower on the food chain—that is, eating more plant foods—involves less waste and has limited environmental impact on our natural resources.

The Drawbacks of Vegetarianism

The vegetarian dietary pattern has several drawbacks. Most may affect vegans. The vegan dietary pattern can provide all the essential nutrients except vitamins D and B_{12}, calcium, and omega-3 fatty acids. These will need to be consumed through carefully selected fortified foods or consumption of supplements as needed.

Most dietary vitamin D is consumed through milk fortified with the vitamin. Because vegans do not consume any dairy products, this source of vitamin D is unavailable.

TABLE 6-1 **Vegetarian Categories**		
Vegan	Includes all plant foods (grains, legumes, fruits, vegetables, seeds, and nuts)	Excludes all animal-derived foods
Lacto-vegetarian	Includes all plant foods plus dairy products (milk, cheese, yogurt, and butter)	Excludes animal meat (meat, fowl, and fish) and eggs
Ovo-lacto-vegetarian	Includes all plant foods, dairy products, and eggs	Excludes animal meat
Pescetarian	Includes all plant foods, dairy products, eggs, and fish	Excludes meat and fowl
Flexitarian	Includes all plant foods, dairy, and eggs with occasional consumption of meat, fowl, or fish	No exclusions but minimal consumption of animal meat

Vitamin D is also available through synthesis during exposure of the skin to direct sunlight; however, many individuals (even those consuming a traditional animal-derived intake) have inadequate levels of vitamin D and should rely on vitamin D–fortified foods or supplements. Factors such as regional limitation to sun exposure, darker skin pigmentation, elderly, cultural clothing customs that conceal the body, and regular use of sunscreen increase the risk of vitamin D deficiency for child and adult vegans.

Reliable sources of vitamin B_{12} are all animal related. Excluding animal-derived foods, including milk, means that sources of B_{12} are simply not available. Even ovo-lacto-vegetarians may have low levels of vitamin B_{12}. Symptoms of vitamin B_{12} deficiency take years to appear and may cause permanent damage to the central nervous system. Individuals who restrict their intake of or exclude animal foods should take B_{12} supplements or consume foods fortified with vitamin B_{12} such as fortified soy milk to ensure adequate intake (Craig, et al, 2009).

Other nutrients that could be deficient in vegans are iron and zinc, minerals usually consumed in meat, fish, and poultry. Calcium levels may also be low if dairy products are excluded; few plants are good sources of calcium. These nutrients are available in a well-planned vegan diet of whole foods. Nonetheless, care must be taken to consume sufficient amounts of calcium during pregnancy and growth periods; supplements will be necessary. If the vegan dietary pattern is poorly implemented and depends on refined and processed foods, nutrients may be lacking.

Another drawback pertains to the dimension of social health. *Social health* is the ability to interact with people in an acceptable manner and to sustain relationships with family members, friends, and colleagues. People following a vegetarian dietary pattern often find themselves rationalizing their behaviors to others. It can sometimes be tricky to do so without alienating others—especially while seated at a steak dinner. Perhaps the simplest approach is to emphasize the health benefits gained by adopting a vegetarian dietary pattern.

Ensuring that a vegetarian dietary pattern is healthful necessitates learning about protein complementing and new ways of preparing meatless dishes. Simply replacing meat with a lot of cheese won't have any health benefits. In fact, the fat content of a cheese dish is probably higher than that of a lean meat dish. The most helpful approach is to read vegetarian cookbooks that not only provide recipes but also include vegetarian nutrition information. MyPlate includes support for vegetarian dietary patterns. The food group recommendations for age, sex, and activity levels provide adequate energy and nutrient intake for vegetarianism if a variety of nutrient-dense foods are chosen. Guidance is available at the MyPlate website (www.choosemyplate.gov).

Contemporary Vegetarianism

Other terms have evolved to describe semivegetarian dietary patterns. The most inclusive term is the *flexitarian* approach. Flexitarians primarily consume vegetarian foods with occasional meat, chicken, or fish consumption. This pattern enables an individual to decrease meat consumption without totally eliminating it. Another approach is *pescetarian,* which adds fish to vegetarian selections. These concepts do not reflect the original ideals of vegetarianism. Instead, they represent new, contemporary dietary patterns evolving in response to current health issues. These health issues center on the risk for development of one or more of the chronic diet-related diseases: CVD, cancer, type 2 diabetes mellitus, and hypertension. Risk is reduced as dietary fat intake is lowered. A major source of fat in our diets is our consumption of animal protein foods. Reducing levels of this category of dietary fat lowers risk for chronic diet-related diseases. Doing so allows one to achieve the health promotion goals of *Healthy People 2020.*

DIETARY PATTERNS OF PROTEIN

So what should we eat for protein? No longer do we need to be confined to a meat and potatoes mentality when it comes to protein. The healthiest approach is to eat mixed sources of protein—animal and plant sources. (See the *Cultural Considerations* box Rituals for Animal-Derived Protein for a discussion of the religious aspects of protein consumption.) The mix provides an excellent assortment of EAAs plus sufficient building block materials for constructing NEAAs. Eating fewer animal protein foods reduces dietary fat intake, and eating more plant protein foods increases dietary fiber.

Restructuring the Dinner Plate

If you were asked to plan a balanced meal, what would the plate look like? Perhaps it would have animal protein (meat, fish, or poultry), vegetables (broccoli, potato, and a salad), and a grain (bread). But how much room on the plate would each portion take?

Before learning about MyPlate, a person's plate would most likely look like that in Figure 6-5. Notice how meat is the centerpiece that takes up the most space on the plate. Such a large portion of chicken, however, is not necessary. A 6-ounce serving of chicken provides about 53 g of protein. Add to that amount the protein in the bread (3 g), potato (4 g), broccoli (2 g), salad (1 g), and skim milk (8 g), and the total protein intake from one meal alone is 71 g. Because we eat protein throughout the day, no one meal needs to provide all our protein. Instead, the balance of the meal needs to be restructured. Because each component of the meal contains protein, whether from animal or plant sources, portion sizes can shift and still provide plenty of protein. An adequate serving of meat is about the size of a deck of cards or the size of an adult's palm. Notice in Figure 6-6 how the chicken, now reduced to 3 ounces, is no longer the focus of the plate. All items occupy more equal spaces on the plate. The protein total is still high at 48 g.

Spreading protein intake throughout the food groups allows the objectives of MyPlate to be met. The first plate (see Figure 6-5) provides the following:
- 1-oz (whole) grains
- 3-cups vegetables
- 0-cups fruit

Rituals for Animal-Derived Protein

Most religions identify foods with specific holidays and rules regarding consumption. Two predominantly Western religions, Judaism and Islam, have rules regarding the daily preparation and consumption of foods; most of these directions focus on consumption of animal-derived protein foods.

Kashrut, Jewish Dietary Laws

The rules of *kashrut* were presented in the Torah, or bible of the Jewish people. *Kosher* means "fit" and is the concept referring to the Jewish dietary laws. Although most of the rules can be explained on the basis of physical health benefits, the foundation and observance of the restrictions are driven by spiritual health rather than physical. By observing the kosher dietary laws, one is respecting God, oneself, and other Jews. There are about eight laws regarding consumption of animal-derived protein. They are briefly described as follows:

1. Only certain animals may be eaten. Only mammals with cloven hooves that chew the cud may be eaten and their milk consumed; this allows cattle, deer, goats, and sheep to be consumed but not pigs. Birds must also meet specific criteria; acceptable birds (and their eggs) include chickens, ducks, geese, and turkey. In addition, fish must have fins and scales to be consumed; therefore all shellfish, eel, and catfish are not permitted. Acceptable foods are viewed as coming from "clean" animals, and unacceptable foods are viewed as "unclean."
2. Animals must be slaughtered in a specific manner that is quick and painless and that causes most blood to drain from the carcass.
3. Slaughtered animals must be free of any bruises or diseases to be consumed.
4. Only certain parts of permitted animals may be consumed. Animal blood from any animal and layers of solid fat may not be consumed.
5. Meat must be prepared for consumption in specific procedures. Blood must be completely drained, and cuts of meat must avoid certain nerves and animal parts. Specially trained "kosher" butchers prepare animals foods according to *kashrut.*
6. Meat and dairy are not consumed together. Consequently, separate cooking utensils, plates, and eating utensils are maintained for meat consumption and dairy consumption. Some foods are considered neither meat nor dairy and may be eaten with either category. These foods are called *pareve.*
7. Products from unclean animals may not be consumed. The exception is honey. Although bees may not be consumed, honey is acceptable.
8. Foods are examined for insects and worms that may not be consumed but may be on vegetables, fruits, and grains.

To ensure that these rules are followed, product preparation is supervised by rabbis (spiritual teachers), after which point the product may then display special logos to that effect. Most often it is a "K" that appears on product packaging.

Halal, Islamic Dietary Laws

The Islamic rules of *halal* or permitted foods, presented in the Koran (bible of Islam), regard food consumption as an aspect of worship. Consequently, eating is viewed as a way to keep one's body healthy. Food should not be consumed excessively and is to be shared with others. All food is permitted unless specifically prohibited. Specific rules concerning foods that may not be consumed include the following:

- Swine (pigs) and birds of prey may not be consumed.
- Animals that are not slaughtered according to specific Muslim procedures may not be consumed. These rules are similar to those of Jewish laws regarding the exact means of slaughter and blood drainage.
- Alcoholic beverages and drugs that affect consciousness, unless required for medicinal purposes, may not be consumed. Coffee and tea, because they contain the stimulant caffeine, are discouraged.

Application to nursing. In nursing practice it is valuable to be knowledgeable and thereby respectful of the possible dietary restrictions of clients. Assistance can then be given as to the best dietary pattern to ensure wholesome nutrient intakes and the alternative medications or treatment available. For example, because observant Jews and Muslims do not consume pigs or products derived from pigs, the source of insulin (usually from pigs) may be problematic for Jewish or Muslim patients with diabetes.

FIG 6-5 A balanced meal. (From Joanne Scott/Tracy McCalla.)

FIG 6-6 A restructured meal. (From Joanne Scott/Tracy McCalla.)

FIG 6-7 A deck of cards is a simple visual tool to judge the size of a protein food.

FIG 6-8 Children suffering from kwashiorkor *(left)* and marasmus *(right)* as a result of inadequate energy intake. (Courtesy Professor R. Hendricksen. In McLaren DS: *A colour atlas and text of diet-related disorders,* ed 2, London, 1992, Mosby Europe Limited.)

- 1-cup milk (low-fat or fat-free)
- 6-oz meat and beans
  The second plate (see Figure 6-6) provides the following:
- 2-oz (whole) grains
- 4-cups vegetables
- ½-cup fruit
- 1-cup milk (low-fat or fat-free)
- 3-oz meat and beans

The new plate provides more complex carbohydrates from grains, fruits, and vegetables while still providing sufficient amounts of protein.

Use the concept of the deck of cards and the restructured meal to visually display appropriate animal-protein portion sizes for clients (Figure 6-7).

PROTEIN AND MALNUTRITION

Malnutrition, the imbalance of nutrient intake, encompasses conditions that range from overconsumption of nutrients to extreme underconsumption. This discussion concerns the conditions related to underconsumption of nutrients, particularly protein. Underconsumption can result in nutrient deficiencies that range from marginal to severe starvation. Marginal deficiencies occur when lower than recommended levels of nutrients are regularly consumed. Although obvious signs of specific nutrient deficiencies may not be visible, the level of wellness and the ability to function at an optimum level are compromised. As the other nutrient categories of vitamins and minerals are studied in Chapters 7 and 8, specific symptoms of deficiencies will be explored.

Starvation has become a catch-all term. Although we may say "I'm starving" when we've missed a meal, our starvation in no way compares with that experienced by those who truly do not have access to sufficient quantities of high-quality food. The technical term for starvation is protein energy malnutrition (PEM). PEM is an umbrella term for malnutrition caused by the lack of protein, of energy, or both.

In young children, PEM can cause permanent disabilities because most brain growth occurs during the early years of life. Extreme PEM results in the conditions *marasmus* and *kwashiorkor* (Figure 6-8). These disorders can be fatal because of decreased resistance to infections; the body, lacking protein, is unable to create sufficient quantities of antibodies to support the immune system. A brief discussion of marasmus and kwashiorkor follows.

Marasmus is malnutrition caused by a lack of sufficient energy (kcal) intake. An individual with marasmus is extremely thin; skin seems to hang on the skeletal bones. Fat stores that normally fill out the skin have been used for energy to maintain minimum body functioning. Muscle mass is also reduced, having also been used for energy, and nutrients are not available to rebuild it. If the condition continues, damage may occur to major organs such as the heart, lungs, and kidneys. Marasmic children will not grow. If the condition occurs between 6 and 18 months of age, the time during which the most brain development occurs, permanent brain damage may result.

In contrast to marasmus, the symptoms of kwashiorkor give the appearance of more than sufficient fat stores in the stomach and face. Kwashiorkor is defined as malnutrition caused by protein deficiency even though adequate energy is consumed. The swollen belly and full cheeks of kwashiorkor are caused by edema (water retention). Edema occurs because protein levels in the body are so low that protein is not available to maintain adequate water balance in the cells, and fluid accumulates unevenly. When adequate nutrition is provided, the fluid is no longer retained. Instead of a full belly and round cheeks, the loss of fat stores becomes apparent, and the skin hangs loosely, similar to marasmus. Without sufficient protein, lipids produced by the liver are unable to leave and thus accumulate there. The liver becomes fatty and unable to function well. An individual with kwashiorkor is apathetic and experiences muscle weakness and poor growth.

Although the extremes of PEM are rare in the United States, health care professionals may encounter patients experiencing nutritional risk from hunger related to lack of access to sufficient quantities of food or malnutrition due to physiologic stress from injury or illness. Clinical issues related to patient care are discussed in Chapter 11.

Malnutrition Factors

Malnutrition is often caused by several factors that affect food availability. Although poverty tends to be a dominant influence, other forces also affect the development of malnutrition. These include biologic, social, economic, and environmental factors (Box 6-6).

Biologic factors affect the ability of the body to use nutrients. Economic effects encompass the ability to purchase food

and also consider the structure of a country's economy and access to employment. Environmental factors directly affect the availability of food as related to crop production and food safety. Lack of education, social isolation, and the rippling effects of underemployment seem to be malnutrition factors throughout the world, regardless of the overall wealth of nations. Health and economic support systems provided throughout the life cycle may prevent the development of factors affecting food availability.

Groups at Risk in North America

Most people in North America are well nourished, although growing numbers of homeless individuals living in shelters or other temporary sites are at risk for varying levels of malnutrition. Without access to cooking facilities or the funds to purchase adequate quantities of foods, these individuals are at nutritional risk. In response to this crisis, food pantries and soup kitchens have been established by nonprofit and charitable groups to distribute food and meals (see the *Social Issues* box Hunger All Around: How to Help). Also at risk are the working poor, whose incomes barely cover the basic expenses of housing, utilities, and health care, leaving little for food purchases. Programs providing support services to these populations also can arrange nutrition education on making healthier choices when buying and preparing economical meals. Societal and personal changes may interrupt family ties, causing the loss of recipes and opportunities to share skills of preparation of low-cost, nutritious meals.

Older adults also are at risk. Although their nutritional concerns are covered in depth in Chapter 10, consider that the physical and financial limitations of older adults may reduce their ability to purchase and prepare wholesome meals. When these issues are compounded by social isolation, the situation of older adults becomes serious.

Chronic Hunger

Although famines and wars affect the nutritional status of people throughout the world, the population of North America has not experienced these extremes of deprivation. Instead, chronic hunger, defined as a continual experience of undernutrition (not enough food to eat), has become the norm for a subset of our population. This subset is growing as the economies of North America tighten, causing government food and welfare programs to be unable to provide an appropriate safety net to prevent and alleviate chronic hunger. Instead, more individuals and families are faced with a consistent lack of opportunities to improve their standard of living and, most important, their health. (See the *Personal Perspectives* box An Unexpected Kitchen: The George Foreman Grill for a unique and interesting story about dealing with chronic hunger.)

TOWARD A POSITIVE NUTRITION LIFESTYLE: CHAINING

Chaining refers to the linking of two behaviors. If two actions consistently occur together, they often become linked or tied

---

BOX 6-6   Malnutrition Factors

Biologic Factors
- Maternal malnutrition before or during pregnancy and/or lactation
- Infections that may affect nutrient absorption
- Chronic diarrhea as both a cause and an effect of malnutrition
- Toxins such as aflatoxin
- Lack of food, particularly protein

Social Factors
- Ignorance of nutrient needs of children, resulting in inappropriate weaning foods
- Child abuse and neglect
- Eating disorders, particularly anorexia nervosa
- Drug abuse affecting the ability to care for oneself appropriately
- Social isolation of older adults, leading to an inability to purchase and prepare adequate quantities of food
- Alcoholism (kcal from alcohol replace consumption of nutrient-dense foods)
- Wars/civil strife disrupting normal social and food production systems

Economic Factors
- Poverty and socioeconomic status
- Unemployment
- Little education
- Political strife affecting distribution of wealth and land ownership

Environmental Factors
- Polluted water, which reduces food production and directly affects the health of populations
- Famine caused by droughts or crop failures
- Improper farming techniques

SOCIAL ISSUES

Hunger All Around: How to Help

"Finish all that food on your plate. Children in India are starving." Parents often said this to their children at the dinner table, causing countless numbers of children to try to figure out how finishing their own vegetables would help feed the children in a faraway land. Of course, parents wanted their children not to waste food and to appreciate their good fortune. However, many children probably believed that by finishing their food they were somehow helping those hungry children.

Because of today's technology, we can have no illusions about the plight of others. We get complete, immediate reports of devastation caused by wars and famines. Reports of hunger among the homeless and older adults are televised. If only finishing the food on our plates would help.

So what can we do? Here are some ideas:

As Individuals

- Be well informed. Learn about hunger in your neighborhood. All communities have people who are in need.
- Volunteer to help in a local soup kitchen.
- Create a food drive at holidays; donate foods to a food bank.
- Let local politicians know of your concerns; give a voice to the voiceless. Send an e-mail to local and state officials.

Campus Organizations (Political, Social, and Religious)

- Include a service component in the group's mission.
- Support World Food Day, which is sponsored by the United Nations and other organizations.
- Ask representatives from local anti-hunger agencies to speak to campus groups.
- Incorporate volunteer time as part of an initiation process or as a commitment of all members of sororities, fraternities, and social clubs.

Data adapted from Food First, Institute for Food and Development Policy: *Hunger at home: The growing epidemic,* Oakland, CA, 2006, Author.

PERSONAL PERSPECTIVE

An Unexpected Kitchen: The George Foreman Grill

The Hidden Kitchens project, created by The Kitchen Sisters— Nikki Silva and Davia Nelson—finds hidden makeshift kitchens across the country. To broaden their search, they began a National Public Radio hotline asking listeners, "What food traditions are disappearing from your life? Who glues your community together through food? What should be captured and documented before it disappears or changes beyond recognition?" The responses were overwhelming. The following story, about the George Foreman grill, was passed on through the Chicago Coalition for the Homeless and is one of several Personal Perspectives boxes throughout this textbook that chronicle some of the responses.

Jeffrey Newton is 57 years old. Until recently, he lived in a refrigerator box, part of a makeshift cardboard community tucked in around trash cans and restaurant loading docks hidden under Chicago's Wacker Drive.

"Me and Smokey found the George Foreman grill at the shelter," Jeffrey remembers. Someone had donated one, broken, without a plug, so the two guys jury-rigged it. "Then you just get you a long extension cord and hookup. There's a lot of electrical plugs on the poles down there. You'd come home in the evening, and you'd fire up your Foreman. Some of us had jobs. Some of us had food stamp Link cards. You put anything in that thing: bologna, hamburgers, grilled cheese sandwiches. We used to take an iron and do that, too, press down, hot on the bread and cheese. You'd be inventive like that."

[At a later time …] George Foreman, two-time heavyweight champion of the world, Olympic gold medalist, former street preacher, and "King of the Grills," is in a radio studio in Houston, Texas …. [W]e tell George what we've been hearing about his grill. The story hits a nerve.

"Whoa … what a story! I've never considered it all," he says, "how homeless people and low-income people, wanting to cook but not being able to, how that little grill afforded them a kitchen. I'm just happy that it's helped so many people. It helped me, of course.

"Growing up in Houston, my whole life was spent trying to get enough to eat. Having seven kids, and my mother raising all of us by herself, there just was never enough food for me. I always dreamed not about a car, not about a beautiful home, but about having enough to eat." Sometimes George's mother would come home with a cheeseburger and try to divide it among her seven kids. "I remember the taste of the mustard. It was the most supreme thing in our family when she'd come home with a burger."

The grill lets Americans grill indoors on a rainy day or in a college dorm, and it gives the homeless a way to have hot bologna and cheese. It gave George and his brother Roy the means to open the George Foreman Youth Center. Foreman has never forgotten the central lesson of the Job Corps (the federal program that saved him from a life of crime): All that most kids need is a chance. He still imagines what his life might have become, and so he holds out the same chance he got to kids who are hungry, and angry.

From Silva N, Nelson D: *Hidden kitchens: Stories, recipes, and more from NPR's The Kitchen Sisters,* New York, 2005, Rodale Books.

to each other. They become one behavior and a habit. Many of us already practice chaining; unfortunately, the results often have a negative impact on our dietary intake patterns. Frequently eating potato chips while studying can link these two actions—eating chips and studying. The chain requires that whenever studying takes place, chips need to be eaten. Chaining, however, can also be used to improve nutritional status.

Consider the following chains:

- When you eat a sandwich, eat a fruit, too. Instead of linking chips and a sandwich (or hoagie, grinder, or sub), this practice links a sandwich to a fruit.

- Have a glass of skim milk with the midday meal regularly to increase calcium intake. Skim milk becomes chained to lunch.
- At home, weigh portions of meat, fish, and poultry. Compare the size of an appropriate portion to the size of a deck of cards. Are they similar? Weigh portions regularly, and consciously compare sizes. Animal protein portion sizes will be linked to the deck of cards, and portion control can be achieved without weighing.

These are just a few chains related to protein consumption. Chaining can be applied to other nutrition and wellness situations of our clients as well.

SUMMARY

- Proteins consist of chains of organic compounds composed of carbon, hydrogen, oxygen, and nitrogen called amino acids.
- All proteins are made from 20 amino acids.
- Nonessential amino acids (NEAAs) can be created by the liver.
- Essential amino acids (EAAs) must be consumed in food.
- All amino acids are available to cells through the amino acid pool to allow proteins to be synthesized.
- Complete proteins contain all nine EAAs, whereas incomplete proteins lack one or more EAAs.

- During digestion, food protein is broken down to amino acids. Once absorbed, the amino acids circulate in the blood to build new proteins.
- The new proteins perform numerous functions, including growth and maintenance, creation of essential substances, immune system response, fluid regulation, acid-base balance, and transportation of nutrients and other substances in the body.
- Chronic hunger and malnutrition such as protein energy malnutrition (marasmus and kwashiorkor) continue to be of global concern.

◎ THE NURSING APPROACH

Case Study: Protein (Wound Healing)

Roy, a 69-year-old homeless man, came to a neighborhood mobile van health clinic with a leg ulcer. Roy said the ulcer had been there for several months, and it had gradually gotten bigger. He was obviously poorly nourished. He said he ate what he could find on the street and sometimes went to the city food center for a hot meal. The nurse cleaned Roy's leg ulcer, and the physician ordered laboratory tests.

Assessment
Subjective (from patient statements):
- Minimal intake of meat, eggs, or other protein foods
- Fatigue and weakness

Objective (from physical examination):
- Height 6'2", weight 140 pounds
- Muscle atrophy in extremities bilaterally
- Decreased muscle strength
- Poor skin turgor
- Hair is dull and thin
- Slight ankle edema bilaterally
- Left lower leg ulcer 4 cm in diameter, stage II
- Serum albumin 2.7 g/dL (norm 3.4 to 4.8 g/dL)

Diagnoses (Nursing)
1. Imbalanced nutrition: less than body requirements related to lack of food availability, as evidenced by minimal intake of

protein foods, 74% ideal body weight (IBW), albumin 2.7 g/dL, delayed healing of lower left leg ulcer
2. Impaired skin integrity related to inadequate nutrition, as evidenced by stage II left lower leg ulcer 4 cm, present for several months and increasing in size

Planning
Patient Outcomes
Short term (at the end of this visit):
- Roy will identify foods high in protein, appropriate portion sizes (such as a deck of cards), and state the importance of protein in healing wounds.
- Roy will verbalize intention to eat high-protein foods at least once each day.
- Roy will demonstrate how to clean his wound.
- He will agree to come to clinic for follow-up twice a week.

Long term (after 2 months):
- Roy will report he ate several appropriate portions of high-protein foods each day.
- Roy's ulcer will heal within 2 months.
- He will gain four pounds in 2 months

Nursing Interventions
1. Teach Roy about the importance of protein in wound healing.
2. Discuss resources for obtaining high-protein food.
3. Provide wound care as ordered by the physician.

THE NURSING APPROACH—cont'd

Implementation

1. Discussed with Roy the role of protein in wound healing.
   Protein is needed for tissue repair and resistance to infection. Sufficient kcal are needed to spare use of proteins for energy.
2. Discussed dietary sources of protein.
   Soy and foods from animals contain complete proteins. Plant foods must be combined in order to have complete proteins.
3. Supplied Roy with cans of high-protein and vitamin supplements at each clinic visit.
   Adequate protein, calories, water, and vitamins are needed for tissue repair. Vitamins A and C and zinc are particularly helpful in wound healing. Vitamin C is needed for collagen formation. Vitamin A is an antioxidant and an important helper in wound healing. Zinc increases tensile strength of the healing wound.
4. Applied wet-to-damp dressing and antibiotic ointment to leg ulcers during clinic visits twice a week.
   Wet-to-damp dressings maintain moisture for healing and help débride wounds. Antibiotics help prevent infection.
5. Encouraged Roy to move into a homeless shelter affiliated with the clinic until the leg ulcer heals.
   A shelter can provide cleanliness, rest, and nutritious food, an environment conducive to healing.
6. Encouraged Roy to eat at least one meal per day in the shelter.
   Nutritious food can help an individual heal wounds and regain weight.

Evaluation

Short term (at the end of the first visit):
- Roy identified several foods high in protein and thanked the nurse for the supplements to help his ulcer heal.
- He said he would try to eat at least one meal per day at the shelter.
- Roy said he would return to the clinic twice a week for follow-up.
- Short-term goal met.

Long term (in 1 month):
- Roy said he had eaten at least one meal each day at the shelter on most of the days and was thinking about moving to the shelter.
- His leg ulcer measured 2 cm.
- He had gained 2 pounds.
- Long-term goal partially met.

Discussion Questions

1. What resources are available in your community to help the homeless and hungry?
2. If Roy has little money for food, what should he buy? Consider nutrient density, food preparation needed, and cost.

APPLYING CONTENT KNOWLEDGE

Karen and her husband, Roger, want to reduce their intake of fat and increase their fiber intake. Both grew up in families that prided themselves as being the "meat and potatoes" type. Suggest three strategies they could adopt to restructure their dinner plates to meet MyPlate goals.

WEBSITES OF INTEREST

Nutrition.gov

www.nutrition.gov
Functions as an entry for consumers to trustworthy food and nutrition information from all federal websites and agencies.

The Vegetarian Nutrition Dietetic Practice Group of the Academy of Nutrition and Dietetics

vegetariannutrition.net
Provides evidence-based research tools to create vegetarian meals for all age groups and fitness levels to enhance health and well-being.

National Institute of Medicine of the National Academies

www.iom.edu
Offers impartial and respected recommendations based on evidence from studies conducted for the government and independent organizations regarding health decisions affecting the nation. Functions as an independent, nonprofit organization.

REFERENCES

Craig WJ, Mangels AR; American Dietetic Association: Position of the American Dietetic Association: Vegetarian diets, *J Am Diet Assoc* 109:1266–1282, 2009.

Matthews DE: Proteins and amino acids. In Ross CA, et al, editors: *Modern nutrition in health and disease*, ed 11, Philadelphia, 2014, Lippincott Williams & Wilkins.

National Research Council: *Dietary reference intakes: The essential guide to nutrient requirements*, Washington, DC, 2006, The National Academies Press.

Rodriguez NR, et al: Position of the American Dietetic Association, Dietitians of Canada, and the American College of Sports Medicine: Nutrition and athletic performance, *J Am Diet Assoc* 109:509–527, 2009.

Vitamins

Knowledge of the existence of vitamins is recent; the discovery of vitamins slowly evolved, beginning in the early part of the twentieth century.

http://evolve.elsevier.com/GRODNER/FOUNDATIONS

LEARNING OBJECTIVES

- Define vitamins.
- Describe the differences between water-soluble and fat-soluble vitamins.
- List the water-soluble vitamins and their functions.
- List the fat-soluble vitamins and their functions.
- Discuss how water-soluble and fat-soluble vitamins are absorbed.
- Explain the level of risk from consuming an excess of water-soluble vitamins and fat-soluble vitamins from foods and from supplements.

ROLE IN WELLNESS

Vitamins seem to have a magical aura. Take enough and you'll have more energy and be healthier, smarter, and even better looking. If only it were that easy. Although vitamins are essential for life, they are only one of many factors required for wellness.

Knowledge of the existence of vitamins is recent; the discovery of vitamins slowly evolved, beginning in the early part of the twentieth century. The focus of research was to discover the amounts of vitamins needed to prevent deficiency symptoms and diseases that undermine the health and well-being of populations throughout the world.

The scientific view of vitamins, however, is in flux. Additional effects of vitamin use are surfacing as more is learned about the functions of vitamins as antioxidants and hormone-like substances. Some vitamins and related substances such as carotenoids may reduce the risk for development of certain chronic diseases. New information points to relationships between consuming foods high in vitamins and a lower incidence of certain diseases.

The Dietary Reference Intake (DRI) considers the concern of providing nutrient requirements necessary to prevent deficiencies and toxicity from overdoses and accounting for the value of nutrient intake as a means of reducing disease risk (National Research Council [NRC], 2006). Recommendations within the DRI documents include the use of fortified foods or supplements for particular nutrients, such as folic acid for women of childbearing age to ensure proper neural tube formation of the fetus during pregnancy.

Vitamins are organic molecules required in very small amounts for cellular metabolism. Each vitamin performs a specific metabolic function. Vitamins, except for vitamin D, are not synthesized by our bodies and thus are essential nutrients that must be provided through dietary intake (see the *Personal Perspectives* box Joseph Aguilar's Mercado [San Antonio]: A Street Kitchen Vision). Vitamin D is the only vitamin created by the human body.

Vitamins are vital to life and therefore to the physical, intellectual, emotional, social, spiritual, and environmental dimensions of health. Vitamins are essential nutrients without which the body cannot continue functioning within the *physical dimension*. Dietary recommendations to eat at least five fruits and vegetables per day throughout the life span are made to reduce the risk of diet-related diseases in the future. *Intellectual health* skills are used to envision future benefits that accrue from food choices today. Deficiencies of several B vitamins can produce irritability, confusion, and paranoia, thereby affecting the *emotional health* dimension. Older adults may be at risk for deficiencies because of their inability to get to the store to buy fruits and vegetables; the physical health of older adults may depend on their *social health* in relation to neighbors who may provide assistance with shopping needs. Sometimes following religious teachings may jeopardize health, as noted by the development of rickets, the vitamin D deficiency disorder, among some African American children of families following the dietary and dress customs of the Islamic faith. *Spiritual health* is interdependent with the other dimensions of health. Since the best sources of vitamins are a variety of foods, the *environmental health* dimension includes having adequate access to grocery stores and the financial means to purchase wholesome foods.

As vitamins are discussed, note that some are referred to by specific names or by letters and numbers. Each vitamin

PERSONAL PERSPECTIVES

Joseph Aguilar's Mercado (San Antonio): A Street Kitchen Vision

Following is another excerpt from the Hidden Kitchens project. The Kitchen Sisters, Nikki Silva and Davia Nelson, are visiting San Antonio, Texas. Most of us buy our fruits and vegetables in large supermarkets, but not everyone finds these markets to be convenient. In the midst of a drab urban area, The Kitchen Sisters find a small shop bursting with colorful produce.

We were walking ... to find some remnant of what had once been San Antonio's vital commercial hub. ... But there's not much commerce on West Commerce anymore. It's one way with no parking on the street, blocks of mostly empty buildings with no shop windows to look in, and no people, except the homeless and those standing at a bus stop waiting to go someplace else.

Then, amid the endless gray, a beacon of bananas glows in a doorway. A tiny storefront with a scale hanging out front surrounded by a basket of ripe mangoes, nopales cactus, deep green chilies, brilliant red tomatoes. We pick up our pace, pulled in by the life force.

As we approach, a horn honks. A middle-aged man darts out of the store, runs up to a car idling out front, hands off a plastic bag, grabs a bill, and runs back inside as the car pulls out into the fast-moving traffic. The man is Joseph Aguilar, owner of West Commerce Mercado.

"Everything we do here is illegal," he tells us. "But it's not bad illegal. I don't sell beer. I don't sell cigarettes—just produce. A little produce stand. A family thing."

"I just delivered a snack bag. That's what we call them. A bag with a banana, apple, orange, and a pear for a dollar. Cars come up and just honk. They don't even get out of their seats. We already know who they are and what they want. It's illegal because this is a bus line in front of our store. It's kind of exciting."

A handsome man with salt-and-pepper hair and a thick mustache, 57-year-old Joseph Aguilar proudly takes us through his tiny market. It has everything "from salsa to sweet peaches." Old-fashioned wooden shelves display hot sauce with lemon and dry pepper that he's selling for a friend who lives in Mexico; crisp tortillas wrapped the old traditional way in paper, imported from a family in Chicago; beautifully packaged species and herbs....

"My customers are downtown working people, senior citizens, and 'the criminal element' who are coming in for food. The courthouse and probation office are nearby. A lot of them are pretty good people; it's just that they had bad luck and got caught."

When Joseph started up his little business, he spent $2,000 to have the windows in his market set back off the sidewalk so he could display his produce outside "so people could see the beauty of how produce looks outside your little store."

From Silva N, Nelson D: *Hidden Kitchens: Stories, recipes, and more from NPR's The Kitchen Sisters*, New York, 2005, Rodale Books.

has a history that affects how we refer to it today. In 1929 Henrik Dam in Copenhagen, Denmark, discovered vitamin K. It was the only substance capable of halting a hemorrhagic disease in which blood does not coagulate. Dam named the vitamin *K* for the Danish word *koagulation.*

In another case, several B vitamins were isolated into the same test tube labeled B, and we therefore have vitamins numbered B_1, B_2, and B_3. In the 1970s the science community decreed that all vitamins should be called by their formal biochemical titles. The public and many health professionals still refer to the simpler letter and number names for vitamins. Both the formal and informal names are used in this chapter.

This chapter lists vitamin DRIs. Because *DRI* is an umbrella term that includes Recommended Dietary Allowance (RDA), Adequate Intake (AI), and Tolerable Upper Intake Level (UL), applicable standards will be identified. Because RDAs and AIs differ with age, gender, and physiologic need, only those for men and women ages 19 to 30 are included for each vitamin, unless special circumstances surrounding the need for a vitamin warrant discussion. The DRI tables are *located inside the front cover of this book* or can be accessed from http://fnic.nal.usda.gov/dietary-guidance/dietary-reference-intakes.

A *primary* deficiency of a vitamin occurs when the vitamin is not consumed in sufficient amounts to meet physiologic needs. A *secondary* deficiency develops when absorption is

impaired or excess excretion occurs, limiting bioavailability. Most deficiencies are detected through clinical and biochemical assessment; specific diagnostic and laboratory procedures are beyond the scope of this text, and their descriptions are available elsewhere (Pagana and Pagana, 2012).

Although vitamin deficiencies are no longer common among Americans, subgroups are at risk. Because of their greater needs, pregnant women are often at risk for marginal deficiencies of essential vitamins. Older adults may also be at risk because of decreased absorptive ability and limited economic and physical resources affecting food availability. Poverty has an overwhelming negative effect on the nutritional status of children and adults. Chronic alcohol and drug abuse not only alters psychologic and mental capacities but also limits the body's ability to absorb and use essential vitamins.

Health professionals can also take into account other special circumstances that may initiate vitamin deficiencies. Individuals dealing with long-term chronic disorders that affect the total body response, such as acquired immunodeficiency syndrome (AIDS) and liver and kidney disorders, have special vitamin concerns because the metabolic processes of the body may be compromised by these disorders and by the medications prescribed. Deficiencies have been documented that were possibly caused by the effects of cancer treatment, use of multiple alternative therapies, and lifestyle behaviors. These deficiencies were at first misdiagnosed because vitamin deficiencies were no longer thought to occur (Fain, et al, 1998; Gessner, et al, 1997; Wood, et al, 1998).

Toxicities of vitamins rarely occur naturally from food consumption. Instead, inappropriate use of supplements may be toxic to our bodies. Vitamins have been studied for their physiologic effect or because of the basic need for health maintenance (Box 7-1). The recommended levels reflect this knowledge. Use of vitamin supplements at megadose levels is equivalent to a pharmacologic effect, with potential druglike physical responses. Some vitamins have ULs; for others, a megadose (i.e., 10 times the RDA for a specific nutrient) of a vitamin is considered the highest amount of the nutrient that will not cause adverse health effects. Because most vitamins have not been studied to determine function and safety at these megadose levels, their extensive use without guidance can be problematic.

VITAMIN CATEGORIES

Vitamins are divided into two categories on the basis of their solubility in solutions. *Water-soluble vitamins* dissolve or disperse in water; they are the B complex vitamins (thiamin, riboflavin, niacin, pyridoxine, folate, vitamin B_{12}, biotin, and pantothenic acid), choline, and vitamin C. *Fat-soluble*

BOX 7-1 Considering Vitamins and Minerals Through Function

Vitamins and minerals are discussed as two separate nutrient categories in Chapters 7 and 8. Although each is discussed individually, they are not grouped on the basis of their functions in the body. Following are the vitamins and minerals required for the specific body functions blood health, bone health, energy metabolism, and fluid and electrolyte balance. Additional functions of individual vitamins and minerals may be found in Tables 7-3, 7-6, 8-3, and 8-4.

Blood Health
Blood is *the* body fluid, supplying tissues with oxygen, nutrients, and energy through circulation within the cardiovascular system. It is composed of water, red and white blood cells, oxygen, nutrients, and other formed substances. Always moving, blood gathers and distributes nutrients and oxygen to all cells and disposes of waste products. Deficiency of any of these nutrients will affect overall blood health. Only the blood-related functions of the vitamins and minerals are listed.

VITAMIN*	FUNCTION	MINERAL[†]	FUNCTION
Cobalamin (B₁₂)	Transport/storage of folate needed for heme and cell formation and other functions	Iron	Distributes oxygen in hemoglobin and myoglobin
Folate (folic acid, folacin, PGA)	Coenzyme metabolism (synthesis of amino acid, heme, deoxyribonucleic acid [DNA], ribonucleic acid [RNA]) and other functions	Zinc	Cofactor for more than 200 enzymes, including enzymes to make heme in hemoglobin, genetic material, and proteins
Pyridoxine (B₆)	Hemoglobin synthesis and other functions	Copper	Helps with iron use
Vitamin K Active form: menaquinones	Cofactor in synthesis of blood clotting factors; protein formation		

Bone Health
As living tissue, bone requires nutrients to maintain cellular structure. Blood circulates through bone capillaries, delivering nutrients while removing waste materials no longer needed by cells. Hormones regulate the use of minerals either for storage and structural purposes in bone or for controlling body processes. Specific vitamins and minerals are indispensable for these functions to occur.

VITAMIN*	FUNCTION	MINERAL[†]	FUNCTION
Vitamin D Precursor: 7- dehydrocholester Active form: cholecalciferol	Bone mineralization	Calcium	Bone and tooth formation
		Phosphorus	Bone and tooth formation (component of hydroxyapatite)
Vitamin K Active form: menaquinones	Protein formation for bone mineralization; cofactor for blood clotting factors	Magnesium	Bone structure
Vitamin A Precursors: carotenoids Preformed vitamin: retinoids	Bone growth; maintains epithelial cells; regulation of gene expression	Fluoride	Bone and tooth formation; increases stability of bone

Energy Metabolism
In order to metabolize carbohydrates, lipids, and protein for energy and other needs, the body depends on many nutrients to support the process, create new cells, and implement various related functions.

BOX 7-1 Considering Vitamins and Minerals Through Function—cont'd

VITAMIN(S)*	FUNCTION	MINERAL†	FUNCTION
Thiamin (B₁)	Coenzyme energy metabolism; muscle nerve action	Iodine	Thyroxine synthesis (thyroid hormone) regulates growth and development; basal metabolic rate (BMR) regulation
Riboflavin (B2)	Coenzyme energy metabolism	Chromium	Carbohydrate metabolism, part of glucose tolerance factor
Niacin (B₃) (nicotinic acid and niacinamide) Precursor: tryptophan	Cofactor to enzymes involved in energy metabolism; glycolysis and tricarboxylic acid (TCA) cycle synthesis	Phosphorus Sulfur Iron	Energy metabolism (enzymes) Component of protein structures Distributes oxygen in hemoglobin and myoglobin
Pyridoxine (B₆)	Forms coenzyme pyridoxal phosphate (PLP) for energy metabolism	Zinc	Carbohydrate metabolism (insulin function); cofactor to more than 200 enzymes
Folate (folic acid, folacin, PGA)	Coenzyme metabolism (synthesis of amino acid, heme, DNA, RNA)		
Cobalamin (B₁₂)	Metabolism of fatty acids/amino acids		
Pantothenic acid	Part of coenzyme A		
Biotin	Metabolism of carbohydrate, fat, and protein		

Fluid and Electrolyte Balance

Life systems depend on fluid and electrolyte balance within the body. Electrolytes consist of mineral salts that maintain cellular fluid balance. The acid-base balance of body fluids is buffered by other minerals.

MINERAL†	FUNCTION
Sodium	Major extracellular electrolyte for fluid regulation; body fluid levels; acid-base balance; nerve impulse and contraction; blood pressure/volume
Potassium	With sodium and chloride, major intracellular electrolyte for fluid regulation; muscle function
Chloride	Acid-base balance
Phosphorus	Acid-base balance

*See text for additional information on vitamins.
†See Chapter 8 for additional information on minerals.

---

vitamins dissolve in fatty tissues or substances; they are vitamins A, D, E, and K.

Solubility characteristics affect how vitamins are absorbed and transported in the body. Water-soluble vitamins are easily absorbed in the small intestine and then pass into the bloodstream for circulation throughout the body. Fat-soluble vitamins follow the more complicated route of other fat-containing substances; bile is required for their absorption from the small intestine. Fat malabsorption problems may also lead to potential deficiencies of fat-soluble vitamins.

The water solubility of the B vitamins and vitamin C allows for minimal storage of any excess vitamin consumed; tissues may be saturated with these vitamins, but they usually are not stored. Deficiencies can develop quickly—within weeks—so we need to consume these vitamins on a daily basis. Excesses are generally not toxic and are simply excreted in urine. However, damage may result if vitamin levels are high over the long term because of supplementation.

If we consume more than the daily requirement of a fat-soluble vitamin, our bodies store the excess rather than excrete it (Box 7-2). The DRIs for fat-soluble vitamins take into account this storage capacity. Although storage is expected in organs such as the liver and spleen, other fatty tissues in the body can also retain excessive amounts of fat-soluble vitamins. Overloading the storage capabilities can be toxic and produce illness; toxicity comes rarely from excessive dietary intake but rather from improper use of vitamin supplements.

FOOD SOURCES

Vitamins are in almost all foods, yet no one food group is a good source of all vitamins. Fresh fruits and vegetables are particularly rich sources. Others are legumes, whole grains, and animal foods—meat, fish, poultry, eggs, and dairy products. Even the almost pure fats of vegetable oils and butter provide vitamins E and A, respectively. Although this does not mean we should consume these products for their vitamin content, it does mean we have a wide range of foods from which to choose for our vitamin nutrition.

It is always best to consume vitamins from food sources. Although synthetic forms of vitamins will perform vitamin

BOX 7-2   MyPlate: Fruits

The health benefits of eating fruits overlap with those of eating vegetables. Both the fruit and vegetable categories of MyPlate provide rich sources of vitamins and are valuable components of an overall healthy diet, providing nutrients essential for the health and maintenance of our bodies (see also Box 8-5). Health benefits of eating fruits and vegetables as part of an overall health diet include reduced risk for stroke, coronary artery disease, and type 2 diabetes mellitus; protection against some cancers (mouth, stomach, colorectal cancer); and, as an excellent source of fiber, possible decreased risk of several chronic diet-related disorders. The recommendation is to eat at least 2 cups of fruits every day.

What Counts as a Cup of Fruit?

In general, 1 cup of fruit or 100% fruit juice, or ½ cup of dried fruit can be considered 1 cup from the fruit group. The specific amounts listed in the following table count as 1 cup of fruit (in some cases equivalents for ½ cup are also shown) toward your daily recommended intake.

FRUIT	AMOUNT THAT COUNTS AS 1 CUP OF FRUIT	AMOUNT THAT COUNTS AS ½ CUP OF FRUIT
Apple	3¼ large (3¼-inch diameter) 1 small (2½-inch diameter) 1 cup sliced or chopped, raw or cooked	½ cup sliced or chopped, raw or cooked
Applesauce	1 cup	1 snack container (4 oz)
Banana	1 cup sliced 1 large (8-9 inches long)	1 small (less than 6 inches long)
Cantaloupe	1 cup diced or melon balls	1 medium wedge (⅛ of a medium melon)
Grapes	1 cup whole or cut-up grapes 32 seedless grapes	16 seedless grapes
Grapefruit	1 medium (4-inch diameter) 1 cup sections	½ medium (4-inch diameter)
Mixed fruit (fruit cocktail)	1 cup diced or sliced, raw or canned, drained	1 snack container (4 oz), drained = 3/8 cup
Orange	1 large (3 3/16-inch diameter) 1 cup sections	1 small (2⅜-inch diameter)
Orange, mandarin	1 cup canned, drained	
Peach	1 large (2¾-inch diameter) 1 cup sliced or diced; raw, cooked, or canned; drained 2 halves canned	1 small (2-inch diameter) 1 snack container (4 oz), drained = ⅜ cup
Pear	1 medium (2½ per lb) 1 cup sliced or diced; raw, cooked, or canned; drained	1 snack container (4 oz), drained = ⅜ cup
Pineapple	1 cup chunks; sliced or crushed; raw, cooked, or canned; drained	1 snack container (4 oz), drained = ⅜ cup
Plum	1 cup sliced, raw or cooked 3 medium or 2 large	1 large
Strawberries	Approximately 8 large 1 cup whole, halved, or sliced; fresh or frozen	½ cup whole, halved, or sliced
Watermelon	1 small wedge (1-inch thick) 1 cup diced or balls	6 melon balls
Dried fruit (raisins, prunes, apricots, etc.)	½ cup dried fruit is equivalent to 1 cup fruit (½ cup raisins, ½ cup prunes, ½ cup dried apricots)	¼ cup dried fruit is equivalent to ½ cup fruit (1 small box raisins [1½ oz])
100% fruit juice (orange, apple, grape, grapefruit, etc.)	1 cup	½ cup

Modified from U.S. Department of Agriculture, Center for Nutrition and Promotion: *ChooseMyPlate.gov: What counts as a cup of fruit?* Accessed January 26, 2014, from www.choosemyplate.gov/printpages/MyPlateFoodGroups/Fruits/food-groups.fruits-counts.pdf.

functions, there may be other factors in foods that provide benefits. For instance, broccoli and other cruciferous vegetables contain a wide variety of chemicals, including sulforaphane, which is a phytochemical (Box 7-3). **Phytochemicals** are nonnutritive substances in plant-based foods that appear to have disease-fighting properties. Sulforaphane appears to block the growth of tumors in animals. Broccoli, along with onions and grapes, also contains flavonols, which seems to reduce the risk of cardiovascular disease (CVD) and cancer while having an anti-inflammatory effect (Heiss, et al, 2010; Hwang, et al, 2012).

BOX 7-3 Phytochemicals and Functional Foods: The Value of Food

Nutrition tends to focus on the nutrients required for the health and well-being of the human body. Other food components exist that may have other health benefits but do not qualify as a nutrient.

Phytochemicals are nonnutritive substances in plant-based foods that appear to have disease-fighting properties. The health-promoting value of these substances is best obtained by eating a diverse assortment of vegetables, fruits, legumes, grains, and seeds. Green tea, soy, and licorice also contain phytochemicals with healthful qualities. *Functional foods* provide physiologic health benefits beyond the nutrients they contain. Phytochemicals and functional foods are of great interest because they may assist in preventing or treating chronic diseases such as diabetes, coronary artery disease, cancer, and hypertension. Even osteoporosis, arthritis, and neural tube defects may be reduced by adequate consumption of these substances. Onions and garlic not only taste good but also contain allylic sulfides—phytochemicals—that improve immune function, enhance excretion of cancer-inducing substances, decrease blood cholesterol levels, and reduce spread of tumor cells—quite a long list of benefits for foods that taste so good. Tomatoes provide lycopene, which appears to have the ability to limit the spread of cancer cells. Consequently, consumption of cooked tomatoes has been related to a decreased risk of certain cancers. Soy contains isoflavones, which also decrease blood cholesterol levels and flavonoids that may reduce menopausal symptoms.

A number of products already use soy-derived ingredients and others are in development. Consumers can gain health benefits while consuming familiar foods that have added soy ingredients. The availability of other functional food products continues to expand. Factors influencing this expansion consist of: increasing health care costs, aging population, changing food regulations; increasing sense of self-efficacy and health care autonomy; and enhancing personal health among the general population.

Perhaps a significant means of disease prevention has always been available to us: consumption of adequate amounts of whole foods such as fruits and vegetables, along with less processed grains and legumes, possibly topped off with a few cups of green tea.

Data from Hasler CM, Brown AC; American Dietetic Association: Position of The American Dietetic Association: Functional foods, *J Am Diet Assoc* 109:735-746, 2009.

WATER–SOLUBLE VITAMINS

Thiamin (B₁)

For centuries, a mysterious disease afflicted people of all ages and status throughout Asia. The disease so wasted muscles that Thai sufferers who tried to stand would cry out, *"Beri, beri,"* meaning "I can't! I can't!" This phrase, **beriberi**, became the name of a serious disease due to thiamin deficiency. In the 1890s it was discovered that beriberi resulted from consumption of hulled (white) rice and that eating unhulled (brown) rice prevented or cured it. Later, researchers found that the thiamin in the hulls of whole grains prevents or cures beriberi.

Function

The main function of thiamin is to serve as a **coenzyme**, a substance that activates an enzyme, in energy metabolism; it also has a role in nerve functioning related to muscle actions.

Recommended Intake and Sources

The RDA for thiamin is 1.2 mg for men and 1.1 mg for women. The amount of thiamin required increases as the metabolic rate rises. Those engaged in rigorous physical activity burn more energy, so they require more thiamin.

Lean pork, whole or enriched grains and flours, legumes, seeds, and nuts are good sources of thiamin. Because it is a water-soluble vitamin, some thiamin can be lost in food processing or when foods are cooked at home. Thiamin may be leached into cooking fluid or destroyed by heat. Generally, however, most of us consume sufficient amounts of thiamin.

Deficiency

Thiamin deficiency alters the nervous, muscular, gastrointestinal (GI), and cardiovascular systems. In beriberi, a severe, chronic deficiency results, characterized by **ataxia** (muscle weakness and loss of coordination), pain, anorexia, mental disorientation, and **tachycardia** (rapid beating of the heart). **Wet beriberi** manifests as edema, affecting cardiac function by weakening the heart muscle and vascular system. **Dry beriberi** affects the nervous system, producing paralysis and extreme muscle wasting. Marginal deficiencies may occur, producing psychologic disturbances, recurrent headaches, extreme tiredness, and irritability (Bemeur and Butterworth, 2014).

Beriberi still occurs in areas of the world, such as Asia, where the staple food is highly polished rice, which is low in thiamin. The practice of repeatedly washing the milled rice results in further loss of thiamin. Very high intakes of raw fish can also produce beriberi. Raw fish naturally contains an enzyme, thiaminase, that destroys thiamin. The presence of this enzyme does not affect those of us who occasionally enjoy sushi or sashimi, Japanese specialties of raw fish.

In the United States, enrichment of refined flour has virtually eliminated thiamin deficiency. However, thiamin deficiency may develop in people who are chronic alcohol users because of decreased food intake and reduced intestinal absorption coupled with an additional need for thiamin by the liver to detoxify alcohol (see the *Cultural Considerations* box, Cuban Crisis).

CULTURAL CONSIDERATIONS

Cuban Crisis

In the spring of 1993 a harsh economy and natural disasters played havoc with Cuba's food supply. The breakup of the Soviet Union dissipated a valuable trade network for Cuba. This event, combined with the devastating effects of a tropical storm, severely limited the variety of foods available. The consequence? A disease resulting in vision loss and a numbness caused by nerve damage spread primarily among men. The *New York Times* headlines were startling: "26,000 Cubans Partly Blinded."

There is speculation that the epidemic was caused by nutritional deficiencies of thiamin and/or folate. These deficits were exacerbated by consumption of home-brewed rum. The rum required thiamin to detoxify the alcohol, further decreasing the thiamin available for body functions. Folate levels declined as supplies of folate-containing foods diminished. Increased reliance on naturally available foods, such as cassava root, and the popularity of cigarettes among 95% of Cuban men further affected folate availability. Both cassava root and cigarettes are high in cyanide, the processing of which uses up folate stores in the body. The epidemic was eventually brought under control when the Cuban government distributed vitamin supplements to provide the missing nutrients.

A follow-up epidemiologic study reveals that the Cuban male population is still at risk for vitamin B deficiencies, suggesting the need to continue recommendation of preventive vitamin supplementation and increased consumption of fruits and vegetables containing an assortment of B vitamins.

Application to nursing. Unusual circumstances may precipitate unexpected conditions. We often expect disorders to be the result of new variations of bacteria or viruses, but sometimes simple deficiencies may be the cause. Note that this chapter also discusses instances of unexpectedly occurring rickets (vitamin D deficiency disorder) and pellagra (niacin deficiency disorder). All factors affecting health should be considered in the determination of the true cause of symptoms.

Data from Altman LK: 26,000 Cubans partly blinded; cause is unclear, *New York Times,* May 21, 1993, A7; Arnaud J et al: Vitamin B intake and status in healthy Havanan men, 2 years after the Cuban neuropathy epidemic, *Br J Nutr* 85(6):741–748, 2001; and Community Nutrition Institute: Epidemic, *Nutrition Week Newspaper* 22:8 (June 11), 1993.

A severe deficiency of thiamin may cause a cerebral form of beriberi called Wernicke-Korsakoff syndrome. It is the most common disorder of the central nervous system, being the neuropsychiatric effect of chronic excessive alcohol intake on nutritional status. Individuals with severe GI disease, those with human immunodeficiency virus (HIV), and those receiving improper parenteral glucose solutions are also at risk for this syndrome (Bemeur and Butterworth, 2014). The effects of this thiamin deficiency syndrome may cause the loss of memory, extreme mental confusion, and ataxia exhibited by people with chronic excessive alcohol ingestion. Clinically, care must be taken when a malnourished person is given parenteral fluids containing dextrose. Parenteral fluids should contain a mix of B vitamins; otherwise, the marginal thiamin levels of nutritionally depleted individuals, combined with a sudden increase of glucose to the brain, can initiate Wernicke-Korsakoff syndrome, regardless of the level of alcohol intake.

Others at risk for thiamin deficiency include patients who are undergoing dialysis because of renal disease, who are receiving parenteral nutrition, who are HIV positive or have AIDS, or who have persistent vomiting (hyperemesis gravidarum), anorexia nervosa, gastrectomy, or genetic disorders that affect thiamin use (Bemeur and Butterworth, 2014). As the number of gastric bypass procedures increases, instances of peripheral neuropathy from thiamin deficiency may increase as well.

Toxicity

Excess thiamin is excreted in urine. Although thiamin is nontoxic, there is no rationale for supplementation in healthy people. In acute care settings, supplemental thiamin and other B vitamins may be recommended for individuals with chronic excessive alcohol consumption. In general, the best advice is to take a daily multivitamin containing B vitamins.

Riboflavin (B₂)

Have you ever wondered why milk is sold in opaque cardboard or nontransparent plastic containers? These containers protect riboflavin from exposure to light. Riboflavin is sensitive to ultraviolet rays in sunlight and artificial light; much of the riboflavin is destroyed if milk, an excellent source of riboflavin, is sold in clear glass or clear plastic receptacles. Why risk loss of a valuable vitamin?

Function

Like that of thiamin, the main function of riboflavin is as a coenzyme in the release of energy from nutrients in every cell of the body.

Recommended Intake and Sources

The RDA for riboflavin is 1.3 mg for men and 1.1 mg for women. The body's need is related to total kcal intake, energy needs, body size, metabolic rate, and growth rate. Conditions requiring increased protein also require increased riboflavin, such as during wound healing and the growth periods of childhood, pregnancy, and lactation.

Riboflavin is found in both plant and animal foods. In the United States, however, milk is a major source, with small amounts coming from other foods such as enriched grain. Good plant sources are broccoli, asparagus, dark leafy greens, whole grains, and enriched breads and cereals. Rich sources of animal origin include dairy products, meats, fish, poultry, and eggs.

As mentioned, riboflavin is sensitive to light and irradiation. It also can be lost in cooking water but is heat stable.

Deficiency

Ariboflavinosis is the name for a group of symptoms associated with riboflavin deficiency. The lips become swollen, and cracks develop in the corners of the mouth (cheilosis). The tongue becomes inflamed, swollen, and purplish red (glossitis), a common symptom of riboflavin and other B vitamins. Seborrheic dermatitis, a skin condition characterized by greasy scales, may occur in the regions of the ears, nose, and mouth. Riboflavin deficiency may also affect the availability and use of pyridoxine and niacin.

Nutritional deficiencies tend to be multiple rather than single, and it is difficult to separate symptoms. If an individual is deficient in a nutrient such as riboflavin, more than likely a deficiency of other nutrients is also present. For example, esophageal cancer is associated with deficiencies of riboflavin and zinc, particularly in Africa, Iran, and China. In the United States, riboflavin deficiency may be related to congenital heart disease, chronic excessive alcohol ingestion, and some cancers (Said and Ross, 2014) as well as to anorexia nervosa and lactose intolerance—all of which are associated with potential multiple nutritional deficiencies.

Toxicity

Toxicity to riboflavin has not been reported. Absorption of riboflavin tends to be limited under normal circumstances; excessive absorption is extremely unlikely (Said and Ross, 2014).

Niacin (B₃)

Niacin occurs naturally in two forms: nicotinic acid and niacinamide. It's hard to imagine, but before niacin was identified, people who were actually suffering from niacin deficiency were so psychologically disoriented that they were sent to mental institutions for treatment. Niacin deficiency can bring on a psychosis that dissipates once sufficient quantities are consumed.

Function

Niacin is involved as a coenzyme for many enzymes, especially those involved in energy metabolism; it is critical for glycolysis and the tricarboxylic acid (TCA) cycle.

Recommended Intake and Sources

Niacin is available in foods as the active vitamin or as its precursor, the amino acid tryptophan. That is, tryptophan can be converted to niacin, and some niacin can be provided this way. Diets adequate in protein tend to be adequate in niacin.

Niacin requirements are measured in niacin equivalents (NEs), reflecting the body's ability to convert tryptophan to niacin. To form 1 mg of niacin, 60 mg of tryptophan is needed, both of which equal 1 mg NE. The RDA recommends that men and women consume 16-mg NE and 14-mg NE per day, respectively. The DRI for niacin includes a UL of 35-mg NE per day because of the adverse reactions experienced when excess amounts are taken in supplement form (see later section titled "Toxicity").

FIG 7-1 Dermatitis in a patient suffering from pellagra. (From McLaren DS: *A colour atlas and text of diet-related disorders,* ed 2, London, 1992, Mosby.)

Protein-containing foods are good sources of both niacin and tryptophan. Meats, poultry, fish, legumes, enriched cereals, milk, and even coffee and tea are sources of niacin.

Deficiency

Pellagra, the niacin deficiency disorder, is characterized by the three D's, as follows (Kirkland, 2014):

Dermatitis: A symmetric scaly rash occurs only on skin exposed to the sun (Figure 7-1).

Dementia: As the central nervous system becomes affected in severe deficiencies, confusion, anxiety, insomnia, and paranoia develop.

Diarrhea: Damage to the GI tract affects digestion, absorption, and excretion of food, leading to glossitis, vomiting, and diarrhea.

In the early 1900s, pellagra was common in the southern United States among the poor, who subsisted on corn-based diets. The niacin in corn is in a bound form unavailable for absorption, and many people subsisting on low incomes had such a limited intake of protein food that neither tryptophan nor preformed niacin was available. In addition, consumption of white flour increased deficiencies of niacin. The incidence of pellagra decreased dramatically when refined wheat flour (white flour) was required to be enriched with niacin. Niacin is naturally found in whole wheat flour, but is lost when processed into refined white flour.

In the United States, health professionals need to be vigilant to recognize the symptoms of vitamin deficiencies among patients undergoing specialized treatments or experiencing disorders that may negatively affect their nutritional status.

For example, pellagra may develop among people with chronic excessive alcohol ingestion, particularly if combined with homelessness and failure to eat regularly (not using shelter-based meal programs) (Kertesz, 2001). Several cases have been reported in which dermatitis was not recognized as a symptom of pellagra. In one situation, the simultaneous use of several alternative remedies initiated pellagra, although the individual consumed sufficient dietary niacin (Wood, et al, 1998). Pellagra may even occur secondary to anorexia nervosa (Prousky, 2003). In contrast, in Africa and Asia, pellagra still occurs among the general population.

Toxicity

The UL for niacin is 35-mg NE per day. When preformed niacin and nicotinic acid (but not niacinamide) are consumed in levels greater than the UL, the vascular system is affected, producing a flushing effect throughout the body. Niacin has been used therapeutically because megadoses may lower total cholesterol and low-density lipoprotein (LDL) cholesterol and increase high-density lipoprotein (HDL) cholesterol (Kirkland, 2014). These therapeutic doses, however, must be medically administered to guard against liver damage and related gout and arthritic reactions.

Pyridoxine (B$_6$)

Vitamin B$_6$ and *pyridoxine* are generic terms representing a group of related chemicals. The three main members are pyridoxine, pyridoxal, and pyridoxamine. All three forms can be converted to the coenzyme PLP for use in the body.

Function

The major function of vitamin B$_6$, in the form of PLP, is to act as a coenzyme in the metabolism of amino acids and proteins. These reactions are involved in the formation of neurotransmitters and are essential for proper functioning of the nervous system. PLP is essential for hemoglobin synthesis. It is required for the conversion of tryptophan to niacin. It also serves as a coenzyme for fatty acid and carbohydrate metabolism.

Recommended Intake and Sources

The RDA for vitamin B$_6$ is 1.3 mg for men and women. These amounts are based on protein intake. Vitamin B$_6$ is found in a wide variety of foods. Particularly good sources are whole grains and cereals, legumes, and chicken, fish, pork, and eggs.

Deficiency

A deficiency of vitamin B$_6$ rarely occurs alone; it normally accompanies low intakes of other B vitamins. Symptoms include dermatitis, altered nerve function, weakness, poor growth, convulsions, and microcytic anemia (small red blood cells deficient in hemoglobin).

Of the numerous drugs affecting the bioavailability and metabolism of vitamin B$_6$, oral contraceptive agents (OCAs) may be among the most widely used. Prolonged use of such drugs as isoniazid (for tuberculosis), penicillamine (for lead poisoning, cystinuria, Wilson's disease, sclerosis, and rheumatoid arthritis), cycloserine (for tuberculosis), and hydralazine (for hypertension) may require vitamin B$_6$ supplements to reduce neurologic side effects and prevent deficiency during treatment (DaSilva, et al, 2014).

Toxicity

Vitamin B$_6$ has sometimes been prescribed to relieve the symptoms associated with premenstrual syndrome (PMS); however, there are no adequate data to support this treatment. Although doses of 10 mg, an amount often prescribed, are most likely not harmful (even considering the RDA, 1.3 mg), long-term supplementation in megadose gram quantities has been reported to cause ataxia and sensory neuropathy. The UL of B$_6$ is 100 mg per day.

Folate

Folate, like other B vitamins, actually consists of several similar compounds. One of these compounds was originally extracted from spinach and was given the name *folic acid,* from the Latin word *folium,* meaning "leaf." Folic acid was discovered in 1945 during the search for the nutritional factor responsible for control of pernicious anemia. We now know that vitamin B$_{12}$, rather than folate, is the nutrient that cures pernicious anemia. Folate and its related compounds, however, play a role in other essential biologic processes. The terms *folate, folic acid, folacin,* and *pteroylglutamic acid (PGA)* are often used interchangeably. Folate is the form of this vitamin found naturally in foods. Folic acid is a synthetic form used in vitamin supplements and for food fortification. Folic acid is actually more available for absorption by the body.

Function

Folate acts as a coenzyme in reactions involving the transfer of one-carbon units during metabolism. As such, it is required for the synthesis of amino acids, which are the building blocks of protein, and for the synthesis of deoxyribonucleic acid (DNA) and ribonucleic acid (RNA). Blood health also depends on folate to form the heme portion of hemoglobin. For the active form of folate to be maintained for use in the body, vitamin B$_{12}$ must be available.

Folate has a role in the proper formation of fetal neural tubes. Neural tube birth defects affect brain and spinal cord development, resulting in the disorders spina bifida and anencephaly. Spina bifida is a congenital neural tube defect caused by the incomplete closure of the fetus's spine during early pregnancy. It may involve incomplete development of the brain, spinal cord, and/or their protective coverings, resulting in a range of disabilities, including paralysis and incontinence (Figure 7-2). In cases of anencephaly, a congenital defect in which the brain does not develop, death may occur shortly after birth. Although these disorders result from a combination of genetics and environment, adequate folate levels during the first month after conception appear to greatly reduce their incidence. Unfortunately, women of childbearing age are sometimes marginally

FIG 7-2 Jean Driscoll is an Olympian, Paralympian, author, and advocate for persons with disabilities around the world who happened to be born with spina bifida. (More information about Jean Driscoll can be found on her website: www.jeandriscoll.com.) (Copyright 1995 PVA Publications, Sports 'N Spokes, Phoenix.)

TABLE 7-1 Food Sources of Folate			
FOOD	**SERVING SIZE**	**AMOUNT (μg)**	**% DAILY VALUE***
Chicken liver	3.5 oz	770	193
Breakfast cereals	½ to 1½ cups	100-400	25-100
Braised beef liver	3.5 oz	217	54
Lentils, cooked	½ cup	180	45
Chickpeas	½ cup	141	35
Asparagus	½ cup	132	33
Spinach, cooked	½ cup	131	33
Black beans	½ cup	128	32
Burrito with beans	2	118	30
Kidney beans	½ cup	115	29
Baked beans with pork	1 cup	92	23
Lima beans	½ cup	78	20
Tomato juice	1 cup	48	12
Brussels sprouts	½ cup	47	12
Orange	1 medium	47	12
Broccoli, cooked	½ cup	39	10
Fast-food French fries	Large order	38	10
Wheat germ	2 Tbsp	38	10
Fortified white bread	1 slice	38	10

*Based on daily value for folate of 400 μg.
Data from U.S. Department of Agriculture, Agricultural Research Service, Nutrient Data Laboratory: 2012. *USDA national nutrient database for standard reference* (Release 26), 2012. Accessed May 22, 2014, from www.ars.usda.gov/ba/bhnrc/ndl.

deficient in folate. They may not know they are pregnant during the first few crucial weeks, when the neural tube of the fetus forms.

Recommended Intake and Sources

The RDA reflects that some folate is stored in the liver, but generally, daily supplies are needed. The RDA is 400 μg for men and women. Physiologic state greatly affects folate need. During pregnancy, a woman's blood supply increases. This increase of blood and the growth of other tissues necessitate a greater need for folate. Consequently, the RDA jumps to 600 μg during pregnancy. During lactation, nutrient needs are elevated because of the nutrient content of the human milk being produced. Therefore, the RDA for folate is 500 μg for lactation needs.

It is recommended that women of childbearing age increase their folate intake to include 400 μg of synthetic folic acid to reduce the risks of birth defects, including spina bifida. The increased levels could be provided by natural sources, fortified foods, or supplements (Table 7-1). To ensure adequate access to folic acid, the U.S. Food and Drug Administration (FDA) mandates that cereal-grain products be fortified with 140-μg folic acid per 100 g of enriched flour and uncooked cereal grains. This means that manufacturers of enriched breads, flours, cornmeal, rice, pastas, and other grain products are required to add folate to their products (Stover, 2014). Fortified product labels may include the claim that adequate intake of folic acid may reduce the risk of neural tube defects.

Although this folic acid fortification assists in meeting the recommended levels for women of childbearing age, health care professionals must be prepared to individualize nutrition guidance to ensure daily optimal consumption of folate and folic acid. Clients and patients need to understand that simply consuming fortified cereals and grains does not necessarily provide sufficient amounts of folate. Dietitians should be consulted to ensure the appropriateness of dietary recommendations.

Concern has been expressed regarding the risks and benefits of this fortification to other age groups. In particular, the effects on older adults may be an issue because an excess of folate can mask a B_{12} deficiency, for which older adults are at risk. Requiring vitamin supplements that contain folic acid to also contain vitamin B_{12} can reduce this risk. This decreases the risk that the larger folate intakes would overshadow possible deficiencies of B_{12}. Overall, the benefits appear to outweigh the risk.

Folate is widely available in foods, particularly in leafy green vegetables, legumes, ready-to-eat cereals, and some fruits and juices. Folate is affected by heat, oxidation, and ultraviolet light; processing and cooking of fresh foods reduce the amount of folate available. Folate is found in many foods that contain ascorbic acid (vitamin C), such as oranges and orange juice. Ascorbic acid protects folate from oxidation. Diets deficient in folate often are deficient in vitamin C, and vice versa.

Deficiency

Cells whose normal activities require rapid cell growth and division are particularly sensitive to folate deficiency. Examples include red blood cells and the cells that line the GI tract. Folate deficiency results in megaloblastic anemia. This is a form of anemia characterized by large red blood cells that cannot carry oxygen properly. Other deficiency symptoms are glossitis, diarrhea, irritability, absent-mindedness, depression, and anxiety (Stover, 2014).

Deficiency may result from any condition that requires cell division to speed up, including infection, cancer, burns, blood loss, GI damage, growth, and pregnancy. Currently, about one third of pregnant women worldwide are affected by folate deficiency. Other groups at risk include people with a limits on intake and variety of food, including older adults with low incomes and people with chronic excessive alcohol ingestion. Alcoholic cirrhosis often results in both liver damage (which interferes with storage and metabolism of folate) and excessive losses of the vitamin in feces and urine (Stover, 2014).

Numerous medications may affect folate absorption or may be antagonistic to folate. These drugs include anticonvulsants, oral contraceptives, aspirin, cancer chemotherapy agents, sulfasalazine, nonsteroidal anti-inflammatory drugs, and antacids. Long-term use of any medication may affect the body's use of nutrients; folate is one that is particularly vulnerable.

Before folic acid supplementation is administered, the absence of vitamin B_{12} deficiency must be established. Therapy with folic acid in the presence of vitamin B_{12} deficiency will favorably improve blood profiles, decreasing megaloblastic anemia, while damage to the central nervous system from lack of B_{12} continues.

Toxicity

Excess folate or folic acid intake is not recommended or warranted. Consuming amounts beyond the UL of 1000-μg folic acid (for men and women) has not been studied. Such high levels may mask the presence of pernicious anemia, discussed later in the next section.

Cobalamin (B_{12})

Cobalamin and *vitamin B_{12}* are used as generic terms to refer to a group of cobalt-containing compounds. The common pharmaceutical name, used widely in supplements, is *cyanocobalamin.*

Function

Two cobalamins function as vitamin B_{12} coenzymes in humans. Vitamin B_{12} plays a role in folate metabolism by modifying folate coenzymes to active forms to support metabolic functions, including the synthesis of DNA and RNA. The metabolism of fatty acids and amino acids also requires vitamin B_{12}. In addition, this vitamin develops and maintains the myelin sheaths that surround and protect nerve fibers.

Recommended Intake and Sources

Absorption of vitamin B_{12} relies on an intrinsic factor. The intrinsic factor is produced by stomach mucosa. Both vitamin B_{12} and the intrinsic factor must be present for absorption. Recommended vitamin B_{12} levels take into account that some of the vitamin is stored in the liver. The RDA for young adults is 2.4 μg. Foods of animal origin are the only reliable sources of vitamin B_{12}; meat, fish, poultry, eggs, and dairy products are all good sources. For example, one glass of skim milk provides 0.93 μg of vitamin B_{12}. The vitamin has been reported to be found in legumes (nodules on roots) because of bacteria formation in soil, but they are not a reliable source. Vegans must supplement their intake with vitamin B_{12} supplements or use fortified products.

Deficiency

Deficiencies of B_{12} are usually secondary. Pernicious anemia (from lack of intrinsic factor for vitamin B_{12} absorption) or megaloblastic anemia (from related folate dysfunction) occurs. Additional neurologic effects develop because of damage to the spinal cord as the breakdown of myelin sheath synthesis affects brain, optic, and peripheral nerves (Carmel, 2014).

Older adults are more at risk for deficiency because of a naturally occurring reduction in production of the intrinsic factor by the stomach mucosa. Most older adults, however, maintain vitamin B_{12} levels within normal range. For those who do become deficient, injections to bypass intestinal absorption are warranted. Particularly noted in this population are neuropsychiatric symptoms, including delusions and hallucinations, which may occur in the absence of anemia. These symptoms can be misdiagnosed as senility or other illnesses. To alleviate this risk, the recommendations include that adults older than 50 years consume foods fortified with vitamin B_{12} or take a B_{12} supplement to ensure adequacy of the RDA for B_{12}. Vitamin B_{12} is more absorbable in this form because it is already separated from food.

As discussed, folate levels may disguise a vitamin B_{12} deficiency. Hematologic damage is masked by folate, but neurologic damage continues.

Toxicity

Toxicity of vitamin B_{12} has not been noted, but there are no benefits to large doses unless deficiency exists.

Biotin

Humans need biotin, a member of the B vitamin complex, in tiny amounts.

Function

Biotin assists in the transfer of carbon dioxide from one compound to another, playing an important role in carbohydrate, fat, and protein metabolism.

Recommended Intake and Sources

Biotin is synthesized in the lower GI tract by bacterial microorganisms. However, the amount produced and its bioavailability are unknown. Although biotin is produced in the body, it is still an essential nutrient. (The human body does not produce biotin, but bacteria hosted in the gut do.) It must also be consumed in foods.

The AI for biotin is 30 µg per day. Biotin is widespread in foods. The richest sources are liver, kidney, peanut butter, egg yolks, and yeast.

Deficiency

Deficiency of biotin is unknown among people eating a typical North American diet. When it is experimentally produced, symptoms include a scaly red rash, hair loss, loss of appetite, depression, and glossitis (Mock, 2014).

Biotin deficiency has been produced by consumption of large amounts of avidin, a protein in raw egg whites that binds biotin. A person would need to consume many raw egg whites for this to occur; salmonella poisoning would probably strike first. Avidin is denatured by heat, so cooked egg whites pose no problem to biotin status.

Antibiotics are known to reduce the number of biotin-producing bacteria. In addition, clients receiving long-term intravenous feeding are prone to biotin deficiency; therefore, their feeding mixtures should contain biotin.

Toxicity

There is no known toxicity for biotin.

Pantothenic Acid

Pantothenic acid gets its name from its presence in all living things (from the Greek *pantothen*, meaning "from all sides").

Function

The principal active form of pantothenic acid functions as part of coenzyme A (CoA for short); therefore, it is required for the metabolism of carbohydrates, fats, and protein.

Recommended Intake and Sources

The AI for pantothenic acid is 5 mg per day. Pantothenic acid is widespread in foods and easily consumed in whole grain cereals, legumes, meat, fish, and poultry.

Deficiency

Deficiencies in pantothenic acid do not naturally occur in humans.

Toxicity

Doses of up to 10 g daily have been administered with no ill effects. Researchers have reported that daily doses of 10 to 20 g may produce diarrhea or water retention.

Choline
Function

Choline is needed for the synthesis of acetylcholine, a neurotransmitter, and lecithin, the phospholipid.

Recommended Intake and Sources

The body can actually make choline from the amino acid methionine, but this process does not produce enough choline to meet the needs of the body. Consequently, food sources are still required. This requirement qualifies choline as an essential nutrient. The AI is 550 mg per day for men and 425 mg per day for women, with a UL of 3500 mg per day for adults.

Food sources include many commonly consumed foods with rich sources, such as milk, eggs, and peanuts.

Deficiency

Deficiency of choline is rare.

Toxicity

Symptoms of choline toxicity include sweating, fishy body odor, vomiting, liver damage, reduced growth, and low blood pressure (hypotension).

Vitamin C

Vitamin C is almost a household word. It's hard to believe that it was isolated as a nutrient only around 1930. The discovery of vitamin C is associated with the search for the cause of scurvy, a potentially fatal disease that weakens the body's connective tissues and causes inflammation of them. As early as the eighteenth century, it was known that eating certain foods, particularly citrus fruits, could control scurvy, but the actual substance responsible for "gluing" the cells together was not determined until Albert Szent-Gyorgyi and Glen King isolated it in 1928 and 1930, respectively (Levine and Padayatty, 2014). One of the two active forms of vitamin C is ascorbic acid (*ascorbic* meaning "without scurvy").

Function

Vitamin C functions as an antioxidant and as a coenzyme. It can perform different functions in various situations. Collagen formation for bone matrix, teeth, cartilage, and connective tissue depends on ascorbic acid. Vitamin C provides the cement that holds structures together. Wound healing, which necessitates the formation of new tissue, also requires vitamin C.

As an antioxidant, vitamin C protects folate, vitamin E, and polyunsaturated substances from destruction by oxygen as they move throughout the body. An antioxidant is a compound that guards others from damaging oxidation by being oxidized itself. Vitamins C and E also work together as antioxidants to destroy substances released as cells age, are oxidized, or become damaged. Their work may prevent damage by free radicals to vascular walls, thereby limiting the development of atherosclerotic plaques.

Among its other functions, vitamin C enhances the absorption of nonheme iron, which is found in plant foods. Thyroid and adrenal hormone synthesis requires vitamin C. Several conversion processes depend on vitamin C; these include tryptophan to serotonin, cholesterol to bile, and folate to its active form.

Vitamin C may have a role in reducing the risk of cancer development. Epidemiologic studies have uncovered an association between levels of dietary intake of vitamin C and incidence of cancer in the stomach, esophagus, and colon. Because these studies are of dietary intakes of populations, it is not yet known whether the effects are caused by vitamin C or to other, as yet unidentified, components of foods containing vitamin C.

It is a common myth that vitamin C can prevent the common cold. Unfortunately, the bulk of evidence does not support the theory that vitamin C reduces the incidence of the common cold. Taking supplemental vitamin C for a limited time, however, can decrease the duration and reduce the severity of the symptoms. The UL, though, should always be observed.

Recommended Intake and Sources

The RDA for vitamin C has varied from 45 mg to 60 mg for adults. Currently, the RDA is 90 mg for men and 75 mg for women. Recommendations vary worldwide; the minimum daily requirement to prevent symptoms of scurvy is 10 mg. However, the amount recommended daily to provide enough circulating vitamin C for tissue saturation for good health is open to interpretation.

As more is learned about vitamin C functions, recommendations customized to specific diseases and lifestyle behaviors will be determined. For example, cigarette smokers have lower circulating levels of vitamin C than nonsmokers, regardless of their dietary intake of vitamin C. The metabolic use of vitamin C by smokers is twice that of nonsmokers. Recognition of this deficit, has led to the advice that smokers increase their vitamin C intake from the 90 mg RDA to 125 mg daily.

Fruits and vegetables provide 95% of the vitamin C we consume. Many foods are excellent sources; some of them are citrus fruits, red and green peppers, strawberries, tomatoes, potatoes, broccoli, and other green leafy vegetables. Serving sizes to meet the RDA are listed in Table 7-2.

Some foods and drinks are fortified with vitamin C. Ready-to-eat cereals have added vitamin C (about 25% of the daily values) and other vitamins not naturally found in grains. Additional vitamin C, often 100% of the daily values, is added to the small amounts naturally found in apple and grape juice.

Vitamin C is destroyed by air, light, and heat. Fruit juices should be stored in an airtight container that holds only the amount that can be consumed in a short time. The vitamin

TABLE 7-2 Recommended Dietary Allowance Serving Sizes of Vitamin C*

FOOD	SERVING SIZE	VITAMIN C (mg)
Orange juice	¾ cup	93
Orange	1 medium	80
Kiwifruit	1 medium	75
Cantaloupe	1¼ cups	68
Peppers, green or red	¾ cup	64
Strawberries	1 cup	64
Broccoli	¾ cup	58
Brussels sprouts	¾ cup	48
Grapefruit	½ fruit	47

*Recommended Daily Allowance = 75-90 mg.
Data from U.S. Department of Agriculture, Agricultural Research Service, Nutrient Data Laboratory: *USDA national nutrient database for standard reference* (Release 26), 2012. Accessed May 22, 2014, from www.ars.usda.gov/ba/bhnrc/ndl.

C contents of cooked foods can be maximized by cooking in the minimal amount of water or, even better, by microwaving (see the *Teaching Tool* box Vegetable Victories).

✳ TEACHING TOOL
Vegetable Victories

Every health recommendation proposes that we (and our clients) significantly increase our intake of vegetables. But how? This Teaching Tool provides several resources to be shared with clients, by providing information about websites to locate local farmers' markets, Community Supported Agriculture (CSA), teaching handouts about buying and preparing vegetables, and more.

LocalHarvest; www.localharvest.org/: Website that provides info about locations of local farmers' markets and CSAs (a group of individuals and/or families joining together to purchase shares of the harvest of a nearby farmer); offers additional strategies for preparing produce for immediate consumption or for storing through the winter.

ChooseMyPlate; www.choosemyplate.gov/healthy-eating-tips/ten-tips.html: Access to The Ten Tips Nutrition Education Series for consumers and health professionals, which are easy-to-implement strategies that can be easily printed.

Fruits & Veggies—More Matters; www.fruitsandveggies morematters.org/: A health initiative to increase Americans' consumption of fruits and vegetables; includes tools for buying, nutrition, storage, and selection.

Deficiency

Although vitamin C deficiency is rare in developed countries in the West, it may still occur among chronic alcohol and drug users, smokers, and those whose dietary intakes are poor. Older adults may have marginal intake because of difficulty in obtaining and preparing fresh foods. These at-risk groups may experience other vitamin and mineral deficiencies as well.

Scurvy represents the extreme result of vitamin C deficiency. The symptoms are tied to the functions of vitamin C in the body. When the gluelike substance collagen is not replaced, tissues throughout the body degenerate. Gingivitis causes gums to bleed, and teeth to come loose. Joints and limbs ache from muscle degeneration and lack of new connective tissue formation. Bruising and hemorrhages occur as the vascular system weakens, and plaques form as a result of the vascular damage. Death ultimately occurs as functioning of all body systems disintegrates.

Marginal deficiency may manifest as gingivitis with soreness and ulcerations of the mouth, poor wound healing, inadequate tooth and bone growth or maintenance, and increased risk of infection as the integrity of tissues throughout the body becomes compromised.

Toxicity

Toxicity from foods high in vitamin C does not occur even if we consume cups of fresh strawberries washed down with a quart of orange juice. Long-term supplement intakes of megadoses from 1 to 15 g may result in cramps, diarrhea, nausea, kidney stone formation, and gout. The effects of anti-clotting medication may also be affected (NRC, 2006).

Taking supplements of vitamin C seems benign, but the body adapts to protect itself from harm. If continually inundated with excessive vitamin C, the body develops a mechanism that destroys much of the extra vitamin C circulating within it. A rebound effect may occur if, after taking megadoses for several months or more, an individual abruptly stops supplementation and consumes a quantity closer to the RDA. The protective mechanism of the body is still in gear

and continues to destroy vitamin C. An individual may experience symptoms of scurvy even though consuming the RDA. A newborn exposed to vitamin C megadoses *in utero* may experience this rebound effect. Although the rebound effect may not occur in every case, withdrawal from vitamin C megadoses should be gradual, over a period of 2 to 4 weeks. Consequently, there is a UL of 2000 mg for adults and 400 to 1800 mg for children and adolescents.

Table 7-3 provides a quick reference to water-soluble vitamins.

TABLE 7-3 Water-Soluble Vitamins

VITAMIN	FUNCTION	CLINICAL ISSUES (DEFICIENCY/TOXICITY)	RECOMMENDED DAILY INTAKES	FOOD SOURCES
Thiamin (B₁)	Coenzyme energy metabolism; muscle nerve action	Deficiency: beriberi (ataxia, disorientation, tachycardia); wet beriberi (edema); dry beriberi (nervous system); Wernicke-Korsakoff syndrome. Marginal deficiency: headaches, tiredness	Men: 1.2 mg Women: 1.1 mg	Lean pork, whole or enriched grains and flours, legumes, seeds, and nuts
Riboflavin (B₂)	Coenzyme energy metabolism	Deficiency: ariboflavinosis with cheilosis, glossitis, seborrheic dermatitis	Men: 1.3 mg Women: 1.1 mg	Milk/dairy products; meat, fish, poultry, and eggs; dark leafy greens (broccoli); whole and enriched breads and cereals
Niacin (B₃) (nicotinic acid and niacinamide) Precursor: tryptophan	Cofactor to enzymes involved in energy metabolism; glycolysis and TCA cycle	Deficiency: pellagra. Toxicity: vasodilation, liver damage, gout, and arthritic reactions	Men: 16 mg NE Women: 14 mg NE (UL 35 mg NE)	Meats, poultry, and fish; legumes; whole and enriched cereals; milk
Pyridoxine (B₆)	Forms coenzyme pyridoxal phosphate (PLP) for energy metabolism; CNS; hemoglobin synthesis	Deficiency: dermatitis, altered nerve function, weakness, anemia; OCAs decrease B₆ levels. Toxicity: ataxia, sensory neuropathy	Men: 1.3 mg Women: 1.3 mg (UL 100 mg)	Whole grains/cereals legumes, poultry, fish, pork, eggs
Folate (folic acid, folacin, PGA)	Coenzyme metabolism (synthesis of amino acid, heme, DNA RNA); fetal neural tube formation	Deficiency: megaloblastic anemia; many drugs affect folate use. Toxicity: megadoses may mask pernicious anemia	Men: 400 μg Women: 400 μg Pregnancy: 600 μg Lactation: 500 μg (UL 1000 μg)	Widely available leafy green vegetables, legumes, ascorbic acid-containing foods
Cobalamin (B₁₂)	Transport/storage of folate; metabolism of fatty acids/amino acids	Deficiency: pernicious anemia, CNS damage	Adults: 2.4 μg	Animal sources
Biotin	Metabolism of carbohydrate, fat, and protein	Deficiency: produced by avidin and long-term antibiotics	Adults: 30 μg AI	Liver, kidney, peanut butter, egg yolks, intestinal synthesis
Pantothenic acid	Part of coenzyme A	Deficiency: not possible	Adults: 5 mg AI	Widespread in foods
Choline	Synthesis of acetylcholine and lecithin	Deficiency: rare. Toxicity: body odor, liver damage, hypotension	Men: 550 mg Women: 425 mg (UL 3500 mg)	Widespread—milk, eggs, peanuts
Vitamin C	Antioxidant, coenzyme, collagen formation, wound healing, iron absorption, hormone synthesis	Deficiency: scurvy. Toxicity: cramps, nausea, kidney stone formation, gout (1-15 g), rebound scurvy	Men: 90 mg Women: 75 mg (UL 2000)	Fruits/vegetables (citrus fruits, tomatoes, peppers, strawberries, broccoli)

AI, Adequate Intake; *CNS,* central nervous system; *DNA,* deoxyribonucleic acid; *NE,* niacin equivalent; *OCAs,* oral contraceptive agents; *PGA,* pteroylglutamic acid; *RNA,* ribonucleic acid; *TCA,* tricarboxylic acid; *UL,* Tolerable Upper Intake Level.

FAT-SOLUBLE VITAMINS

Vitamin A

Each year approximately 250,000 children enter a world of permanent darkness. The cause? Vitamin A deficiency. Extreme vitamin A deficiency is so damaging to corneas that blindness occurs. Although this could be prevented with just a few cents' worth of vitamin A per year, there is little money for preventive health measures in areas of the world where food is scarce.

Function

Vitamin A is a group of compounds that function to maintain skin and mucous membranes throughout the body. Specific activities depending on vitamin A are vision, bone growth, functioning of the immune system, and normal reproduction. Our eyes depend on visual purple, technically called *rhodopsin,* to be able to adjust to light variations. Rhodopsin is formed from retinal, a vitamin A substance, and opsin, a protein. Without enough vitamin A, rhodopsin cannot be formed, and the retina cannot easily respond to light changes. As a result, night blindness develops. Bone growth involves a process of remodeling that reshapes and enlarges the skeleton. Reshaping requires vitamin A to undo existing bone. Vitamin A also maintains the integrity of epithelial tissues throughout the body, providing protection against infections and ensuring optimum function. Hormone-like effects of vitamin A appear to be tied to cell synthesis for reproductive purposes.

Recommended Intake and Sources

Vitamin A is measured as retinol activity equivalents (RAE). The RDA, based on providing optimum storage of vitamin A in the liver, is 900-μg RAE for men and 700-μg RAE for women. RAE incorporates both the preformed, active forms of vitamin A, called *retinoids* (found in animal foods), and the precursor forms of vitamin A, called *carotenoids* (found in plant foods). The carotenoid beta carotene is the primary source of vitamin A from plant foods.

Because vitamin A (a fat-soluble vitamin) is stored in the body, daily doses are not necessary, but they are desirable. Deficiency of other nutrients affects the absorption and use of vitamin A (Ross, 2014). Nutrients are interdependent, and imbalances of specific nutrients affect the functioning of others.

Natural preformed vitamin A is found only in the fat of animal-related foods; these include whole milk, butter, liver, egg yolks, and fatty fish. Carotenoids are found in deep green, yellow, and orange fruits and vegetables. The best sources are broccoli, cantaloupe, sweet potatoes, carrots, tomatoes, and spinach (Table 7-4). High consumption of carotenoids, particularly beta carotene, has been associated with decreased risk of certain cancers and other chronic diseases. This may be due to their action as anti-oxidants. Table 7-5 lists other nutrients that also function as anti-oxidants.

When fats are removed from animal-related foods, preformed vitamin A is also lost. To maintain traditional sources

TABLE 7-4 Vitamin A/Beta Carotene Sources*

FOOD	SERVING SIZE	CAROTENE (RAE)
Liver (beef)	3½ oz	10,000
Sweet potato	1 whole, baked	2488
Carrots	1 whole, raw	2025
	½ cup, cooked	1915
Spinach	½ cup, cooked	737
Butternut squash	½ cup, cooked	714
Cantaloupe	1 cup	516
Red pepper	1 whole	422
Apricots	3 medium	277

*RDA = 900 RAE for men; 700 RAE for women.
RAE, retinol activity equivalent.
Data from U.S. Department of Agriculture, Agricultural Research Service, Nutrient Data Laboratory: *USDA national nutrient database for standard reference* (Release 26), 2012. Accessed May 22, 2014, from www.ars.usda.gov/ba/bhnrc/ndl.

of the vitamin, low-fat, skim, and nonfat milks are fortified with vitamin A. Other fortified products include margarine (which often replaces butter, a natural source of vitamin A), and ready-to-eat cereal, a staple food product commonly fortified with many nutrients.

Deficiency

Vitamin A deficiency is either primary, caused by lack of dietary intake, or secondary, the result of chronic fat malabsorption. As liver storage becomes depleted, symptoms develop. The effects are closely tied to vitamin A functions. Ocularly, xerophthalmia incorporates a range of problems, from night blindness (the inability of the eyes to readjust from bright to dim light) progressing to a hard, dry cornea (keratinization) or keratomalacia, resulting in complete blindness. The degeneration of the epithelial tissues protecting the eye itself leads to the effects of xerophthalmia. Compromised epithelial tissues also result in the development of hard white lumps of keratin on hair follicles (hyperkeratosis), respiratory infections, diarrhea, and other GI disturbances. Overall, the immune system is endangered; for deficient children especially, a minor illness or a bout of measles may be deadly. Growth is inhibited because of lack of vitamin A–dependent proteins for bone growth.

In the United States, individuals experiencing chronic fat malabsorption are at risk for vitamin A deficiency and deficiencies of other fat-soluble vitamins. These nutrients are incorporated into their overall nutrition plans. Although marginal vitamin A deficiency is possible, overt deficiencies are rare.

Deficiency is a health threat in parts of the world where food availability is limited. To counteract this threat in areas where rice is a staple food, Golden Rice has been genetically transformed to accumulate increased amounts of provitamin A. Public health efforts are being made to distribute Golden Rice to farmers and to further increase the nutrient value of the grain (Tang, et al, 2009).

TABLE 7-5 **Antioxidants**				
ANTIOXIDANT	**ANTIOXIDANT FUNCTIONS**	**MAJOR FOOD SOURCES**	**ADULT RDA**	**DAILY RECOMMENDED SUPPLEMENTATION**
Beta carotene (provitamin A vitamin A)	May decrease risk of some cancers and CVD	Sweet potatoes, winter squash, carrots, red bell peppers, dark green vegetables, apricots, mangos, cantaloupe	No RDA (1 sweet potato = 15 mg, 1 carrot = 10 mg)	6-15 mg; nontoxic; higher doses may give skin a harmless orange cast (not recommended for smokers)
Vitamin C	May decrease risk of certain cancers and CVD	Kiwi, citrus fruits, berries, cantaloupe, honeydew, bell peppers, tomatoes, cabbage family vegetables	75-90 mg (1 kiwi = 150 mg, 1 cup broccoli = 115 mg, 1 orange = 70 mg)	250-500 mg, more may cause diarrhea (UL 2000 mg)
Vitamin E	May decrease risk of cancer; may also prevent or delay cataracts	Vegetable oil, nuts, seeds, margarine, wheat germ, olives, leafy greens, avocado, asparagus	15-mg α-TE (1 Tbsp oil = 9 mg, 1 Tbsp margarine or 1 oz nuts = 2 mg)	300-600 mg (200-400 international units) daily* for all adults; higher doses may cause headaches and diarrhea (UL 1000 mg)
Selenium	Prevents cell and lipid membrane damage	Meat, fish, eggs, whole grains	55 µg	Same as RDA; not more than 200 µg; higher levels very toxic, causing severe liver damage, vomiting, diarrhea, metallic aftertaste (UL 400 µg)

α-TE, Alpha-tocopherol; *CVD,* cardiovascular disease; *RDA,* Recommended Dietary Allowance; *UL,* Tolerable Upper Intake Level
*Contraindicated for those who have hypertension or who take warfarin (Coumadin) and other drugs to inhibit blood clots.

Toxicity

Hypervitaminosis A occurs only from preformed vitamin A from either a short- or long-term intake of supplements. Most food sources of preformed A do not contain high enough levels to ever result in toxicity. The only exception noted is polar bear liver and the livers of other large animals. Explorers who feasted on polar bear liver experienced hypervitaminosis A; in fact, the way we learned about the toxic effects of vitamin A was through their misfortune. Apparently, the livers of hibernating animals store an extraordinary quantity of vitamin A to provide sufficient amounts for a long winter without nourishment. When humans consume the preformed vitamin A of these livers, the quantity is toxic.

Toxicity does not occur from the carotenoid precursor in foods. If carotenoids are consumed in excess, either from foods or supplements, the skin takes on an orange hue, which dissipates when carotenoid consumption is reduced.

Immediate symptoms of vitamin A toxicity include blistered skin, weakness, anorexia, vomiting, headache, joint pain, irritability, and enlargement of the spleen and liver; long-term effects include bone abnormalities and liver damage (Ross, 2014).

Vitamin A supplements taken internally will not cure or improve acne and are toxic in excess. Even prescription medications can be problematic. The acne medications sotretinoin (Accutane) and isotretinoin (oral forms) are nonnutritive sources of vitamin A that cause birth defects when used by pregnant women. Women who take either of these drugs should be advised to use a highly reliable method of birth control.

Vitamin D

With sufficient exposure to ultraviolet light or sunshine, the body can manufacture its own supply of vitamin D. The exposure of skin to ultraviolet light begins the conversion process of the vitamin D precursor 7-dehydrocholesterol (found in our skin) to cholecalciferol, the active form of vitamin D. Because the body can produce vitamin D, it is technically a hormone. However, when vitamin D is supplied by the diet, it is technically a vitamin. Regardless of how it is classified, vitamin D is a substance necessary for a variety of the body's regulating processes as well as normal development of bones and teeth.

Function

Intestinal absorption of calcium and phosphorus depends on the action of vitamin D. This vitamin also affects bone mineralization and mineral homeostasis by helping to regulate blood calcium levels.

Vitamin D also has potential effects on growth and regulation, cardiovascular function and immunological performance.

Recommended Intake and Sources

The RDA for vitamin D is 15 µg (600 international units [IU]). For newborns through 1 year, an AI of 10 µg (400 IU) is recommended. The RDA for people ages 70 and older jumps to 20 µg (800 IU). This level reflects the lesser efficiency of older adults to synthesize vitamin D from sun exposure. If these amounts are not consumed from foods or obtained from sunlight, supplement use may be appropriate.

The UL for vitamin D is 100 µg (4000 IU). The effects of intakes higher than the UL are discussed in the section on toxicity.

The current recommendations for optimal vitamin D intakes are based on preventing bone disease and providing sufficient biologically active vitamin D for the other potential effects.

Vitamin D is available through body synthesis or from dietary sources. Cholecalciferol, the active form of vitamin D, can be synthesized. Ultraviolet irradiation from sunlight affects the vitamin D precursor 7-dehydrocholesterol in our skin, and this cholesterol derivative is transformed by the liver and kidneys into its hormonal form, calcitriol. The amount of vitamin D produced depends on length of exposure to ultraviolet irradiation, atmospheric conditions, and skin pigmentation. Geographic regions and seasons that are particularly cloudy and rainy diminish the quantity of vitamin D synthesized. Darker skin pigmentation also reduces the effect of radiation on the skin, as do sunscreen and concealing clothing. Aging may lessen the amount of vitamin D formed from sunlight exposure.

The few sources of natural preformed vitamin D are the fat of the animal-related foods butter, egg yolks, fatty fish, and liver. Milk, although containing fat, is not a good source; it is, however, a good vehicle for vitamin D fortification because it contains calcium and phosphorus, which need vitamin D for absorption. Because vegans consume no animal foods, they may require supplements or regular sunlight exposure to ensure formation of cholecalciferol. Appropriate guidance should be sought from a primary health care provider or dietitian.

Deficiency

A deficiency of vitamin D can lead to the disorders **rickets** (Figure 7-3) and **osteomalacia**; the extent of vitamin D deficiency among children and adults in the United States may be more widespread than previously suspected (Jones, 2014). Because of insufficient mineralization of bone and tooth matrix, rickets in children leads to malformed skeletons, characterized by bowed legs unable to bear body weight, oddly angled rib bones and chests, and abnormal tooth formation. In adults, osteomalacia, or "bad bones," is characterized by soft demineralized bones that are at risk for fractures. It may be due to vitamin D or calcium deficiency.

It has been thought that rickets occurs rarely among well-nourished populations. However, reports now reveal that the risk of rickets has increased among breastfed dark-skinned infants and toddlers of African and Asian descent, especially in northern areas such as Canada and Alaska. The increased risk for these children is caused by several factors, including darker pigmentation, use of heavier clothing by children that limits exposure of the skin to vitamin D synthesis, and limited consumption of dietary sources of fortified vitamin D dairy products by children or by women who are breastfeeding infants (Jones, 2014). Consequently, Canadian and U.S. pediatric medical associations recommend vitamin D supplementation of 10 µg (400 IU) per day. Use of rice milk or soy milk,

FIG 7-3 Rickets. This child has characteristic bowed legs. (From McLaren DS: *A colour atlas and text of diet-related disorders*, ed 2, London, 1992, Mosby.)

neither of which is fortified with vitamin D and other nutrients found in human breast milk from well-nourished mothers and in infant formulas, may lead to severe nutrient deficiencies such as rickets. Children are also at risk for rickets as a result of chronic lipid malabsorption or continuous anticonvulsive therapy (Hollick, 2006).

Among older adults who may have a diminished ability to produce vitamin D, osteomalacia may develop when marginal intakes of vitamin D or calcium exist for a number of years. Calcium absorption may also be affected by the aging process and may contribute to osteomalacia risk. Older women are more at risk than older men because of the effects of repeated pregnancies and lactation on bone density. Symptoms of osteomalacia include weakness, rheumatic-like pain, and an awkward gait. Because bones are weakened, fractures of the spine, hips, and limbs may occur.

Another disorder of the skeleton is **osteoporosis**. Osteoporosis is a condition in which bone density is reduced and the remaining bone is brittle and breaks easily. Because vitamin D is crucial for absorption of calcium and the mineralization of bone, chronic vitamin D deficiency may be one of the risk factors for this disorder. Osteoporosis is discussed in detail in Chapter 8.

Vitamin D deficiency is associated with increased risk of CVD, rheumatoid arthritis, cancers, type 1 diabetes mellitus, and multiple sclerosis.

Outright deficiency of vitamin D is thought to be rare in the United States because milk and related food products are fortified. But the amounts recommended for dietary consumption assume that greater amounts are produced by our bodies. Deficiency, however, is a concern when a lack of exposure to sunlight occurs as a result of (1) environmental limitations, (2) cultural clothing customs that conceal the body, or (3) the inability of older adults or people with disabilities to get outdoors or to the store, resulting in malnourishment. These conditions may require vigilance in the consumption of fortified dietary sources, or supplements may be appropriate. When dietary intake and blood levels of vitamin D are assessed, many more Americans are found to have marginal vitamin D status.

Toxicity

High intakes of vitamin D can result in hypercalcemia (high calcium level in blood) and hypercalciuria (high calcium level in urine), which affect kidneys and may cause cardiovascular damage. Toxicity symptoms occur when dietary intake of vitamin D is just above the UL of 100 µg or 4000 IU.

Vitamin E

During the 1970s, vitamin E supplements were a popular aphrodisiac. Male virility, in particular, was thought to be enhanced by taking extra vitamin E. There was only one problem. Vitamin E increased the libido of male rats but not that of humans. Research conducted on rats about the effects of vitamin E noted that the rats were able to reproduce better with additional intake of vitamin E. Although research conducted on rats is often applicable to humans, in this instance the results could not be generalized to humans. However, vitamin E is an essential nutrient that performs vital functions; we are still learning about its role in relation to disease prevention.

Function

Vitamin E acts as an antioxidant, protecting polyunsaturated fatty acids and vitamin A in cell membranes from oxidative damage by being oxidized itself. This function is particularly important in protecting the integrity of lung and red blood cell membranes, which are exposed to large amounts of oxygen. Other antioxidative functions of vitamin E are performed as part of a system in conjunction with selenium and ascorbic acid (vitamin C).

Recommended Intake and Sources

Plants contain a family of compounds called *tocopherols*. Vitamin E requirement is met by a particular tocopherol, alpha-tocopherol, which is the most widely occurring form and the most active. The RDA for vitamin E is 15 mg for men and women (the older measurement, IU, may still be in use on dietary supplements: one IU equals .67 mg alpha-tocopherol). A positive relationship exists between dietary intake of polyunsaturated fats and vitamin E requirements. As our dietary intake of polyunsaturated fats increases, we

need more vitamin E to protect the integrity of these fats from oxidation.

The best sources of vitamin E are vegetable oils (e.g., corn, soy, safflower, canola, and cottonseed) and margarine. Whole grains, seeds, nuts, wheat germ, and green leafy vegetables also provide adequate amounts of vitamin E. Processing of these foods may decrease the final vitamin E content.

Deficiency

A primary deficiency of vitamin E is rare. Secondary deficiencies occur in premature infants and in other people who are unable to absorb fat normally. Some chronic fat absorption disorders in which deficiencies may occur are **cystic fibrosis, biliary atresia** (blocked bile duct), other disorders of the hepatobiliary system, and liver transport problems. Symptoms of vitamin E deficiency are neurologic disorders resulting from cell damage and anemia caused by hemolysis of red blood cells (hemolytic anemia) (Traber, 2014).

Toxicity

There is no evidence of toxicity associated with excessive intake of vitamin E. Intakes of about 70 to 530 mg (100 to 800 IU) per day appear to be tolerated, but the value of such doses has not been determined. Megadoses of vitamin E can exacerbate the anticoagulant effect of drugs taken to reduce blood clotting; vitamin E supplementation is not recommended in people who are undergoing anticoagulant therapy, have a coagulation disorder, or have a vitamin K deficiency. A UL of 1000-mg alpha-tocopherol has been set.

Vitamin K

As previously mentioned, vitamin K was discovered by a Danish scientist and was called *koagulationsvitamin* for its blood-clotting properties. Later research revealed that vitamin K is several related compounds with similar functions in the body.

Function

Vitamin K's main function is as a cofactor in the synthesis of blood-clotting factors, including prothrombin. Protein formation in bone, kidney, and plasma also depends on the actions of vitamin K.

Recommended Intake and Sources

The AI for vitamin K is 120 µg per day for men and 90 µg for women. This amount provides for sufficient storage of vitamin K in the liver. Vitamin K actually consists of compounds in different forms in plant and animal tissues. All are converted by the liver to the biologically active form of menaquinone called vitamin K.

Vitamin K is available through dietary sources and can be synthesized by microflora in the jejunum and ileum of the digestive tract. From plants, vitamin K is consumed as phylloquinone; bacterial synthesis produces vitamin K homologues as forms of menaquinones. As noted, phylloquinone and vitamin K homologues are converted to the active form of menaquinone—vitamin K—by the liver.

Vitamin K is still an essential nutrient, although bacteria residing in the intestinal tract can synthesize it. The key distinction is that bacteria hosted by the human body produce the vitamin. Additionally, not enough vitamin K is produced by the microflora to ensure adequate levels for total blood-clotting needs; dietary intake is still required (Suttie, 2014).

Primary food sources for vitamin K are dark green leafy vegetables. Lesser amounts are found in dairy products, cereals, meats, and fruits.

Deficiency

Deficiency of vitamin K inhibits blood coagulation. Deficiencies may be observed in clinical settings related to malabsorption disorders or medication interactions. Long-term intensive antibiotic therapy destroys the intestinal microflora that produce vitamin K. As with the other fat-soluble vitamins, any barrier to absorption affects the quantity of fat-soluble vitamin absorbed.

Premature infants and newborns are unable to immediately produce vitamin K; their guts are too sterile, free of the microflora necessary to produce vitamin K. Hospitals in the United States routinely give newborns an intramuscular dose of vitamin K to prevent hemorrhagic disease. Infants born in nonhospital settings (such as at home) may not receive the recommended dose of vitamin K. Intracranial bleeding and other symptoms consistent with abuse may actually be due to vitamin K deficiency (Brousseau, et al, 2005).

Because vitamin K also has a role in bone metabolism, research is investigating whether vitamin K has a function in the treatment of osteoporosis. Although insufficient data exist to support vitamin K as a formal treatment component for osteoporosis (Suttie, 2014), they do highlight the need to regularly consume at least the AI.

Toxicity

Consumption of foods containing vitamin K produces no problems of toxicity. Certain medications may be affected by vitamin K. The effectiveness of anticoagulant medications such as warfarin (Coumadin) and other blood-thinning drugs can be reduced by high intakes of vitamin K from either foods or supplements. Clients should be advised to moderate their consumption of foods containing vitamin K.

Vitamin K supplements should be used only if advised by a registered dietitian/nutritionist or primary health care provider. Because vitamin K has a role in blood clotting, excess amounts may decrease clotting time, thereby increasing the risk for stroke.

Table 7-6 provides a summary of fat-soluble vitamins.

AMERICANS AND VITAMIN SUPPLEMENTATION

Why do vitamins capture the attention of Americans? We generally do not suffer from vitamin deficiencies, and any problems of vitamin toxicity tend to be self-imposed. Considered through a wellness perspective, vitamin consumption is just one of many factors for achieving optimum health. Yet sales of dietary supplements continue to significantly increase. More than half the adult American population uses these products (Marra and Boyer, 2009).

Perhaps vitamins are an easier target on which to focus when one is emphasizing good health. If a person is concerned about vitamin intake, he or she can always take a vitamin pill. That's a lot easier than the dietary and behavior modifications required to meet other health factors, such as decreasing fat intake or increasing physical activities. There are, though, circumstances that may warrant supplementation.

Rethinking Vitamin Supplementation

Recommendations for vitamin supplementation intend to improve the nutritional status of at-risk groups of the population. These have included adolescent girls, pregnant and lactating women, individuals with limited economic resources, older persons, alcohol-dependent individuals, and possibly those following vegetarian or vegan food patterns. Additionally, individuals with increased nutrient needs due to medication interaction with nutrients and/or chronic health conditions may require vitamin supplementation. Another subgroup at risk are people experiencing food insecurity, whose intake may have nutrient gaps. Folate, vitamins A and C, and the minerals iron, calcium, and zinc tend to be consumed in inadequate amounts by these at-risk groups.

The purpose of recommendations for these groups is to address basic deficiency issues. If adequate levels are not consumed as a result of social, cultural, or economic reasons, then it is the role of health professionals to provide guidance as to how to achieve these levels.

Recommendations are beginning to move beyond the level of nutrient adequacy to issues of health promotion and prevention of disease. For example, folate requirements are vitally important for the development of a healthy fetus. Should the whole population receive folic acid through fortification when only potentially pregnant women have the additional requirement?

The DRI addresses the issue of availability of vitamin B_{12} and older adults. It recommends that adults older than 50 years use a vitamin B_{12} supplement or foods fortified with the vitamin to ensure adequate bioavailability to prevent potential deficiencies. But what foods should be fortified that older adults are sure to eat? The DRI has also recommended that the level of vitamin D be increased above the levels usually consumed, suggesting the use of vitamin D supplements. This recommendation marks a significant change in philosophy, because supplements of vitamin D had been discouraged because of toxicity issues. Other important questions for health professionals to consider are how will older adults know of these vitamin B_{12} and vitamin D recommendations, and how should the recommendations be implemented?

Nutrition education regarding the use of functional (fortified) foods and appropriate use of supplements is one means of teaching a target population about nutrient needs. When such education is implemented on a broad scale to the public at large, other segments of the population learn of the

TABLE 7-6 Fat-Soluble Vitamins

VITAMIN	FUNCTION	CLINICAL ISSUES DEFICIENCY/TOXICITY	REQUIREMENTS	FOOD SOURCES

Vitamin A
Precursors:
  carotenoids
Preformed vitamin:
  retinoids
	Maintains epithelial tissues (skin and mucous membranes); rhodopsin formation for vision; bone growth; reproduction	Deficiency: xerophthalmia; night blindness; keratomalacia; degeneration of epithelial tissue; inhibited growth (respiratory and gastrointestinal disturbances)
		Toxicity: hypervitaminosis A (from supplements) with blistered skin, weakness, anorexia, vomiting, enlarged spleen and liver
			Men: 900-µg RAE
			Women: 700-µg RAE
			UL 3000-µg RAE
				Deep green, yellow, and orange fruits and vegetables; animal fat sources: whole milk, fortified skim, and low-fat milk; butter; liver; egg yolks, fatty fish

Vitamin D
Precursor:
  7-dehydrocholesterol
Active form:
  cholecalciferol
	Calcium and phosphorus absorption; bone mineralization	Deficiency: bone malformation, rickets (children), osteomalacia (adults)
		Toxicity: hypercalcemia, hypercalciuria
			Adults: 5-µg AI
			(<51 yr 10 µg)
			(<70 yr 15 µg)
			UL 50 µg
				Animal (fat) sources: butter, egg yolks, fatty fish, liver, fortified milk; body synthesis

Vitamin E α-Tocopherol	Antioxidant for polyunsaturated fatty acid and vitamin A; antioxidant with selenium and ascorbic acid	Deficiency: primary deficiency rare; secondary deficiency (caused by fat absorption) neurologic disorders Toxicity: none, but supplements contraindicated with anticoagulation drugs	Adults: 15-mg α-TE UL 1000-mg α-TE	Vegetable oil, whole grains, seeds, nuts, green leafy vegetables
Vitamin K Active form: menaquinones	Cofactor in synthesis of blood clotting factors; protein formation	Deficiency: blood coagulation inhibited; hemorrhagic disease (infants) Toxicity: therapeutic vitamin K (menadione form) reactions in neonates, causing hemolytic anemia and hyperbilirubinemia	Men: 120-µg AI Women: 90-µg AI	Green leafy vegetables, intestinal synthesis

α-TE, Alpha-tocopherol equivalent; AI, Adequate Intake; RAE, retinol activity equivalent; UL, Tolerable Upper Intake Level.

nutrient value. For example, women should be taught the value of folic acid during pregnancy, but men can also be aware of this value so that they can support the implementation of the folic acid goal by the women in their lives. In addition, younger women can become aware of the special nutrient needs of the pregnancy years before they enter them, so that the importance of nutrition during pregnancy is not something new or an afterthought when they are older.

Functional foods may increase the amount of a nutrient in the food supply. Through careful selection of the foods to which specific nutrients are added, increased consumption of the nutrient can be achieved with little effort by the target group. This is a public health approach that affects the community at large. Folic acid fortification provides a safety net for women of childbearing age but only if they consume foods containing the additional folic acid. Supplements may still be warranted.

A third approach to nutrient supplements is an individualized one. Individuals take the supplements on their own. Ideally, a qualified health professional such as a registered dietitian/nutritionist, licensed nutritionist, or primary health

care provider guides the individual as to the need and quantity of the nutrient supplements to be regularly taken. This approach requires the individual to take the responsibility for continued consumption of the supplement, if appropriate.

The optimal approach is the use of all three approaches to achieve nutrient adequacy that takes into account the special needs of subgroups.

Role of the Health Practitioner

Recommendations for use of nutrient supplements should be determined by dietetic professionals such as registered dietitians or by informed primary health care providers. Their counseling evaluates the client's current nutrient intake and assesses his or her dietary supplementation practices and possible interactions with prescribed medical treatments and medications. Foremost in importance is that dietary adequacy should first be met by eating a diverse selection of whole foods while following the basic dietary guidelines of MyPlate with awareness of portion (moderation) sizes.

The role of other health professionals, such as nurses, is to guide the client to the appropriate nutritional counseling to determine the client's actual nutrient status. After counseling has been completed, nurses can support the recommendations of the dietitian through teaching strategies such as how to incorporate more fruits and vegetables into the diet and how to reinforce the understanding of potential drug-nutrient interactions.

TOWARD A POSITIVE NUTRITION LIFESTYLE: SOCIAL SUPPORT

Social support extends throughout the life span; it goes beyond having friends and family with whom to socialize. For families with young children, social support may be cooperative meals when illness strikes (e.g., during a flu epidemic) and cooking time becomes compromised. The term *cooperative* may mean cooking double portions to feed a friend's family during bouts of the croup or childhood ear infections. The kindness would then be reciprocated in the future. Both families gain nutritious meals at times when merely thinking about cooking seems overwhelming.

Support for older adults, as mentioned earlier in this chapter, may mean assistance with food shopping or food delivery. Neighbors or relatives may provide this social support. In some communities, local Red Cross chapters and other charitable organizations have developed car or bus services specifically to provide transportation for older residents. This measure enables individuals to safely shop in food stores and have the convenience of being driven to their homes and helped with carrying groceries into their kitchens. Health care professionals working with older clients should be aware of these services or perhaps help community organizations initiate similar programs.

▮ SUMMARY

- Vitamins are organic molecules that perform specific metabolic functions.
  - Essential nutrients are required in very small amounts.
- Vitamins are divided into water soluble and fat soluble.
  - Solubility of vitamins affects the processes of their absorption, transportation, and storage in our bodies.
- Water-soluble vitamins are vitamin C, choline, and the B complex vitamins (thiamin, riboflavin, niacin, folate, pyridoxine [B_6], vitamin B_{12}, pantothenic acid, and biotin).
  - B vitamins function as coenzymes.
  - Choline is part of a neurotransmitter and lecithin.
  - Vitamin C serves as an antioxidant in addition to its coenzyme ability.

- Water-soluble vitamins are easily absorbed into blood circulation.
  - Excesses are excreted; toxicity is less likely; however, it may occur with pyridoxine and vitamin C.
- Fat-soluble vitamins are vitamins A, D, E, and K.
  - These serve structural and regulatory functions.
- Fat-soluble vitamins are absorbed the same as lipids; bile is required, and the nutrients enter the lymphatic system.
  - These are retained in fatty substances of the body; toxicity from supplemental fat-soluble vitamin intakes is possible.

◎ THE NURSING APPROACH

Case Study: Vitamins and Chronic Alcohol Use

Brad, age 24, worked in a manufacturing plant. His supervisor had been concerned about his frequent absences from work, declining productivity, and noticeable weight loss. When Brad came to work today, he looked unkempt and thin. With alcohol on his breath, he was slurring his words and having difficulty with balance. His coworker reported that Brad had a longtime drinking problem. His supervisor, worried about safety, took Brad to the occupational nurse on site.

Assessment
Subjective (from Patient Statements)

- "Maybe I drank a little too much last night, but I am not an alcoholic."
- "I can't remember how long I have worked here. Am I in trouble because I was late today? Where am I anyway?"
- Complained of headache
- Says he has lost weight, is not interested in eating because food doesn't taste good and his mouth is sore

Objective (from Physical Examination)
- Height 5'10", weight 135 lb
- Blood pressure 110 mm Hg systolic/70 mm Hg diastolic, temperature 98°F, pulse 92 bpm, respirations 21 breaths/min
- Ataxia (muscle weakness and loss of coordination)
- Alcohol on breath, speech slurred
- Stomatitis (inflamed mouth and gingiva)
- Pale conjunctiva

Diagnoses (nursing)
1. Imbalanced nutrition: less than body requirements related to probable chronic alcohol use and inadequate food intake as evidenced by alcohol on breath, reported weight loss, 81% ideal body weight (IBW), ataxia, stomatitis, and pale conjunctiva
2. Probable ineffective coping related to chronic alcohol use

◎ THE NURSING APPROACH—cont'd

Planning
Patient Outcomes
Short term (at the end of this visit):
- Brad will eat at least two meals per day and take a multiple vitamin with minerals each day.
- He will identify foods he can eat without irritation to his mouth.

Long term (at follow-up visit in 1 month):
- Brad will report that he took a multiple vitamin with minerals every day, and he will participate in a more thorough nutrition assessment.
- He will weigh at least 2 more pounds.
- He will have no alcohol on his breath, stable balance, less inflammation in his mouth, and pink conjunctiva

Nursing Interventions
1. Encourage Brad to decrease or avoid alcohol intake.
2. Encourage him to increase food intake and take a multiple vitamin with minerals every day.

Implementation
1. Sent a blood sample to the lab for complete blood count and hemoglobin and hematocrit, ferritin, and albumin measurements.
   Pale conjunctiva could indicate anemia. Weight loss and muscle weakness could be a result of inadequate food intake and toxicity from alcohol.
2. Recommended that Brad stop drinking alcohol and start taking a multiple vitamin with minerals every day.
   Alcohol inhibits the absorption of thiamin while increasing the need for it. Insufficient thiamin can lead to decreased mental alertness, short-term memory loss, and ataxia (muscle weakness and loss of coordination). Lack of riboflavin can cause stomatitis. Lack of vitamin B₆, folate, and iron can cause anemia. Vitamin supplements ensure adequate intake of vitamins when diets are not consistently well balanced.
3. Encouraged him to eat small frequent meals high in protein, vitamins, and calories.

Small, frequent meals are more easily absorbed than large meals and are easier to tolerate when a person has anorexia. Protein, vitamins, and sufficient calories are needed for healing and weight gain.

4. Gave him a list of nonirritating dietary sources of protein and vitamins (especially B vitamins).
   Milk products are high in protein. Cold, smooth foods are soothing to a sore mouth: puddings, eggnog, milkshakes, ice cream, yogurt, cottage cheese, instant breakfast drinks, and supplements like Ensure. Soy milk could be substituted if Brad has lactose intolerance. Other foods that would help provide vitamins include bland fruits without peelings, soft-cooked vegetables; refined enriched breads, cereals, and pasta; and tender pork, tuna, and chicken.
5. Set up an appointment for a follow-up visit in 1 month.
   Follow-up is needed to evaluate health status and changes made.
6. Encouraged Brad to see a counselor to help him reduce his alcohol intake.
   An alcohol rehabilitation program is likely indicated.

Evaluation
Short term (at the end of the visit):
- Brad said he could take a vitamin each day and eat ice cream more often. He couldn't remember any other dietary recommendations but did take the list of foods.
- He declined to see a counselor about his alcohol intake but said he would come back in a month to see the nurse again.

Short-term goals partially met. Brad did not return for a follow-up visit in the nurse's office.

Discussion Questions
1. How could the nurse encourage Brad to come to the nurse's office for follow-up?
2. What additional information would the nurse need to obtain in order to confirm or rule out her nursing diagnoses?
3. How does alcoholism contribute to malnutrition? What food could provide the vitamins that Brad may be lacking?

❓ APPLYING CONTENT KNOWLEDGE

Mark, age 3, is having his yearly health examination. His mom, rather proudly, tells you that Mark eats one apple and carrot sticks every day. She says that means he gets all the vitamins he needs. How do you respond?

▌ WEBSITES OF INTEREST

MedlinePlus
www.nlm.nih.gov/medlineplus/
Provides reliable data about diseases, conditions, and wellness including nutrition. Created by the National Institutes of Health as a service of the U.S. National Library of Medicine.

U.S. Food and Drug Administration Center for Food Safety and Applied Nutrition
www.cfsan.fda.gov
Supplies FDA policies, rules, and FDA Talk Papers pertaining to supplements and health claims on foods.

WebMD
www.webmd.com
Offers strategies for managing health by providing accurate health and medical reference information, including online community interaction.

REFERENCES

Bemeur C, Butterworth RF: Thiamin. In Ross AC, et al, editors: *Modern nutrition in health and disease*, ed 11, Philadelphia, 2014, Lippincott Williams & Wilkins.

Brousseau TJ, et al: Vitamin K deficiency mimicking child abuse, *J Emerg Med* 29(3):283–288, 2005.

Carmel R: Cobalamin (vitamin B₁₂). In Ross AC, et al, editors: *Modern nutrition in health and disease*, ed 11, Philadelphia, 2014, Lippincott Williams & Wilkins.

DaSilva VR, et al: Vitamin B₆. In Ross AC, et al, editors: *Modern nutrition in health and disease*, ed 11, Philadelphia, 2014, Lippincott Williams & Wilkins.

Fain O, et al: Scurvy in patients with cancer, *BMJ* 316:1661–1662, 1998.

Gessner BD, et al: Nutritional rickets among breast-fed black and Alaska Native children, *Alaska Med* 39(3):72–74, 1997.

Heiss C, et al: Flavanols and cardiovascular disease prevention, *Eur Heart J* 31(21):2583–2592, 2010.

Hollick MF: Resurrection of vitamin D deficiency and rickets, *J Clin Invest* 116(8):2062–2072, 2006.

Hwang SL, et al: Neuroprotective effects of citrus flavonoids, *J Agric Food Chem* 60(4):877–885, 2012.

Jones G: Vitamin D. In Ross AC, et al, editors: *Modern nutrition in health and disease*, ed 11, Philadelphia, 2014, Lippincott Williams & Wilkins.

Kertesz SG: Pellagra in 2 homeless men, *Mayo Clin Proc* 76(3):315–318, 2001.

Kirkland JB: Niacin. In Ross AC, et al, editors: *Modern nutrition in health and disease*, ed 11, Philadelphia, 2014, Lippincott Williams & Wilkins.

Levine M, Padayatty SJ: Vitamin C. In Ross AC, et al, editors: *Modern nutrition in health and disease*, ed 11, Philadelphia, 2014, Lippincott Williams & Wilkins.

Marra MV, Boyar AP: American Dietetic Association: Position of the American Dietetic Association: Nutrient supplementation, *J Am Diet Assoc* 109:2073–2085, 2009.

Mock DM: Biotin. In Ross AC, et al, editors: *Modern nutrition in health and disease*, ed 11, Philadelphia, 2014, Lippincott Williams & Wilkins.

National Research Council (NRC): *Dietary reference intakes: The essential guide to nutrient requirements*, Washington, DC, 2006, The National Academies Press.

Pagana KD, Pagana JT: *Mosby's diagnostic and laboratory test reference*, ed 11, St Louis, 2012, Mosby.

Prousky JE: Pellagra may be a rare secondary complication of anorexia nervosa: a systematic review of the literature, *Altern Med Rev* 8(2):180–185, 2003.

Ross AC: Vitamin A. In Ross AC, et al, editors: *Modern nutrition in health and disease*, ed 11, Philadelphia, 2014, Lippincott Williams & Wilkins.

Said HM, Ross AC: Riboflavin. In Ross AC, et al, editors: *Modern nutrition in health and disease*, ed 11, Philadelphia, 2014, Lippincott Williams & Wilkins.

Stover PJ: Folic acid. In Ross AC, et al, editors: *Modern nutrition in health and disease*, ed 11, Philadelphia, 2014, Lippincott Williams & Wilkins.

Suttie JW: Vitamin K. In Ross AC, et al, editors: *Modern nutrition in health and disease*, ed 11, Philadelphia, 2014, Lippincott Williams & Wilkins.

Tang G, et al: Golden Rice is an effective source of vitamin A, *Am J Clin Nutr* 89(6):1776–1783, 2009.

Traber MG: Vitamin E. In Ross AC, et al, editors: *Modern nutrition in health and disease*, ed 11, Philadelphia, 2014, Lippincott Williams & Wilkins.

Wood B, et al: Pellagra in a woman using alternative remedies, *Australas J Dermatol* 39(1):42–44, 1998.

CHAPTER 8

Water and Minerals

An ever-circulating ocean of fluid bathes all the cells in our bodies; this fluid allows for chemical reactions, transmission of nerve impulses, and transportation of nutrients and waste products throughout the body.

http://evolve.elsevier.com/GRODNER/FOUNDATIONS

LEARNING OBJECTIVES

- List the functions of water.
- Describe dietary sources of water.
- Explain the diverse roles of minerals.
- List and define major and trace minerals.

- Discuss plant and animal food sources of minerals.
- Explain the different levels of bioavailability of the food sources of minerals.

ROLE IN WELLNESS

An ever-circulating ocean of fluid bathes all the cells in our bodies; this fluid allows for chemical reactions, transmission of nerve impulses, and transportation of nutrients and waste products throughout the body. The fluid is not simply water, although water is its primary constituent. Some fluid in the body is used to form blood, lymph, and structure for cells. Minerals circulating in our body fluids create the setting for biochemical reactions to occur.

Water and minerals affect every system of our bodies, as well as our six dimensions of health. *Physical health* dimension depends on adequate levels of these nutrients. *Intellectual health* dimension is compromised when iron levels are low; iron deficiency affects cognitive abilities and thus diminishes the ability to learn. *Emotional health* may rely on our being sufficiently hydrated with fluids; cases of fluid volume deficit or dehydration have been mistaken for senility when the thirst acuity of older adults diminishes. *Social health* dimension may be affected if older adults become debilitated by bone fractures or osteoporosis caused by chronic calcium deficiencies; social mobility may be limited as their physical movement is inhibited. Vegans who consume no animal-derived foods because of spiritual health beliefs need carefully designed eating plans that provide adequate levels of zinc, iron, and calcium to avoid deficiencies. The *environmental health* dimension impacts access to safe and plentiful sources of water, a nutrient essential to health.

Although water and minerals are primary components of body fluids, they perform other functions as well. This chapter explores water and minerals in the context of their nutritional requirements and physiologic roles in achieving nutritional wellness.

WATER

We can live several weeks without food but can survive only a few days without water or fluids. Although our bodies use stored nutrients to fuel energy needs, a minimum intake of water is required for cell function and as a solution through which waste products of the body are excreted in urine.

We need water in our diets every day.

Food Sources

If we drank only water and no other liquids, we could meet our body's need for fluid. Most of us, however, consume fluids in addition to water throughout the day. Some fluids also contain other nutrients. Consider the wealth of nutrients found in milk (skim or whole), fruit juices, and soups. Some fruits and vegetables contain as much as 85% to 95% water. Watermelon, grapes, oranges, lettuce, tomatoes, and zucchini have high water content. Most foods contain water, but some are better sources of fluids than others. Generally, we depend on beverages as our main source of fluids.

The Adequate Intake (AI) recommendations for water are about 13 cups a day for men and 9 cups a day for women. This amount is in addition to fluids from foods consumed throughout the day, such as fruits and vegetables (National Research Council [NRC], 2006). Although the minimum amount needed by healthy adults may be about 4 cups, higher amounts are optimum, considering an individual's physiologic status and energy output.

Our primary source of water should be the liquids we drink (Table 8-1). Notice that coffee, tea, alcohol, and soft drinks are not listed as primary sources. Although they do contain water, coffee, tea, and alcohol act as diuretics, which cause an increase in water loss via the kidneys as urine. Soft drinks add fluid to the body, but they contain solutes (sugar, salt, various chemicals) that must be diluted as they enter the bloodstream. Drinking a soda increases the concentration of these solutes in the blood. The body responds by pulling fluid from the cells into the bloodstream to dilute the sugar and salt. The body loses the increased fluid in the bloodstream when it is excreted as urine. In addition, the body responds to the increased solutes and decreased fluid content by once again triggering the thirst mechanism.

Bottled water has become a mainstay in U.S. beverage selections and an economic force. Sales of bottled water have reached to more than $11 billion (Beverage Marketing Corporation, 2013). Products range from imported sparkling mineral waters to spring waters to waters treated from nearby reservoirs. Although the price range is equally broad, the common denominator is that Americans enjoy the convenience of water as a beverage when available in portable containers and single portions.

Water Quality

The minerals found naturally in water vary. Hard water refers to water that contains high amounts of minerals such as calcium and magnesium. Drinking this water can provide a significant amount of these nutrients. Non–nutrition-related problems from hard water can develop; mineral deposits may damage appliances and other machinery that interacts with water, and soap suds are reduced. To diminish these problems, a filtration process can be installed to soften water by replacing some minerals with sodium chloride (salt). Soft water containing sodium, however, can be a problem for sodium-sensitive individuals, such as those at risk for hypertension. To prevent health problems, water softeners may be

TABLE 8-1 Foods as Sources of Water (by Percentage)

FOOD	PERCENTAGE WATER
Dairy Products	
Milk	88-91
Cheddar cheese	37
Cottage cheese	79
Ice cream, ice milk	61-66
Fruits	
Apples	84
Grapefruit (whole or juice)	90
Grapes	81
Melons	90
Oranges (whole or juice)	88
Vegetables	
Asparagus	91
Carrots	88
Cucumber	96
Lettuce	96
Potato	75
Spinach	90
Sweet potato	73
Tomatoes	94
Miscellaneous	
Beans (cooked)	60-70
Bread	30-40
Fruit punch	88
Gelatin	84
Meats	50-60
Oatmeal (cooked)	85
Poultry	65
Soups	85-98

Data from U.S. Department of Agriculture, Agricultural Research Service, Nutrient Data Laboratory: *USDA national nutrient database for standard reference* (Release 26), 2012. Accessed May 24, 2014, from www.ars.usda.gov/ba/bhnrc/ndl.

used on only the hot tap in kitchens, leaving the cold tap unsoftened for consumption.

Another aspect of water quality is contamination. For example, many older buildings have pipes with lead solder joints that can release lead into the water that sits in or runs through them. If the level of lead in water is more than 15 parts per billion (ppb), pregnant women, infants, and children are advised to drink bottled water because even low levels of lead can seriously impair normal development. The local health department can recommend a competent laboratory that tests household water quality.

To reduce the chance that lead will leak into drinking and cooking water, do the following:

- Run the water for 2 minutes after it has been standing in the pipes.
- Use only cold water for drinking, cooking, and preparing baby formula (cold water absorbs less lead than hot).

Water treatment processes can remedy some contamination concerns. Others, such as industrial pollution, can be difficult to identify. Complications of bacterial contamination or inadvertent exposure of water to carcinogenic industrial substances can lead to health problems that range from simple gastroenteritis to cancer. Municipal and regional water processing plants take great care to ensure the safest water supply possible. Some water sources (private wells, surface water, springs, and cisterns), however, may exceed the maximum contaminant levels set by the Environmental Protection Agency (EPA).

The most severe water-related threats, such as cholera and typhoid, are no longer public health hazards in North America. Other potential industrial and environmental pollutants, however, can enter our water supply and endanger our health. Small suppliers may not have the financial means to improve technologic surveillance.

Poorer countries throughout the world continue to struggle with unsafe water supplies (see the *Cultural Considerations* box Do Not Take Water for Granted). Without the financial and technologic knowledge and resources, many people become ill by consuming bacteria-contaminated water. Increased incidence of stomach cancer is associated with exposure to *Helicobacter pylori*, which is sometimes found in contaminated waters.

Water as a Nutrient in the Body
Structure

The structure of water—two hydrogen atoms bonded to one oxygen atom—allows it to provide a base for biochemical reactions in the body and to easily move through the various compartments of cells and body systems. As the basis of body fluids, water can host other substances of different electrical charges and characteristics. Intracellular fluids (within the cell) are composed of water plus concentrations of potassium and phosphates. Interstitial fluids (between the cells) contain concentrations of sodium and chloride. Extracellular fluids consist of interstitial fluid and encompass all fluids outside cells, including plasma and the watery components of body organs and substances (Box 8-1).

Digestion and Absorption

Because water is inorganic, it is not digested. It passes quickly to the small intestine. Once there, most water is absorbed; the

---

🌐 **CULTURAL CONSIDERATIONS**

Do Not Take Water for Granted

Here in our highly developed system, we have access to safe and plentiful water for drinking, bathing, and all of the other countless uses for water to maintain our way of life. Much of the world is not as fortunate. The following, from the World Health Organization (WHO) of the United Nations, is the FACT FILE on global water scarcity. Review these facts and consider how such limitations affect the lives of people throughout the world.

FACT FILE: Water Scarcity

Fact 1: Water scarcity occurs even in areas where there is plenty of rainfall or freshwater. How water is conserved, used, and distributed in communities and the quality of the water available can determine whether there is enough to meet the demands of households, farms, industry, and the environment.

Fact 2: Water scarcity affects one in three people on every continent of the globe. The situation is getting worse as needs for water rise along with population growth, urbanization, and increases in household and industrial uses.

Fact 3: Almost one fifth of the world's population (about 1.2 billion people) live in areas where the water is physically scarce. One quarter of the global population also live in developing countries that face water shortages due to a lack of infrastructure to bring water from rivers and aquifers.

Fact 4: Water scarcity forces people to rely on unsafe sources of drinking water. It also means they cannot bathe or clean their clothes or homes properly.

Fact 5: Poor water quality can increase the risk of such diarrheal diseases as cholera, typhoid fever and dysentery, and other water-borne infections. Water scarcity can lead to diseases such as trachoma (an eye infection that can lead to blindness), plague, and typhus.

Fact 6: Water scarcity encourages people to store water in their homes. This practice can increase the risk of household water contamination and provide breeding grounds for mosquitoes—which are carriers of dengue fever, malaria, and other diseases.

Fact 7: Water scarcity underscores the need for better water management. Good water management also reduces breeding sites for such insects as mosquitoes that can transmit diseases and prevents the spread of water-borne infections such as schistosomiasis, a severe illness.

Fact 8: A lack of water has driven up the use of wastewater for agricultural production in poor urban and rural communities. More than 10% of people worldwide consume foods irrigated by wastewater that can contain chemicals or disease-causing organisms.

Fact 9: Millennium Development Goal* number 7, target 10, aims to halve, by 2015, the proportion of people without sustainable access to safe drinking water and basic sanitation. Water scarcity could threaten progress to reach this target.

Fact 10: Water is an essential resource to sustain life. As governments and community organizations make it a priority to deliver adequate supplies of quality water to people, individuals can help by learning how to conserve and protect the resource in their daily lives.

Modified from World Health Organization (WHO): *10 facts about water scarcity.* Accessed February 2, 2014, from www.who.int/features/factfiles/water/water_facts/en/index.html.
*The United Nations established eight goals for international development, called Millenium Development Goals, in 2000.

BOX 8-1   Body Fluid Compartments

Intracellular Fluid (65% of Body Water)	Extracellular Fluid (35% of Body Water)
Enzymes	Antibodies
Hemoglobin	Bicarbonate ions
Magnesium	Blood proteins
Minerals	Carbohydrates
Phosphorus	Chloride
Potassium	Glucose
Proteins	Minerals
	Proteins
	Lipids
	Lipoproteins
	Sodium

BOX 8-2   Functions of Water

Provides shape and rigidity to cells
Helps regulate body temperature
Acts as a lubricant
Cushions body tissues
Transports nutrients and waste products
Acts as a solvent
Provides a source of trace minerals
Participates in chemical reactions

---

rest is regulated by the colon and is either absorbed or excreted with feces.

Metabolism

Although not metabolized or broken down by gastrointestinal (GI) tract processes, water is an integral component of metabolic processes. In some reactions, the water of metabolism is water released as a byproduct of oxidative reactions; in others, water may be a part of the process to release energy from adenosine triphosphate (ATP), which is discussed in greater detail in Chapter 9. The released water may be excreted as waste or used elsewhere in the body. Glycogen in muscle and the liver contains water in the structure of glycogen molecules. When glycogen is used for energy, the water becomes available for body functions.

Functions

Water performs a variety of vital functions in the body (Box 8-2). It is an important structural component of the body, giving shape and rigidity to cells. It assists in regulating body temperature. Water conducts heat, absorbing and distributing it throughout the body, keeping body temperature stable from day to day. Water also helps cool the body by evaporating invisibly from the lungs and the surface of the skin, carrying off excess heat. This type of water loss is called **insensible perspiration**.

Water acts as a lubricant in the form of joint fluid and mucous secretions. It forms a shock-absorbing fluid cushion for body tissues such as the amniotic sac, spinal cord, and eyes.

Water is a major component of blood, lymph, saliva, and urine. As such, it delivers nutrients and removes waste products. Acting as a **solvent**, it enables minerals, vitamins, glucose, and other small molecules to be moved throughout the body.

Water may also supply trace minerals such as fluoride, zinc, and copper. Sometimes it is a source of too many minerals, including potentially toxic metals such as lead, cadmium, and incidental substances from pesticides and industrial waste products.

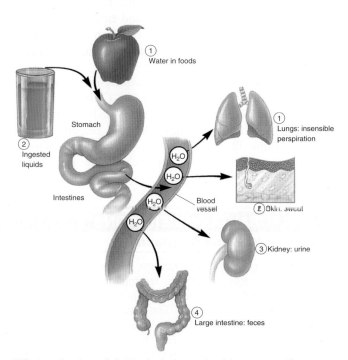

FIG 8-1 Intake of fluids is balanced with output. (Courtesy Joan Beck. Modified from Thibodeau GA, Patton KT: *The human body in health and disease*, ed 2, St Louis, 1997, Mosby.)

In addition to serving as a medium for biochemical reactions, water also participates as a reactant. A **reactant** is a substance that enters into and is altered during a chemical reaction. For example, large molecules such as polysaccharides, fats, and protein are split into smaller molecules; water participates in and is changed by the process.

Ultimately, no growth or cell renewal occurs without water; it is part of every cell and is necessary as a medium for reactions and transporter of supplies.

Regulation of Fluid and Water in the Body

Our bodies have delicate but efficient mechanisms for maintaining appropriate fluid levels. The intake of fluids is balanced with the output through urine, sweat, feces, and insensible perspiration (Figure 8-1). Regulation of fluid in the body is of physiologic importance because water makes up 50% to 60% of the weight of an average adult; the percentage is are even higher for an infant, whose body weight is 75% to 80% water (Figure 8-2). Fortunately, all we need to do is take

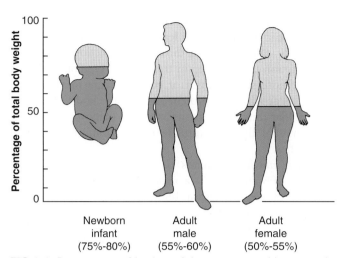

FIG 8-2 Percentage of body weight represented by water in infants compared with that in adults. (From Rolin Graphics. In Thibodeau GA, Patton KT: *Structure and function of the body,* ed 10, St Louis, 1997, Mosby.)

in enough fluids and our bodies' natural systems take care of the rest.

Homeostasis (physiologic equilibrium) is maintained by electrolytes that include minerals and blood proteins. Two of the most important minerals are sodium and potassium. The extracellular distribution of fluid depends on sodium, and potassium influences intracellular water. Water moves within and between the cells in interstitial fluids in response to the levels of these minerals. An imbalance is corrected by mechanisms that cause thirst and regulate the ability of the kidneys to release or retain fluids.

Thirst, a dryness in the mouth, stimulates the desire to drink liquids. We often ignore our thirst until mealtimes. The thirst mechanism is controlled by the hypothalamus and involves several steps. The sodium and solute levels in blood rise as the water level in the body gets low. This causes water to be drawn from the salivary glands to provide more fluid for the blood. The mouth then feels dry because less saliva, which keeps the mouth moist, is produced. This sensation, thirst, stimulates the drinking process. If the thirst mechanism is faulty, as it may be during illness, physical exertion, or aging, hormonal mechanisms also help conserve water by reducing urine output.

The mechanisms of the kidneys regulate the amounts of water excreted. Obligatory water excretion of at least 500 mL (1 pint) must be performed daily, regardless of the amount ingested, to clear the body of waste products. The mechanism relies on the combined actions of the brain, kidneys, pituitary gland, and adrenal gland. When fluid in the body becomes low, the hypothalamus stimulates the pituitary gland to release antidiuretic hormone (ADH). ADH is secreted in response to high sodium levels in the body or too-low blood pressure or blood volume. The target organ of the hormone is the kidney. The kidneys then conserve water by decreasing excretion of water, and the retained fluid is recycled for use throughout the body.

When the sodium concentration in the kidneys gets high (too much fluid excreted), another process kicks in to counteract the lowered blood volume and pressure. The kidneys release renin, an enzyme that activates the blood protein angiotensin. Angiotensin raises blood pressure by narrowing blood vessels; it is a vasoconstrictor. Angiotensin also prompts the adrenal gland to release the hormone aldosterone. The target organ of aldosterone is the kidney. The effect is to decrease excretion of sodium, causing the kidneys to respond by retaining fluid in the body.

Fluid and Electrolytes

Dissolved in body fluids are minerals and other organic molecules required for the regulation of both intracellular and extracellular fluid distribution. Fluids follow salt concentrations; this means that cells can control fluid balance by directing the movement of mineral salts.

Electrolytes are minerals that carry electrical charges or ions (particles) when dissolved in water. These minerals separate into positively charged ions (cations) or negatively charged ions (anions). The primary extracellular electrolytes in body fluids are sodium (Na^+/cation) and chloride (Cl^-/anion), and the primary intracellular electrolyte is potassium (K^+/cation). To maintain fluid balance, cells control the movement of electrolytes. Water will follow sodium concentration. Moving electrolytes in and out of the cell membrane requires transport proteins. The sodium/potassium pump is a transport protein that works to exchange sodium from within the cells for potassium. Other ions are also exchanged.

In addition to water regulation, the kidneys also regulate electrolyte levels. If body levels of sodium are low, aldosterone directs the kidneys to reabsorb or retain more sodium. This in turn results in excretion of potassium so the balance of electrolytes is maintained.

Imbalances

What happens when our regulatory mechanisms are unable to maintain the balance? Abnormal shifts in fluid balance may cause a deficit or excess in fluid volume.

Fluid volume deficit. In fluid volume deficit (FVD), a person experiences vascular, cellular, or intracellular dehydration. FVD can occur from diarrhea, vomiting, or high fever—symptoms often experienced with stomach and intestinal viral infections and influenza. Other causes of excessive fluid loss are sweating, diuretics, and *polyuria* (excessive urination). Whenever we lose fluid and have difficulty taking in additional fluids, we are at risk for FVD.

Determining whether symptoms are caused by dehydration or illness can be difficult. Characteristics of FVD include infrequent urination, decreased skin elasticity, dry mucous membranes, dry mouth, unusual drowsiness, lightheadedness or disorientation, extreme thirst, nausea, slow or rapid breathing, and sudden weight loss. The person with FVD is less able to maintain blood pressure immediately after rising from a sitting or lying position (called *orthostatic hypotension*). A primary health care provider should be consulted for any illness that lasts more than a few days and causes loss of body fluids. In moderate or severe FVD, intravenous (IV) therapy is indicated to replace fluids.

FVD can also happen when we are not ill. Strenuous physical activity, either athletic or work-related, that causes excessive sweating can lead to FVD. Hot, dry weather also can overwork the body's cooling mechanisms. Drinking fluids throughout the day despite a low level of thirst sensation can alleviate these risks.

Older adults and infants are the groups most at risk for FVD. Older adults have decreased fluid reserves and diminished thirst mechanism acuity. FVD symptoms may be misdiagnosed as senility. Reminding older clients to drink even when they are not thirsty is appropriate to ensure adequate intake of fluids. In infants, water makes up a larger percentage of body weight than in adults, and a greater percentage is extracellular fluid; dehydration from fluid loss can occur rapidly. In addition to other signs of FVD, an infant may have a depressed fontanelle (soft spot) in the skull.

Fluid volume excess. Fluid volume excess is a condition in which a person experiences increased fluid retention and edema. It is associated with a compromised regulatory mechanism, excess fluid intake, or excess sodium intake.

Edema is excess accumulation of fluid in interstitial spaces caused by seepage from the circulatory system, which results in the retention of about 10% more water than normal. Some of us may notice that when we eat meals that are particularly high in sodium, we feel bloated, and our weight may even rise a few pounds the next day. This weight gain is not true weight gain but simply water retention that occurs in response to the excess intake of sodium. Within a few days, weight and water levels in the body return to their usual levels.

Edema can be a symptom of a health risk in certain situations. Sodium-sensitive individuals not only retain fluid when consuming high levels of sodium but also experience an increase in blood pressure, leading to hypertension. Reducing excess water retention through a reduction in sodium consumption is a first step in treating this type of hypertension. A more serious form of edema occurs in victims of kwashiorkor when the protein levels in the body are so low that cellular fluid levels are imbalanced. Inappropriate levels of interstitial fluid accumulate in the stomach, face, and extremities.

Water intoxication refers to the consumption of large volumes of water within a short time, which results in a dilution of electrolytes in body fluids. It causes muscle cramps, decreased blood pressure, and weakness. Water intoxication is also possible if there is extensive loss of electrolytes because of dehydration and rehydration is accomplished using only water, without the addition of replacement electrolytes. This condition is relatively rare but tends to occur when athletes continually hydrate without equivalent loss of fluid while participating in slower-paced events such as runs lasting longer than 4 hours or extended triathlons, or they rehydrate after a strenuous event with excessive amounts of water. Nonetheless, fluid volume deficit, dehydration, is much more common and more dangerous for athletes.

MINERALS

Minerals serve a variety of functions in our bodies (Box 8-3). Structurally, minerals provide rigidity and strength to the teeth and skeleton; the skeletal mineral components also serve as a storage depot for other needs of the body. Minerals, allowing for proper muscle contraction and release, influence nerve and muscle functions. Other functions of minerals are acting as cofactors for enzymes and maintaining proper

---

BOX 8-3   Considering Vitamins and Minerals Through Function

Vitamins and minerals are discussed as two separate nutrient categories in Chapter 7 and this chapter. Although each essential vitamin and mineral is discussed individually, they are not grouped together on the basis of their functions for the body. The information here provides vitamins and minerals required for the specific body functions blood health, bone health, energy metabolism, and fluid and electrolyte balance. Additional functions of individual vitamins and minerals may be found in Tables 7-3, 7-6, 8-3, and 8-4.

Blood Health

Blood is *the* body fluid, supplying tissues with oxygen, nutrients, and energy through circulation within the cardiovascular system. It is composed of water, red and white blood cells, oxygen, nutrients, and other formed substances. Always moving, blood gathers and distributes nutrients and oxygen to all cells and disposes of waste products. Deficiency of any of these nutrients will affect overall blood health. Only the blood-related functions of the vitamins and minerals are listed.

VITAMIN*	FUNCTION	MINERAL†	FUNCTION
Cobalamin (B₁₂)	Transport/storage of folate needed for heme and cell formation and other functions	Iron	Distributes oxygen in hemoglobin and myoglobin
Folate (folic acid, folacin, PGA)	Coenzyme metabolism (synthesis of amino acid, heme, DNA, RNA) and other functions	Zinc	Cofactor for more than 200 enzymes, including enzymes to make heme in hemoglobin, genetic material and proteins
Pyridoxine (B₆)	Hemoglobin synthesis and other functions	Copper	Helps with iron use
Vitamin K Active form: menaquinones	Cofactor in synthesis of blood clotting factors; protein formation		

BOX 8-3   Considering Vitamins and Minerals Through Function—cont'd

Bone Health

As living tissue, bone requires nutrients to maintain cellular structure. Blood circulates through bone capillaries, delivering nutrients while removing waste materials no longer needed by cells. Hormones regulate the use of minerals either for storage and structural purposes in bone or for controlling body processes. Specific vitamins and minerals are indispensable for these functions to occur.

VITAMIN*	FUNCTION	MINERAL[†]	FUNCTION
Vitamin D Precursor: 7-dehydrocholester Active form: cholecalciferol	Bone mineralization	Calcium	Bone and tooth formation
Vitamin K Active form: menaquinones	Protein formation for bone mineralization; cofactor for blood-clotting factors	Phosphorus	Bone and tooth formation (component of hydroxyapatite)
Vitamin A Precursors: carotenoids Preformed vitamin: retinoids	Bone growth; maintains epithelial cells; regulation of gene expression	Magnesium Fluoride	Bone structure Bone and tooth formation; increases stability of bone

Energy Metabolism

In order to metabolize carbohydrates, lipids, and protein for energy and other needs, the body depends on many nutrients to support the process, create new cells, and implement various related functions.

VITAMIN(S)*	FUNCTION	MINERAL[†]	FUNCTION
Thiamin (B$_1$)	Coenzyme energy metabolism; muscle nerve action	Iodine	Thyroxine synthesis (thyroid hormone) regulates growth and development; basal metabolic rate (DMN) regulation
Riboflavin (B$_2$)	Coenzyme energy metabolism	Chromium	Carbohydrate metabolism, part of glucose tolerance factor
Niacin (B$_3$) (nicotinic acid and niacinamide)	Cofactor to enzymes involved in energy metabolism; glycolysis and tricarboxylic acid (TCA) cycle synthesis	Phosphorus Sulfur Iron	Energy metabolism (enzymes) Component of protein structures Distributes oxygen in hemoglobin and myoglobin
Precursor: tryptophan			
Pyridoxine (B$_6$)	Forms coenzyme pyridoxal phosphate (PLP) for energy metabolism		
Folate (folic acid, folacin, PGA)	Coenzyme metabolism (synthesis of amino acid, heme, DNA, RNA)		
Cobalamin (B$_{12}$)	Metabolism of fatty acids/amino acids	Zinc	Carbohydrate metabolism (insulin function); cofactor to more than 200 enzymes
Pantothenic acid	Part of coenzyme A		
Biotin	Metabolism of carbohydrate, fat, and protein		

Fluid and Electrolyte Balance

Life systems depend on fluid and electrolyte balance within the body. Electrolytes consist of mineral salts that maintain cellular fluid balance. The acid-base balance of body fluids is buffered by other minerals.

MINERAL[†]	FUNCTION
Sodium	Major extracellular electrolyte for fluid regulation; body fluid levels; acid-base balance; nerve impulse and contraction; blood pressure/volume
Potassium	With sodium and chloride, major intracellular electrolyte for fluid regulation; muscle function
Chloride	Acid-base balance
Phosphorus	Acid-base balance

*See Chapter 7 for additional information on vitamins.
[†]See text for additional information on water and minerals.

BOX 8-4   Essential Minerals in the Human Body

Major	Trace
Calcium	Chromium
Chloride	Copper
Magnesium	Fluoride
Phosphorus	Iodine
Potassium	Iron
Sodium	Manganese
Sulfur	Molybdenum
	Selenium
	Zinc

acid-base balance in body fluids. Minerals are also required for blood clotting and for tissue repair and growth.

Mineral Categories

On the basis of the amount of each mineral in the composition of our bodies, the 16 essential minerals are divided into two categories: major and trace minerals. To maintain body levels of major minerals, the minerals must be consumed daily from dietary sources in amounts of 100 mg or higher. In contrast, trace minerals are required daily in amounts less than or equal to 20 mg (Box 8-4). Although the required amounts differ greatly between the major and trace minerals, each is absolutely necessary for good health.

The Dietary Reference Intakes (DRIs) listed in this chapter for minerals are those for young adults ages 19 to 30 years (NRC, 2006). Levels for other groups are noted when special mention is needed. Keep in mind that because nutrition is a relatively young science, new functions of minerals as nutrients in the human body are still being discovered.

Food Sources

The prime sources of minerals are both plant and animal foods. Valuable sources of plant foods include most fruits, vegetables, legumes, and whole grains. Animal sources consist of beef, chicken, eggs, fish, and milk products. The discussions of individual minerals highlight the best food choices (Box 8-5).

In contrast to vitamins, minerals are stable when foods containing them are cooked. As inorganic substances, they are indestructible. Minerals may leach into cooking fluids but can still be absorbed if the fluid is consumed.

Although plants may contain an abundance of various minerals, some minerals in plants are not easily available to the human body. *Bioavailability* refers to the level of absorption of a consumed nutrient and is of nutritional concern. Binders such as phytic and oxalic acids may bind some minerals to the plant fiber structures. *Binders* are substances in plant foods that combine with minerals to form indigestible compounds, making them unavailable for our use. The amount of plant minerals available for absorption may depend on minerals in soils in which the plants are grown.

Minerals from animal foods do not have the same bioavailability issues. In fact, minerals from animal foods can be absorbed more easily than those from plants. However, fat content may be an issue for some animal foods. Lower-fat sources of dairy and meat products are usually available and provide the same levels of minerals at a higher nutrient density. Liver is often cited as a good source of minerals such as iron and zinc. But liver is also high in cholesterol and saturated fats and may contain toxins to which the animal may have been exposed. These factors, combined with liver's somewhat unusual taste, often leave the impression that good nutrient intake depends on eating healthy food that tastes bad. Other sources of each nutrient may be more appealing and equally as nutritious.

Food processing may reduce the amount of minerals available for absorption. Processing oranges into orange juice does not affect potassium levels naturally contained in oranges. However, processing whole-wheat flour into white flour does cause significant loss of minerals because the whole grain is not used. Iron is the only mineral returned to white flour through enrichment; zinc, selenium, copper, and other minerals are permanently lost.

Because we have difficulty obtaining high enough levels of some minerals naturally, fortification of manufactured foods has become commonplace. It is through fortification that food processing can serve the nutrient needs of consumers while still addressing the issues of convenience and taste appeal. Salt fortified with iodine is available; dry cereals have added minerals such as iron and an assortment of vitamins and other minerals.

Minerals as Nutrients in the Body

Structure

Minerals are inorganic substances. As elements, they are found in the rocks of the earth. Their tendency to gain or lose electrons makes them electrically charged. Thus, they have special affinities for water, which itself carries positive and negative charges. As we consume plant and animal foods containing minerals, we can incorporate them into our body structures (bones), organs, and fluids.

Digestion and Absorption

During the process of digestion, minerals (as inorganic substances) are separated from the foodstuffs in which they entered our bodies. Digestion does change the valence states of some minerals, thereby changing their ability to be absorbed. However, their structure is not changed so they can be absorbed.

As noted, bioavailability affects the level of minerals we actually absorb. Generally, consuming a variety of whole foods ensures an adequate intake of minerals. Mineral deficiencies for which Americans tend to be at risk are those of iron, calcium, and zinc. Concerns and strategies for consuming appropriate amounts of these nutrients are discussed later in this chapter.

BOX 8-5 MyPlate: Vegetables

As noted in Chapter 7, the health benefits of eating vegetables overlap with those of eating fruits. Both fruit and vegetable MyPlate categories provide rich sources of minerals and are valuable components of an overall healthy diet, providing nutrients essential for the health and maintenance of our bodies (also see Box 7-2). Health benefits of eating vegetables and fruits as part of an overall health diet include reduced risk for stroke, coronary vascular disease (CVD), and type 2 diabetes mellitus; protection against some cancers (mouth, stomach, colorectal); and, because they are excellent sources of fiber, possible decrease in risk of several chronic diet-related disorders. The recommendation is to eat at least 2½ cups of vegetables every day.

What Counts as a Cup?

In general, 1 cup of raw or cooked vegetables or vegetable juice, or 2 cups of raw leafy greens can be considered 1 cup from the vegetable group. The following lists specific amounts count as 1 cup of vegetables (in some cases equivalents for ½ cup are also shown) toward your recommended intake.

VEGETABLE	AMOUNT THAT COUNTS AS 1 CUP OF VEGETABLES	AMOUNT THAT COUNTS AS ½ CUP OF VEGETABLES
Dark Green Vegetables		
Broccoli	1 cup, chopped or florets 3 spears, 5 inches long, raw or cooked	
Greens (collards, mustard greens, turnip greens, kale)	1 cup cooked	
Spinach	1 cup cooked 2 cups raw = 1 cup	1 cup raw = ½ cup
Raw, leafy greens: spinach, romaine, watercress, dark green leafy lettuce, endive, escarole	2 cups raw = 1 cup	1 cup raw = ½ cup
Orange vegetables		
Carrots	1 cup; strips, slices, or chopped; raw or cooked 2 medium 1 cup baby carrots (approximately 12)	1 medium Approximately 6 baby carrots
Sweet potato	1 large, baked (2¼ inches or more in diameter) 1 cup sliced or mashed, cooked	
Winter squash (acorn, butternut, hubbard)	1 cup cubed, cooked	¾ acorn squash, baked = ¾ cup
Dry beans and peas		
Dry beans and peas (such as black, garbanzo, kidney, pinto beans; soybeans; black-eyed, split peas)	1 cup whole or mashed, cooked	
Tofu	1 cup - ½-inch cubes (approximately 8 oz)	1 piece, 2½ inches × 2¾ inches × 1 inch (approximately 4 oz)
Starchy vegetables		
Corn, yellow or white	1 cup 1 large ear (8-9 inches long)	1 small ear (approximately 6 inches long)
Green peas	1 cup	
White potatoes	1 cup diced, mashed 1 medium boiled or baked potato (2½ to 3 inches in diameter) French-fried: 20 medium to long strips (2½ to 4 inches long) (contains discretionary calories)	
Other vegetables		
Bean sprouts	1 cup cooked	
Cabbage, green	1 cup, chopped or shredded, raw or cooked	
Cauliflower	1 cup, pieces or florets, raw or cooked	

Continued

BOX 8-5   MyPlate: Vegetables—cont'd

VEGETABLE	AMOUNT THAT COUNTS AS 1 CUP OF VEGETABLES	AMOUNT THAT COUNTS AS ½ CUP OF VEGETABLES
Celery	1 cup, diced or sliced, raw or cooked	
	2 large stalks (11-12 inches long)	1 large stalk (11-12 inches long)
Cucumbers	1 cup raw, sliced or chopped	
Green or wax beans	1 cup cooked	
Green or red peppers	1 cup chopped, raw, or cooked	1 small pepper
	1 large pepper (3 inches in diameter, 3¾ inches long)	
Lettuce, iceberg or head	2 cups raw, shredded or chopped = 1 cup	1 cup raw, shredded or chopped = ½ cup
Mushrooms	1 cup raw or cooked	
Onions	1 cup chopped, raw or cooked	
Tomatoes	1 large raw, whole (3 inches)	1 small raw, whole (2¼ inches)
	1 cup chopped or sliced; raw, canned, or cooked	1 medium, canned
Tomato or mixed vegetable juice	1 cup	½ cup
Summer squash or zucchini	1 cup cooked, sliced or diced	

Modified from U.S. Department of Agriculture, Center for Nutrition and Promotion: *ChooseMyPlate.gov: What counts as a cup of vegetables?* Accessed February 2, 2014, from www.choosemyplate.gov/printpages/MyPlateFoodGroups/Vegetables/food-groups.vegetables-counts.pdf.

Metabolism

Because minerals are inorganic and do not provide energy, they are not metabolized by the human body. Instead, some minerals assist as cofactors of metabolic processes.

MAJOR MINERALS

Calcium

Function

Calcium is the most abundant mineral in the body. Almost all of the calcium in the body, about 99%, is found in our bones, serving structural and storage functions. The other 1% of body calcium is released into body fluids when blood passes through bones; this constant interaction of blood with bone allows calcium to be distributed throughout the body. Other functions that depend on calcium include (1) the central nervous system, particularly nerve impulses; (2) muscle contraction and relaxation, when needed; (3) formation of blood clots; and (4) blood pressure regulation. Continuing research supports that increased levels of calcium (and vitamin D) intakes may be protective for colorectal cancer (Weaver and Heaney, 2014).

Regulation

Our dietary intake of calcium influences the deposition of calcium in our bones. Blood calcium levels, however, do not depend on a daily dietary calcium intake. Instead, the skeletal supply of calcium provides the source of calcium to be distributed throughout the body through the circulatory system. If calcium blood levels get too low, three actions can occur to reestablish calcium homeostasis: bones release calcium, intestines absorb more calcium, and kidneys retain more calcium.

Hormones that regulate the level of calcium in body fluids control the release of calcium from bones. Hormones affecting blood levels include parathormone (parathyroid hormone), calcitriol (active vitamin D hormone), and calcitonin. Parathormone is secreted by the parathyroid gland in response to low blood calcium levels. It raises blood calcium levels by stimulating all three ways of providing calcium to body fluids. Vitamin D has a hormone-like effect as calcitriol and increases blood calcium levels by acting on all three systems. The third hormone involved, calcitonin, is released by the special C cells of the thyroid gland. Calcitonin reacts in response to high blood levels of calcium by lowering both calcium and phosphate in the blood.

Reactions of very low or extremely high blood levels can occur if regulatory mechanisms are hindered by a lack of vitamin D or hormone malfunction. If calcium blood levels get too high, calcium rigor (with symptoms of hardness or stiffness of muscles) may occur. Conversely, if levels are too low, a person may experience calcium tetany, with spasms caused by muscle and nerve excitability.

Recommended Intake and Sources

Calcium AI for men and women ranges from 1300 mg per day (ages 9 through 13) to 1000 mg (ages 19 through 50). Levels increase to 1200 mg for men and women older than 50 years. The AI during pregnancy and lactation is 1000 mg.

Concerns have been raised regarding the calcium intake of those most at risk for deficiency: youths ages 11 through 24 and pregnant and lactating women. During adolescence, pregnancy, and lactation, calcium needs are still high, although actual consumption of calcium may decrease. For many Americans, meeting these recommendations means increasing the number of servings of calcium-rich foods to at least three or more a day (Box 8-6). Other issues surrounding calcium intake and children are discussed in Chapter 10.

Primary sources of calcium are dairy products, mainly milk (whole, low-fat, and skim) and milk-based products

BOX 8-6 MyPlate: Milk

MyPlate focuses on the milk group of foods as a source of the minerals calcium and potassium and vitamin D and protein. These nutrients can also be obtained from non–milk-derived foods, but milk products are rich sources and are a traditional part of the dietary intake of most Americans.

Health benefits of consuming foods in the milk group include assisting the building and maintaining of bone mass during the life span, particularly during childhood and adolescence; possible reduced risk of osteoporosis; and overall higher quality of nutritional intake. The recommendation is to consume 3 cups or servings daily of milk or milk products. If milk products are not consumed because of lactose intolerance, lactose-reduced products, calcium-fortified foods, and other naturally good sources of calcium can be chosen instead.

What Counts as a Cup?

In general, 1 cup of milk, yogurt, or soymilk (soy beverage), 1½ ounces (oz) of natural cheese, or 2 oz of processed cheese can be considered 1 cup from the dairy group.

The table lists specific amounts that count as 1 cup in the dairy group towards your daily recommended intake.

	AMOUNT THAT COUNTS AS A CUP IN THE DAIRY GROUP	COMMON PORTIONS AND CUP EQUIVALENTS
Milk (choose fat-free or low-fat milk)	1 cup milk 1 half-pint container milk ½ cup evaporated milk	
Yogurt (choose fat-free or low-fat yogurt)	1 regular container (8 fluid oz) 1 cup yogurt	1 small container (6 oz) = ¾ cup 1 snack size container (4 oz) = ½ cup
Cheese (choose reduced-fat or low-fat cheeses)	1½ oz hard cheese (cheddar, mozzarella, Swiss, Parmesan) ⅓ cup shredded cheese 2 oz processed cheese (American) ½ cup ricotta cheese 2 cups cottage cheese	1 slice of hard cheese is equivalent to ½ cup milk 1 slice of processed cheese is equivalent to ⅓ cup milk ¼ cup of cottage cheese is equivalent to ¼ cup milk
Milk-based desserts (choose fat-free or low-fat types)	1 cup pudding made with milk 1 cup frozen yogurt 1½ cups ice cream	1 scoop of ice cream is equivalent to ⅓ cup milk
Soymilk (soy beverage)	1 cup calcium-fortified soymilk 1 half-pint container calcium-fortified soymilk	

Key Consumer Message: *Switch to fat-free or low-fat (1%) milk.*

Modified from U.S. Department of Agriculture, Center for Nutrition and Promotion: *ChooseMyPlate.gov: What counts as a cup in the dairy group?* Accessed February 2, 2014, from www.choosemyplate.gov/food-groups/dairy-counts.html.

---

such as ice cream, ice milk, yogurt, frozen yogurt, cheeses, and puddings (Figure 8-3). Although butter, cream cheese, and cottage cheese are dairy products, they are not good sources of calcium; butter and cream cheese are predominantly fat, and cottage cheese loses calcium through processing. Non-dairy sources include green leafy vegetables (broccoli, kale, and mustard greens), small fish with bones (sardines and salmon canned with processed edible bones), legumes, and tofu processed with calcium. In addition, a variety of calcium-fortified foods are available, ranging from fortified orange juice to bread products. Box 8-7 lists foods that boost calcium intake, and the *Teaching Tool* box Visualizing the Calcium

Values of Foods provides calcium education strategies for working with clients who have low literacy skills.

Some leafy green vegetables—in particular, spinach, collards, Swiss chard, and escarole—contain oxalic acid, a binder that reduces the calcium absorbed. Plant foods containing oxalic acid cannot be considered a trustworthy source of calcium. Tea contains oxalic acid as well as tannins (also found in coffee), both of which may affect the absorption of calcium in foods consumed with tea. With the increased consumption of iced tea beverages, this effect should be considered, particularly for female adolescents and young adults.

FIG 8-3 Calcium can be consumed in many different foods, including beans, milk (animal-derived or fortified), yogurt, cheese, canned sardines and salmon, broccoli, kale, and other leafy greens.

✳ TEACHING TOOL

Visualizing the Calcium Values of Foods

Food charts that show the calcium values of different foods may be helpful to most people, but they may be meaningless to clients who cannot read English or have minimal literacy skills. Consider this innovative teaching strategy for visualizing the calcium content of commonly consumed foods (e.g., skim milk, yogurt, hard cheese), as follows:

1. Select four calcium-rich foods and four low-calcium foods (e.g., cottage cheese, broccoli, pinto beans).
2. Fill plastic resealable bags with small marshmallows to represent the calcium content of each of the selected foods. Each marshmallow can represent 10 mg of calcium. In addition, fill a large plastic resealable bag with 100 marshmallows (1000 mg or 100% Daily Value) as a reference.
3. Match the bag of "calcium" with the appropriate food model (or picture). Have the participants do the matching.
4. Distribute a pictorial representation of this activity with additional foods along with their bags of "calcium."

Courtesy Gayle Coleman, MS, RD, when employed at State University Extension, East Lansing.

Many adults are lactose intolerant. Lactose intolerance occurs when the body does not produce enough lactase, an enzyme necessary for the digestion of lactose, the carbohydrate found in milk. (Lactose intolerance is detailed in Chapter 4.) People experiencing lactose intolerance need to regularly incorporate sources of calcium other than dairy products into their dietary patterns. For some people, calcium supplements may be indicated; a registered dietitian or qualified nutritionist may be consulted.

Some calcium supplements are poorly absorbed because they don't dissolve in the stomach. If a calcium tablet doesn't readily dissolve when stirred into cider vinegar, it probably will not dissolve in the body.

BOX 8-7 Suggestions For Boosting Calcium Intake

Dairy
Melted cheese added to broccoli
Calcium-fortified milk and cottage cheese
Powdered milk added to baking mixes, soups, puddings, gravies, hamburgers, and meat loaves
Eating cheese wedges with sliced apples and pears
Smoothies (fruit drinks made with milk, yogurt, and fruits)
Soups made with low-fat or skim milk

Nondairy
Bean burritos
Bean soups (split pea or lentil soup)
Breads fortified with calcium
Chicken cacciatore (chicken with bones cooked in tomato sauce; acid of tomatoes pulls calcium from bones)
Juices fortified with calcium
Soy milk and soy products fortified with calcium
Tofu (made with calcium carbonate), fresh or in frozen meals and desserts

Absorption Factors

Our bodies absorb calcium on the basis of physiologic need. During childhood growth phases, we may absorb up to 75% of calcium consumed, compared with absorption rates of 30% to 60% once we complete our primary growth years. Similarly, during pregnancy and lactation, percentages of absorption are higher as dictated by physiologic need (Weaver and Heaney, 2014). In addition to physiologic need, other factors also seem to enhance the levels of calcium absorbed, including the following (Box 8-8):

Lactose: Found naturally in milk (an excellent source of calcium), lactose appears to increase calcium absorption.

Sufficient vitamin D: Vitamin D is involved in the synthesis of a protein that allows calcium to pass through the intestinal wall into the bloodstream.

Acidity of digestive mass: Calcium is more soluble in acidic substances, so it is better absorbed when ingested as part of a meal. Generally, enough hydrochloric acid passes from the stomach to the intestine for calcium absorption. As we age, the amount of hydrochloric acid in digestive juices may decrease, causing less calcium to be absorbed.

Binders: Naturally occurring substances in plant foods may bind with calcium in plant foods; two common calcium binders are phytic and oxalic acids (also called *phytates* and *oxalates,* respectively). Human digestive processes may be unable to separate calcium from the binder; both are then excreted, reducing the calcium available for absorption.

Dietary fat: Dietary fat can form insoluble soaps with calcium; the insoluble soaps are harder to digest, making calcium less accessible for absorption. Moderate and low dietary fat intakes discourage the formation of this insoluble mass.

High-fiber intake and laxatives: Excessive fiber consumption or laxative abuse results in food stuff moving through the

BOX 8-8 Factors Favoring and Hindering Calcium Absorption

Factors Favoring Calcium Absorption
Acidity of digestive mass
Body's need for higher amounts (as in pregnancy)
Lactose
Sufficient vitamin D

Factors Hindering Calcium Absorption
Aging
Binders such as phytic acid and oxalic acid
Dietary fat
Dietary fiber
Drug use
Excessive phosphorus intake
Laxative use
Sedentary lifestyle

Typical posture in osteoporosis. (From Shipley M. *A colour atlas of rheumatology*, ed 3, London, 1993, Mosby-Year Book Europe Limited. By permission of Mosby International Ltd.)

GI tract too quickly for minerals, particularly calcium, to be absorbed.

Excessively high intakes of phosphorus or magnesium: Excessively high intakes of these minerals disturb the balance of calcium in the body. Calcium is best absorbed when moderate or recommended levels of phosphorus and magnesium are ingested in proportion to calcium intake.

Sedentary lifestyle: Being a couch potato has its consequences. A physically inactive lifestyle leads to less bone density. In contrast, weight-bearing exercise that pulls the muscle against the bone enhances calcium deposits in the bone matrix. This action occurs during running, brisk walking, biking, and strength training.

Drugs: Some medications, including anticonvulsants, tetracycline, cortisone, thyroxine, and aluminum-containing antacids, are associated with reduced calcium absorption.

Deficiency

Deficiency of calcium primarily affects bone health. During the growing years, inadequate intake of calcium reduces the density of bone mass and, if severe, can stunt growth. For adults, long-term calcium deficiency may be one of the risk factors for *osteoporosis*, a multifactorial systemic skeletal disorder. This condition takes many years to develop, and overt symptoms appear late in life. Osteoporosis is a condition in which bone density is reduced and the remaining bone is brittle and breaks easily.

One of the most recognizable characteristics of osteoporosis is the dowager's hump; as vertebrae in the spine collapse from weakness, the spine is no longer able to support the weight of the head. The back bows and the head angles down. Most significantly, the internal organs affected by the curvature are unable to function efficiently, and other health difficulties develop.

In contrast to *osteomalacia*, osteoporosis is multifactorial, and all the factors are tied to bone mineral density. These factors include genetics, diet, and lifestyle determinants. Bone density builds through early adulthood. Peak bone density is reached by about age 20, although some additional bone mineralization continues into the 30s. The more density built early in life, the less potential risk encountered. Factors that affect bone density but cannot be modified include genetic determinants of race and gender and family history, as follows:

Race: Osteoporosis is more common in white and Asian women than among African and African American women. The reason is racial differences in the skeletal density, possibly caused by hormonal differences.

Gender: Men have greater bone density than women and enter the later years, when bone demineralization begins, with a larger storage of calcium. The fact that men have more lean body mass or muscularity may cause more calcium to be deposited and retained in comparison with women. Women lose greater amounts of bone calcium during the first few years after menopause. The drop in estrogen levels appears to initiate the calcium loss. To slow the loss and to provide additional protection against heart disease, many primary health care providers prescribe hormone (estrogen) replacement therapy for postmenopausal women.

Family history: A predisposition to lower bone density may be genetically passed between generations, particularly from mother to daughter. If a close family member is diagnosed with osteoporosis, one should take care to reduce the effects of other risk factors.

Osteoporosis, however, does occur in men and women. For men, osteoporosis tends to be a result of secondary causes that affect peak bone mass development or speed the loss of bone density. These causes are steroid therapy, chronic alcoholism, hypogonadism, skeletal metastasis, multiple myeloma, gastric surgery, and anticonvulsant treatment (Jacobs-Kosmin, 2013). Men and women who undergo organ transplantation are more at risk for osteoporosis, particularly during the first year after surgery. The loss of bone density is probably caused by the medications used to prevent organ rejection, such as glucocorticoids, that disturb bone and mineral homeostasis. Osteoporosis prevention can begin before transplantation if bone density is marginal, or therapy can be implemented immediately following transplantation (Fratianni, 2013).

Factors related to development of osteoporosis that can be adjusted include nutrition, particularly calcium intake, and lifestyle determinants, as follows:

Nutrition/calcium intake: Dietary calcium intake is of concern throughout the life span. In particular, the growth years (when calcium is deposited in the bone matrix) and the postmenopausal years of bone mineralization loss are periods when calcium intake appears crucial. Although the AI for calcium provides sufficient amounts, many individuals consume less than these levels. Female adolescents often consume levels of kcal and nutrients well below the AI while attempting to control body weight. These eating patterns often continue through adulthood. This long-term marginal deficiency of calcium may set the stage for future bone disorders. The issue is even more complicated for older adults. When they consume calcium-containing foods, they may absorb less calcium because of decreased gastric acidity and lower levels of available vitamin D.

Alcohol: Long-term excessive intake of alcohol appears to reduce bone density. Alcohol may directly depress bone formation or may take the place of more nutritious foods, producing marginal deficiencies.

Smoking: Cigarette smoking has been associated with a higher risk of osteoporosis. Smokers tend to be of lower weight (less bone density) than nonsmokers, and women who smoke appear to lose more bone mineralization after menopause than those who don't.

Caffeine: Caffeine consumption has been tied to urinary excretion of calcium. Reasonable use of caffeinated beverages, however, may be acceptable. More than likely, the relationship of caffeine to lower levels of body calcium concerns replacement by caffeinated beverages of those containing calcium, such as skim milk and other calcium-fortified beverages. Although caffeinated coffee consumption may affect bone density of postmenopausal women, adequate calcium intake can overcome these effects (Tucker and Rosen, 2014)

Sedentary lifestyle: A physically active lifestyle not only enhances calcium absorption but also helps maintain bone matrix mineralization. However, excessive exercise that results in extremely low body fat levels for women may be detrimental to bone density. If amenorrhea (abnormal cessation of menses) occurs because of excessive exercise, the resulting premature drop in estrogen may limit or decrease bone mineralization during the prime growth periods. Similarly, girls and women experiencing anorexia nervosa lose significant bone density within a year of onset and have a greater risk of hip fracture later in life. Boys and men with anorexia nervosa are at similar risk for osteoporosis and its complications (Coughlin, et al, 2014).

Although the risk factors for osteoporosis may seem overwhelming, several can be reduced by following basic recommendations for achieving wellness. Consuming the serving amounts recommended by MyPlate and engaging in regular physical exercise can minimize most of the risk. The *Teaching Tool* box Calcium: By Any Means Possible provides tips on educating clients on appropriate calcium intake.

Low levels of calcium intake are also associated with an increased risk of colon cancer and hypertension.

Toxicity

Calcium toxicity from consuming foods that contain calcium is not a concern. Problems may occur when supplements of calcium and other nutrients are used instead of foods. Over-supplementation may cause constipation, urinary stone formation affecting kidney function, and reduction in absorption of iron, zinc, and other minerals (Weaver and Heaney, 2014). The general guideline for calcium supplements is that levels should not exceed the AI for calcium. In addition, a Tolerable Upper Intake Level (UL) of 2500 mg has been established.

Phosphorus
Function

Most of the phosphorus in the body (85%) is in our bones and teeth as a component of hydroxyapatite, a natural mineral structure. The other 15% of body phosphorus has functions (1) in energy transfer; (2) as part of the genetic material of deoxyribonucleic acid (DNA) and ribonucleic acid (RNA); (3) as a buffer in the form of phosphoric acid, which balances body acid-base levels; and (4) as a component of phospholipids used for transportation and structural functions.

Recommended Intake and Sources

The Recommended Dietary Allowance (RDA) for phosphorus is 700 mg per day for men and women aged 19 years and older. Phosphorus is widely available in foods. Particularly good sources are protein-rich foods such as dairy foods, eggs, meat, fish, poultry, and cereal grains. Because of the processing of convenience foods and soft drinks, both are also sources of phosphorus.

Deficiency

Deficiency of phosphorus is unknown. It is part of the genetic material of every cell of the body.

Toxicity

Excessive amounts of phosphorus, usually possible only from phosphorus supplements, cause calcium excretion from the body. Very high phosphorus intakes could affect the calcium/phosphorus ratio, possibly reducing the amount of calcium

✳ TEACHING TOOL

Calcium: By Any Means Possible

The adequate intake (AI) for calcium ranges from 1000 to 1300 mg per day, depending on a person's age. The best sources are calcium-rich foods. But what if a client is lactose-intolerant or just doesn't like many calcium-containing foods?

Because the potential ramifications of chronic calcium deficiency are serious—fractures and other complications of osteoporosis—calcium supplementation may be appropriate. Following are some suggestions and cautions for client education:

- Calcium supplementation may increase the dietary intake of calcium, but it does not alleviate other risk factors associated with osteoporosis. Other nutrients and lifestyle behaviors also affect the level of risk. Popping a calcium pill does not mean a person is osteoporosis-free.
- Many people have problems with compliance; the regularity of calcium intake, not an occasional dose, builds dense bones. It is better to rely on food sources.
- The source of calcium affects the amount of actual calcium available. Tablets composed of calcium carbonate contain more elemental calcium (often 500-600 mg) than those made of calcium citrate or lactate (usually 200 mg per tablet), and it takes fewer pills to achieve the AI. Calcium citrate, however, is more easily absorbed by the digestive tract, even if more pills are needed.

- Be aware that calcium is always combined with another substance to form the tablet. A tablet may contain 1200 mg of calcium carbonate but only 500 mg of elemental calcium. The supplements to avoid are those made from dolomite, bone meal, and oyster shell; they may be contaminated with lead and other toxic metals.
- Although the tablets are supplementing dietary intake, it's best to take them with meals. The acid of the digestive process also helps in the breakdown and absorption of the calcium tablet(s), and tying the supplement to meals works as a reminder system. This also helps to spread supplementation throughout the day. One large dose will not be absorbed as well as two or three smaller doses.
- Calcium supplements often contain added vitamin D. The new vitamin D recommendation doubles after age 50 and triples after age 70, so the added vitamin D may be age appropriate. If other sources provide sufficient amounts of vitamin D, such as multivitamin/mineral supplements or foods or cereals fortified with 100% of the daily value for vitamin D, then the added D is not necessary.
- Before starting a supplement, keep track of sources and amounts of dietary calcium for several days. Intake may be adequate. If not, first contemplate ways to increase intake with foods, and then consider supplementation.

absorbed. This is a problem only if calcium intake is inadequate. Because phosphorus-containing soft drinks and convenience foods have replaced milk beverages and less processed foods for many American teens and adult women, this may be a dietary concern. A UL of 4000 mg has been determined for phosphorus.

Magnesium

Function

As with calcium and phosphorus, most of the magnesium in the body is found in our bones, providing structural and storage functions. Magnesium assists hundreds of enzymes throughout the body. It also regulates nerve and muscle function, including the actions of the heart, and has a role in the blood clotting process and in the immune system.

Recommended Intake and Sources

The RDAs for magnesium are 400 mg per day for men (420 mg for men 31 years and older) and 310 mg for women (320 mg for women 31 years and older). Many commonly eaten foods contain magnesium. Particularly good sources are most unprocessed foods, including whole grains, legumes, broccoli, leafy green vegetables, and other vegetables. Hard water can be a significant source of magnesium.

Deficiency

Magnesium deficiency tends to be related to secondary causes rather than due to a primary lack of magnesium consumption. These secondary causes include excessive vomiting and

diarrhea caused by pathologic conditions. A GI tract disorder may affect magnesium absorption, or kidney disease may inhibit retention of the mineral. Malnutrition and alcoholism may also have a negative impact on magnesium levels in the body. Similarly, drug interference or artificial feeding solutions deficient in magnesium may influence total body levels of magnesium. Whenever body fluids are lost, so is magnesium. Individuals on long-term regimens of diuretic agents are also at risk for deficiency.

In addition, if magnesium intake levels are borderline and intake of calcium is high, such as from calcium supplements, magnesium absorption may be limited.

Symptoms of magnesium deficiency include twitching of muscles, muscle weakness, and convulsions. In children, magnesium deficiency also may be associated with growth failure.

Toxicity

Toxic effects of magnesium are rare but serious and are due to nondietary sources such as supplements and mineral salts. A UL of 350 mg pertains to nonfood sources. Self-supplementation with calcium tablets containing magnesium while also taking magnesium supplements adds up to an excess that is not seriously toxic but is excessive enough to cause long-term diarrhea and deficient fluid volume (dehydration). This situation is an example of why all medications and dietary supplements should be reported to health care providers before invasive and/or costly procedures are conducted to determine the cause of symptoms. Simply stopping the magnesium supplementation will most likely restore proper function of the large intestine.

Sulfur

Function

Sulfur is a component of protein structures. It is present in every cell of the body and is part of several amino acids, thiamine, and biotin. Sulfur is also involved in maintaining the acid-base balance of the body.

Recommended Intake and Sources

No DRI has been established for sulfur. Diets adequate in protein provide sufficient amounts of sulfur. Sulfur is found in all protein-containing foods.

Deficiency

Deficiencies of sulfur do not occur; sulfur is so basic to the structure of the human cell that deficiencies cannot develop.

Toxicity

Toxicity to sulfur is not a health issue.

ELECTROLYTES: SODIUM, POTASSIUM, AND CHLORIDE

Electrolytes are minerals circulating in blood and other body fluids that carry an electrical charge. Maintaining a balance of these minerals is important because of their effect on body processes such as the amount of water in the body, blood pH, and muscle action. Electrolytes travel in blood as acids, bases, and salts and include sodium, calcium, potassium, chlorine, magnesium, and bicarbonate. Laboratory studies of blood serum determine electrolyte values.

Sodium, potassium, and chloride are major electrolytes of the body. As electrolytes, these minerals serve specific functions. The acid-base balance of body fluids depends on regulated distribution of these minerals, proteins, and other electrolytes. Electrolytes also have a role in the normal functioning of nerves and muscles. In addition, each mineral serves other specific functions in the body.

Sodium

Function

Sodium performs a variety of important functions in the body. Blood pressure and volume are maintained by the characteristics of sodium as the major cation in extracellular fluid. Transmission of nerve impulses relies on body sodium levels. As the major extracellular electrolyte, sodium has a role in the regulation of body fluid levels in and out of cells. This movement affects blood volume as well, which is tied to the thirst mechanism and total body fluid levels. The blood proteins, such as albumin, that prevent the development of some types of edema also regulate blood volume.

Recommended Intake and Sources

The AI for sodium is 1500 mg per day for adults or about ¾ teaspoon of salt (sodium chloride). The AI lowers to 1300 mg

FIG 8-4 Daily salt intakes: Adequate Intake of sodium (1500 mg) equals ¾ tsp salt (*on the left*); excessive consumption of processed and fast food products may result in an intake of sodium that equals 3 tsp salt (6000 mg) (*on the right*). The UL for sodium (2,300 mg) equals about 1 tsp, while the average American intake (3,300 mg) equals 11/2 tsp salt.

for adults 51 to 70 years of age. This dietary recommendation is based on the known adequate intake required for good health (Figure 8-4).

The average American adult consumes about 3300 mg of sodium a day, much higher than the AI for all ages. Professional health organizations such as the American Medical Association, the American Public Health Association, and the American Heart Association and other scientific groups support reduction of our dietary sodium intake. To achieve that goal, recommendations are to reduce daily intake to less than 2300 mg. For individual 51 years old and older, African Americans, and people with hypertension, chronic kidney disease, and/or diabetes, a goal of 1500 mg is suggested (Institute of Medicine, 2013).

Most sodium enters our diet as sodium chloride (table salt). Sodium occurs naturally in many foods. It is also added to foods as salt during the cooking process and right before consumption (see the *Cultural Considerations* box A [Cooking] History of Salt). Processing of foods, particularly quick-serve foods, often adds substantial amounts of sodium, as listed in Table 8-2. Processed foods are carriers for other additives that often contain sodium. The sodium adds flavor that may be lost in processing.

Do you salt your food first, and then taste it? Some habits are hard to break but are worth the effort. However, breaking the salt-shaker habit will reduce sodium intake only 15% for most Americans; most of the sodium eaten comes from processed foods.

The more a foodstuff is processed, the higher the sodium content becomes (see Box 8-8). More nutrients are also lost along the way. Which is saltier, or to be more exact, which contains more sodium—a bowl of corn flakes or a large order of fast-food fries? The corn flakes win, containing 290 mg of sodium compared with 200 mg for the fries. Of course, the fries contain a lot more fat and calories.

TABLE 8-2 Effects of Processing on Sodium Content of Foods

FOOD PRODUCT	TOTAL SODIUM CONTENT (mg)
Potatoes	
Baked potato (1)	16
French-fried potatoes (10 strips)	108
Scalloped potatoes from dry mix (1 cup)	835
Chicken	
Baked chicken (3 oz)	64
Batter-fried chicken (3 oz)	231
Chicken nuggets (6 pieces)	542
Oats	
Oatmeal prepared with water (1 cup)	2
Oatmeal bread (1 slice)	124
Ready-to-eat cereal (1 cup)	307
Apples	
Apple (1)	Trace
Applesauce (1 cup)	8
Apple pie (1 slice)	476

Data from U.S. Department of Agriculture, Agricultural Research Service, Nutrient Data Laboratory: *USDA national nutrient database for standard reference* (Release 26), 2012. Accessed May 24, 2014, from www.ars.usda.gov/ba/bhnrc/ndl.

🌐 CULTURAL CONSIDERATIONS

A (Cooking) History of Salt

The course of history has been influenced by salt. Nations explored the world in search of salt because of its value in preserving foods. Bacterial and mold cells are inhibited from growing when placed in a concentrated salt solution, thus decreasing food spoilage. Though salt is no longer needed to preserve foods, we continue to value its ability to transform the taste of a dish from bland to sublime. Salt's importance to the human body cannot be denied because we have specialized taste buds to identify its consumption. Salt as a compound of sodium chloride contains two essential minerals without which the human body cannot survive.

Recognition of the importance of salt to human life began early. In the Old Testament of the Bible, salt was identified as an offering to God. Later on, Roman soldiers were given a stipend, called *salarium,* to buy salt. Today we can buy salt with our "salaries," a term that is derived from *salarium.* "Salt of the earth" was a phrase used by Jesus to describe his followers who were pure and of the earth.

Application to nursing. Although salt has its virtues, it also has drawbacks. Health professionals continue to recommend moderate intakes of sodium to reduce the risk of hypertension. The amounts recommended for cooking vary because an amount that is pleasing to one person may vary for another. Amounts of salt listed in a recipe can usually be modified to suit the health and taste requirements of the cook and the eaters.

Data from McGee H: *On food and cooking: The science and lore of the kitchen,* New York, 1997, Firestone; and O'Neill M: Let it pour, *New York Times Magazine,* Oct 22, 1995, p. 77.

Consider the potato. A plain baked potato contains only 16 mg of sodium. Prepared at a local fast-food restaurant, a baked potato with cheese sauce and broccoli skyrockets to having more than 400 mg of sodium and lots of fat. A cheese or sour cream mix prepared at home is even higher in sodium—close to 600 mg. The sodium in plain mashed potatoes from a mix (dehydrated and then reconstituted) jumps from 8 mg in its original whole form to more than 300 mg, and that's without butter or gravy. The point is that processing foods adds invisible sodium as sodium chloride; in fact, it's so invisible that we can no longer taste the saltiness.

Sodium enjoys widespread use in the American diet as a flavoring agent (sodium chloride, monosodium glutamate [MSG], sodium saccharin), dough conditioner (baking powder, baking soda), and preservative (sodium sulfite). Because of consumer demand, lower-sodium versions of many products are available. Nutrition labeling information must include sodium content. This is powerful information that allows for comparing the sodium contents of similar products.

Deficiency

Depletion of sodium can develop through dehydration or excessive diarrhea. Because of concern over the relationship between sodium and hypertension, some people may overly restrict sodium and thus be at risk for deficiency. Typical athletic activity or physical labor that produces excessive sweating may cause dehydration and sodium loss, but drinking fluids and consuming foods containing sodium soon restore body levels of sodium. Salt tablets, once a common remedy, are not recommended and may be dangerous.

Symptoms of sodium deficiency include headache, muscle cramps, weakness, reduced ability to concentrate, and loss of memory and appetite. For most people, sodium deficiency is unlikely to occur because we get enough sodium naturally from foods. These symptoms are similar to those of fluid volume deficit, which is more common.

Hyponatremia, or low blood sodium, may occur. The symptoms are the same as for sodium intake deficiency. Hyponatremia may be acute, as a one-time episode due to specific factors, or chronic—that is, a recurring condition. Acute hyponatremia is of concern for endurance athletes. Athletes completing endurance events or slower runners in marathon races who continually drink fluid without an equivalent loss of fluid through sweat or urination may so overhydrate as to experience hyponatremia. This condition is rare, but awareness is important, because medical treatments for fluid volume deficit and acute hyponatremia are different even though the symptoms are the same. Blood testing determines the cause of the symptoms. Chronic hyponatremia may occur because of secondary disorders such as neurologic and kidney disorders that affect the fluid regulatory mechanisms of the body. Blood levels of sodium decrease as excess fluid is retained or too much sodium is excreted by the kidneys. Drug and dietary treatments may address chronic hyponatremia (Bailey, et al, 2014).

Toxicity

The UL for sodium is 2300 mg. An excess sodium intake is difficult for the body to handle. The kidneys have the primary responsibility to flush out the excess sodium. Some individuals are sodium sensitive and may experience hypertension and edema in response to high intake of sodium. Levels consumed in diets based on highly processed foods and high-sodium foods may be enough to initiate hypertension in sodium-sensitive individuals. Although others may not experience negative ramifications of high-sodium intakes, there are no benefits either. This is one of the few nutrients that we can overdose on from foods we consume.

An occasional very salty meal may produce edema but not hypertension. The best remedy for occasional edema is simply to drink more water to equalize the sodium concentration of body fluids. The kidneys take care of the rest by filtering out the excess sodium.

Potassium

Function

Although sodium as a cation maintains the fluid levels extracellularly, potassium, as the primary intercellular cation, maintains fluid levels inside the cells. Potassium is also crucial for normal functioning of nerves and muscles, including the heart.

Recommended Intake and Sources

The AI for potassium is 4700 mg per day. Even though the AI is higher than most Americans consume now, it should lower blood pressure, decrease the negative effects of sodium chloride on blood pressure, reduce the risk of kidney stones, and possibly reduce bone loss. The best sources for potassium for these purposes are the forms found naturally in fruits and vegetables (NRC, 2006).

Sources of potassium include whole unprocessed foods, white potatoes with skin, sweet potatoes, tomatoes, bananas, oranges, other fruits and vegetables, dairy products, and legumes.

Deficiency

Like magnesium deficiency, potassium deficiency may be caused by dehydration from vomiting or diarrhea, diuretics, and misuse of laxatives. If long-term use of diuretics is warranted to reduce edema associated with hypertension, particular attention should be paid to consuming adequate levels of potassium from foods. Some diuretics are potassium wasting; some are potassium sparing. Potassium supplementation with use of a potassium-sparing diuretic could be dangerous. Potassium supplements should be taken only when prescribed by a primary health care provider.

Most often, bananas and oranges are suggested to patients at risk for potassium deficiency. These fruits may not be the best sources according to nutrient content, satiety, and economy. Whereas an *edentulous* (toothless) older person with congestive heart failure who is taking potassium-wasting diuretics and is on a low-income budget can make a meal out of a whole baked potato, he or she cannot be equivalently satisfied with a banana. A baked potato eaten with the skin contains 844 mg of potassium, whereas a whole banana contains 891 mg. A whole orange yields only 326 mg. A potato stores easily without refrigeration for much longer than a banana, and somewhat longer than an orange, and fits better into a tight budget. Yet foods like a simple potato may not be suggested to patients. Nurses can create patient education nutrient/food lists that consider factors such as satiety and economy to enhance compliance.

Symptoms associated with potassium deficiency include muscle weakness, confusion, decreased appetite, and in severe cases, cardiac dysrhythmias.

Toxicity

In general, potassium toxicity occurs only from supplements, not from consuming excess from foods. Toxicity doesn't usually occur with foods as long as a person has properly functioning kidneys. For individuals with renal disease, high-potassium foods are toxic. Even patients undergoing dialysis may still be at risk for potassium toxicity. Symptoms of toxicity are similar to those of a deficiency. They include muscle weakness, vomiting, and at excessively high levels, cardiac arrest.

Chloride

Function

As the key anion of extracellular fluids, chloride assists in maintaining fluid balance inside and outside cells. In addition, chloride is a component of hydrochloric acid, an indispensable gastric juice produced by the stomach.

Recommended Intake and Sources

The AI for chloride is 2300 mg per day for adults. For adults more than 50 years old, the AI is 2000 mg, and for those older than 70 years, 1800 mg. These requirements are easily met by consumption of sodium chloride; foods containing sodium usually provide chloride as well.

Deficiency

Deficiency of chloride is rare; adequate amounts are easily consumed. Although chloride deficiency is possible, it would occur from the same circumstances as sodium deficiency or from excessive vomiting.

Toxicity

Chloride toxicity may occur because of dehydration, which can cause an imbalance of chloride with the other electrolytes. However, the other effects of dehydration are more severe than those of chloride toxicity.

Table 8-3 provides a summary of the major minerals.

TRACE MINERALS

Trace minerals as a group of nutrients function primarily as cofactors by performing metabolic and transport functions.

TABLE 8-3 Major Minerals

MINERAL	FUNCTION	CLINICAL ISSUES DEFICIENCY/TOXICITY	RECOMMENDED DAILY INTAKES*	FOOD SOURCES	ABSORPTION ISSUES
Calcium (Ca)	Bone and tooth formation; blood clotting; muscle contraction/relaxation; central nervous system; blood pressure	Deficiency: reduced bone density; osteoporosis Toxicity: constipation; urinary stones; reduced iron and zinc absorption	AI: Adults: 1000-1200 mg Pregnancy/ lactation: 1000 mg UL: 2500 mg	Milk (whole, low-fat, skim), milk-based products, green leafy vegetables legumes	Absorption based on need: increased by vitamin D; decreased by binders, inactivity, coffee/tea
Phosphorus (P)	Bone and tooth formation (component of hydroxyapatite); energy metabolism (enzymes); acid-base balance	Deficiency: rare Toxicity: increased calcium excretion	RDA: Adults: 700 mg Pregnancy/ lactation: 700 mg UL: 4000 mg	Dairy foods, egg, meat, fish, poultry	Absorbed with calcium
Magnesium (Mg)	Structure/storage; cofactor; nerve and muscle function; blood clotting	Deficiency: secondary with muscle twitching, weakness, convulsions from FVD	RDA: Men: 420 mg Women: 320 mg Pregnancy/ lactation: 320-360 mg UL: 350 mg	Whole grains, legumes, green leafy vegetables (broccoli), hard water	—
Sulfur (S)	Component of protein structures	Deficiency: only with protein malnutrition	Protein-adequate diets contain adequate levels	Protein-containing foods	—
Sodium (Na)	Major extracellular electrolyte for fluid regulation; body fluid levels; acid-base balance; nerve impulse and contraction; blood pressure/volume	Deficiency: FVD with headache; muscle cramps, weakness, decreased concentration, memory and appetite loss Toxicity: sodium-sensitive hypertension	AI: Adults: 1200-1500 mg	Table salt; natural in many foods; processed foods	—
Potassium (K)	Major intracellular electrolyte for fluid regulation; muscle function	Deficiency: muscle weakness, confusion, decreased appetite, cardiac dysrhythmias caused by FVD from vomiting/diarrhea or diuretics Toxicity: from diet or supplements if renal disease present	AI: Adults: 4700 mg	Unprocessed foods, fruits, vegetables, dairy products, meats, legumes	—
Chloride (Cl)	Acid-base balance; gastric hydrochloric acid for digestion	Deficiency: FVD caused by vomiting/diarrhea	AI: Adults: 1800-2300 mg	Table salt	—

AI, Adequate Intake; *FVD*, fluid volume deficit; *RDA*, Recommended Dietary Allowance; *UL*, Tolerable Upper Intake Level.
*Ages 19-30 years.

Iron

Function

Iron is responsible for distributing oxygen throughout our bodies. Oxygen depends on the iron in the hemoglobin (an oxygen-transporting protein) of red blood cells (erythrocytes) to bring oxygen to all cells. Myoglobin (an oxygen-transporting protein) holds oxygen in the muscle cells for quick use when needed. Because of its ability to change ionic charges, iron also assists enzymes in the use of oxygen by all cells of the body.

Iron is conserved and recycled by the body. When red blood cells are old or damaged, the spleen removes their iron component. Some iron is kept in the spleen for later use, and the rest is sent to the liver for processing. From the liver, iron is transported as transferrin to bone marrow and recycled for use in new red blood cells. Some iron is lost through the shedding of tissue cells in urine and sweat and when bleeding occurs; this lost iron must be replaced by dietary sources.

Recommended Intake and Sources

When red blood cells break down, the iron in the hemoglobin is recycled to the liver and used to form new red blood cells. Whenever blood is lost from the body, iron is lost as well and cannot be recycled. Internal bleeding, such as from acute ulcers, can be a deceptive cause of iron loss. More obvious is the loss of blood by women from menstruation. On the basis of this monthly loss and the greater iron demands of pregnancy, women's overall need for iron is higher than men's. The RDA for men is 8 mg, and that for women is 18 mg. During pregnancy the requirement is 27 mg; the blood supply of a pregnant woman is 1.5 times greater than her normal level.

The RDA allows for the unusual absorption rate of dietary iron. Only about 10% to 15% of dietary iron consumed is absorbed; this amount increases up to 20% if body levels are deficient. Higher percentages are absorbed during pregnancy and during periods of growth.

Intestinal mucosal cells contain two proteins that assist in absorption of dietary iron. One protein, *mucosal transferrin*, moves iron to a protein carrier in blood transferrin. This allows for the movement of iron through blood to bone marrow and tissues as needed. The second, *mucosal ferritin*, stores iron in the mucosal cells as a reserve if iron is needed. If not used, mucosal cells are replaced every few days so a continuous short-term supply of iron is available.

The RDA is also set to provide adequate storage levels of iron in the liver; iron is also stored in the spleen and bone marrow. In these organs, iron is contained in the proteins ferritin and hemosiderin. Ferritin is always being made and is easily available as an iron source. Hemosiderin is made when iron levels are high. Although it is a source of iron, hemosiderin must be moved from storage to be used by the body, so it isn't as readily available as ferritin.

Iron is found in both plant and animal sources (Figure 8-5). **Heme iron**, found in animal sources of meat, fish, and poultry, is more easily absorbed than nonheme iron found in plant foods. Animal sources of iron also contain nonheme iron in addition to heme iron. Although egg yolks contain iron, the iron in them is not absorbed as well as other heme from other sources. **Nonheme iron** plant sources include vegetables, legumes, dried fruits, whole-grain cereals, and enriched grain products, especially iron-fortified dry cereals.

Increased absorption of iron occurs when dietary sources are consumed with foods containing ascorbic acid (vitamin C). For example, drinking orange juice or eating slices of cantaloupe with meals increases the amount of nonheme iron absorbed. Absorption of nonheme iron increases in the presence of heme iron. This means that consuming iron from several sources improves absorption of the total iron amounts of heme and nonheme iron.

Another way to increase dietary iron intake is to cook foods in cast-iron skillets. Iron in the skillet leaches into the foods, providing an easy means of boosting iron intake.

FIG 8-5 An assortment of foods containing iron includes chicken, spinach, and beans in black bean soup.

Factors that inhibit iron absorption include consumption of foods that contain binders (e.g., phytates and oxalates) that keep the dietary iron from separating from plant sources. Tannins in plants, most notably in teas and coffee, can also interfere with iron absorption. Continual use of antacids and excessive intake of other minerals competes with the absorption sites for iron. Pica, the consumption of nonnutritive substances, creates health problems. When the nonnutritive substances are excreted from the body, minerals are also excreted, decreasing mineral absorption. Pica is discussed in the next section.

Deficiency

Iron deficiency has been a public health problem for many years. Although the incidence has decreased in the United States, most likely because of greater fortification of foods with iron, it is still common for iron deficiency and iron-deficiency anemia to occur among young children, teenage girls, and women of childbearing age. These disorders are more common among minority women of low income who have had many children. In other parts of the world, it is still the most widespread nutrient deficiency, primarily in the developing world. Children and women of childbearing age are most at risk. The effects of iron deficiency can be subtle and may be ascribed to other causes. A range of symptoms accompanies different degrees of deficiency. All levels of iron deficiency affect the availability of oxygen throughout the body.

Iron deficiency occurs when there is reduced supply of iron stores available in the liver. If neither the diet nor body stores can supply the iron needed for hemoglobin synthesis, the number of red blood cells in the bloodstream decreases. The blood hemoglobin concentration also falls. When both the percentage of red blood cells (called *hematocrit*) and the hemoglobin level fall, a health care provider should suspect iron deficiency.

In severe deficiency, the hemoglobin and hematocrit levels fall so low that the amount of oxygen carried in the blood is decreased and the person is pale, tired, and anemic. Iron deficiency anemia is characterized by microcytes or small, pale red blood cells. Physical activity or work may be difficult to perform because not enough oxygen is available for use by the muscles. Cognitive functioning is compromised. In children, developmental delays and learning problems may develop; an iron-deficient child is easily distracted and unable to focus on learning tasks. A person may have a sensation of always feeling cold, as if body temperature cannot be regulated appropriately. The immune system is compromised as well, reflected in decreased wound-healing ability. During pregnancy, iron-deficiency anemia due to inadequate dietary intake is associated with greater risk of premature delivery and low birth weight.

Because infants have received more iron during the past 3 years, a decline in iron-deficiency anemia among American children has occurred. However, prevalence has remained constant among women of childbearing age. The Centers for Disease Control and Prevention (CDC) has made guidelines for use by primary health care providers to prevent, detect, and treat iron deficiency. The guidelines focus on adequate iron nutrition for infants and young children, screening for anemia among women of childbearing age, and the value of low-dose iron supplements for pregnant women.

A form of anemia called *sports anemia* occurs among endurance athletes. As the body adapts to aerobic development from intense exercise, the individual's volume of blood expands. This expansion lowers hemoglobin concentration, producing an appearance of anemia. This condition, however, is not an illness but a positive adaptation of the body.

To alleviate iron deficiency, the cause of the deficiency (either internal loss of blood or lack of dietary intake) needs to be addressed. Children may lack sufficient intake of iron foods. Iron-deficiency anemia may develop in toddlers from drinking too much milk, a poor source of iron, which fills them up and keeps them from eating other iron-containing foods. Women tend to be doubly at risk because of dieting habits and female physiology. Long-term dieting may affect the intake of iron-rich foods; loss of blood through menses and the high iron demands of pregnancy combine to greatly increase female iron requirements. The recent increased consumption of iced tea as a popular soft drink may also affect women's iron levels. The tannin in tea reduces iron absorption. For adults in the United States, iron deficiency is rarely caused by dietary deficiency; instead, it usually results from

the blood loss of menstrual bleeding or internal bleeding in the GI tract, perhaps from bleeding ulcers or hemorrhoids.

An unusual behavior associated with iron deficiency is pica. Pica is characterized by a hunger and appetite for nonfood substances, including ice, cornstarch, clay, and even dirt. These substances contain no iron, and their consumption may even lead to loss of additional minerals, particularly when clay and dirt are consumed. Although *geophagia* (pica of clay or dirt) and *amylophagia* (pica of cornstarch and laundry starch) are primarily recognized among women of rural lower socioeconomic groups, *pagophagia* (excessive ice consumption) has been noted among all socioeconomic levels (Kushner and Shanta, 2005). Of particular concern is the practice of pica during pregnancy, when the risk and implications of iron-deficiency anemia are most severe. A challenge to obstetric nurses is to elicit information about this type of dietary behavior when assessing clients.

If increases in dietary sources of iron-rich foods do not raise hematocrit levels, supplements may be prescribed. Determination of dose is based on physiologic requirements, as assessed by primary health care providers. Long-term compliance is necessary to adequately restore iron storage levels in the body. Client education and support from nurses are advantageous.

Strategies to enhance absorption of iron supplements are simple. Drinking a glass of orange juice when taking an iron supplement will maximize iron absorption. Avoid taking iron supplements with milk because the calcium in milk interferes with absorption. Use of iron supplements may cause stools to turn black and constipation to result.

Toxicity

Hemosiderosis, storing too much iron in the body, is a health concern. This condition may be caused either by hemochromatosis, a genetic disorder that allows more dietary iron to be absorbed than usual, or by consumption of very high levels of iron-containing foods, perhaps through iron fortification. The resulting iron overload can damage tissue cells when excess iron is stored. Bacterial microorganisms may thrive on the excessive amounts of iron circulating in the blood. These effects manifested as vague symptoms such as weakness and fatigue. More specific symptoms include liver and heart damage, diabetes, arthritis, and discoloration of skin (Needs and George, 2006).

Those at risk include men, people with chronic excessive alcohol consumption, and individuals who are genetically at risk for hemochromatosis. Because men lose no iron through menstruation or childbirth and may consume more foods fortified with iron, their bodies can potentially store more iron than needed. Excessive consumption of alcohol puts people at risk because their livers are affected by alcohol and may malfunction, absorbing too much iron. Individuals with diabetes may also be at higher risk (Needs and George, 2006).

Hemochromatosis alters iron metabolism, allowing excess iron to be absorbed from food and supplements. Treatment for hemochromatosis is blood removal by giving blood regularly and by decreasing dietary intake of iron-containing foods. This disorder is sometimes misdiagnosed as diabetes or as liver disorders. Although both of these disorders are caused by hemochromatosis, they are treated as individual ailments, and the underlying iron overload is not addressed. However, awareness of hemochromatosis is increasing among primary health care providers and other health professionals. Screening during regular checkups is recommended for those older than 30 years, particularly if they have diabetes. Screening is achieved with a blood test to assess transferrin saturation.

A final concern about iron toxicity is less a nutritional issue and more of a public health and safety issue. Accidental iron poisoning of a child who consumes iron supplements or vitamin or mineral supplements containing iron is a medical emergency. As few as 6 to 12 pills can be lethal, depending on the dose and the age of the child. All supplements, even the fruit-flavored shapes formulated for children, should be treated as medicinal drugs and be kept out of the reach of children.

Zinc
Function

More than 200 enzymes throughout the body depend on zinc. Zinc affects our growth process, taste and smell ability, healing process, immune system, and carbohydrate metabolism by assisting insulin function.

Recommended Intake and Sources

The zinc RDAs for men and women are 11 mg and 8 mg per day, respectively. During pregnancy and lactation, suggested levels for women increase to 11 to 12 mg.

Zinc-containing foods include meat, fish, poultry, whole grains, legumes, and eggs. In the United States, a variety of zinc sources are easily available. In parts of the world where animal foods are not regularly consumed and grains are a primary zinc source, deficiencies may develop because of the low bioavailability of zinc from fibrous whole-grain plant foods. Grains contain phytic acid, which remains bound to zinc in the intestinal tract; human digestive juices cannot break this bond. Use of leavening agents such as yeast to prepare whole-grain food products breaks this bond, making zinc available. Zinc deficiency still occurs in parts of the world where food sources may be limited and whole grains are consistently consumed as unleavened breads.

Deficiency

Deficiency symptoms are related to zinc's functions in the body. Symptoms include impaired growth, reduced appetite, and immunologic disorders. Severe zinc deficiency during the growth years may result in dwarfism and hypogonadism (reduced function of gonads), leading to delayed sexual development. Reduced appetite is most likely related to a diminished ability to taste (hypogeusia) and smell foods (hyposmia). The difficulty is that once appetite is reduced, fewer potential sources of zinc may be consumed, causing the zinc deficiency to worsen. Marginal deficiencies among children categorized as picky eaters have been noted to negatively

affect height status. Among older adults, inadequate dietary intake resulting in reduced zinc intake appears to affect wound healing, taste and scent ability, and immune functions.

Toxicity

Zinc toxicity from inappropriate supplementation produces GI distress, leading to vomiting and diarrhea, fever, and exhaustion. The symptoms appear similar to those of the flu. Continual use of supplements decreases iron and copper levels in the body and reduces levels of high-density lipoprotein (HDL) cholesterol, thereby increasing risk of coronary artery disease. Intake should be no higher than the RDA unless directed by a primary health care provider; individuals should not self-medicate. Consequently, the UL of 40 mg should be observed.

Iodine
Function

Iodine is part of the hormone thyroxin produced by the thyroid gland. Thyroxin is involved with regulating growth and development, basal metabolic rate, and body temperature.

Recommended Intake and Sources

The RDA for iodine is 150 μg per day for both men and women. Many sources of iodine provide inconsistent amounts. Water may contain some iodine, but the amounts vary. Seafood is a good source, and dairy products and eggs may contain some iodine depending on the feed the animals consumed. Surprisingly, sea salt does not contain iodine; the iodine is lost in processing. The amount of iodine in plant foods depends on the amount in the soil in which the food is grown. Incidental sources of iodine are cleaning products whose residues adhere to cooking and baking equipment and dough conditioners. To ensure the population receives adequate amounts of this nutrient, salt in the United States may be purchased fortified with iodine.

Deficiency

Iodine deficiency reduces the amount of thyroxine produced. Symptoms of iodine deficiency then reflect the effects of reduced thyroxine, including sluggishness and weight gain. Severe iodine deficiency during pregnancy causes cretinism of the fetus, resulting in permanent mental and physical retardation.

Goiter, enlargement of the thyroid gland, occurs during extended iodine deficiency (Figure 8-6). The thyroid gland works to compensate for the low iodine levels and expands; the goiter frequently remains even after iodine intake is again sufficient.

The incidence of goiter in certain populations is endemic or regionally defined. In the past, a goiter belt existed in the Midwestern states. Iodine was unavailable in the soil and water of the area because this region is untouched by oceans, which provide a natural source of iodine. Since then, fortification of salt with iodine and the wider availability of seafood

FIG 8-6 Goiter caused by iodine deficiency. (From Swartz MH: *Textbook of physical diagnosis history and examination,* ed 3, Philadelphia, 1998, Saunders.)

because of improvements in refrigeration and transportation systems reduced this deficiency. Goiter, although extremely rare in North America, may still occur in parts of Europe, Africa, and South and Central America. To eliminate iodine deficiency globally, the United Nations Joint Commission on Health Policy recommends universal salt iodization in countries in which iodine deficiency is a public health concern.

Goiter may also be caused by the action of goitrogens. When consumed as staple components of dietary intake, goitrogens (substances in the root vegetable cassava and in cabbage) suppress the actions of the thyroid gland. Although the thyroid gland swells as in iodine deficiency goiter, the iodine level is not the initiating agent; instead, substances in these vegetables suppress the actions of the thyroid gland. To control these iodine deficiency disorders (IDDs) in areas such as southern Ethiopia, programs are conducted to teach villagers how to prepare using safer methods of preparing cassava.

Toxicity

Too much iodine can cause iodine-induced goiter called thyrotoxicosis; therefore, the UL is set at 1100 µg per day.

Fluoride
Function

Fluoride increases resistance to tooth decay and is part of tooth formation. Skeletal health also depends on fluoride for bone mineralization.

Recommended Intake and Sources

The AI for fluoride is 4 mg per day for men and 3 mg for women.

Sources of fluoride vary. The most consistent is fortified water to which fluoride has been added. Tea, seafood, and seaweed are other reliable sources. Unfortunately, these are not regularly consumed, particularly by children during tooth-formation years.

An inadvertent source of fluoride is toothpaste. Most toothpaste has fluoride added as a topical agent to strengthen tooth enamel. However, some fluoride is ingested during the rinsing process, providing a kind of dietary source of fluoride. Children can ingest a lethal dose of fluoride if a tube of toothpaste is consumed.

Deficiency

Low levels of fluoride raise the risk of dental caries. Factors such as hygiene, food choices, and possibly genetics also affect plaque and subsequent dental caries.

Toxicity

Too much fluoride causes fluorosis. Fluorosis consists of mottling or brown spotting of the tooth enamel; severe fluorosis may also cause pitting of the teeth. A UL of 10 mg per day reduces the risk of toxicity.

Selenium
Function

Selenium is part of an enzyme that acts as an antioxidant. Vitamin E and selenium work together to prevent cell and lipid membrane damage from oxidizing substances. Selenium is also associated with thyroid function. It is found extensively throughout the body.

Recommended Intake and Sources

The RDA for selenium ranges from 55 to 70 µg per day. Meats, fish, eggs, and whole grains are good sources of selenium. It is a nutrient for which the RDA is easily met.

Deficiency

Deficiency of selenium may predispose individuals to heart disease, particularly Keshan disease. Keshan disease was first noted in China, primarily in children and women of childbearing age. The symptoms of the disease include cardiomyopathy and other features common to selenium deficiency, including muscle pain and tenderness. It is difficult, however, to separate other environmental factors specific to China that may also affect long-term nutritional status. Deficiencies of nutrients other than selenium may have a role in the etiology of Keshan disease. Keshan disease differs from the form of heart disease common in the United States because the myocardium of the heart is affected. In the United States, most heart disease is coronary artery disease. Therefore, selenium deficiency is probably not a factor affecting the American incidence of heart disease.

However, low dietary levels of selenium or reduced blood levels of selenium may be associated with an increased risk of cancer among Americans. The relationship of cancer to selenium consumption is probably caused by selenium's antioxidant functions combined with those of other antioxidants in the body. This relationship continues to be explored.

Toxicity

Selenium can be toxic at levels as low as five times the RDA, which is 55 µg per day. The most common symptoms of chronic toxicity are hair and nail brittleness and loss. Other effects are severe liver damage, vomiting, and diarrhea. Additional symptoms include metallic aftertaste, respiratory distress with lung edema and bronchopneumonia, and garlic-scented breath and sweat. Chronic toxicity is not likely to occur in the U.S. population, because food is consumed from many regional areas, a pattern that dilutes consumption of food grown in naturally occurring high-selenium areas.

The toxicity of selenium highlights the delicate nature of the body's use of trace minerals. Although selenium is proposed as an antioxidant supplement, the amounts suggested are those of the RDA for selenium. To avoid toxicity, a UL of 400 µg per day is established.

Copper
Function

Although the body requires minute amounts of it, copper performs many functions. Some roles of copper are its actions as (1) a coenzyme involving antioxidant reactions and energy metabolism, (2) a component of wound healing, (3) a constituent of nerve fiber protection, and (4) a required element for iron use.

Recommended Intake and Sources

The RDA for copper is 900 µg per day for adults. Good sources include organ meats (liver), seafood, green leafy vegetables, legumes, whole grains, dried fruits, and water that flows through copper pipes.

Deficiency

Copper deficiency causes bone demineralization and anemia; this form of anemia can also be caused by zinc toxicity, which reduces body levels of copper. Copper deficiency does not occur in the United States.

Toxicity

Copper toxicity occurs from supplementation. A common toxic response consists of vomiting and diarrhea. Wilson's disease, an inherited disorder, results in the excessive accumulation of copper in the liver, brain, and cornea of the eye (see the *Personal Perspectives* box "Wilson" Joins the Family). Eventually the disorder can lead to cirrhosis, chronic hepatitis, liver failure, and neurologic disorders. Worldwide, the incidence of copper toxicity appears tied to the use of brass and copper pots to prepare and store foods. Nutritional treatment for copper toxicity, whether caused by Wilson's disease or dietary sources, consists of dietary restrictions and chelation therapy that initiates excretion of excess copper from the body (Collins, 2014). In addition, 10 mg per day is the UL for copper.

Chromium
Function

Chromium has a role in carbohydrate metabolism as a constituent of the glucose tolerance factor (GTF) that facilitates the reaction of insulin.

Recommended Intake and Sources

The AI of chromium is 35 µg per day for men and 25 µg for women. In adults older than 50 years, the AI is 30 µg for men and 20 µg for women. Found in animal-related foods, eggs, and whole grains, chromium is lost in food processing, particularly when wheat is refined to white flour.

Studies are exploring the effects of chromium supplementation on increasing HDL cholesterol levels and decreasing glucose and insulin levels. The findings may have implications for populations who consume refined foods and for those who are exposed to stressors that increase the need for chromium; such stressors include infections, trauma, and diets high in simple sugars.

Deficiency

Although chromium is lost through food processing, outright deficiencies of chromium are unusual. Inadequate chromium status may be responsible in part for some cases of impaired glucose tolerance, hyperglycemia, hypoglycemia, and unresponsiveness to insulin.

Toxicity

Chromium toxicity has been noted from environmental contaminants in industrial settings rather than from excessive dietary intake.

Other Trace Minerals

The amount needed of the following trace minerals is so low that it is easy to meet these amounts through ordinary consumption of foods. All are problematic in large doses; supplements are contraindicated.

Manganese is a component of enzymes involved in metabolic reactions. The AI for manganese is 2.3 mg per day for men and 1.8 mg for women. The mineral is found in whole grains, green vegetables, legumes, and other foods, and manganese deficiency in humans is unknown. The UL for manganese is 11 mg.

Molybdenum functions as a coenzyme. The RDA, 45 µg per day, is easily consumed through typical dietary selections. Deficiencies have not been recorded except under medical circumstances in which dietary intakes have been greatly altered. The UL for molybdenum is 2000 µg per day.

Other trace minerals found in our bodies that may have a role in human health are *silicon, boron, nickel, vanadium, lithium, tin,* and *cadmium*. The amounts required are so small that we naturally consume enough and are never deficient in these nutrients. Table 8-4 provides a quick reference to the trace minerals.

PERSONAL PERSPECTIVES

"Wilson" Joins the Family

I've never heard the whole story, but apparently my sister Natalie begged my parents for a sibling. Nine and a half years later, I came along. To me, Natalie was a mother, sister, and friend all rolled into one. When my sister was 39 years old—a full-time IT manager, wife, and mother—I was 30, a stay-at-home mom with a daughter and a newborn baby boy. Everything seemed perfect, until my sister started feeling tired and came down with a fever.

Everyone assumed she was run-down and tired. This was in September 2005. She was diagnosed with bronchitis. After 2 weeks of antibiotics, her fever had not gone down and she felt worse.

Natalie consulted my husband, Gary, an emergency room (ER) doctor, who ran a battery of tests. In the next few weeks, she met with an infectious disease specialist, as well as her own doctor, all of whom ordered test after test. From blood work to CT scans to ultrasounds, all her test [results] were negative. She did not have mononucleosis or Epstein-Barr virus. Her blood was negative for hepatitis and a host of other diseases. She was told to stop taking her birth control pills and not to take Tylenol or other medications in case she was having a weird reaction to medications.

By mid-October, my sister's stomach swelled like she was 4 months pregnant. Gary suggested she come for another CT scan even though she just had one 2 weeks prior. [*The results were shocking.*] In the space of 2 weeks, my sister's liver started to go into failure. She already reached the point at which she would need a liver transplant!

Natalie was immediately transported from Jersey Shore Medical Center in New Jersey to the Hospital of the University of Pennsylvania [Philadelphia, Pennsylvania], known for its liver transplant teams. Natalie spent 4 days in a general room, waiting for some news as to what was wrong. Her skin was yellow and her stomach grew to enormous proportions. This was a woman who up until 2 months ago was young, vibrant, and beautiful. Now she was deteriorating.

Finally, on the fourth day, an important liver biopsy was performed. The biopsy results came back. Apparently, my sister has *Wilson's* disease. What is Wilson's disease? Why had no one thought of this? What disease changed all of us forever?

Now five years later, my family is well versed on Wilson's disease. This [genetic] disease releases excess copper into the liver [also brain and cornea of the eye], eventually leading to hepatic failure. But this is not the whole story. The way my sister presented with this disease only affects 5% of Wilson's disease patients. Most have extreme symptoms, such as neurologic disturbances (psychotic episodes, seizures) and other obvious physical ailments. Natalie did not. She did have obsessive-compulsive disorder, difficulty conceiving, and periods of mood swings. At times, her liver functions were elevated, but not too [seriously]. During the battery of tests performed at the beginning of her illness, Natalie's blood was tested for Wilson's disease but the result was negative. Now we know there is a point when the copper leaves the blood and travels into the liver, becoming undetectable in simple blood tests. A urine test would have showed the excess copper in her body but was never ordered. The signs were there but not obvious enough.

Wilson's disease is a genetic disorder. Natalie has had it her *whole* life, dormant. What set it off at this point is still not known. Because Wilson's is a genetic disorder, I was tested as well.

I collected a urine sample for 24 hours, to be tested for copper level. I also gave blood for a genetic test as well. What would my results show?

The test results were borderline normal. However, to the Wilson's disease specialist we consulted in New York City, the results predicted that my genetic test would be the same as my sister's—detecting the identical genetic defects. Sure enough, he was right. I, too, have this disease. It has been diagnosed so early that the simple treatment is to take zinc pills three times a day for the rest of my life. I can take what is essentially a mineral and be a healthy person. The zinc will counteract the copper. [*The zinc competes with the copper for absorption receptor sites.*] Unfortunately, Wilson's experts are very few, and genetic testing is new and very expensive. There is simply not enough education about this disease.

Little did my parents know that when my sister begged to have a sibling, she would end up saving her sibling's life. If my sister had not gone into hepatic failure, I would have at some point. It was only a matter of time. If more was known about this disease and its abstract symptoms, maybe my sister would have been diagnosed earlier and able to take zinc, just as I am.

Tanya Popovetsky
Marlboro, N.J.

Tanya's sister received a liver transplant within a few days of diagnosis and continues her recovery while taking many medications, adjusting to a life much different from the one she knew.

TOWARD A POSITIVE NUTRITION LIFESTYLE: PROJECTING

Projection is placing responsibility for our own unacceptable feelings or behaviors on others. In relation to health, we may attribute our poor eating patterns to hectic schedules and possibly to roommates or family members who don't want to shop for food or prepare meals. We project our unacceptable behaviors on others rather than take responsibility for our own health.

One mineral for which projection sometimes occurs is iron. Because iron deficiency often manifested as tiredness, paleness, and frequent infections, it is commonly self-diagnosed as the pathologic cause of poor health. Accurate diagnosis of iron deficiency is based on blood analysis, not on self-reporting. As an aspect of client education, we can

TABLE 8-4 Trace Minerals

MINERAL	FUNCTION	CLINICAL ISSUES DEFICIENT/TOXICITY	RECOMMENDED DAILY INTAKES	FOOD SOURCES	ABSORPTION ISSUES
Iron (Fe)	Distributes oxygen in hemoglobin and myoglobin; growth	Deficiency: microcytic anemia (children and women at risk) Toxicity: hemosiderosis; hemochromatosis	RDA: Men: 8 mg Women: 18 mg Pregnancy: 27 mg Lactation: 9 mg UL: 45 mg	Heme sources: meat, fish, poultry, egg yolks Nonheme sources: vegetables, legumes, whole grains, enriched grains	Conserved and recycled; only 10%-15% of dietary iron consumed is absorbed
Zinc (Zn)	Cofactor for more than 200 enzymes; carbohydrate metabolism (insulin function)	Deficiency: decreases wound healing; decreases taste and smell; impaired sexual and physical development; immune disorders Toxicity: similar to flu with vomiting/diarrhea/fever/exhaustion	RDA: Men: 11 mg Women: 8 mg UL: 40 mg	Meat, fish, poultry, whole grains, legumes, eggs	Binders may decrease absorption in whole grains
Iodine (I)	Thyroxine synthesis (thyroid hormone) regulates growth and development; regulation of basal metabolic rate	Deficiency: decreases thyroxine, causing sluggishness and weight gain, goiter, cretinism (if during pregnancy) Toxicity: thyrotoxicosis	RDA: Adults: 150 mcg UL: 1100 mcg	Iodized salt, seafood	—
Fluoride (Fl)	Bone and tooth formation; increases resistance to decay; increases mineralization	Deficiency: increases dental caries Toxicity: fluorosis	AI: Men: 4 mg Women: 3 mg UL: 10 mg	Fluoridated water, tea, seafood, seaweed	—
Selenium (Se)	Antioxidant cofactor with vitamin E; prevents cell and lipid membrane damage	Deficiency: possible Keshan disease/cancer Toxicity: liver damage, vomiting, diarrhea	RDA: Adults: 55 µg UL: 400 mcg	Meat, fish, eggs, whole grains	—
Copper (C)	Coenzyme in antioxidant reactions and energy metabolism; wound healing; nerve fiber protection; iron use	Deficiency: bone demineralization and anemia (not in U.S.) Toxicity: Wilson's disease or with supplements producing vomiting/diarrhea	RDA: Adults: 900 µg UL: 10,000 µg	Organ meats (liver), seafood, green leafy vegetables	—
Chromium (Cr)	Carbohydrate metabolism, part of glucose tolerance factor	Deficiency: possible link with cardiovascular disorders; hypoglycemia, hyperglycemia, and unresponsive insulin	AI: Men: 35 µg Women: 25 µg	Animal food, whole grains	—
Manganese (Mn)	Part of metabolic reaction enzymes	Deficiency: unknown	AI: Men: 2.3 mg Women: 1.8 mg UL: 11 mg	Whole grains, green leafy vegetables, legume	—
Molybdenum (Mo)	Coenzyme	Deficiency: unknown	RDA: Adults: 45 µg UL: 2000 µg	Many foods	—

AI, Adequate Intake; *RDA,* Recommended Dietary Allowance; *UL,* Tolerable Upper Intake Level.

help clients clarify the actual causes of their symptoms if they are not clinically iron deficient. Often these symptoms are caused by poor health habits: not enough sleep, irregular meals, and too little exercise. Rather than blaming ill health on the mineral iron, clients can take responsibility and modify their own health behaviors.

SUMMARY

- Water and minerals are primary components of body fluids, and each performs other functions as well.
- Water supports a variety of functions: It is a structural component of the body, a temperature regulator, a lubricant, a fluid cushion, a transportation vehicle, a source of trace minerals, and a medium for and participant in biochemical reactions.
- Sources of water include beverages and foods with high water content; the best source is pure water.
- Minerals have diverse roles: provide structural rigidity and strength to teeth and skeleton, allow for proper muscle contraction and release, influence nerve function, assist enzymes, maintain proper acid-base balance of body fluids, and are required for blood clotting and wound healing.
- The 16 essential minerals are divided into two categories: major minerals (needed daily in amounts of 100 mg or higher) and trace minerals (needed daily in amounts less than or equal to 20 mg).
  - Major minerals are calcium, phosphorus, magnesium, sulfur, and the electrolytes sodium, potassium, and chloride.
- Trace minerals include iron, zinc, iodine, fluoride, selenium, copper, chromium, manganese, and molybdenum.
- Prime food sources of minerals include both plants and animals.
  - Plant sources include most fruits, vegetables, legumes, and whole grains.
  - Animal sources consist of beef, chicken, eggs, fish, and milk products.
- Minerals are stable when cooked.
- The bioavailability of some minerals may be limited, depending on the source.
  - Some plant minerals are not easily available to the human body because of binders inhibiting absorption.
  - Generally, minerals from animal foods can be absorbed more easily than those from plants.
- Dietary patterns consisting primarily of whole foods provide an adequate supply of minerals.

◎ THE NURSING APPROACH

Case Study: Deficient Fluid Volume

Ben, an 8-month-old infant, had a rectal temperature of 101.2° F. His mother suspected he had a viral infection and brought him to the emergency department, worried he might be getting dehydrated.

It was November, and the nurse suspected Ben had rotavirus. After interviewing the infant's mother, the nurse did a physical examination, and Ben was admitted to the rapid treatment unit. The physician ordered lab tests, including a stool culture, white blood count, and hematocrit, and electrolyte measurements. Prescriptions were written for acetaminophen given per rectum every 6 hours, Pedialyte by mouth as tolerated, and lactated Ringer's solution given intravenously.

Assessment
Subjective (from Mother's Statements)
- For 24 hours Ben vomited whenever his mother attempted to give him a bottle of formula.
- Ben had been crying and seemed weak.
- Ben had several loose brown stools in his diaper and probably urinated less than usual.
- One of his brothers also has had diarrhea and vomiting.

Objective (from Physical Examination)
- Dry skin and oral mucous membranes
- Sunken fontanelle
- Skin flushed and warm
- Temperature of 101.2° F (rectal)
- Rapid pulse and respirations
- Abdomen soft
- Bowel sounds hyperactive
- Urine concentrated

Diagnoses (Nursing)
1. Deficient fluid volume related to diarrhea and vomiting as evidenced by report of mother, dry mucous membranes, sunken fontanelle, and concentrated urine
2. Hyperthermia related to infection and dehydration as evidenced by temperature 101.2° F, skin flushed and warm

Planning
Patient Outcomes
Short term (within 24 hours):
- No further fluid loss, and fluid balance restored
- Temperature of 100° F or less

Continued

◎ THE NURSING APPROACH—cont'd

Nursing Interventions
- Carry out physician's orders.
- Monitor health status hourly.

Implementation
1. Sent a stool specimen from the diaper to the lab.
   A stool culture can lead to identification of microorganisms, a correct diagnosis, and appropriate treatment.
2. Gave acetaminophen per rectum as ordered.
   Acetaminophen (Tylenol) can lower the temperature. Aspirin is not given to children because of its association with Reye's syndrome (an uncommon but potentially lethal complication).
3. Offered sips of Pedialyte in a baby bottle every hour.
   Pedialyte, containing glucose, water, and electrolytes, helps replace fluids and electrolytes lost through diarrhea and vomiting. Clear liquids minimize peristalsis and are better tolerated than formula when diarrhea and vomiting are present.
4. Administered intravenous fluids (IV), regulated by an IV pump.
   Intravenous fluids can immediately replace lost fluids. Rate must be carefully controlled to prevent fluid overload.
5. Checked vital signs hourly.
   Monitoring vital signs frequently aids early detection of complications and evaluation of health status.
6. Recorded intake and output and monitored for signs of dehydration.
   Once stabilized, intake (IVs and fluids by mouth) should be approximately equal to output (vomitus, diarrhea, urine). Diapers are weighed to determine amounts of urine.
7. Monitored lab reports.
   White blood count is commonly elevated by infections. Increased hematocrit can indicate a loss of fluids. Electrolyte levels are diminished by vomiting and diarrhea.

Evaluation
Short term (within 24 hours):
- A stool specimen was sent to the lab. Ben drank 2 ounces of Pedialyte, but then vomited. An IV was administered, and urination increased. Oral mucous membranes were moist, and fontanelle was flat.
  - Goal partially met. Plan: Continue to offer Pedialyte hourly. Continue IVs until Ben is taking fluids well by mouth.
- Temperature dropped to 100.8° F after acetaminophen was given. Pulse rate and respirations decreased.
  - Goal partially met.

Discussion Questions
1. Why is it important to keep Ben hydrated?
2. How does Pedialyte help balance electrolytes as well as fluids? At what temperature should it be given?
3. What drinks and/or foods would be best for decreasing diarrhea in Ben's older brother?

❓ APPLYING CONTENT KNOWLEDGE

Dorothy, a 77-year-old woman with a history of heart failure, presents to the hospital with shortness of breath. During your assessment you find that she has +3 edema on her lower extremities, bilateral lower lung crackles, and dyspnea on exertion, and she mentions she has gained 2 pounds since last week. The doctor orders a potassium-wasting diuretic to remove excess fluid. What are the signs and symptoms of potassium deficiency? What foods would you recommend Dorothy consume to prevent a potassium deficiency?

WEBSITES OF INTEREST

Centers for Disease Control and Prevention
www.cdc.gov/healthywater/
Offers many resources about water uses and safety.

Food and Nutrition Information Center
fnic.nal.usda.gov/food-composition
Provides resources on individual macronutrients, phytonutrients, vitamins and minerals. Created by U.S. Department of Agriculture, National Agriculture Library.

National Osteoporosis Foundation (NOF)
www.nof.org
Offers resources on causes, prevention, detection, and treatment of osteoporosis.

REFERENCES

Bailey JL, et al: Water, electrolyte, and acid-base metabolism. In Ross AC, et al, editors: *Modern nutrition in health and disease*, ed 11, Philadelphia, 2014, Lippincott Williams & Wilkins.

Beverage Marketing Corporation (BMC): *U.S. bottled water sales totaled $11.8 billion in 2012*. From: www.bevnet.com/news/2013/u-s-bottled-water-sales-totaled-11-8-billion-in-2012. Accessed February 2, 2014.

Collins JF: Copper. In Ross AC, et al, editors: *Modern nutrition in health and disease*, ed 11, Philadelphia, 2014, Lippincott Williams & Wilkins.

Coughlin JW, et al: Behavioral disorders affecting food intake: Eating disorders and other psychiatric conditions. In Ross AC, et al, editors: *Modern nutrition in health and disease*, ed 11, Philadelphia, 2014, Lippincott Williams & Wilkins.

Fratianni CM: Osteoporosis in solid organ transplantation: Overview of treatment (updated: September 3, 2013), *eMedicine/Medscape*. From: emedicine.medscape.com/article/128108-overview#aw2aab6b2. Accessed December 26, 2013.

Institute of Medicine: *Sodium intake in populations: Assessment of evidence* (Report Brief), Washington, DC, 2013, The National Academies Press.

Jacobs-Kosmin D: Osteoporosis (updated October 4, 2013), *eMedicine/Medscape*. From: emedicine.medscape.com/article/330598-overview#showall. Accessed December 26, 2013.

Kushner RF, Shanta RV: Emergence of pica (ingestion of non-food substances) accompanying iron deficiency anemia after gastric bypass surgery, *Obes Surg* 15(10):1491–1495, 2005.

National Research Council: *Dietary reference intakes: The essential guide to nutrient requirements*, Washington, DC, 2006, The National Academies Press.

Needs S, George DK: Haemachromatosis: Testing and management, *Gastrointest Nurs* 4(1):27–31, 2006.

Tucker KL, Rosen CJ: Prevention and management of osteoporosis. In Ross AC, et al, editors: *Modern nutrition in health and disease*, ed 11, Philadelphia, 2014, Lippincott Williams & Wilkins.

Weaver CM, Heaney RP: Calcium. In Ross AC, et al, editors: *Modern nutrition in health and disease*, ed 11, Philadelphia, 2014, Lippincott Williams & Wilkins.

9 | CHAPTER

Energy, Weight, and Fitness

All people—the fat, the thin, and the in between—can benefit from adopting attitudes and behaviors that over time should promote the body composition appropriate to each individual's genetic makeup and contribute to true wellness.

ⓔ http://evolve.elsevier.com/GRODNER/FOUNDATIONS

LEARNING OBJECTIVES

- Compare and contrast the two energy pathways.
- State the three major components of daily energy requirements.
- Define a healthy weight.
- List factors that influence body fat levels.
- Describe methods for assessing body fat composition and body weight.
- Discuss nutritional needs of athletes.

ROLE IN WELLNESS

This chapter explores the issues of energy, weight, and fitness. Synergistic effects of energy intake and energy output are mediated by genetically defined physiology and behavioral options as influenced by environment. Body weight reflects factors within our control plus factors outside our control that are unable to be modified.

The meanings of weight and fatness in our contemporary culture and how they relate to wellness are considered. Because it is body fat that is really the issue, our focus is on fat rather than on weight. In addition, we use the approach *management of body composition, specifically body fat levels,* rather than achievement of ideal body fatness. In this context, *management* is defined as the use of available resources to achieve a predetermined goal. This definition recognizes that individuals differ in the resources available to them and in the goals they set.

Consideration of the physical, intellectual, emotional, social, spiritual, and environmental dimensions of health guides our understanding of the value of energy supply, fitness, and their potential impact on healthy body weight. Dietary intake and regular physical activity are essential to the achievement of optimal *physical health* and fitness. Exercise affects all muscles; even the muscles of our gastrointestinal tract function better when we exercise regularly. Managing body composition levels by decreasing or increasing body fat or lean body mass is, if appropriate, also an aspect of the *physical* dimension of health. Adequate levels of body fat allow the body to function most efficiently.

To strengthen our *intellectual health* dimension, the old saying "A sound body makes for a sound mind" still holds true. By being physically fit, we may be able to devote our full intellectual capacity to our work. The *intellectual* dimension of health also provides the skills to understand and critique the role of society in molding our attitudes to our levels of fitness and the shapes of our bodies.

The *emotional health* dimension may be supported by fitness because for some people, depression seems to lift if they regularly engage in sustained aerobic activities. Even if we are not depressed, our general state of mind improves with daily physical exercise. Regardless of body size, our *emotional* health depends on our developing positive self-esteem.

Group sports provide an excellent opportunity for social activity while pursuing healthful goals that enhance *social health.* A sense of belonging and sharing occurs whether the group is a formal organization, such as a running club, or consists of friends who bike together. The *social* dimension of health may not be affected by body fat levels, although those at either extreme of body size may need to develop a circle of friends and family who accept their size differences.

Respecting and caring for our bodies by engaging in regular physical activity reflects the understanding of the unique nature of the human body, which in turn reflects *spiritual health* (see the *Personal Perspectives* box Detecting a Deficiency). The spiritual dimension of health is sometimes tested as a belief in a higher being, providing support for some individuals who are struggling with behavior changes related to food consumption.

PERSONAL PERSPECTIVES

Detecting a Deficiency

George Sheehan, MD, was as comfortable writing articles as medical editor for Runner's World *magazine as he was practicing medicine. His running habit began at age 45, "a decisive age, an age for change." He was responsible for inspiring many to find the athlete within themselves to achieve their own personal best. His message was that physical excellence leads to achievements in other arenas of life. Here is an excerpt from his book* Personal Best.

Are you feeling run-down, sluggish, low in energy? Is simply getting to school or work becoming too much for you? Are you exhausted by three o'clock in the afternoon? Do you feel depressed? Have you lost your initiative?

If you answer yes, you may be suffering from a lifestyle disease that, surveys tell us, affects about one-half of all Americans. It is called exercise deficiency, it is undoubtedly a leading cause of ill health, and no household is exempt.

Exercise deficiency—the sweat deficit—is a self-inflicted disease. It is an old and familiar story: Our greatest tendency is to cheat on ourselves. We think we can enjoy the fullness of life without paying for it. But that is not the way the world works—or the human machine, either: Nothing is free.

Full-blown exercise deficiency states are evident to the most inexperienced observer—sufferers are manifestly out of shape. These extreme cases usually fatigue easily and early and spend most of the day in physical and mental torpor. They are much too tired when they get home at night to even consider taking any physical exercise. For them, repose is the natural state, and any activity is an effort.

Many people with exercise deficiency are unaware that they have it. They expect no more from their bodies than they are getting. They believe their lack of energy and enthusiasm goes with age. They think they are normal. The reality: They are average, because it's average to slow down, average to become less productive, average to have less energy—and since that's exactly what happens to most of us, we confuse the two. But average is not normal. Normal is the best you can be.

The notion that loss of physical vigor is inevitable usually comes in the mid-thirties. At the FBI Academy, where recruits are placed in a fitness program to get them back in condition, one aspirant complained to the director, "I'm 35; I'm too old for this stuff."

But we are never too old to be fit, and never too young to start preserving fitness. We need to be physically fit whether we are 20 or 35 or even 70. Being unfit at any age is settling for less than your best and is a classic example of the sort of thinking that is behind the widespread incidence of exercise deficiency.

Fortunately, the movement toward fitness is equally widespread. Half the people in this country now realize the need for physical exercise. They know there is no need to lose the gleam in their eye, the bloom in their cheek, the lift in their walk, and the life in their day.

And all it takes is sweat.

From Sheehan G: *Personal best: The foremost philosopher of fitness shares techniques and tactics for success and self-liberation,* Emmaus, PA, 1989, Rodale Press.

The *environmental health* dimension may be key to defusing the impact of *obesogenic* settings. Maintaining healthy levels of fitness and weight is significantly affected by the physical environments surrounding us. Are there safe areas in which to exercise outside? Are affordable gym memberships available, whether at a commercial facility or at the local community center? Are there supermarkets in the neighborhood that provide fresh produce and wholesome products at reasonable prices?

Obesogenic environments entice by limiting our need to be physical as well surround us with inexpensive food selections that are high in calories, fat, refined carbohydrates, and simple sugars. Considering ways to modify our environments to improve our individual and community health is a major contemporary health challenge (see Box 9-2).

ENERGY

The abilities to perform work, produce change, and maintain life all require energy. Energy exists in many forms—mechanical, chemical, heat, electrical, light, and nuclear energies. The laws of thermodynamics tell us that each type of energy can be converted from one form to another. As our bodies function, chemical energy from food is converted to mechanical energy and heat.

The ultimate source of energy is the sun. Sunlight is used by plants to produce chemical energy in the form of carbohydrates, proteins, or fats. These foods possess stored energy. People are not capable of doing this. We must convert the chemical energy from the foods we eat into forms usable by the human body.

The energy released from food is measured in kcal (thousands of calories), or calories. Technically, a *calorie* is the amount of heat necessary to raise the temperature of a gram of water by $1°C$ $(0.8°F)$. As first noted in Chapter 1, to ensure accuracy, the term *kilocalories* is used throughout this text, abbreviated as *kcal*.

Two methods are used to determine the energy a food contains. One is through the use of a bomb calorimeter (Figure 9-1). This instrument is designed to burn a food while measuring the amount of heat or energy released. It provides an estimate of the energy available to humans. Because the bomb calorimeter method is more efficient than the human body, the kcal value assigned to a food item is adjusted to reflect the limitations of the human system. Amounts listed in food tables reflect this adjustment.

FIG 9-1 Cross section of a bomb calorimeter. To determine energy, a dried portion of food is burned inside a chamber charged with oxygen that is surrounded by water. As the food is burned, it gives off heat. The heat raises the temperature of the water surrounding the chamber. The increase in water temperature indicates the number of kcal contained in the food. One kcal equals the amount of heat needed to raise the temperature of 1 kilogram of water by 1°C (0.8°F).

The other method of assessing food energy is proximate composition, which determines the grams of carbohydrates, proteins, and fats of a food item. The grams are then multiplied by the energy value of each (carbohydrates 4 kcal/g; proteins 4 kcal/g; fats 9 kcal/g). The sum of these calculations equals the total energy content of a specific food.

Energy Pathways

The processes of digestion, absorption, and metabolism for each of the three energy-supplying nutrients—carbohydrates, fats, and proteins—have been presented in previous chapters. (Alcohol also provides energy but is not considered a nutrient category.) Carbohydrate digests to glucose, triglycerides (fats) to fatty acids and glycerol, and protein to amino acids. Here we continue to follow their journey as they are used for energy in individual cells.

The nutrients release energy when they are catabolized (broken down), forming carbon dioxide and water. The released energy becomes caught within adenosine triphosphate (ATP), the fuel for all energy-requiring processes in the body (Figure 9-2).

Carbohydrate as a Source of Energy

Glucose releases energy and is converted to carbon dioxide and water through three processes: glycolysis, tricarboxylic acid (TCA) cycle, and oxidative phosphorylation. These complicated processes are reviewed in general here; the intricate details are beyond the scope of this text.

Through glycolysis, which results in the conversion of glucose to carbon compounds, a glucose molecule produces pyruvic acid and ATP. Part of this process depends on niacin and other B-complex vitamins. Oxygen is not needed for glycolysis to occur because it is an anaerobic pathway. The anaerobic pathway provides energy for sprint or speed-type exercise such as soccer, basketball, and football. We also depend on this energy source to run for the train, chase after toddlers, or bound across the room to answer the phone. This type of exertion is limited because oxygen is not available quickly enough to continue its support. Instead, the incomplete use of glucose causes the pyruvic acid to be converted to lactic acid. As lactic acid builds up, the muscles become sore and stiff. Consequently, the exertion ceases because of pain. Within a few minutes, enough oxygen is available to break down the lactic acid, relieving the physical discomfort. The effect is called oxygen debt.

Anaerobic glycolysis takes place in the cell cytoplasm, but oxygen-dependent aerobic glycolysis (the aerobic pathway) occurs in the mitochondria of the cell. In the mitochondria, pyruvic acid (made without oxygen) reacts with coenzyme A (CoA) to create acetyl CoA. The energy process continues as acetyl CoA reaches the TCA cycle. The reactions that are part of that cycle lead to the formation of additional ATP and carbon dioxide. The aerobic pathway is the primary energy source for exercises that are low enough in intensity to be carried on for at least 5 minutes. They include endurance-type exercise (e.g., swimming, bicycling, running), as well as walking and most of our daily activities.

The last process of glucose conversion to energy is oxidative phosphorylation. A number of actions lead to the release of hydrogens in the forms of water and additional energy that is captured in ATP. The term *oxidative* reflects the combination of hydrogen with oxygen to form water; *phosphorylation* is the creation of the phosphate bond to form ATP.

Fat as a Source of Energy

The first step in the use of fat for energy is the hydrolysis into glycerol and three fatty acids. Glycerol is changed into pyruvic acid and is used for energy. The fatty acids undergo a an irreversible process known as *beta-oxidation,* which involves the breakdown of the fatty acids into acetyl CoA molecules, which then enter the TCA cycle and proceed like the acetyl CoA from carbohydrate (glucose).

Protein as a Source of Energy

Amino acids are first catabolized through deamination, as described in Chapter 6. Whereas the liver and kidneys process the nitrogen-containing amino acid groups, the other amino acid components enter the energy metabolism pathway, with each component entering at a different location. Some of the amino acid components are converted to pyruvic acid; others become intermediaries of the TCA cycle or part of the acetyl groups. If sufficient energy is available, amino acids are used for protein synthesis rather than for energy.

It is important to note that just as all three nutrients (carbohydrate, protein, and fat) can be used for energy when consumed in excess, they can also be stored as fat in the body. Likewise, when too little energy is consumed, these processes

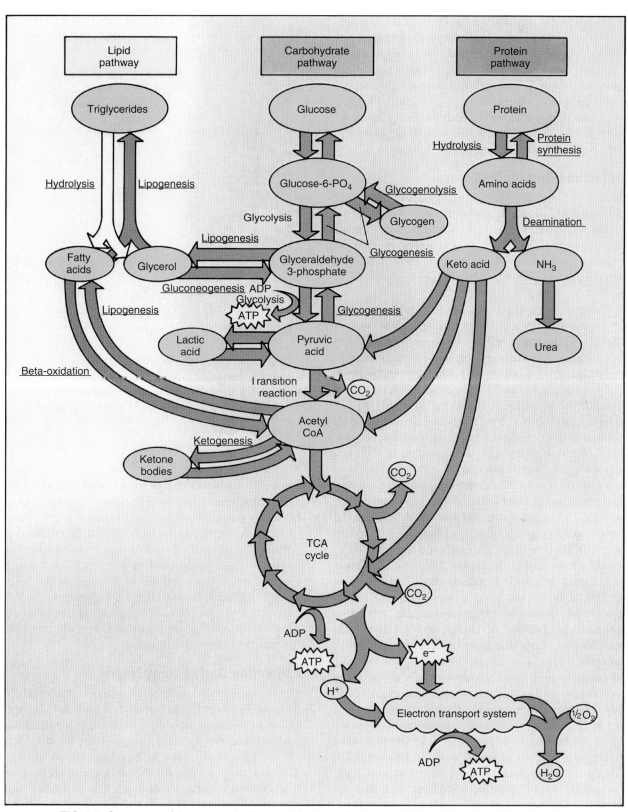

FIG 9-2 Summary of key steps in the metabolism of glucose, fatty acids, glycerol, and amino acids. *ADP,* Adenosine diphosphate; *ATP,* adenosine triphosphate; *CoA,* coenzyme A; *TCA,* tricarboxylic acid cycle. (From Thibodeau GA, Patton KT: *Anatomy and physiology,* ed 4, St Louis, 1999, Mosby.)

reverse. Energy that is consumed is used immediately, regardless of its source. The first stored energy used is glycogen, followed by the energy reserve of body fat in adipose cells. Blood-borne glucose must be available to the brain. Only a small portion of triglycerides (glycerol) can yield glucose, and continuous use of this source results in a buildup of ketones and the potential imbalance of the body pH (see Chapter 6). The body prefers to spare protein for its more important functions: building and repairing cells and tissues.

Anaerobic and Aerobic Pathways

How do anaerobic and aerobic energy pathways work together to supply energy? For the first minute or two of exertion, oxygen has not arrived at the muscles, and therefore energy must come from anaerobic sources. After several minutes the aerobic pathway takes over. However, as the exertion or exercise continues, there is a constant interchange or use of energy sources.

The energy source that muscles use during exercise depends on the intensity and length of exercise, the person's fitness level, and the foods eaten. Short-term, high-intensity activities such as sprinting rely mostly on the anaerobic pathway for energy, and only carbohydrates (primarily from muscle glycogen) can be used. On the other hand, exercise of low to moderate intensity is supported primarily by the aerobic system, and both carbohydrates and fats are used. Fats are an important energy source during exercise because, unlike carbohydrates, fatty acids are abundant in the body and their use spares muscle glycogen.

The length of activity also determines what type of fuel the muscles will use during exercise. As the duration of exercise increases, glycogen stores become depleted, and fat becomes the primary source of energy (Figure 9-3). A sedentary person breaks down glycogen faster and as a result accumulates more lactic acid in the tissues. The lactic acid causes muscle fatigue. A physically fit person has a higher aerobic capacity (the ability of the heart to supply oxygen) so that oxygen is available sooner and in greater quantity; this allows use of the aerobic pathway of energy, avoiding lactic acid buildup. This also means that more fat than glycogen can be used for fuel.

If we eat a diet high in carbohydrates, more glycogen can be stored as energy. The amount of carbohydrate stored in the body depends on how much carbohydrate we consume and our level of fitness. Endurance training increases the capacity of the muscles to store glycogen, but there is still a limit to the total amount of energy that can be stored. The more glycogen that we store, the more energy we have available for all kinds of everyday activities, not just for marathons.

ENERGY BALANCE

To maintain a healthy weight, we should consume only as much energy as we expend. Because of our sedentary lifestyles, some of us may need less energy than standard energy requirement charts recommend. In contrast, the serious

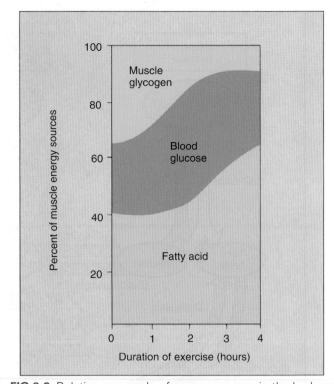

FIG 9-3 Relative use made of energy sources in the body as exercise continues. (From Guthrie HA, Picciano MF: *Human nutrition,* New York, 1995, McGraw-Hill, with permission from Helen A. Guthrie.)

competitive athlete's energy intake must support a training and competition schedule that allows the athlete to achieve his or her personal best.

Individuals who are acutely ill and hospitalized or are adapting to chronic disorders may require energy intake levels specifically calculated to meet their changing physiologic needs. Consultation with a registered dietitian/nutritionist may be warranted for patients, their family members, and other caregivers. Misconceptions about energy needs can be eliminated by nutrition counseling regardless of the nature of the health disorder.

Estimating Daily Energy Needs

The recommended energy allowances published by the National Research Council appear in Table 9-1. These energy values are based on individuals with a light to moderate activity level. The average daily energy intake for the referenced 19- to 24-year-old man is 2900 kcal, or 40 kcal/kg. It is 2200 kcal or 38 kcal/kg for the same age-referenced woman. If a person is more active or of a larger or smaller body size, further adjustments must be made. Most important, these levels are simply guidelines; the only accurate recommendation for individuals is one that supports healthy weight levels.

Many different formulas have been developed to estimate energy expenditure, some of which are complicated. An easy way to determine kcal need is to multiply weight by one of the numbers in Table 9-2. For example, a 77-kg (170-pound) man who participates in moderate exercise needs about

TABLE 9-1 Estimated Calorie Needs per Day by Age, Gender, and Physical Activity Level*

AGE (years)	MALE SEDENTARY[†]	MALE MODERATELY ACTIVE[†]	MALE ACTIVE[†]	FEMALE[‡] SEDENTARY[†]	FEMALE[‡] MODERATELY ACTIVE[†]	FEMALE[‡] ACTIVE[†]
2	1000	1000	1000	1000	1000	1000
3	1200	1400	1400	1000	1200	1400
4	1200	1400	1600	1200	1400	1400
5	1200	1400	1600	1200	1400	1600
6	1400	1600	1800	1200	1400	1600
7	1400	1600	1800	1200	1600	1800
8	1400	1600	2000	1400	1600	1800
9	1600	1800	2000	1400	1600	1800
10	1600	1800	2200	1400	1800	2000
11	1800	2000	2200	1600	1800	2000
12	1800	2200	2400	1600	2000	2200
13	2000	2200	2600	1600	2000	2200
14	2000	2400	2800	1800	2000	2400
15	2200	2600	3000	1800	2000	2400
16	2400	2800	3200	1800	2000	2400
17	2400	2800	3200	1800	2000	2400
18	2400	2800	3200	1800	2000	2400
19-20	2600	2800	3000	2000	2200	2400
21-25	2400	2800	3000	2000	2200	2400
26-30	2400	2600	3000	1800	2000	2400
31-35	2400	2600	3000	1800	2000	2200
36-40	2400	2600	2800	1800	2000	2200
41-45	2200	2600	2800	1800	2000	2200
46-50	2200	2400	2800	1800	2000	2200
51-55	2200	2400	2800	1600	1800	2200
56-60	2200	2400	2600	1600	1800	2200
61-65	2000	2400	2600	1600	1800	2000
66-70	2000	2200	2600	1600	1800	2000
71-75	2000	2200	2600	1600	1800	2000
76+	2000	2200	2400	1600	1800	2000

Reproduced from http://www.cnpp.usda.gov/Publications/USDAFoodPatterns/EstimatedCalorieNeedsPerDayTable.pdf.

*Estimated amounts of calories needed to maintain calorie balance for various gender and age groups at three different levels of physical activity. The estimates are rounded to the nearest 200 calories for assignment to a U.S. Department of Agriculture Food Pattern. An individual's calorie needs may be higher or lower than these average estimates.

Estimated calorie needs are based on Estimated Energy Requirements (EER) equations, using reference heights (average) and reference weights (healthy) for each age-gender group. For children and adolescents, reference height and weight vary. For adults, the reference man is 5 feet 10 inches tall and weighs 154 pounds. The reference woman is 5 feet 4 inches tall and weighs 126 pounds. EER equations are from the Institute of Medicine: *Dietary reference intakes for energy, carbohydrate, fiber, fat, fatty acids, cholesterol, protein, and amino acids*, Washington, DC, 2002, The National Academies Press.

†*Sedentary* means a lifestyle that includes only the light physical activity associated with typical day-to-day life. *Moderately active* means a lifestyle that includes physical activity equivalent to walking about 1.5 to 3 miles per day at 3 to 4 miles per hour, in addition to the light physical activity associated with typical day-to-day life. *Active* means a lifestyle that includes physical activity equivalent to walking more than 3 miles per day at 3 to 4 miles per hour, in addition to the light physical activity associated with typical day-to-day life.

‡Estimates for females do not include women who are pregnant or breastfeeding.

3060 kcal a day. Remember that these numbers represent averages. Some people need fewer kcal; others need more.

Components of Total Energy Expenditure

Our daily energy requirement depends on many variables, including basal metabolism, physical activity, and the thermic effect of food. Basal metabolism represents the amount of energy required to maintain life-sustaining activities (e.g., breathing, circulation, heartbeat, secretion of hormones) for a specific period. Basal metabolic rate (BMR) is the rate at which the body spends energy to keep all these life-sustaining

processes going. BMR is measured in the morning on awakening, before any physical activity, and again at 12 to 18 hours after the last meal. Two methods are used. One consists of placement of the human subject in a chamber; the body heat the subject gives off changes the temperature of the chamber, reflecting the energy used by the body for the most basic functions. The second method, *indirect calorimetry,* uses a calorimeter. The calorimeter measures the respiratory quotient or exchanges of gases as a person breathes into the mouthpiece of the machine. This quotient determines the amount of oxygen used and carbon dioxide (CO_2) expired.

TABLE 9-2 Factors For Estimating Daily Energy Allowances at Various Levels of Physical Activity for Men and Women (Ages 19 to 50)

LEVEL OF ACTIVITY	ACTIVITY FACTOR* (× REE)	ENERGY EXPENDITURE† (kcal/kg per day)
Very Light		
Men	1.3	31
Women	1.3	30
Light		
Men	1.6	38
Women	1.5	35
Moderate		
Men	1.7	41
Women	1.6	37
Heavy		
Men	2.1	50
Women	1.9	44
Exceptional		
Men	2.4	58
Women	2.2	51

*Based on examples presented by World Health Organization (1985).
†Resting energy expenditure (REE) is the average of values for median weights of people ages 19 to 24 and 25 to 74 years: men, 24 kcal/kg; women, 23.2 kcal/kg.

Several factors affect BMR, including age, body size, sex, body temperature, fasting/starvation, stress, menstruation, and thyroid function. BMR varies with the amount of lean tissue in the body; higher levels of lean body mass increase BMR. For example, men have higher BMRs than women because of larger body size and more lean body tissue. The BMR of adults slowly lowers after age 35 because of decreases in lean body tissue associated with aging. The BMR of a physically fit person may not slow down as much with age as that of a physically unfit person. The process of sustaining fitness maintains the muscle mass of lean body tissue and slows the loss caused by aging. It is never too late to develop fitness; with the approval of a primary health care provider, exercise is appropriate at any age.

BMR also depends on thyroid function. The thyroid hormone *thyroxine* is a key BMR regulator; the more thyroxine produced in the body, the higher the BMR. Of course, production of too much thyroxine is not desirable either.

Many scientists, however, prefer to use a more practical measurement called *resting energy expenditure (REE)*. REE is the energy a person expends in a normal life situation while at rest, and it includes some energy the body uses following meals and exercise. It accounts for approximately 60% to 75% of our total energy needs, similar percentages to those of BMR (Figure 9-4).

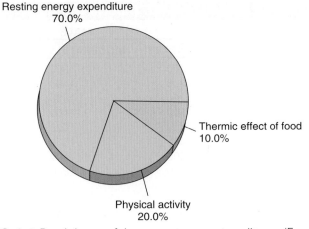

FIG 9-4 Breakdown of human energy expenditure. (From Rolin Graphics.)

Physical Activity

The second largest component of energy expenditure after REE (or BMR) is physical activity. Physical activity is any body movement produced by skeletal muscles that results in energy expenditure. It demands about 20% to 30% of our total energy needs. Of all the components, it varies the most among people. The amount of energy we expend depends on the intensity and duration of the activity. Walking requires more energy than sitting, and walking for 60 minutes uses more energy than walking for 15 minutes. Thus, even a moderate activity can become one of high energy if it is carried on for a long time.

Body size affects energy expenditure more than any other single factor. A heavier person uses more energy to perform a given task than a lighter person. Table 9-3 shows the number of kcal burned per hour for two individuals, one weighing 205 pounds and the other 125 pounds, as they engage in various activities.

Thermic Effect of Food

The third component of energy output is the energy required for our body to digest, absorb, metabolize, and store food. When we eat, the body's cells increase their activities. This increase in cellular activity is called the thermic effect of food (TEF), or diet-induced thermogenesis. The thermic effect is relatively small, accounting for approximately 7% to 10% of a person's total energy needs.

Adaptive Thermogenesis

Adaptive thermogenesis is the energy used by our bodies to adjust to changing physical and biologic environmental situations. This includes energy used to adapt to coldness, extreme changes in kcal intake (of several days' duration), and physical and emotional trauma. This category of energy need incorporates additional demands from illness and the process of recovery. Because the expenditure depends on individualized variables, it is not calculated into average energy requirements.

TABLE 9-3 Approximate Calories Used Per Hour in Various Athletic Activities

| ACTIVITY | CALORIES/HOUR | | ACTIVITY | CALORIES/HOUR | |
	BY A 125-lb PERSON	BY A 205-lb PERSON		BY A 125-lb PERSON	BY A 205-lb PERSON
Baseball:			Skiing:		
Infield or outfield	234	382	Downhill	483	789
Pitching	299	488	Level, 5 mph	586	956
Basketball:			Soccer	447	730
Moderate	352	575	Swimming:		
Vigorous	495	807	Backstroke:		
Bicycling:			20 yd/min	194	316
On level ground, 5.5 mph	251	409	40 yd/min	418	682
13 mph	537	877	Breaststroke:		
Dancing:			20 yd/min	241	392
Moderate	209	341	40 yd/min	482	786
Vigorous	284	464	Butterfly	586	956
Football	416	678	Crawl:		
Golf—twosome	271	443	20 yd/min	241	392
Horseback riding:			50 yd/min	532	869
Walk	165	270	Tennis:		
Trot	338	551	Moderate	347	565
Mountain climbing	503	820	Vigorous	488	797
Rowing:			Volleyball:		
Pleasure	251	409	Moderate	285	565
Rowing machine or sculling 20 strokes/min	684	1116	Vigorous	488	797
Running:			Walking:		
5.5 mph	537	887	2 mph	176	286
7 mph	669	1141	4.5 mph	331	540
9 mph level	777	1269	Wrestling, judo, or karate	643	1049
Skating:					
Moderate	285	465			
Vigorous	513	837			

Total energy expenditure has a direct impact on the maintenance of a healthy weight. Sustaining a healthy weight as influenced by energy input (consumption of food) and energy output (BMR/REE, voluntary physical activity, and TEF) is explored next.

HEALTHY WEIGHT

A healthy weight is a weight at which a person can physically move comfortably, maintain without undue restriction of food intake (but following healthy eating guidelines) or without excessive exercise, and live without experiencing any weight-related associative disorders such as diabetes, hypertension, coronary artery disease, or high blood lipid levels. If associative disorders do develop, lifestyle changes can be initiated to achieve a healthier weight. The definition of *healthier weight* involves a weight loss of 10 to 16 pounds accompanied by healthy lifestyle behaviors.

In response to increasing concerns about weight-related health disorders, similar concepts of healthier weight are being incorporated into many health promotion programs to change perspectives regarding healthy weight and management of body composition. These programs focus not on encouragement of dieting and weight loss but rather on prevention of obesity and promotion of healthy eating and exercise lifestyles. Thus, as more such programs are launched by government health departments, hospitals, and nonprofit health organizations, good prevention campaigns may lead toward greater acceptance of individual differences in body size, shape, and fatness (Box 9-1).

Measuring Body Fatness

Body weight is the most common way to estimate fatness. Weight is used even though our bodies are made up not only of fat but also bone, muscle, and other nonfat tissue known as *lean body mass*. Weighing works fairly well as a means to determine fatness because usually the lean body mass changes slowly. Therefore, we assume if the scale shows we are a pound heavier this week than last week, the change is probably caused by a gain of fat.

There are several situations in which weight is not a good measurement of fatness. One involves fluctuations in body fluid; fluid retention that occurs before menstruation or during hot weather may be interpreted as fat gain, and losses in a sauna may appear to be fat losses. In these circumstances, normalizing the fluid balance makes the apparent fat change

BOX 9-1	**Health Care Bill of Rights**

1. To have a policy in the health care system against discriminating practices based on weight, size, or health status.
2. To have access to affordable quality medical care, social services, and adequate physical accommodations, equipment, and testing facilities in the health care setting.
3. To have access to affordable and appropriate health insurance.
4. To have complete and accurate explanations of all treatments.
5. To have a full say in the modality of treatment, including the areas of analgesia and anesthesia.
6. To have the right to refuse treatment.
7. Access and treatment should not hinge on the acceptance or enrollment in any type of weight loss program.
8. To have or provide access to a patient advocate, either an individual or organizational representative of our choice, to play an active role in our medical care.
9. All caregivers are to act in a professional manner free of ridicule, coercion, and harassment, and they should be informed about the latest research in the areas of bariatrics, nutrition, metabolism, and genetics with regard to "obesity."
10. To privacy and confidentiality of all medical records, following federal and local laws.

From National Association to Advance Fat Acceptance: *Healthcare bill of the [sic] rights.*
Copyright 2008 NAAFA, P.O. Box 22510, Oakland CA 94609.
Telephone: (916)558-6880.
Accessed from http://www.naafaonline.com/dev2/education/brochures/Healthcare_Bill_of_Rights–EDITED.pdf.

promptly disappear. On the other hand, the scale is also misleading for anyone whose amount of lean body mass deviates from what is expected. A bodybuilder has a higher portion of lean body mass than the average person and thus will weigh more at the same height. Someone who suffers from a wasting disease has less lean tissue.

Because weighing is so convenient, it remains a useful assessment. However, to determine body composition (lean body mass plus body fat), other means, which generally involve other measurements of the size of the body (anthropometric measurements) or assessments that distinguish between fat and other body components on the basis of their physical differences, are used. Of the latter group, underwater weighing (**densitometry**) is the most widely accepted and is often used as a standard to assess the validity of other measures. Unfortunately, densitometry apparatus is bulky and expensive, and not everyone is willing or able to be submerged.

A practical alternative is **bioelectric impedance analysis (BIA)**, a method often offered at health fairs and health and fitness centers. This method for better accuracy uses four electrodes placed at the wrists and ankles to monitor the ease of passage of a mild electrical current. (Two electrodes for foot-to-foot passage are not as accurate but are more available to consumers.) Fat is a poor conductor of electricity; the

conductivity occurs through the nonfat parts of the body. BIA actually estimates the amount of lean body mass, and then the amount of fat is calculated from the difference between the lean body mass and the total weight. BIA is safe, inexpensive, easily performed, and reasonably accurate, but it is not considered sensitive enough to detect day-to-day changes experienced by someone trying to gain or lose fat. Hydration levels, though, may affect accuracy of the BIA readings. Other methods of assessing fat level are triceps skinfold and mid–upper arm circumference, but likewise these are unable to detect day-to-day changes.

Interpreting Weight

A convenient way to interpret weight is to determine body mass index (BMI). BMI is calculated by dividing the weight in kilograms by the square of the height in meters. This calculation yields a value that can be interpreted without further reference to height. BMI can be determined and related to the associated health risk by consulting the information shown in Table 9-4. BMI levels apply equally well to men and women without adjustment. BMIs in the normal to lower overweight category are associated with the least health risks (Rodriguez, et al, 2009). Although some controversy exists as to whether the standards should be increased with age, health risk evidence supports relaxation of the recommended range for older adults. Mortality is higher for individuals at the lowest BMI and highest BMI levels, whereas those in the mid-range appear less at risk (Wellman and Kamp, 2012).

Bear in mind that although BMI is widely used and convenient, it is still a measure of weight and has all the shortcomings of using weight to estimate fat. When both weight and fat are measured on the same men and women, there are usually some individuals who have weight-to-height ratios considered normal but levels of body fat that are beyond what is recommended; they are normal weight for their height but obese. On the other hand, there are other individuals who are overweight but not "overfat"; this group is most likely to include very physically active persons.

HEALTHY BODY FAT

Functions of Fat

Body fat serves a number of vital functions. As discussed in Chapter 5, we could not live without some body fat. For most people, the major portion of body fat is storage fat. A layer of this fat under our skin provides protection from extremes of environmental temperatures, and cushions of fat defend many internal organs against physical trauma. Storing fat provides an efficient means of stockpiling energy so we can endure moderate fasts. In addition to this storage fat, there is a small amount of fat that serves vital functions such as membrane integrity; this minimal amount of fat is termed *essential*. Although there are individual differences, essential fat in men seems to be 3% to 8% of their body weight. When appropriate amounts of storage fat are added to essential fat for men, the recommended range for total fat is 15% to 20%

TABLE 9-4 Body Mass Index Table

HEIGHT (INCHES)								BODY WEIGHT (POUNDS)											
58	91	96	100	105	110	115	119	124	129	134	138	143	148	153	158	162	167
59	94	99	104	109	114	119	124	128	133	138	143	148	153	158	163	168	173
60	97	102	107	112	118	123	128	133	138	143	148	153	158	163	168	174	179
61	100	106	111	116	122	127	132	137	143	148	153	158	164	169	174	180	185
62	104	109	115	120	126	131	136	142	147	153	158	164	169	175	180	186	191
63	107	113	118	124	130	135	141	146	152	158	163	169	175	180	186	191	197
64	110	116	122	128	134	140	145	151	157	163	169	174	180	186	192	197	204
65	114	120	126	132	138	144	150	156	162	168	174	180	186	192	198	204	210
66	118	124	130	136	142	148	155	161	167	173	179	186	192	198	204	210	216
67	121	127	134	140	146	153	159	166	172	178	185	191	198	204	211	217	223
68	125	131	138	144	151	158	164	171	177	184	190	197	203	210	216	223	230
69	128	135	142	149	155	162	169	176	182	189	196	203	209	216	223	230	236
70	132	139	146	153	160	167	174	181	188	195	202	209	216	222	229	236	243
71	135	143	150	157	165	172	179	186	193	200	208	215	222	229	236	243	250
72	140	147	154	162	169	177	184	191	199	206	213	221	228	235	242	250	258
73	144	151	159	166	174	182	189	197	204	212	219	227	235	242	250	257	265
74	148	155	163	171	179	186	194	202	210	218	225	233	241	249	256	264	272
75	152	160	168	176	184	192	200	208	216	224	232	240	248	256	264	272	279
76	156	164	172	180	189	197	205	213	221	230	238	246	254	263	271	279	287
BMI	**19**	**20**	**21**	**22**	**23**	**24**	**25**	**26**	**27**	**28**	**29**	**30**	**31**	**32**	**33**	**34**	**35**
NORMAL							*OVERWEIGHT*					*OBESE*					

Modified from NHLBI Obesity Education Initiative Expert Panel on the Identification, Evaluation, and Treatment of Obesity in Adults (US). *Clinical guidelines on the identification, evaluation, and treatment of overweight and obesity in adults: The evidence report* (NIH Publication No. 98-4083, Bethesda, MD, 1998, National Heart, Lung, And Blood Institute. Accessed on March 4, 2014, from www.nhlbi.nih.gov/guidelines/obesity/bmi_tbl.pdf. *NOTE:* Additional BMI categories may be accessed from this site.

of body weight. In women the concept of essential fat must be expanded to include gender-specific fat in their breasts, pelvic region, and buttocks, which is apparently an evolutionary feature providing energy during childbearing and lactation. Thus, for women, the minimum levels of fatness compatible with health are based on the essential fat plus the gender-specific fat and are in the range of 12% to 14% of body weight; healthy levels of total fat range from 25% to 30% (Figure 9-5).

Sometimes athletes and dancers may strive for body fat levels below these ranges. There is concern that low body fat levels may be responsible for the menstrual irregularities experienced by many athletic women. Amenorrhea (lack of menstruation) is associated with bone loss and increased risk of fractures. The fat level associated with the best athletic performance may not be the best level for all around long-term health. Working to achieve a lower level of body fat can be tempting; the desirability of doing this should be carefully assessed, with consideration of the effect on strength, general health, menstruation, and other individual factors.

Body Fat Distribution

From both a health and an appearance perspective, it is not only the amount of fat but also its location that is important. Spend a few minutes at a popular swimming pool and notice the diverse patterns of fat distribution. Differences related to gender, age, and stage of development become apparent. Fat patterns may also vary among ethnic groups. These distinctions are genetically determined, and although the amount of

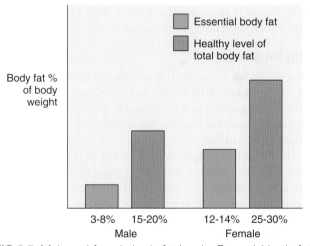

FIG 9-5 Male and female body fat levels. Essential body fat, minimum level of body fat for biologic functions; total body fat, range of level of body fat that provides for biologic functions but that does not have potential to negatively affect health. (From Rolin Graphics.)

exercise can affect the tone of the underlying muscle, it cannot change the pattern of distribution.

Imagine the various adult shapes seen at the swimming pool; try to classify them as either apples or pears. Apples (android body type) are biggest around the waist, and pears (gynoid type) are biggest in the hips, buttocks, and upper thighs. Although some evenly proportioned people will fit neither category, probably most of the pears are women and most of the apples are men and older women. Although this swimming pool visualization may seem frivolous, it focuses attention on the location of fat, which largely determines its effect on health. Fat that is visceral in the abdominal cavity seems to be much more dangerous than subcutaneous such as lower-body fat or the fat under the skin in the abdominal area.

Although some sophisticated techniques accurately assess fat distribution patterns, a good estimate can be made by comparing waist circumference to hip circumference (Figure 9-6). For men it is healthier to have a waist-to-hip ratio of less than 0.95 to 1, whereas women should have a ratio of 0.8 or less. The diameter of your waist alone provides a good estimate of the fat in your abdominal area; people with waist measurements more than 40 in. (102 cm) for men and more than 35 in. (88 cm) for women are at greater risk for the various chronic diseases associated with obesity (Rodriguez, et al, 2009). (For those of Asian descent, higher risk is associated with waist measurements more than 36 in. [91 cm] for men and more than 32 in. [81 cm] for women.) When waist-to-hip measurements are combined with BMI ranges, the level of disease risk is further assessed (Table 9-5).

The two types of fat distribution also differ in their rate of turnover, with visceral fat being much more easily lost and also more quickly regained than subcutaneous abdominal fat or lower-body fat. This is one of the factors contributing to men's apparent greater ease in losing and regaining fat. It is ironic that although the typical female fat pattern of lower-body obesity is more benign, women tend to be more concerned with their fatness than men.

Body Fat Storage

Most of the fat in our bodies is stored in special cells called **adipocytes**. Each of these cells has a nucleus, mitochondria, and other organelles just as other cells do, but these features are usually squeezed over to the side to make room for the droplet of stored fat.

The fat in this droplet is in the form of triglycerides, the same type of molecule making up most of the fat we eat. These triglycerides are synthesized from glucose, glycerol, fatty acids, and some amino acids that are carried to the adipocyte by the bloodstream. The stored fat is in a constant state of flux, with some triglycerides breaking down while others are built. The net effect of this flux—that is, how much fat is in storage—is the result of our energy balance at that time. If we need energy, the balance shifts to favor breakdown and release of fatty acids and glycerol to be transported to various cells, where they are oxidized or converted to other needed molecules. When we have a ready supply of energy, especially shortly after a meal, the balance tilts toward storage.

At birth most of us have relatively small numbers of adipocytes, but during the next few years, these cells increase in number (a type of growth known as **hyperplasia**) and in size (**hypertrophy**). Hypertrophy occurs whenever we continue in positive energy balance for any time. Hyperplasia, however, is more specialized, occurring during the growth spurts that accompany normal development. These growth-related times

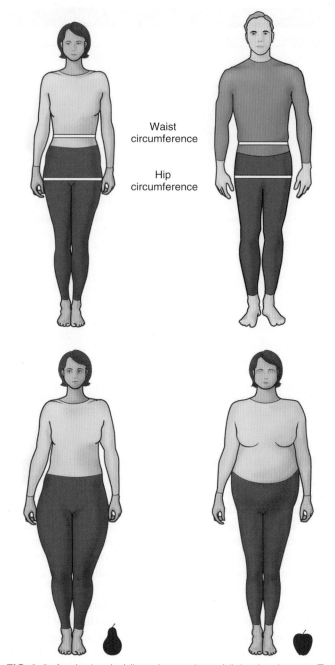

FIG 9-6 Apple (android) and pear (gynoid) body shapes. To estimate your fat distribution, measure the circumferences of your waist and your hips. Divide your waist measurement by your hip measurement. You are an apple if you are a man and your waist-to-hip ratio is greater than 0.95 to 1 or if you are a woman and your waist-to-hip ratio is greater than 0.8. You are a pear if you are a woman and your waist-to-hip ratio is less than 0.8.

of hyperplasia occur during infancy, the preschool years, adolescence, and pregnancy. The adolescent increase in the number of fat cells is much more pronounced among girls than in boys, and it results in the higher level of body fat normal for girls and women.

Most evidence indicates that once these cells form the process of adipocyte hyperplasia, there is no natural means

TABLE 9-5 **Potential Health Concerns Associated with or at Greater Risk for Obese Individuals**	
Cancer	Colon cancer
	Endometrial cancer
	Esophageal cancer
	Gallbladder cancer
	Kidney cancer
	Postmenopausal breast cancer
Metabolic disease	Cardiovascular disease
	Hyperlipidemia
	Hypertension
	Nonalcoholic fatty liver
	Stroke
	Type 2 diabetes
Reproductive disorders	Birth defects
	Cesarean section
	Fetal macrosomia
	Infertility
	Maternal death
	Miscarriage
	Preeclampsia
	Stillbirth
Other	Asthma
	Depression
	Osteoarthritis
	Sleep apnea

Adapted from Power ML, Schulkin J: *The evolution of obesity*, Baltimore, MD, 2009, The Johns Hopkins University Press.

of reducing the number. Knowing there are predictable times of adipocyte hyperplasia, scientists once thought if we carefully controlled our energy balance during those critical periods, we would have lifetime insurance against becoming too fat. Unfortunately, we now know this is not true. If conditions are right, new adipocytes can form at any stage of life.

If more energy is consumed than expended, fat storage will go on until the fat droplet reaches its maximum size. If the positive energy balance continues, the body will make new adipocytes, thereby expanding the storage capacity. The stored fat is relatively equally divided, so all cells contain less than their maximum capacity. The body is then able to continue to expand our storage capacity as long as the positive energy balance persists.

When fat is lost, whether through reduced intake, increased physical activity, or illness, fat is mobilized from adipocytes to meet energy needs. This reduces the size of the droplet of stored fat, producing a smaller adipocyte.

If we have been obese and then lose a lot of fat, our adipocytes may become quite tiny—smaller than the cells of people who were never fat. Our bodies seem to monitor the size of adipocytes, interpreting the shrunken cells as evidence of imminent starvation. We may then feel compelled to eat more. Although the response mechanisms are not fully understood, the effects on metabolism and drive to eat clearly developed as a means to reverse the threat of further loss. This

set of responses is a major part of the theory of set point, discussed later in this chapter.

REGULATION OF BODY FAT LEVEL

Our bodies form fat as a way of storing energy between eating episodes. When excess energy is available, we synthesize triglycerides and store them in adipose cells. When there is a shortage of energy, those stored triglycerides break down and the stored energy is used. Thus, the bottom line in adjustment of body fat levels is the status of the body's energy balance: When energy intake exceeds expenditure, we gain fat; when it is less than expenditure, we lose fat. Sounds simple, doesn't it? But in fact, it's not simple at all. Our bodies are much more complex than the teeter-totter that is often used to illustrate energy balance. Many factors affect the rate of energy intake and expenditure. We all are familiar with the concept that some cars get good gas mileage and others don't. Humans have many systems regulating the mileage we get from our food energy.

Changes in Body Fatness

Levels of body fatness change when a disequilibrium in energy balance is established and maintained for a period. A pound of body fat is roughly equivalent to 3500 kcal. Thus a cumulative positive balance of that magnitude should cause an estimated weight gain of 1 pound, whereas a negative balance of the same size should result in the loss of about a pound of fat. Recall that energy balance is determined by the relationship of the energy intake to the energy expenditure. The intake side of the equation is simple: It represents the kcal value of the food and drink consumed. The expenditure side is more complex, including the resting energy expenditure, the energy cost of physical activity and exercise, and the thermic effect of food. The levels of these expenditures are major factors in determining whether we will gain weight, lose weight, or stay the same weight with a given level of intake.

Earlier this chapter discussed how the effect of changes in one's physical activity alter the energy balance, an important factor when trying to achieve healthy levels of fatness. In addition to the effect of physical activity, the rate of energy expenditure is affected by a number of factors that cause individuals to vary significantly in the efficiency of their energy use. Differences in REE may occur because of ethnicity. African Americans may have lower REEs than whites. This may affect efforts to prevent childhood/adolescent obesity in the former group (Tershakovec, et al, 2002). Although factors affecting basal metabolic rate BMR and TEF are of interest, there is no safe and practical way to alter them. Nevertheless, understanding these influences helps interpret the outcomes of the weight management efforts.

Genetic Influences on Body Size and Shape

Genetic effects on body weight are researched through family studies and investigations of specific genes and their mechanisms. The similarities of BMI values among first-degree family members are best explained by genetic similarity. This accounts for an increased risk of obesity for the first-degree relatives of obese individuals. Family studies reveal that obese children tend to be the offspring of obese parents. However, such studies cannot separate out the intermingled effects of natural genetic factors from those of the environment. Adoptive studies, though, favor the effects of genetics over environment. The adult weights of adoptive children mostly resemble the BMI of their biologic parents rather than of their adoptive parents. This tendency negates or lessens the effects of environment on weight.

Genetic influences related to obesity include the endocrine influence of the hormones leptin and ghrelin. Leptin, produced by adipocytes, has a role in the complex system of the regulation of body weight and fat regulation. Leptin inhibits food intake and regulates long-term appetite. The size of adipose stores is regulated through messages transmitted by leptin between the brain and leptin receptors. Mutations in functions of leptin and leptin receptors may have a role in the development of obesity. This association is more theoretical than diagnosable (Polsky, et al, 2014). In addition, leptin has a role in supporting functions of the body requiring substantial amounts of energy such as reproduction and puberty. Leptin regulates these actions according to the adequacy of nutrient stores (Hussain, et al, 2014).

Another hormone of interest is ghrelin, which is produced by the stomach and increases the appetite or food intake of humans (and rodents). When weight is lost, changes in appetite and energy use occur. Ghrelin, which circulates in plasma, makes up part of the adaptive response of the body to weight loss by leading the body to regain lost weight. As such, it acts as a long-term regulator of body weight. Consequently, depending on genetic predisposition, ghrelin may make maintaining weight loss harder—especially when the weight loss is accomplished through restrictive dieting. Its effect is less when weight loss occurs through the severe gastric bypass surgical intervention (see Chapter 13), probably because the stomach, under that circumstance, produces less ghrelin.)

Studies of leptin and ghrelin are ongoing. Such studies significantly contribute to the understanding of the chemistry of appetite control and demonstrate that there are genetic factors associated with obesity. The work also serves to remind us that human fatness is complex, influenced by the interaction of many factors, both genetic and environmental.

The efforts of the scientists conducting these studies reveal that the role of genetics in fatness levels is complex. There is no single gene for human fatness or thinness. Therefore, fatness must be considered a *multifactorial phenotype*; that is, the displayed characteristic (phenotype) is the product of numerous genetic (DNA), epigenetic (potentially heritable traits that do not alter DNA), and environmental factors. The main genetic influences come from susceptibility genes— genes that do not in themselves produce a certain characteristic but rather affect the susceptibility to other factors (Figure 9-7). Interactions between genes and gene-environmental influences as well as nongenetic influences complete the

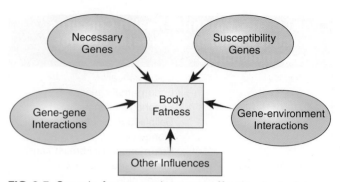

FIG 9-7 Genetic factors and causes affecting body fatness levels. (Modified from Bouchard C: Genetic factors and body weight regulation. In Dalton S, editor: *Overweight and weight management,* Gaithersburg, MD, 1997, Aspen.)

scheme of factors contributing to differences in body fatness levels.

Regardless of one's genetic makeup, one's fatness is also influenced by nutritional, psychologic, economic, and social factors. In addition, there are many different types of obesity and thinness. When a family is characterized by a marked degree of fatness or thinness, casual observations are unable to distinguish among the effects of a shared environment, those of shared genetics, and both. By extensive study of large numbers of people, geneticists have learned that a significant amount of the influence on one's fatness (and characteristics such as metabolic efficiency contributing to fatness) is genetic. Somewhat more influence comes from cultural or environmental influences shared by a family, and the remaining influence is related to factors beyond the shared genes and shared environment within a family (Box 9-2; see the *Cultural Considerations* box Field Trips to Fast Food Restaurants?).

How would genes affect the amount and distribution of fat? Research suggests there is a strong genetic influence on certain components making up the energy balance equation: BMR or resting metabolic rate, TEF, and the energy cost of light exercise. Investigators also found genetic influences on the ability to use ingested fat for energy, on taste preferences, and on the ability to achieve a high level of physical conditioning. These findings help explain why people differ in the ease of gaining or losing weight. Nevertheless, for almost every component studied, there were not only genetic but also environmental factors involved. Although genetics plays a part in the level of body fatness, it is not the only factor. The extent of its influence probably varies from person to person.

Set Point and Body Fatness

Many of our body characteristics are regulated so they are maintained at a constant level or within a narrow range. This is true of body temperature, the level of glucose in our blood, blood pressure, the acidity of body fluids, and many other features. Departure from the usual levels of these variables is usually a clear indication that something is wrong. Usually when the problem is corrected, the characteristic returns to

BOX 9-2 Obesogenic Environments

Obesogenic environments refers to factors and conditions that increase the risk of development of obesity. Even if obesity does not occur, such environments may still have a negative impact on our health. During the past 50 years, so many aspects of life have changed, with many of those changes leading us to consume more dense foods in greater quantities while utilizing the ever-evolving technologies that keep us "plugged in" with one another, without needing to leave our homes our rooms, our chairs but also near the fridge! Add to this situation frenetic stressful work and/or school responsibilities leaving no time for physical activity, and we may find ourselves caught in lifestyle behaviors that keep us from achieving our personal health goals.

This is happening not just in the United States. Throughout the world, "globesity" is occurring in countries where a generation ago, hunger and malnutrition were of concern. Now overnutrition in the form of obesity is prevalent among children and adults as abundant cheap, processed, high-calorie foods have replaced traditional sources of nourishment.

In the Social-Ecological Framework for Nutrition and Physical Activity Decisions model shown here, each circle can be considered "an environment" that, depending on the decisions made, could be an obesogenic environment. Consider for yourself or with your clients the influences of each of the social-ecological framework components on the risk that an environment is obesogenic.

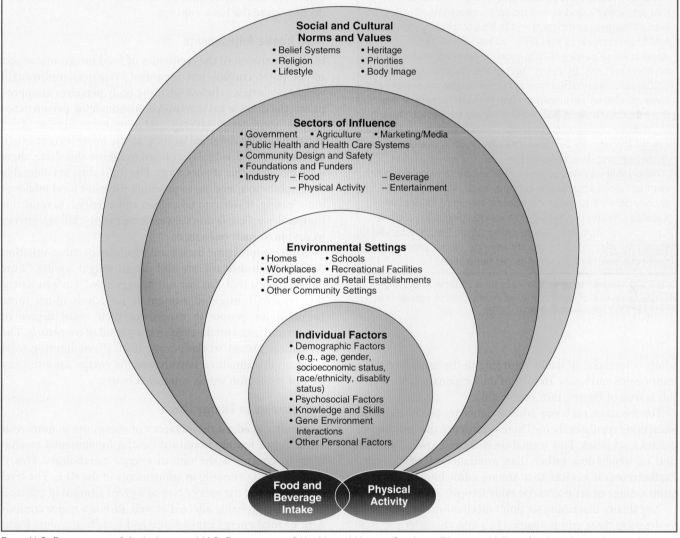

From U.S. Department of Agriculture and U.S. Department of Health and Human Services: *Dietary guidelines for Americans, 2010,* ed 7, Washington, DC, 2010, U.S. Government Printing Office. Accessed March 9, 2014, from www.health.gov/dietaryguidelines/dga2010/DietaryGuidelines2010.pdf.

its usual level. This usual or natural level is called the set point. Actually, this term usually indicates not a single point but rather a narrow range defining the natural level for the characteristic. The adjustments our bodies make to return to the set point are called *defending the set point*. Thus, we can

define set point as a natural level (of some characteristic) that the body regulates or defends.

Because energy is a high priority for the body, the level of energy stores is not left to chance or without regulation. Indeed, as described, the weight (and body fatness) of most

CULTURAL CONSIDERATIONS

Field Trips to Fast-Food Restaurants?

To initiate lifestyle behavior changes among high-risk, ethnically diverse, low-income adults, eight community nursing centers (CNCs) of the Midwest Nursing Centers Consortium conducted a 16-week course titled Wellness for a Lifetime for clients of the centers. The purpose of the course was to promote increased physical activity and to improve the quality of dietary intake of the participants.

Created by a multidisciplinary team, Wellness for a Lifetime was based on health behavior theory and included culturally appropriate content. Each CNC was provided with complete course content, including themes for support group discussions. Course topics were foods and nutrition, stretching and exercising basics, relationship between chronic diseases and diet and activity, and stress reduction strategies. The course was interactive; participants made trips to grocery stores and fast-food restaurants and explored walking routes.

Application to nursing. CNCs provide services within neighborhood settings. By being "part of the neighborhood," each CNC was able to recruit clients for the course who might not have otherwise participated. The physical activity levels of the ethnically diverse populations served increased. Describing the need for exercise may not be enough; actually leading clients through an exercise session or on a walking route models appropriate behaviors.

Although the Wellness for a Lifetime course was developed with culturally appropriate content, each site still needed to modify content to meet the specific needs of its population, such as offering the sessions in various languages (Spanish, Chinese, or Russian). When using other health education tools, we may need to modify aspects of the programs to meet the needs of our own target population.

Data from Anderko L, et al: Wellness for a lifetime: Improving lifestyle behaviors of low-income, ethnically diverse populations, *Ann Fam Med* 3(Suppl 2):S35-S36, 2005.

---

adults is remarkably stable, returning to the usual level after minor gains and losses. In spite of minor gains over the years, this is true of fat and thin people alike.

For the most part, our adult weights are pretty constant. Something regulates them. There is evidence that our bodies defend a set point. This regulation is skewed toward prevention of weight loss rather than avoidance of weight gain. Furthermore, it is clear that among adult humans there is quite a range of set points for body fatness.

Any theory describing set point mechanisms must be able to describe three components: (1) some characteristic that the body monitors, (2) some kind of messenger to carry the information to the central nervous system (CNS), and (3) some mechanism of response to exert the control. Evidence suggests that fatness, lean body mass, and body mass in general are all monitored.

Our attention is on the possible mechanisms of response, the actual regulation. The only options for exerting this control are (1) changing the amount of energy ingested, (2) changing the level of physical activity, or (3) changing the efficiency with which we use ingested and stored energy. These options are exercised through overlapping neural, endocrine, and metabolic mechanisms to exert both short- and long-term adjustments. Defending our bodies' fat stores is a matter of some complexity. Undoubtedly, this complex system with lots of checks and balances and backup schemes reflects the fact that energy is of prime importance to survival.

The concept of a set point for body weight or composition is controversial. Some of the controversy involves the question of set point versus set range. Other experts debate what characteristic (weight, fat, or lean body mass) is under regulation. Still others resist the concept because they feel it discourages individual responsibility for one's own health behaviors. The importance of these controversies is that they do not refute the basic concept.

Food Intake Adjustments

In the discussion of the regulation of food intake, one aspect of set point control was identified. When an individual's weight or fatness is below what the body perceives as appropriate, the drive to eat is activated. Although the person experiences short-term satiety, this long-term hunger drive apparently is maintained as long as the lower weight exists. Although an individual may learn to ignore this drive, there is no evidence that it goes away. The individual is vulnerable to disinhibition, leading to potential excessive food intake or binge eating. It seems to take effort and attention to resist this hunger drive. People don't always have the psychologic energy to devote to such resistance.

Some people come back from a holiday or other situation during which they overate and gained weight, saying, "I ate so much then that I'm just not hungry now." Unfortunately, this type of hunger adjustment is rare. It is much more common for people to experience their usual degree of hunger and usual intake even after a period of overeating. The regulation system works poorly, if at all, in limiting food intake in this situation. Fortunately, the energy use efficiency part of regulation works somewhat better.

Adjustments in Energy Use

The body can adjust the efficiency of energy use in numerous ways; only a few are examined here. A fundamental mechanism of control is the rate of energy metabolism. This is implemented primarily in adjustments in the REE. The level of the TEF and the energy cost of a given amount of physical activity are probably affected as well. REE is a major component of total energy expenditure and usually accounts for at least half of total energy expenditure. Reducing food intake produces an immediate and significant depression in REE, which drops promptly and stays depressed throughout the period of lowered intake. If the reduction in intake is not too great, the drop in REE may be sufficient to prevent weight loss; this is a successful defense of set point. With greater dietary restriction, weight is lost, producing a departure from set point (at least temporarily). When weight is lost, there is less body to use energy; this change also depresses REE. Thus, these adjustments greatly slow the rate of weight loss. Most often the weight is then regained.

NUTRITION : WEIGHT ESSENTIALS

Gaining, Losing, or Maintaining: A Wellness Approach

Although it is untrue that we can mold our bodies to any size or shape we desire, we do have the power to change our attitudes and behaviors if needed so that we can achieve satisfaction and wellness at the body composition most natural for each of us. This section describes some guidelines that are equally applicable to nurses and to their patients who are fat, thin, or just right. This concept is commonly referred to as a *nondiet approach.* All of the behaviors recommended focus on long-term changes. Those who adopt these attitudes and implement these behaviors can expect to feel more comfortable with their bodies and probably better about themselves in general. If we eat well and are physically active, we will look and feel good. Body fatness may or may not change. Although this approach may seem discouraging, the harmful and disheartening effects of diets and other programs that promise a lot but deliver only worse problems will be avoided. Box 9-3 describes dietary procedures for those few people who have a serious health condition that justifies the risks of traditional weight-loss efforts (see also the *Health Debate* box Can "Commercial" Diet Programs Teach Healthy Eating Habits?)

BOX 9-3 Restricted Dietary Patterns

The goal of weight management is weight stabilization through the adoption and maintenance of healthy lifestyle behaviors, including consistent eating patterns. Although these changes in behavior may result in minimal weight changes, health status may improve.

Certain chronic medical conditions are improved by weight loss. Consequently, although kcal-restricted diets are associated with physical and psychologic risks, the benefits outweigh them. Following is a guide for comparison of weight loss programs and brief reviews of the primary weight loss formats of these diets. Programs should be contacted directly to determine current fees. New programs may become available through the Internet and should be judged according to the criteria presented here.

Examples of weight loss programs follow:

Weight Watchers	www.weightwatchers.com 800-651-6000
Jenny Craig	www.jennycraig.com 866-706-4042
Nutri/System	www.nutrisystem.com 800-435-4074
South Beach Diet	www.southbeachdiet.com 866-218-2681
Health Management Resources (HMR)	www.hmrprogram.com 800-418-1367
Registered dietitians/ nutritionists (RDNs)	www.eatright.org 800-877-1600
Physicians practicing alone	Available, but may not be trained to treat obesity

Comparison of Weight Loss Programs
Moderate Restriction of Kilocalories
Kcal restriction should be at least 500 kcal less than the individual's daily requirement for energy; daily intake should not be lower than about 1200 kcal. Adults, depending on their gender, height, and weight, may lose weight at intakes between 1200 and 1500 kcal. Intake below this level cannot provide sufficient amounts of nutrients unless supplements are prescribed. The diet should still follow general dietary guidelines, providing 45% to 65% kcal from carbohydrates, about 10% to 35% kcal from protein, and 20% to 35% kcal from fat.

Very-Low-Calorie Diets (VLCDs)
VLCDs are intended for use by moderately or severely obese individuals (BMI >30) whose attempts with more traditional methods have been unsuccessful and for individuals with BMIs of 27 to 30 or higher whose medical conditions depend on weight loss for improvement. Containing only 200 to 800 kcal, a VLCD causes rapid weight loss but increases the risk of gout, gallstones, and other related symptoms, including cardiac complications. Individuals must be under the complete and regular supervision of a physician. The American Dietetic Association (ADA, 2009) has developed medical nutrition intervention procedures for the use of VLCDs. Maintenance of the weight loss is difficult and depends on nutritional counseling, exercise, and lifestyle changes. Regain of lost weight most often occurs after 5 years even with adjunct support from behavior therapy.

Formula Diets
Developed by pharmaceutical and food manufacturers, diet solutions are available in a variety of forms. Designed to replace meals, they may provide a daily total of about 900 kcal and often contain or may be supplemented by vitamins and minerals (ADA, 2009). Although such diets are helpful for quick weight loss, the loss is rarely maintained because boredom with the solution and the lack of learning new eating approaches soon lead to regaining of the weight.

Pharmacotherapy
The criterion for pharmacotherapy is having a BMI greater than 30 or having comorbidities and a BMI of 27. The pharmacotherapy should be accompanied by medical nutrition therapy and exercise. Generally, starting weight loss is only 5% to 15% of original weight. Weight loss is regained when drug therapy is discontinued.

The use of pharmacologic drugs for obesity intervention is controversial among health professionals because of the lack of data on long-term effects and the possibility of abuse when prescribed to patients who do not meet the criterion for pharmacotherapy.

Data from American Dietetic Association: Weight management, *J Am Diet Assoc* 109:330-346, 2009.

HEALTH DEBATE

Can "Commercial" Diet Programs Teach Healthy Eating Habits?*

With the ever-advancing epidemic of obesity in the United States, health professionals are constantly telling the American population, "Don't gain weight! Lose weight!" But at the same time the health professionals are also saying, "Don't go on a diet! Stay away from those dangerous fad diets advertised on television!" So what is the average person supposed to do? How can we expect nondietary experts to lose weight even while we health professionals struggle with our own weight control? Surely there must be some positive aspects of weight loss programs that we can use in our national "battle of the bulge."

This box presents discussion of healthy food aspects of programs like Weight Watchers—focusing on moderation and portion control; and intake of fruits, vegetables, and fiber— and the South Beach Diet—emphasizing whole grains and fruits and vegetables—as helping individuals normalize eating patterns and food portions, *after* the first 2 weeks of deprivation! Perhaps we need to change our approach to the use of commercial diet programs. Let's consider how to customize a program whether online or through books. This approach applies to men and women.

Portion Sizes

Programs that either provide premeasured food *or* have no limit on portion sizes do us a disservice. After years of eating out of control or even just eating our "usual" servings, we may consume portions that are just too large for our caloric needs. It is better to spend a few weeks with measuring cups, learning that your favorite cereal bowl actually holds three servings of cereal, not just one.

Cooking Skills

Eating out may be convenient, but it is more nutritious and economical to cook simple meals. Some programs include easy-to-follow recipes that taste good to both dieters and non-dieters. Because more families consist of busy two-career parents, and children have many extracurricular activities, children may grow up without learning basic cooking skills. As young adults they can easily teach themselves by following simple directions. Better healthy eating programs provide recipes for novice cooks.

Personal and Time Management

Goal-oriented individuals succeed. They plan and follow through. These skills are woven into the higher-quality weight-management programs. Planning ahead, shopping, and cooking for meals for the week involve time-management skills. Consider whether a particular week includes difficult social events involving food and how to cope with them; some programs are flexible enough to educate participants as to strategies for dealing with such situations.

Food Records

Food records or journaling has become an established means of keeping track of foods eaten. It is a diary of all that is consumed, including portion sizes and time of day. Studies show that more success occurs when someone attempting to normalize food consumption keeps written records of food intake. There are now "blogs" or personal diaries online of individuals' food struggles that all can read. A person's food record may be part of an online program of a commercial weight loss program or may be a free program available on the Internet.

Food for Thought?

When a commercial weight loss program advertises that if we do exactly as the program states, we will lose weight, run the other way! A healthy eating plan to manage body weight should be customized to our individual needs. To achieve this, we must take personal responsibility for creating our own strategy for healthy eating.

What is your opinion? Is there a role for commercial weight loss programs? How would you advise your clients who need to manage their body weight?

*This discussion does not advocate the use of any named commercial diet program.

Establishing Realistic Goals

In setting goals, we should consider two almost opposing factors: (1) our unique and individual values, needs, and characteristics and (2) the limits to the extent of control we have over our bodies and our level of fatness. It is fashionable to deny any limits to this control, but objective observation will reveal the fallacy in that thinking. Aspiring to total control is neither realistic nor healthy for most of us. In goal setting, we need to consider what is practical and feasible.

Changing Behavior

The most important goals are those related to changes in behavior. By choosing appropriate behaviors for change, we can work toward establishing habits that will become almost self-sustaining. The behavioral goals should be related to each person's unique needs. For example, in examining his lifestyle, one person may discover that he is always out of food and running out to grab whatever he can find, usually pizza and convenience store items. He may try to establish a habit of planning and shopping for the next week every Sunday afternoon. For him, this behavior change automatically leads to better food choices. For a different person, this particular goal might be irrelevant.

The *Teaching Tool* box Principles of Behavior Change outlines basic principles of behavioral modification applicable to choosing appropriate changes. In recent decades, it has become popular to make superficial use of the principles of behavioral change in weight loss programs. These techniques had limited success because they were presented as just a list of handy hints (e.g., eat on a smaller plate, put down the fork between bites) rather than the individualized system described in the box. Don't confuse these principles with those hints having little to do with the original concepts.

☀ TEACHING TOOL

Principles of Behavior Change

Set a positive, specific, and achievable objective. It is helpful to frame a goal in terms of the exact behavior to be practiced. Objectives like "I want to eat better" or "I don't want to be so inactive" fail to give you any guidance about how to achieve them and what constitutes success. On the other hand, an objective such as eating vegetarian meals five times a week can orient you in a helpful direction right from the start. It is easier to replace a behavior with a new one than to just stop doing it. Break down major behaviors into smaller, less daunting parts, and try only a few changes at a time.

Establish a system for monitoring the behavior to be changed. This observation helps you assess success in changing the behavior and determine what contributes to and detracts from mastery of it.

Modify the environment so that it supports the change. If you were trying to eat more vegetarian meals, for instance, it would be helpful if the environment included vegetarian cookbooks and ingredients and opportunities to be with vegetarian friends.

Set up a plan for rewarding successes. Be sure to choose rewards that will be appreciated but are appropriate to the magnitude of the achievement. The reward should be as immediate as possible. You can make a long-range reward seem immediate by awarding points that build toward the reward.

Recruit support from friends and family. These people may want to be helpful but may not be skilled at it. Tell them of your objectives and how they can help, but do not make them responsible for your personal behaviors.

Allow enough time for a new behavior to become a habit. A simple new behavior like taking smaller bites, if practiced faithfully for 3 weeks, should be well on the way to becoming habit. More complex lifestyle behaviors take much longer to change, usually at least 4 months. Under stress, most of us revert to old habits, so have a plan for how to deal with this occurrence.

Normalizing Eating

The goal of normalizing eating is to reclaim eating as a comfortable and natural process. It involves being in tune with the needs of one's body and its signals about those needs.

Enjoying eating. Normal eating should be enjoyable. Eating is a very sensual process and has the potential to be highly pleasant. Unfortunately, the ubiquitous dieting mentality dictates a love-hate relationship with food. We tend to label the foods we most love sinful and off-limits. Then we long for them and feel dissatisfied with the more ordinary foods we allow ourselves.

In normalizing eating, we strive to retain the enjoyment of the process. This involves eating with awareness, relaxation, and without guilt, allowing ourselves to eat, in appropriate quantities, all the foods we enjoy. It may also involve expanding our pleasure by learning to enjoy a wider variety of foods.

Enjoyment can be enhanced by keeping meals and snacks simple enough that the true flavors of each item can be tasted.

BOX 9-4 MyPlate: Weight Management

The MyPlate food guidance system can also be used for weight management. Several tools of MyPlate can be used to supervise our own energy in/out equations to maintain, lose, or gain weight depending on our individual health needs. These tools are available through www.MyPlate.gov.

Potential MyPlate Tools

MyPlate Plan: A customized food guide providing recommended number of daily food group serving amounts based on an individual's age, gender, and activity level.

SuperTracker and other tools: The SuperTracker is an online dietary and physical activity personal assessment tool that provides information on diet quality, activity levels, nutrition information based on the assessment, and links to related resources. The Food Calories/Energy Balance feature automatically determines energy balance by subtracting the energy expended through physical activity from food calories/energy consumed. The SuperTracker presents the components of the energy balance equation and allows the user to understand the relationship between good nutrition, regular physical activity, and weight management.

Not only do toppings, sauces, and the like usually involve the addition of extra sugars and fats, but they also obscure flavors.

In spite of all this emphasis on enjoyment, normal eating does not mean depending on food as a major source of pleasure. Just as drinking a tall, cold glass of water is a joy when we are thirsty (but is without appeal when we're not thirsty), eating should be a natural source of pleasure and not a preoccupation. We are not advocating that we all live to eat (Box 9-4).

Letting hunger and satiety guide eating. As discussed earlier, most of us guide our eating not only by physiologic cues to hunger and satiety but also by environmental and cognitive factors. Of these three sets of stimuli, only the physiologic cues are triggered by the body's needs. Therefore, normalizing eating involves letting hunger and satiety guide eating. It means eating when hungry even if it is not a traditional mealtime, and it means stopping with the first signs of satiety even if there is still food on the plate.

Although it would seem that eating this way would be easy, trying to implement this advice is actually challenging. A person may fear that if the cognitive control that tells us what we should be eating is relinquished, all control will be lost and huge amounts eaten. A few people actually do go through such a period—a pretty scary experience. Nevertheless, when they trust that they can eat again as soon as hunger dictates, most find they are no longer driven to continue eating such large quantities.

A great many people actually have a different problem: They have ignored their hunger/satiety cues for so long that they no longer sense them. Reversing this lack of awareness involves relearning how to feel and identify the body's signals for satiety. An individual can start this process by carefully noting feelings when several hours pass without eating. Then the person should interrupt a meal midway through it and examine body sensations for satiety cues. A few minutes will be needed to perceive the satiety. If there are no cues to satiety, eating should continue but be stopped again to assess satiety after a few more bites.

Most people are less aware of their satiety signals than of hunger cues. Eating slowly may enhance awareness of satiety. Keeping meals and snacks simple may help, too. Some research indicates there is a component of satiety tied to specific tastes: The greater the variety, the more food is required to reach satiety because each component is activated by the array of sensations. This relationship may be responsible for eating behaviors at generous buffets (see the *Teaching Tool* box Mindless Eating Revealed).

✴ TEACHING TOOL

Mindless Eating Revealed

On the basis of years of studying the psychology of our food choices and quantities consumed, Brian Wansink, Ph.D., Cornell University professor of psychology, food marketing, and nutrition, and director of the Cornell Food and Brand Lab, has revealed some of the cues and influences that govern our mindless consumption of calories. He notes, "The best diet is the one you don't know you are on." The mindful eating approach may be supportive for clients needing to improve their dietary intake. Dr. Wansink suggests that rather than trying to "eat right," try to "eat better." A summary of his approach follows.

Your Mindful Eating Plan

Your Mindless Margin: By making 100- to 200-calorie changes in your daily intake, you feel deprived and backslide.

Mindless Better Eating: Focus on reengineering small behaviors that will move you from mindless overeating to mindless better eating. Five common places to look (diet danger zones) are meals, snacks, parties, restaurants, and your desk or dashboard.

Mindful Reengineering: To trim your mindless margin, you can use basic diet tips, but a more personalized approach is to use food trade-offs or food policies. Both give you a chance to eat some of what you want without making it a labored decision.

The Power of Three: Design three easy, doable changes that you can mindlessly make without much sacrifice.

Mindless Margin Checklist: Use this daily checklist to help you move from mindless overeating to mindless better eating.

Data from Wansink B: *Mindless eating: Why we eat more than we think,* New York, 2006, Bantam Dell; also available from www.MindlessEating.org.

Sensations of hunger are often confused for those of tiredness, anxiety, relief of anxiety, and other states. Distinguishing the difference may require work. It may be helpful to keep a journal of the various sensations observed.

Minimizing the Use of Food to Meet Emotional Needs

Probably all humans use food and eating to help them deal with emotions. We use food to express positive feelings, to celebrate good fortune, to reward hard work, and to create a sense of companionship. Eating as a means of handling negative emotions such as boredom, frustration, anger, or loneliness is especially problematic for many people. Compared with some other ways of responding to strong emotions, eating may be relatively benign, but when we rely on it as our main means of coping, our consumption patterns may have little or no relationship to our physiologic needs. This emotion-driven eating often is followed by feelings of guilt that may feed into the original negative feelings, creating a destructive cycle.

Minimizing emotional eating requires being aware of feelings and any eating associated with them. For personal understanding or as an adjunct to patient education, a journal or eating record can help achieve this awareness by monitoring feelings, hunger, and eating. Records kept for several weeks catch a range of moods. Examine the records from both the perspective of what triggered eating and of how the feelings were expressed or handled.

When we practice eating in response to hunger, we will probably use food less to meet emotional needs. However, if a pattern of eating in response to feelings rather than to hunger still occurs, or if we regularly use food to deal with certain emotions, we need to learn some alternative ways to respond to emotions. We can often be our own best resource for discovering alternative responses by using the records to identify coping behaviors that are already working and that can be used more often. Books are available that deal with making these kinds of changes. Counseling also can help.

Although we are probably never going to completely give up using food to meet emotional needs, it is worth considering how to do so effectively so that we may increase our awareness of how food consumption and emotions are connected. The following guidelines may help:

- Be aware of the reasons behind food use. Verbalize the intended function of the food. Eat food slowly and with concentration.
- Eat without guilt. If this type of eating occurs only rarely, there is nothing about which to feel guilty.
- Arrange a safe circumstance for eating. If some rich, creamy chocolate is just the thing needed, that's fine. Have some, but make sure there is no danger of overdoing it. Buy just one piece, eat in public, or do whatever is necessary to ensure that you can enjoy a reasonable amount without feeling at risk of bingeing.

Eating Regularly and Frequently

Our bodies have evolved so that we function best when we eat several times a day at times spaced throughout our waking hours. Unfortunately, our modern hurried lifestyle often makes eating balanced meals inconvenient. We tend to snack on what is handy early in the day and do most of our eating between 5 PM and bedtime. This pattern has several undesirable effects, as follows:

- It puts the greatest food intake at the least active time of day. This means that the energy ingested must be stored as fat to await use the next day. Because many individuals do not efficiently mobilize stored fat for energy, they probably feel sluggish and curtail their activity the next day.

- It may mean long stretches of time with little food. During these times we often find it too inconvenient to eat, and therefore we deny our hunger or stave it off with inadequate snacks. By late afternoon our hunger, now joined by tiredness and frustrations of school and work, overwhelms us, and we eat frantically, often far more than we need. Thus, this pattern runs counter to our goal of hunger-directed eating. Furthermore, with little or nothing to break the overnight fast, it's hard to get a good start in the morning.
- The quick meals or snacks we grab during the day usually are high in sodium and fat with little nutritive value.

There is nothing magical about eating three meals a day. Five may be better. Fewer than three results in long fasting times and may induce the problems described earlier. Whatever pattern works best, it should space food throughout active hours and should not produce overwhelming hunger or the drive to consume excessively. For most of us, how often we eat has to reflect the difficulties of providing ourselves with nourishing options throughout the day. Normalizing eating involves planning ahead to ensure that we don't get caught without any alternatives to chips and candy bars.

Adopting an Active Lifestyle

Does physical exercise help maintain a desirable body composition? The conclusions from research are contradictory and confusing. A lot of the confusion disappears when one distinguishes between what is possible in a controlled laboratory experiment and what is probable in the reality of most people's lives. Although exercise is not a panacea, it is one of the few factors consistently associated with success in maintaining a healthy body composition.

NUTRITION: FITNESS ESSENTIALS

Major advances in technology have made the lives of our clients and our own more comfortable and simple. We drive instead of walk, take the elevator instead of the stairs, and ride the lawn mower instead of pushing it. The amount of physical activity performed at work and in the home has declined steadily. How important is physical activity to health, fitness, and total well-being? Let's take a closer look.

Physical activity is defined as any body movement produced by skeletal muscles that requires energy expenditure. It varies by day, time of year, and stage of life. Physical activity is similar to yet different from physical fitness. Physical activity describes the actions or movements that we make, whereas physical fitness describes the limits on the actions that we are capable of making.

Being physically fit is more than just being fast or strong. True physical fitness consists of three major components: flexibility, muscular strength and endurance, and cardiovascular endurance. Flexibility is the ability to move the muscles to their full extent without injury. Muscular strength and endurance describes the ability of the muscles to perform hard or prolonged work. Cardiovascular endurance is the ability of the body to take in, deliver, and use oxygen for physical work. Although flexibility and muscular strength and endurance are important components of health and well-being, cardiovascular endurance is the best physiologic index of total body endurance. Life depends on the strength of the heart and lungs to deliver nutrients and oxygen to the cells.

Health Benefits of Physical Exercise

Much of what we do today will affect our future health. We have many choices to make regarding health behaviors. These choices have positive and negative consequences. The choices include using seat belts, smoking cigarettes, consuming alcohol, nutrition, and frequency of exercise. Our choices reflect our lifestyles; we are responsible for those choices.

Exercise is one of the many lifestyle factors that can be controlled. Increased physical activity leads to improved physical fitness and to other physiologic changes (Box 9-5). It is the combination of these changes that leads to better health. People who exercise regularly often adopt a healthier lifestyle; they may stop smoking, have more energy, handle stress better, and make wiser food choices—all of which improve the quality of life.

Most Americans have little or no physical activity in their daily lives. National surveys indicate that approximately one in four adults have sedentary lifestyles. Inactivity increases with age and is more common among women than men.

Persons with physically disabling conditions also benefit from moderate amounts of physical activity. Although this population tends not to perform regular exercise, it is still at risk for chronic diseases for which risk may be reduced by regular moderate exercise appropriate to the level of physical abilities. Other benefits are increased stamina and muscle strength and improvement of feelings of well-being through potential reduction of anxiety and depression (U.S. Department of Health and Human Services [USDHHS], 2008).

Currently, disparities in physical activity levels exist among American subgroups. Higher numbers of women than men, of African Americans and Hispanic Americans than whites, of older adults than younger, and of less affluent than more affluent Americans report no leisure time physical activity. This means that generally women, African Americans, Hispanic Americans, older adults, and the less affluent are not exercising sufficiently to gain the health benefits associated with physical activity (USDHHS, 2008). Health care providers can reduce these disparities by teaching patients about the benefits of exercise and providing information or referrals for exercise programs.

Physical activity need not be strenuous to achieve healthful benefits. Even people who are usually inactive can improve their health by becoming moderately active on a regular basis. As we counsel clients and patients in community and acute care settings, we can incorporate suggestions for simple fitness activities into care plans. The *2008 Physical Activity Guidelines for Americans* provides recommendations regarding the quantity, intensity, and type of exercise to promote health and reduce risk for major chronic diseases, psychological well-being, and a healthy body weight (USDHHS, 2008).

BOX 9-5 MyPlate: Why Is Physical Activity Important

Regular physical activity can produce long term health benefits. People of all ages, shapes, sizes, and abilities can benefit from being physically active. The more physical activity you do, the greater the health benefits.

Being Physically Active Can Help You:
- Increase your chances of living longer
- Feel better about yourself
- Decrease your chances of becoming depressed
- Sleep well at night
- Move around more easily
- Have stronger muscles and bones
- Stay at or get to a healthy weight
- Be with friends or meet new people
- Enjoy yourself and have fun

When You Are *Not* Physically Active, You Are More Likely to:
- Get heart disease
- Get type 2 diabetes
- Have high blood pressure
- Have high blood cholesterol
- Have a stroke

Physical activity and nutrition work together for better health. Being active increases the amount of calories burned. As people age their metabolism slows, so maintaining energy balance requires moving more and eating less.

Some Types of Physical Activity Are Especially Beneficial:
- *Aerobic activities* make you breathe harder and make your heart beat faster. Aerobic activities can be moderate or vigorous in their intensity. Vigorous activities take more effort than moderate ones. For **moderate activities**, you can talk while you do them, but you can't sing. For **vigorous activities**, you can only say a few words without stopping to catch your breath.
- *Muscle-strengthening activities* make your muscles stronger. These include activities like push-ups and lifting weights. It is important to work all the different parts of the body—your legs, hips, back, chest, stomach, shoulders, and arms.
- *Bone-strengthening activities* make your bones stronger. Bone strengthening activities, like jumping, are especially important for children and adolescents. These activities produce a force on the bones that promotes bone growth and strength.
- *Balance and stretching activities* enhance physical stability and flexibility, which reduces risk of injuries. Examples are gentle stretching, dancing, yoga, martial arts, and t'ai chi.

FOOD AND ATHLETIC PERFORMANCE

Physical activity and nutrition have been associated with health since the time of ancient Greece. Hippocrates said, "All parts of the body which have a function, if used in moderation and exercised in labors in which each is accustomed, become thereby healthy, well-developed, and age more slowly, but if unused and left idle they become liable to disease, defective in growth and age quickly" (Simopoulos, 1989). More than 2000 years later, this advice is still consistent with our knowledge about nutrition, physical fitness, and health.

Physically active people of all ages and levels of competition are seeking information to enhance their training and achieve a competitive edge. They want to know what kinds of foods to eat and specific dietary regimens to follow. The nutritional needs of athletes are basically no different from nonathletes, with the exception of kcal and fluids. A diet that provides a variety of foods supplying 45% to 65% of kcal intake from carbohydrate; 20% to 35% of kcal intake from fat; and 10% to 35% of kcal intake from protein is recommended for health and performance (NRC, 2006). However, some forms of heavy training increase the requirement for certain nutrients. For example, carbohydrates are an important source of energy during endurance exercise, and therefore runners, cyclists, and swimmers may need more carbohydrates (60% to 70% of their total kcal intake) than other individuals.

Nutrition can affect an athlete in many ways. At the most basic level, nutrition is essential for normal growth and development and for maintaining good health. By staying healthy, an athlete will feel better, train harder, and be in better condition. Among comparable athletes, good eating habits can be the factor that determines the winner. However, these good habits do not come from the pregame meal or even from what the athlete eats the week before competition. They are built daily over a long period.

A number of dietary patterns provide good nutrition. The MyPlate program can be a useful outline for athletes of what to eat every day. Each food group provides some—but not all—of the nutrients an athlete needs. Foods in each of the food categories of MyPlate provide kcal from different combinations of carbohydrate, protein, and fat (see www.chooseMyPlate.gov). For example, fruits provide kcal from carbohydrates, and grain products contain carbohydrate, protein, and varying amounts of fat.

Athletes should eat at least the minimum number of servings for each group daily to meet energy needs. Depending on their body size and level of training, some athletes may need more than the larger number of servings.

Nurses and other health professionals should have a basic understanding of the nutritional needs of athletes to provide fundamental information and to conduct a simple assessment or screening of nutritional status as influenced by athletic activities. Referrals to a registered dietitian with expertise in sports nutrition is appropriate for athletes and coaches with more specific concerns, such as the creation of individualized eating plans to support training and competitive needs (Rodriguez, et al, 2009).

Kilocalorie Requirements

As noted earlier, kcal requirements vary greatly from person to person and are affected by activity level, body size, age, and climate. Body size affects kcal requirements more than any

TABLE 9-6 **Recommendations for Adequate Fluid Replacement**		
	WHAT TO DO	**WHAT TO EAT AND/OR DRINK**
Before exercise	Hydrating several hours before exercise allows for fluid absorption and urine output to normalize.	Beverages with sodium and/or salted snacks or small meals with beverages can help stimulate thirst and retain needed fluids.
During exercise	Weighing before and after exercise is useful for determining replacement fluid amounts.	Beverages containing electrolytes and carbohydrates are best.
After exercise	Consuming normal meals and beverages restores average hydration.	Beverages and snacks with sodium help speed recovery by stimulating thirst and fluid retention.

Data from American College of Sports Medicine, et al: American College of Sports Medicine position stand: Exercise and fluid replacement, *Med Sci Sports Exerc* 39(2):377-390, 2007.

other single factor. The smaller the athlete, the lower the kcal requirement.

Some sports demand high-energy expenditure, whereas others do not. A frequently asked question is "how many kcal should I consume?" Athletes are consuming enough kcal if they are maintaining their best competitive yet healthy weight. Ideally, kcal intake should balance energy expended. If intake is consistently more or less than an athlete's requirement, weight gain or weight loss will occur, both of which can affect performance.

Many athletes are concerned about their appearance and thus eat less to keep their body weight and percentage of body fat low. However, restricting kcal can have a negative impact on health and performance. As kcal intake decreases, so does nutrient intake. A minimum requirement for college athletes is 1800 to 2000 kcal a day. Eating less than this amount can leave the athlete feeling weak and listless and may lead to iron deficiency, stress fractures, and, for women, *amenorrhea* and osteoporosis.

On the other hand, increasing kcal intake to gain weight may also be difficult for athletes. Too much food can cause discomfort, especially if a workout takes place soon after eating. Furthermore, for an athlete balancing school, work, and practice, little time is available to eat. Small meals and snacks become an important source of nutrients. How often to snack depends on body size and kcal needs.

Water: The Essential Ingredient

Water is the nutrient most critical to athletic performance. Without adequate water, performance can suffer in less than an hour. Water is necessary for the body's cooling system. It also transports nutrients throughout the tissues and maintains adequate blood volume.

During exercise there is always the risk of becoming dehydrated (fluid volume deficit), especially when the temperature is hot. When athletes sweat, they lose water. Although sweat rates vary among people, losing as little as 2% to 3% of weight via sweat can impair performance (Bardis, et al, 2013). When the water lost via sweat is not replaced, blood volume falls and body temperature rises, causing confusion and loss of coordination. To replace the lost water, athletes must consume extra fluids.

The athlete's sense of thirst is not the best indicator that the body needs water; fluid needs may be greater than thirst

can gauge. Adequate water intake before, during, and after an event or practice session is of utmost importance. Table 9-6 lists recommendations based on evidence statements from the American College of Sports Medicine (ACSM, 2007) to ensure adequate fluid replacement, which leads to optimal performance.

Stress the importance of adequate fluid intake. Clients should weigh themselves nude before and after exercise to determine fluid replacement needs. Sweat loss of 1 pound (2.2 kg) of body weight is equal to 2 cups (480 mL) of water. For every pound lost, an athlete needs to drink 2 cups of fluid. Another criterion of hydration is that urine should be basically clear in color throughout most of the day. (See Chapter 8 for effects of a fluid volume deficit.)

Athletes completing endurance events or slower runners in races who continually drink fluid without an equivalent loss of fluid through sweat or urination may so overhydrate themselves as to experience hyponatremia (low blood sodium). Fluid volume deficit (dehydration) is much more common. Awareness of dehydration and hyponatremia is important because their medical treatments differ even though the symptoms appear similar.

Sport Drinks

Athletes often wonder which is better for replacing fluids during exercise—water or sport drinks. The number one goal is to remain well hydrated. Whether the athlete drinks water or a sport drink is his or her choice. Cool water is what the body really needs during activities lasting less than 1 hour. However, athletes participating in endurance events requiring more than 90 minutes of continuous moderate to heavy exercise, such as distance running or cycling, may benefit from sport drinks that contain carbohydrate and electrolytes (sodium and potassium). Sports drinks provide fluids to keep the athlete well hydrated and provide extra carbohydrates for energy.

A major consideration in fluid replacement is how quickly the fluid empties from the stomach. To hydrate the total body, the fluid needs to leave the stomach quickly to be distributed throughout the body. Although larger volumes of fluid empty more rapidly from the stomach, many athletes cannot exercise with a full stomach. Cool fluids empty faster from the stomach than warm fluids. Kcal content is also important. The greater the kcal content of a beverage, the slower the emptying rate. Fluid recovery choices are most effective if

TABLE 9-7 Some Commonly Used Recovery Fluids and Foods after Exercise

FLUIDS	FOODS
Chocolate milk	Cheerios with milk
Gatorade	Yogurt, flavored
Endurox	Pasta with meat sauce

Data from Clark N: *Nutrition and exercise workshop,* New York City, September 2013.

carbohydrates, protein, and water are provided as a 3:1 or 4:1 ratio of carbohydrate to protein (Clark, 2013). Table 9-7 lists commonly used recovery fluids and foods.

Carbohydrate: The Energy Food

Carbohydrate stores in the body (glycogen) are limited. Low levels of muscle glycogen can impair performance. Consuming carbohydrates before and during exercise will delay the onset of fatigue and allow the athlete to compete longer.

How much carbohydrate should an athlete eat each day to replace muscle glycogen? The amount depends mostly on body size. An athlete with more muscle mass will require more carbohydrate. Carbohydrate requirements also depend on intensity and level of training. Athletes participating in high-energy sports that require short bursts of energy (e.g., basketball, tennis, football, soccer) need about 5 g of carbohydrate per kilogram of body weight daily to maintain muscle glycogen stores. Endurance athletes who train aerobically for more than 90 minutes daily may need a higher intake of carbohydrate per kilogram of body weight to replace glycogen. Individuals who exercise regularly to maintain conditioning do well with the general guidelines of high–complex carbohydrate diets, as represented by MyPlate. The *Teaching Tool* box How Much Carbohydrate Do You Need? shows how to calculate carbohydrate requirements.

✴ TEACHING TOOL

How Much Carbohydrate Do You Need?

1. Divide body weight in pounds by 2.2 lb/kg to determine body weight in kg. For example,
   154 lb ÷ 2.2 lb/kg = 70 kg body weight
2. Multiply each kg of body weight by 5 g to determine the number of g of carbohydrate needed daily. For example,
   70 kg × 5 g = 350 g of carbohydrate daily

Both complex and simple carbohydrates are effective in replenishing glycogen in the muscles. However, complex carbohydrates provide vitamins, minerals, and fiber as well. Examples of complex carbohydrates are whole grains, bread, potatoes, pasta, cereal, fruits, and fruit juices. Simple sugars include maple syrup, molasses, honey, agave nectar, and table sugar.

Carbohydrate Loading

Carbohydrate loading is the process of changing the type of foods eaten and adjusting the amount of training to increase glycogen stores in the muscle. This concept first became of interest around 1939, when scientists studied the effects of dietary manipulation on the ability to perform prolonged hard work. They found that men consuming a high-carbohydrate diet for 3 days could perform heavy work twice as long as men fed a high-fat diet for the same 3 days (Christensen and Hansen, 1939). Since then, researchers have investigated several techniques for increasing glycogen levels in the muscles.

To achieve maximum muscle glycogen stores through carbohydrate loading, athletes should consume a high-carbohydrate diet as part of their regular training program. At least 60% (preferably 60% to 70%) of their total kcal should come from carbohydrate. For the athlete eating 3000 kcal a day, this proportion represents a minimum of 450 g of carbohydrate daily. Three days before competition, exercise should taper off to allow muscles to rest. Dietary carbohydrates should be increased to 60% to 70% of total kcal. This technique of combining rest and increased carbohydrate intake encourages greater glycogen storage. Kcal intake may need to be reduced to compensate for less training.

Carbohydrate loading is usually recommended only for athletes engaged in continuous exercise lasting more than 90 minutes, although benefits may be gained for shorter events as well. It is not recommended for athletes participating in short-term events such as sprints or in sports such as football, baseball, and wrestling; nor should individuals with diabetes or hypoglycemia consider this dietary pattern, which affects carbohydrate metabolism. Furthermore, the degree of benefit from carbohydrate loading varies among individuals. Therefore, athletes should determine before competition the value of this regimen for themselves and should refer to specific resources for detailed recommendations. The potential negative side effects of carbohydrate loading include increased water retention and weight gain, stiffness, cramping, and digestive problems (Williams, et al, 2012).

A more practical concern is whether athletes are eating enough carbohydrate on a daily basis to maintain adequate levels of muscle glycogen for training and workouts. See the Websites of Interest at the end of this chapter for sites that determine adequate carbohydrate intake to maximize muscle glycogen stores.

Protein

The importance of protein for athletes has been a subject of controversy for many years. Many athletes and coaches believe that a high-protein diet supplies extra energy, enhances athletic performance, and increases muscle mass. There is no evidence, however, that eating more protein than needed improves athletic ability.

Although carbohydrate and fat are the major fuels used for energy, studies indicate that protein use increases during exercise, and under certain conditions, protein may contribute significantly to energy metabolism (Williams, et al, 2012). Two factors that influence the use of protein as an energy source are the length of exercise and the carbohydrate content of the diet. The body may depend on protein for an greater percentage of energy in prolonged exercise (more than 90 minutes), particularly when carbohydrate intake is low.

The Dietary Reference Intake (DRI) for protein for sedentary adults is 0.8 g per kilogram of body weight per day. Research suggests that athletes need between 1.5 and 2 g of protein per kilogram of body weight per day. For a 150-pound (68-kg) athlete (runner), this amounts to 102 to 136 g of protein per day. Factors such as kcal intake, protein quality, and type and intensity of the sport are important considerations. The lower the kcal intake, the higher the protein requirements. This is one reason why protein intake is often a concern among female athletes, because many do not consume enough calories.

The type of protein eaten also affects the amount of protein needed. The 1.5 to 2 g of protein per kilogram of body weight recommendation is based on a diet containing animal foods. Athletes who eat meat, fish, poultry, eggs, milk, or cheese will have little problem meeting their protein needs. Strictly vegetarian athletes, however, will need to plan their diets more carefully to ensure that their protein needs are met. Protein bars may be used to supplement protein and energy intakes for athletes. Products should be carefully chosen to avoid excess intake of protein and simple sugars masked as dietary supplement bars.

Protein and Amino Acid Supplements

The use of protein and amino acid supplements is a common practice among athletes. Various combinations of individual amino acids are sold to athletes with the promise that the acids will stimulate the release of growth hormone and thus increase muscle mass. Promoters claim that amino acids can build muscle, aid fat loss, provide energy, speed up muscle repair, and improve endurance. Others claim that they are more readily digested and absorbed than the protein consumed in foods.

The question is: Do athletes need to take these supplements, or can they get the protein they need from food alone? Many athletes eat more than the recommended amount of protein (and thus amino acids) from food alone. Amino acids as building blocks of all proteins are found in a wide variety of foods, from pork chops to bread, from beans and peas to milk and tacos. Because the body cannot store extra protein, excess protein and amino acids are broken down and used for energy or stored as fat. If protein or amino acid supplements provide more nutrients than needed for protein functions, the body treats supplements the same as any excess source of protein.

It is safer and cheaper to take amino acids in a glass of milk, a turkey sandwich, or other protein-rich foods. Muscle size and strength increase only after weeks of work. If athletes want to gain muscle mass, they need to become involved in a resistive strength training program and consume a diet rich in carbohydrates.

Fat

In athletic performance, carbohydrate and fat are the major sources of energy. The amount of fat used during exercise depends on the duration and intensity of exercise, the level of prior training, and the composition of the diet. Exercise performed under aerobic conditions will promote fat use as a source of energy. There is a good reason to increase your body's ability to burn fat as fuel; using fat as a source of energy will spare muscle glycogen.

Athletes need a certain amount of fat in their diets and on their bodies for optimal health and performance. The challenge is eating a diet that provides the right amount. The position of the American Dietetic Association, Dietitians of Canada, and the American College of Sports Medicine recommends moderate energy intake of 20% to 25% energy from fat (Rodriguez, et al, 2009). Because each athlete is different, some may eat less and some slightly more than the recommended range of kcal from fat. Many athletes cannot get the kcal they need without eating a little extra fat. However, fat intakes greater than 35% of total kcal have been associated with increased risk of certain diet-related diseases (e.g., heart disease, obesity, cancer).

To lower fat intake, athletes should choose lean meats, fish, poultry, and low-fat dairy products. Fat and oils should be used sparingly in cooking, and fried foods and high-fat snacks should be eaten in moderation. (See Chapter 5 for strategies designed to lower dietary fat intake.)

Vitamins and Minerals

A balanced diet generally supplies enough vitamins and minerals to meet the needs of most athletes, and consuming more has not been shown to improve performance. Nevertheless, use of supplements by high school and college athletes is common. Their use is even higher among elite athletes. Female athletes tend to use vitamin/mineral supplements more than men, and patterns exist among sport groups; for example, bodybuilders, cyclists, and runners are bigger supplement users than wrestlers and basketball players.

There are reportedly many reasons why athletes take vitamin/mineral supplements, such as for extra energy, to make up for a poor diet, to recover quicker after exercise, and for general well-being. The problem is that athletes may view supplements as "good" and therefore harmless. Such beliefs can lead to excessive intakes. For many athletes, the level of nutrients consumed from food alone is greater than 200% of the DRI. With the addition of a supplement, combined food and nutrient intakes can exceed 1000% of the DRI. Toxicity and adverse health effects can occur from consumption of high doses of vitamins and minerals over a long period.

On the other hand, athletes in "thin-build" sports (e.g., gymnastics, figure skating, wrestling, and distance running) often consume low-calorie intakes and thus are at risk for vitamin and mineral deficiencies. For these athletes, supplementation with a multivitamin/mineral providing 100% of the DRI can be beneficial.

Ergogenic Aids

In athletics, the term ergogenic aids is used to describe drugs and dietary regimens believed by some to increase strength, power, and endurance (Table 9-8). Because winning is often a matter of a split second, it is easy to see why athletes are continuously looking for the competitive edge. The fact that more and more nutritional supplements are marketed to athletes presents a challenge to coaches, trainers, nutritionists,

TABLE 9-8 Ergogenic Aids Marketed to Athletes

SUBSTANCE(S)	DESCRIPTION	CLAIMS	ACTUAL EFFECT
Arginine, lysine, ornithine	Amino acids	Stimulate release of human growth hormone	No proven effect
Antioxidant vitamins C, E, beta carotene	Compounds that may prevent free-radical damage	Prevent muscle damage from oxidation following high-intensity exercise	Some evidence of proven benefit
Caffeine*	Stimulant	Improves performance, increases fatty acid, oxidation, spares glycogen	Some evidence of proven benefit
Carnitine	Facilitates the transfer of long-chain fatty acids into the mitochondria	Enhances energy levels; decreases body fat	No proven effect on body fat
Creatine	Protein/amino acids	Increases intramuscular creatine; increases power output; promotes increase in lean body mass	Some evidence of proven benefit
Dehydroepiandrosterone (DHEA)	Hormone	Increases energy, increases muscle mass, decreases body fat	More research is needed to confirm these observations
Ginseng	Extract of ginseng root	Reduces fatigue and improves endurance, strength, and recovery from exercise	No proven effect
β-hydroxy-β-methylbutyrate (HMB)	Metabolite of the amino acid leucine	Increases lean body mass, decreases body fat, increases strength	More research is needed to confirm these observations

*The use of caffeine is considered a form of doping by the International Olympic Committee (IOC). The IOC has set an upper limit of 12 µg/mL of caffeine content in urine.

and health care providers to provide sound nutrition information.

The nutritional supplements used by athletes constantly change. Often, as athletes find that one doesn't work, they search for another. Today commonly used nutritional aids include creatine monohydrate (a protein), chromium picolinate, β-hydroxy-β-methylbutyrate (HMB), and dehydroepiandrosterone (DHEA). Although the use of DHEA is banned in some states, athletes still use it. With the exception of creatine, research has not shown these supplements to have a significant effect on performance. Despite a lack of scientific basis for the claims associated with these products, their widespread use continues.

Nutritional supplements are a multimillion-dollar business. Athletes are prime targets for the marketers of these products. Athletes make good consumers because, like many Americans, they believe that if a little is good, a lot is better. It is not uncommon for an athlete to consume five or six different supplements a day and to not know what substances are in them. Many of the supplements athletes purchase from specialty nutrition stores and mail-order catalogs are not subject to the regulations established by the U.S. Food and Drug Administration (FDA), presenting another concern. Athletes have no way of knowing whether these nutritional supplements are safe.

Taking several different supplements at one time, or one containing a large amount of one nutrient such as vitamin A, can be toxic. There is also the risk of nutrient-nutrient interactions, in which an excess of one nutrient can interfere with the body's ability to use another nutrient. Such a situation may occur when excessive amounts of one amino acid are consumed, possibly affecting the body's use of other amino acids.

ROLE OF NURSES

Approaches to weight, body composition management, and fitness are being reformulated. Recognition that traditional weight loss approaches to eat less and exercise more are not successful and are often counterproductive is growing and is forcing health professionals to consider alternative and adjunct approaches. Some of these approaches are presented in this chapter. Acceptance of genetic limitations and redefinition of weight management and fitness goals provide health professionals and their clients with potentially achievable objectives to achieve and maintain health.

Within these changes it is important for nurses to understand that the role of the dietitian is evolving from that of a counselor/educator who gives only dietary advice to that of a therapist who practices advanced counseling skills using psychodynamic models of therapy to assist and coach clients. This new view expands nutrition therapy and involves a shift from a short-term to a long-term approach. Weight management is a lifelong process and so incorporates broader lifestyle skills to achieve healthy weight and fitness goals. Dietitians can coach clients about the process of food choice, shifting the responsibility of decision-making about food and portion control to the client, who is then armed with skills and support from dietetic counseling. The goal is to ensure enjoyment of eating while still maintaining a healthy lifestyle. Everyone should be able to enjoy his or her favorite foods but make conscious choices about where, when, and how much of the foods are eaten.

Dietitians are often part of multidisciplinary teams that incorporate primary health care providers, physicians, nurses, behavior therapists, exercise therapists, and psychologists. Nurses can provide support during the formal and informal interactions within the health care system. An important aspect of this support involves nurses' considering their attitudes about their own bodies and about clients who struggle with their weight, body image, and possible associated health concerns. In addition, nurses need to be knowledgeable about the lifestyle changes and food choices needed to achieve long-term body composition management to further support client success. This may required the nurse to further specialize as a member of a multidisciplinary health team.

TOWARD A POSITIVE NUTRITION LIFESTYLE: EXPLANATORY STYLE

In his book *Learned Optimism,* Dr. Martin Seligman, a psychologist and professor, explores applications of explanatory styles to everyday life situations (Seligman, 2006). As a component of personal control, *explanatory style* is the way in which a person regularly explains why events happen. An individual with a pessimistic explanatory style spreads learned helplessness by having a pervasive negative view that no matter what he or she does, nothing will change. In contrast, a person with an optimistic explanatory style feels able to stop the reaction of learned helplessness and understands events in a more positive way. An optimistic person feels competent that he or she can change the course of events.

Explanatory style has been studied in relation to health and wellness. A person's approach to dealing with issues of physical health can be helped or hindered by cognitions about personal control over health conditions and maintenance. Seligman notes the following:

- The way we think, especially about health, changes our health.
- Optimists catch fewer infectious diseases than pessimists do.
- Optimists have better health habits than pessimists do.
- Our immune system may work better when we are optimistic.
- Evidence suggests that optimists live longer than pessimists.

How does this information apply to body fat management? Having an optimistic explanatory style may mean accepting one's body as it is and acting in ways to improve health by attempting to eat well and exercise regularly. A pessimistic explanatory style would judge one's body negatively and would not attempt behaviors to improve body composition because physical attributes would be understood to be permanent and thus unchangeable. Consider other ways that our patients' explanatory styles affect their approach to their illnesses and that our explanatory styles affect the strategies of nursing care.

SUMMARY

- The abilities to perform work, produce change, and maintain life all require energy, which is converted from food eaten into ATP energy.
- The two energy pathways are the aerobic pathway (depends on oxygen) and the anaerobic pathway (functions without oxygen).
- Carbohydrate in the form of glucose is the only fuel to be used anaerobically without oxygen to produce ATP.
- During low- to moderate-intensity exercise, muscle cells mainly use fat for fuel.
- Daily energy requirement depends on three major components: basal metabolism, physical activity, and the thermic effect of food (TEF), or diet-induced thermogenesis.
- Each component is affected directly or indirectly by many factors, including age, gender, and body size.
- A healthy weight is a weight at which a person can physically move comfortably, maintain without undue restriction of food intake or without excessive exercise, and live without experiencing any weight-related associative disorders.
- Lifelong management of body fat levels provides a more holistic health approach to body size than does body weight.
- Goals for body fat levels account for an individual's genetic and family factors as well as those of society and health.
- Ways of measuring body fat composition include densitometry and bioelectric impedance analysis.

- Body mass index (BMI), which is calculated by dividing the weight in kilograms by the square of the height in meters, can relate to the associated health risk for men and women.
- Weight may be maintained by set point, through which the body regulates its most natural weight.
- Individuals at both extremes of fatness—those very thin and those very fat—are at increased risk for certain health-related disorders.
- Physical fitness consists of three major components: flexibility, muscular strength and endurance, and cardiovascular endurance.
- The nutritional needs of athletes are generally no different from those of nonathletes, with the exception of kcal and fluids.
- For athletes, a diet that provides a variety of foods supplying 45% to 65% of kcal intake from carbohydrate, 20% to 35% of kcal intake from fat, and 10% to 35% of kcal intake from protein is recommended for health and performance.
- Eating enough carbohydrates daily maintains adequate levels of muscle glycogen for training and workouts.
- Recommendations for protein intake for athletes, 1.5 to 2 g per kilogram of body weight, are greater than those for of sedentary individuals (0.8 g per kilogram).
- Ergogenic aids are drugs and dietary regimens believed to increase strength, power, and endurance.

◎ THE NURSING APPROACH

Case Study: Nutrition for an Athlete

Tom, an 18-year-old freshman student on the university track team, is preparing for a marathon running event. He has been given instructions about diet from his coach but wants to confirm the information with the nurse at the student health center. He has been training hard and is highly motivated to do his best in the race.

Assessment

Subjective (from Patient Statements)
- "I eat healthy and follow the MyPlate guidelines."
- "How do I carbohydrate load before the marathon?"
- "I would like to know what type of sports drinks I should drink and how much and when I should drink them."
- "Please tell me about protein powders."

Objective (from Physical Examination)
- Height 5'9", weight 140 lb
- Blood pressure 120/80. Temperature 98.4°F, pulse 60, respirations 16
- Lean with well-defined muscles

Diagnoses (Nursing)

Readiness for enhanced nutrition as evidenced by desire to know about carbohydrate loading before a marathon race, sports drinks, and protein powders

Planning

Patient Outcomes
Short term (at the end of this visit):
- Tom will state specific plans for carbohydrate loading, hydration, and protein supplements.
- He will discuss the rationale for each dietary plan.

Nursing Interventions
1. Assess Tom's knowledge of nutrition and teach him about nutrition for athletes.
2. Caution Tom to avoid steroids and other banned or illegal substances.

Implementation
1. Assessed Tom's knowledge of nutrition.
   It is important to know the beliefs of an individual so that his knowledge can be confirmed or corrected. Teaching should proceed from the familiar to new information. Teaching should be centered on the learning needs.
2. Taught him the correct procedure for carbohydrate loading.
   During endurance training, at least 60% of calories should come from carbohydrates. A few days before the endurance event, exercise is tapered down to allow muscles to rest, and carbohydrates are increased to help build glycogen stores in the muscles and liver. On the day of the event, a light carbohydrate meal is consumed before the race.

3. Taught him that hydration is important before the event. About 6 oz of sports drinks should be consumed every 15 to 20 minutes during an event lasting longer than 90 minutes. *Water is needed to cool the body and prevent dehydration. Carbohydrate supplies energy, and sodium and potassium replace electrolytes lost through sweat.*
4. Taught Tom that endurance athletes may have higher protein needs than the general population but probably do not need protein powders.
   Endurance and strength-trained athletes may need 1.5 to 2 g protein/kg body weight per day. These recommendations are usually met through diet alone because most Americans actually consume almost twice the recommended amount of protein. Female athletes, though, may need to be aware of their protein intake in relation to their overall caloric intake.
5. Cautioned him to avoid steroids and other banned or illegal substances.
   Even when not asked about steroids and other banned or illegal substances, the nurse should address the subject for health promotion. Steroids are synthetic hormones that are anabolic and androgenic, taken by some athletes to increase muscle size and strength. They are very dangerous and can cause premature closure of bone growth, liver injury, heart disease, high blood pressure, and sterility, and they many other physical effects. Other banned or illegal substances could disqualify him from participating in sporting events.
6. Referred Tom to a registered dietitian/nutritionist to discuss specific personal diet questions and concerns.
   Although a nurse is qualified to discuss general nutrition, specific individualized diets should be planned by a dietitian.

Evaluation
Short term (at the end of the visit):
- Tom was able to state correct plans for consuming carbohydrates, sports drinks, and protein foods.
- He was able to explain valid rationales for his plans.
- He stated that he does not take steroids and other banned or illegal substances and will continue to avoid them.
  Goals met.

Discussion Questions
Tom went to a registered dietitian/nutritionist to work out a personalized meal plan, and he reported to the registered dietitian/nutritionist after the race. He was able to finish his marathon running event but was not among the fastest runners. He planned to do more training.
1. Describe one prerace dinner meal that would provide high protein and about 60% carbohydrate.
2. Would the basic principles in this case study be the same for a young woman who planned to run a marathon? What might be different?

◎ THE NURSING APPROACH

Case Study: Weight Management

His mother brought 10-year-old Jake to the clinic for a physical examination before the start of Little League baseball season. The mother said she hoped the sport would help control Jake's weight. Concerned about his rapid weight gain during the last year, she indicated that Jake was not very active and that he loved to eat.

Assessment
Subjective (from Patient Statements)
- "My friends tease me. They call me Fat Albert."
- "I get tired easily when I have to run, and I'm always the last one to finish a race."
- "I hope the team won't laugh at me if I run slower than the other boys."
- "I usually spend my time playing computer games or watching TV. I like to eat snacks when I watch TV."
- "We usually eat fast foods two or three times a week. Desserts and French fries are my favorites."

Objective (from Physical Examination)
- Height 55 inches, weight 102 pounds
- Weight at the 95th percentile, BMI 24 (>95th percentile for children his age)
- Blood pressure 120/80 (117/75 is 90th percentile for his age)

Diagnosis (Nursing)
Imbalanced nutrition: more than body requirements related to overeating and inactive lifestyle as evidenced by weight at 95th percentile, frequently eats fast foods, usually sits for activities, friends tease him about his weight, and BP at 90th percentile

Planning
Patient Outcomes
Short term (at the end of this visit):
- Jake will identify healthy foods and state his intent to incorporate them into his diet and reduce his intake of foods high in fat and sugar.
- He will agree to watch less TV, play fewer computer games, and play actively every day.
Long term (phone follow-up after 1 month):
- No weight gain, weight stable

Nursing Interventions
1. Assess Jake's knowledge of healthy food choices.
2. Encourage healthy food choices and activities.
3. Inform Jake and his mother about potential serious health problems caused by obesity.

Implementation
1. Used a picture board to see whether Jake could point to the healthier food choices.
   Assessment of knowledge and skills helps determine learning needs.
2. Showed Jake pictures of foods with equivalent calories—large serving sizes of healthy foods and small servings of high-fat, high-sugar foods. Said it was important to choose nutritious food and limit portion sizes when eating a treat.
   Many people are visual learners. Pictures can communicate comparisons without a lot of words. Portion sizes help determine calories consumed.
3. Gave him a list of the healthier choices at fast-food establishments.
   Information and choice can empower individuals. The child should be encouraged to take responsibility for his own choices when possible.
4. Encouraged Jake's mother to have healthy food on hand for after-school snacks.
   By providing nutritious food choices, parents can help control weight gain and promote good health.
5. Recommended maintaining his weight.
   Weight maintenance rather than weight loss is usually recommended for a child who is overweight or obese. As the child grows taller, he will help even out weight proportionately.
6. Suggested to Jake that he spend less time at the TV and computer and spend more time playing—for example, riding a bike or swimming.
   Active sports will help burn calories and could improve his self-esteem and socialization with friends.
7. Showed Jake and his mother how his weight compared to standard growth charts for boys his age. Reported Jake's high blood pressure for his age group and discussed potential complications of obesity: hypertension, insulin resistance (precursor to type 2 diabetes), high cholesterol levels (precursor to coronary heart disease), joint problems, and sleep apnea.
   Knowledge of potential complications can motivate an individual to adopt a healthy lifestyle.
8. Encouraged his mother to praise Jake for making healthy choices.
   Praise and encouragement reinforce healthy choices.
9. Ordered fasting lab tests, including lipid panel, insulin level, and blood glucose.
   Baseline lab results help determine predisposition to complications and could indicate need for treatment.
10. Referred Jake and his mother to a registered dietitian/nutritionist for a dietary consultation. Asked them to record and bring a 2- or 3-day food journal.
    The registered dietitian/nutritionist can individualize food patterns and make compliance easier.

Evaluation
Short term (at the end of the first visit):
- Jake was able to identify the healthier foods and fast-food choices.
- He stated the intention to try to eat smaller portions and choose food lower in fat and sugar.
- He stated willingness to watch less TV and practice baseball and running.
Goals met.
Long term (in 1 month at a follow-up phone call):
- Jake's mother reported that Jake's weight was stable, and they had met with the registered dietitian.
Goals met.

Discussion Questions
1. Why do you think Jake was not asked to adopt a rigid weight loss plan?
2. List five snacks that you could recommend for the mother to have on hand for Jake.

APPLYING CONTENT KNOWLEDGE

Darren, a college student, just started an aerobic exercise plan to lose some fat. Because he feels tired, he stops by the college health center and chats with a nurse practitioner about his exercise program. He asks, "If my muscles use simple carbohydrates for energy, why isn't it okay for me to have a soda and a candy bar rather than a regular meal? It's all kcal, isn't it?" How might the nurse practitioner respond?

WEBSITES OF INTEREST

President's Council on Fitness, Sports & Nutrition

www.fitness.gov/index.html

Provides comprehensive information on physical activity, nutrition, and obesity and related programs in the United States.

American College of Sports Medicine (ACSM)

www.acsm.org

Encourages developing active lifestyles for people of all ages.

Healthy Weight—It's Not a Diet, It's a Lifestyle!

www.cdc.gov/healthyweight/tools/

Offers strategies and tools for achieving and maintaining a healthy weight. Developed by the Centers for Disease Control and Prevention (CDC).

Shape Up America!

www.shapeup.org

Promotes evidence-based information, educative tools, and strategies for achieving weight management.

REFERENCES

American College of Sports Medicine (ACSM), et al: American College of Sports Medicine position stand: Exercise and fluid replacement, *Med Sci Sports Exerc* 39(2):377–390, 2007.

Bardis CN, et al: Mild hypohydration decreases cycling performance in the heat, *Med Sci Sports Exerc* 45(9):1782–1789, 2013.

Christensen E, Hansen O: Arbeitsfahigkeit and Ernahrung, *Skand Arch Physiol* 81:160–171, 1939.

Clark N: *Nancy Clark's sports nutrition guidebook*, ed 5, Champaign, IL, 2013, Human Kinetics.

Hussain SS, et al: Control of food intake and appetite. In Ross AC, et al, editors: *Modern nutrition in health and disease*, ed 11, Philadelphia, 2014, Lippincott Williams & Wilkins.

National Research Council (NRC): *Dietary reference intakes: The essential guide to nutrient requirements*, Washington, DC, 2006, The National Academies Press.

Polsky S, et al: Obesity: Epidemiology, etiology and prevention. In Ross AC, et al, editors: *Modern nutrition in health and disease*, ed 11, Philadelphia, 2014, Lippincott Williams & Wilkins.

Rodriguez NR, et al: American Dietetic Association (ADA): Position of the American Dietetic Association, Dietitians of Canada, and the American College of Sports Medicine: Nutrition and athletic performance, *J Am Diet Assoc* 109:509–527, 2009.

Seligman MEP: *Learned optimism*, New York, 2006, Alfred A. Knopf.

Simopoulos AP: Opening address: Nutrition and fitness from the first Olympiad in 776 BC to 393 AD and the concept of positive health, *Am J Clin Nutr* 49(5 Suppl):921–926, 1989.

Tershakovec AM, et al: Age, sex, ethnicity, body composition, and resting energy expenditure of obese African American and white children and adolescents, *Am J Clin Nutr* 75(5):867–871, 2002.

U.S. Department of Health and Human Services (USDHHS): *2008 Physical activity guidelines for Americans*, Washington, DC, 2008, U.S. Government Printing Office. From: www.health.gov/paguidelines/guidelines/default.aspx. Accessed January 2, 2014.

Wellman NS, Kamp BJ: Nutrition in aging. In Mahan LK, et al, editors: *Krause's food & the nutrition care process*, ed 13, St. Louis, MO, 2012, Elsevier.

Williams MH, et al: *Nutrition for health, fitness and sport*, ed 10, New York, 2012, McGraw-Hill Science.

CHAPTER 10

Nutrition Across the Life Span

Aging is a gradual process that reflects the influence of genetics, lifestyle, and environment over the course of the life span.

http://evolve.elsevier.com/GRODNER/FOUNDATIONS

LEARNING OBJECTIVES

- Discuss nutrient needs during pregnancy.
- Explain the process of lactation and the benefits of breast-feeding for mother and infant.
- Identify sound nutrition practices during the first year of life.
- Compare and contrast the nutrient requirements, eating styles, food choices, and community supports for childhood, adolescence, and adulthood.

- Describe approaches to prevent food asphyxiation, lead poisoning, overweight/diabetes, and iron deficiency during childhood and adolescence.
- Summarize nutrition strategies to reduce risk of the chronic disorders osteoporosis, cardiovascular disease, hypertension, and obesity.

ROLE IN WELLNESS

This chapter not only addresses the basic nutrition requirements of pregnancy, infancy, childhood, adolescence, and adulthood through older adulthood but also considers the factors that affect health promotion. As presented in Chapter 1, the goal of health promotion is to increase the level of health of individuals, families, and communities. Health promotion strategies often focus on lifestyle changes leading to new, positive health behaviors.

Development of these behaviors may depend on knowledge, techniques, and community supports. *Knowledge* is learning new information about the benefits or risks of health-related behaviors. *Techniques* are strategies used to apply new knowledge to everyday activities. By applying our knowledge, we modify lifestyle behaviors. *Community supports* (environmental or regulatory measures) are available that support new health-promoting behaviors within a social context.

Previous chapters have begun with a discussion of the relationship of the chapter topic to the six dimensions of health. Because this chapter covers the full range of the life span, a more fitting application of the dimensions is covered with the *Cultural Considerations* box, Live Long and Prosper … the Okinawa Way!

NUTRITION DURING PREGNANCY

Although the influence of nutrition on the course of pregnancy was assumed for some time, it was not until the twentieth century that research provided a scientific basis to substantiate such assumptions. Appropriate nutritional intake during pregnancy is integral to a successful pregnancy. Successful pregnancy outcomes include a viable infant of acceptable birth weight, an infant free of congenital defects, and a favorable long-term health outlook for both mother and infant.

Body Composition Changes During Pregnancy

Following conception and continuing until parturition (childbirth), many metabolic, anatomic, hormonal, psychologic, and physiologic changes take place in the mother. This chapter focuses on those most affected by or affecting nutrient intake.

Hormones of Pregnancy

Numerous steroid hormones, peptide hormones, and prostaglandins influence the course of pregnancy. Some of them, such as the placental hormones *human placental lactogen* and *human growth hormone*, are produced only during pregnancy. Others, including insulin, glucagon, and thyroxine, are present in different amounts from those in the nonpregnant state and have profound influences on metabolism throughout gestation.

Progesterone and estrogen have a particularly strong influence on pregnancy. The action of progesterone promotes development of the endometrium (mucous membrane of the uterus) and relaxes the smooth muscle cells of the uterus. This relaxation serves to both help the uterus expand as the fetus grows and prevent any premature contractions of the

🌐 CULTURAL CONSIDERATIONS

Live Long and Prosper ... the Okinawa Way!

Ageism, discrimination against the elderly, would cease to exist if we followed the lifestyles of the "successful-aging" elders of the Japanese island of Okinawa. According to the ongoing Okinawa Centenarian Study that began in 1976, the elders who follow Okinawa traditional ways experience lower levels of heart disease, stroke, and cancer; are generally healthier; and are more physically active for a greater number of years in comparison with other worldwide populations.

Because most of the present Okinawa centenarians are disabled, frail, and physically and/or cognitively impaired, the researchers decided to study the small number of successful-aging centenarians who are able to care for themselves by accomplishing activities of daily living (ADLs) and live independently in their villages. Although findings show genetic factors to be significant for their longevity and wellness, environmental factors may be even more important. The blend of these environmental factors of culture, attitude, and habits as an aspect of wellness may be understood through the definition of health as the blending of the six dimensions of health.

Okinawan Longevity and Wellness through the Six Dimensions of Health

Physical health (efficient body functioning): *Nuchi gusui* and *hara hachi bu* address efficient body functioning through nourishing the body. *Nuchi gusui* means "let food be your medicine" by consuming a plant-based diet of fruits, vegetables, whole grains, sweet potatoes, legumes, fish, tofu, and other soy products. About 15 different foods, in small portions, are eaten every day. *Hara hachi bu* translates as eating in moderation until just about almost full. This approach allows the hypothalamus time to signal the brain that hunger has been satisfied, preventing overconsumption. The healthiest elders tend to be the most physically active, those who work, garden, and pursue interests.

Intellectual health (use of intellectual abilities): Rural Okinawan society views aging as a valuable achievement. Intellectual ability allows for acceptance of the aging process while maintaining one's active role in the community. Birthdays from ages 73 to 100 are observed with symbolic gestures such as elders patting family and friends to impart their good health and good fortunes.

Emotional health (ability to control emotions): *Taygay* represents a calm and relaxed approach to life. Traditional Okinawan society encourages being able to deal with stressors while maintaining appropriate control of one's emotions.

Social health (interactions and relationships with others): *Yuimaru* is the principle of mutual assistance upon which Okinawan society is based. This concept applies to all ages as *moais* (groups of individuals who may be friends or work together) provide support for one another over many years. For the elders, their *moais* are important social links, providing daily interaction over shared pots of tea to discuss the news of the day.

Spiritual health (cultural beliefs about the purpose of life): "*Isha-hanbun, yuta-hanbun*" is a proverb meaning "To best understand your problem, see both a doctor and a shaman." This addresses the balance of life, to be aware of spiritual as well as physical well-being. Okinawan pursuits such as T'ai chi and karate provide both physical and spiritual benefits.

Environmental health (external factors that affect health and well-being): Life is organized around meeting the simple needs of community and personal well-being. The other five dimensions of health are supported within the natural setting of Okinawa.

Application to nursing. Although we may not find ourselves in the semirural environment of the Okinawan villages in which these elders live, we can draw some strategies from their lifestyles to apply to our nursing practice.

We need to be mindful that elderly clients from diverse cultural backgrounds may have lost touch with their *moais*. Perhaps they have recently moved to live with their adult children or have lost a spouse, or both. In addition to medical care, suggestions for seeking out a new *moai* may be most helpful. Art classes, card games, or discussion groups at a local senior center may be helpful in addition to medication for hypertension.

As we advocate for behavior change by our clients, particularly around food choices, consideration of the meaning of food is valuable. Asking an elder to make sweeping food changes is very unsettling. Perhaps introducing the traditional Okinawan concepts of *nuchi gusui* ("let food be your medicine") and *hara hachi bu* (eating in moderation until about almost full) may initiate a lively discussion about food choices and quantities consumed. Your client will remember "that interesting discussion I had with the friendly nurse."

Data from Buettner D: The secrets of long life, *Nat Geogr* 208(5):2-27, 2005; Weil A: Longevity lessons from the Okinawans, *Dr. Andrew Weil's self-healing*, November 2005, p. 8; Suzuki M, et al: Successful aging: Secrets of Okinawan longevity, *Geriatr Gerontol Int* 4:S180, 2004.

uterus. The same effect also influences other smooth muscle cells, such as the gastrointestinal (GI) tract. The resulting slowing of the GI tract during pregnancy may increase the absorption of several nutrients, most notably iron and calcium. One perhaps annoying consequence of this decreased gut motility is the promotion of constipation. Progesterone causes increased renal sodium excretion during pregnancy. The body compensates for this sodium-losing mechanism by increasing aldosterone secretion from the adrenal gland and renin from the kidney. Sodium restriction during pregnancy, once thought to prevent hypertensive disorders of pregnancy, is actually harmful because it reduces plasma volume and cardiac output.

Estrogen promotes the growth of the uterus and breasts during pregnancy and renders the connective tissues in the pelvic region more flexible in preparation for birth.

Metabolic Changes

Profound changes in maternal metabolism occur during pregnancy, and successful adaptation to these changes is necessary for a favorable pregnancy outcome. The basal metabolic rate (BMR) rises during pregnancy, by as much as 15% to 20% by term. This increase is caused by the greater oxygen needs of the fetus and the maternal support tissues. There are alterations in maternal metabolism of protein, carbohydrate, and fat. The fetus prefers to use glucose as its primary energy source. Changes occur in maternal metabolism to accommodate this need of the fetus. The adaptation allows the mother to use fat as the primary fuel source, thus permitting glucose to be available to the fetus (Turner, 2014). Increased macronutrient and micronutrient intake by the mother during pregnancy ensures that these higher metabolic needs are met.

Anatomic and Physiologic Changes

Plasma volume doubles during pregnancy, beginning in the second trimester. Failure to achieve this plasma expansion may result in a spontaneous abortion, a stillbirth, or a low-birth-weight infant. One of the results of this increase in plasma volume is a hemodilution effect, or dilution of the blood. In other words, measured components in the plasma such as hemoglobin, serum proteins, and vitamins will appear to be at lower levels during pregnancy because there is a greater volume of solvent (the plasma) relative to concentrations of solute (the components). Cardiac hypertrophy occurs to accommodate this increased blood volume, accompanied by an increased ventilatory rate.

In the kidneys, the glomerular filtration rate (GFR) increases to accommodate the expanded maternal blood volume being filtered and to carry away fetal waste products. As a result of this increase in GFR, small quantities of glucose, amino acids, and water-soluble vitamins may appear in the urine. Although minor losses may be acceptable, a woman who excretes large amounts of protein may experience a more serious problem called *preeclampsia*, or pregnancy-induced hypertension, which needs strict medical monitoring. Preeclampsia is described in more detail later in the chapter.

As mentioned, progesterone may slow GI motility during pregnancy, leading to constipation, heartburn, and delayed gastric emptying. In late pregnancy, these problems may be exacerbated by the weight of the uterus and fetus as they compress the abdominal cavity.

Weight Gain in Pregnancy

There are three components to maternal weight gain: (1) maternal body composition changes, including increased blood and extracellular fluid volume; (2) the maternal support tissues, such as the greater size of the uterus and breasts; and (3) the products of conception, including the fetus and the placenta. Inadequate weight gain by the mother during pregnancy suggests that she may not have received the proper nutrients during pregnancy. Poor weight gain may then lead to intrauterine growth retardation in the infant. Infants born small for gestational age (SGA) or at low birth weight are more likely to require prolonged hospitalization after birth or to be ill or die during the first year of life. SGA is defined as an infant born at a lower birth weight than expected for the length of gestation, whereas low birth weight is a weight less than 5.5 pounds (2500 g) at birth. Additionally, infant mortality rate, which in part reflects maternal weight gain, is regarded as one measure of a country's health and well-being. Although the 2009 infant mortality rate for the United States (6.39 per 1000 live births) continued an all-time low first reached in 1996 (6.9 per 1000 live births), it still remains far higher than rates in other developed countries (Matthews, 2013). Infant mortality rates are higher among non-Hispanic black infants than among non-Hispanic white and Hispanic infants (Matthews and MacDorman, 2013).

There is strong evidence that the pattern of weight gain is just as important as the absolute recommended weight gains, as shown in Table 10-1. Failure to gain adequately during the second trimester of pregnancy is associated with poor infant birth weight, even if the net gain falls within the recommendations.

TABLE 10-1   New Recommendations for Total and Rate of Weight Gain During Pregnancy, by Prepregnancy Body Mass Index (BMI)

| | TOTAL WEIGHT GAIN | | RATES OF WEIGHT GAIN IN SECOND AND THIRD TRIMESTERS* | |
PREPREGNANCY BMI	RANGE IN kg	RANGE IN lbs	MEAN (RANGE) IN kg/week	MEAN (RANGE) IN lbs/week
Underweight (<18.5 kg/m^2)	12.5-18	28-40	0.51 (0.44-0.58)	1 (1-1.3)
Normal weight (18.5-24.9 kg/m^2)	11.5-16	25-35	0.42 (0.35-0.50)	1 (0.8-1)
Overweight (25.0-29.9 kg/m^2)	7-11.5	15-25	0.28 (0.23-0.33)	0.6 (0.5-0.7)
Obese (≥30.0 kg/m^2)	5-9	11-20	0.22 (0.17-0.27)	0.5 (0.4-0.6)

*Calculations assume a 0.5- to 2-kg (1.1-4.4 lbs) weight gain in the first trimester (based on Siega-Riz AM, et al: Institute of Medicine maternal weight gain recommendations and pregnancy outcome in a predominantly Hispanic population, *Obstet Gynecol* 84(4):565-573, 1994; Abrams B, et al: Factors associated with the pattern of maternal weight gain during pregnancy. *Obstet Gynecol* 86(2):170-176. 1995; Carmichael S, et al: The pattern of maternal weight gain in women with good pregnancy outcomes, *Am J Public Health* 87(12):1984-1988, 1997).
From Institute of Medicine and National Research Council: *Weight gain during pregnancy: Reexamining the guidelines,* Washington, DC, 2009, The National Academies Press.

TABLE 10-2 Dietary Reference Intakes to Meet Needs of Pregnancy and Lactation

	ADULT WOMEN 19-50 YEARS OF AGE	PREGNANT WOMEN THIRD TRIMESTER	LACTATING MOTHERS*
Energy (kcal)	2200	2652	2530
Protein (g)	46	71	71
Vitamin A (retinol equivalent, μg)	700	770	1300
Vitamin D (μg)†	15	15	15
Vitamin E (alpha-tocopherol equivalent, mg)	15	15	19
Vitamin C (mg)	75	85	120
Thiamin (mg)	1.1	1.4	1.4
Riboflavin (mg)	1.1	1.4	1.6
Niacin (niacin equivalent, mg)	14	18	17
Vitamin B$_6$ (mg)	1.3	1.9	2
Folate (μg)	400	600	500
Vitamin B$_{12}$ (μg)	2.4	2.6	2.8
Calcium (mg)†	1000	1000	1000
Phosphorus (mg)	700	700	700
Iron (mg)‡	18	27	9
Zinc (mg)	8	11	12
Iodine (μg)	150	220	290
Selenium (μg)	55	65	75

*During the first 6 months of lactation.
†Adequate Intake.
‡The increased iron requirement for pregnancy cannot be met by the usual American diet or from body stores; thus a supplement of 30 to 60 mg of elemental iron is recommended.
Data from Institute of Medicine, Food and Nutrition Board: *Dietary DRI references: The essential guide to nutrient requirements*, Washington, DC, 2006, The National Academies Press.

A balance must be struck regarding weight gain during pregnancy. Although women who are underweight or normal weight (as defined by body mass index [BMI]) are counseled to eat sufficiently to promote adequate gain, caution must be observed in counseling women who enter pregnancy while overweight or obese. Overweight and obese women should gain enough weight to support the fetus and maternal support tissues but without increasing total body fat. There are increased risks for operative delivery, increased maternal postpartum weight, gestational diabetes, and other long-term health consequences when maternal weight goes beyond the guidelines, particularly among women who are obese before pregnancy (Turner, 2014). In addition, there may be subpopulations, such as minorities and low-income women, who need special guidance regarding weight gain during pregnancy. Figure 10-1 summarizes the possible determinants and the effects of gestational weight gain.

Additional issues arise when women who have undergone gastric bypass surgery become pregnant. Because of smaller stomach size, less food is consumed, and intestinal absorption of nutrients may be compromised. Recommendations are to delay pregnancy until at least a year after bypass surgery and to seek nutrition services to support adequate nutrient absorption and energy intake.

Energy and Nutrient Needs During Pregnancy

The Dietary Reference Intakes (DRIs) recommend increases during pregnancy of all nutrients *except* vitamin D, vitamin E, vitamin K, phosphorus, fluoride, calcium, and biotin (Table 10-2). There are separate dietary recommendations for adolescents who are pregnant.

Energy

It is difficult to estimate the true energy cost of pregnancy, but the best estimates place the total energy cost somewhere between 68,000 and 80,000 kcal. The increase accommodates the rise in maternal BMR during pregnancy as well as the synthesis and support of the maternal and fetal tissues (Turner, 2014). The current recommendation is for a woman to consume an extra 340 kcal per day during the second trimester and 452 kcal per day during the third trimester of pregnancy. Although she appears to be eating for two, the expectant mother need not and should not double her food intake. An extra sandwich, fruit, and a glass of milk can easily provide the additional kcal per day, provided that she was eating well before pregnancy. Personal preference may guide particular food choices to provide the extra kcal, as long as the foods are nutritious.

What happens if a pregnant woman fails to increase her energy intake during pregnancy? The best-known example in the twentieth century occurred in Holland during World War II. Infants born during the famine of 1944 and 1945 had smaller birth weights and birth lengths than infants born either before or after the famine (Smith, 1947). Later research shows that when women who begin pregnancy in energy deficit (e.g., those who are chronically undernourished in developing countries) are provided with energy supplementation throughout the course of pregnancy, there is a positive

WEIGHT GAIN DURING PREGNANCY

FIG 10-1 Summary of the possible determinants and the effects of gestational weight gain. (From the Institute of Medicine and the National Research Council: *Weight gain during pregnancy: Reexamining the guidelines,* Washington, DC, 2009, The National Academies Press.)

BOX 10-1 MyPlate: Pregnancy and Breastfeeding

MyPlate is an accessible source of information for pregnant and breastfeeding women. Below is an example of the interactive MyPlate web page that includes links to resources.

Health & Nutrition Information for Pregnant & Breastfeeding Women

When you are pregnant or breastfeeding, you have special nutritional needs. This site is designed just for you. It has advice you need to help you and your baby stay healthy.

First: Visit your doctor or health care provider if you haven't already. Every pregnant woman needs to visit a doctor regularly. Only he or she can make sure both you and your baby are healthy. Your doctor can also prescribe a safe vitamin and mineral supplement, and anything else you may need.

Next: Get your own Daily Food Plan for Moms. Your Plan will show you the foods and amounts that are right for you. Enter your information for a quick estimate of what and how much you need to eat. Or, enter the foods you eat into the Supertracker to see how your food choices compare to what you need.

Then: Learn more by choosing a topic from the menu below. "Sources of information" will take you straight to the government's best advice on pregnancy and breastfeeding.

For Pregnant Moms

- Nutritional Needs
- Healthy Weight Gain
- Tips for Pregnant Moms

For Breastfeeding Moms
- Nutritional Needs
- Healthy Weight Loss
- Tips for Breastfeeding Moms

Accessed March 10, 2014, from www.choosemyplate.gov/pregnancy-breastfeeding.html.

effect on maternal weight gain and infant birth weight (Bitler and Currie, 2005). On the other hand, some research suggests that women in the United States who are well nourished and do not increase their total energy intake by the recommended extra kcal per day can still have a positive pregnancy outcome. Most likely, in the third trimester, many women decrease their energy expenditure in pregnancy by reducing activity, thereby attaining a net increase in energy intake.

Pregnancy is not a time to restrict kcal or to lose weight, even if the mother begins the pregnancy as overweight. This issue may be particularly important to emphasize to the adolescent population. The mother should be encouraged to eat at least the minimum number of servings recommended during pregnancy from the MyPlate program (Box 10-1). The interactive Daily Food Plan for Moms creates a personalized dietary food pattern based on height, weight, age, and other characteristics. Sample menus can be helpful in showing the pregnant woman how MyPlate can be used (Box 10-2).

Protein

The Recommended Dietary Allowance (RDA) for protein during pregnancy is 71 g per day for adolescent and adult women. Women can easily obtain this amount in the American diet; the use of special protein powder supplements is not recommended. Pregnant patients may be counseled to include appropriate sources of protein that provide vitamins, minerals, and moderate amounts of fat. Clients from low-income populations may need counseling or other assistance to ensure that their protein intake is sufficient; these clients may qualify for food vouchers through the Special Supplemental Nutrition Program for Women, Infants, and Children (WIC)

of the U.S. Department of Agriculture (USDA) (see the *Social Issues* box, Providing the Essentials).

SOCIAL ISSUES
Providing the Essentials

Nutrient-dense foods are the foundations for healthy expectant mothers and their offspring. Women at low socioeconomic levels may have difficulty affording these essentials. One way to ensure adequate nutrition is through a federal government program, such as the U.S. Department of Agriculture's Special Supplemental Nutrition Program for Women, Infants, and Children (WIC). More than 9.2 million women, infants, and children receive the benefits of WIC.

The WIC program began in 1974 and currently operates through approved clinics in all 50 states. Eligible participants must live in an area served by WIC, meet federal income guidelines (income no greater than 185% of U.S. poverty level), and have a nutritional risk factor such as anemia, poor weight gain during pregnancy, previous low-birth-weight infant, or inadequate diet. Pregnant and postpartum women (up to 12 months' postpartum if breastfeeding, 6 months if not) are eligible to participate, as well as infants and children up to 5 years of age.

WIC provides vouchers for foods, including fresh fruits and vegetables high in protein, vitamin C, vitamin A, iron, and calcium—nutrients having shown to be lacking in this population. Participants are offered nutrition education or nutrition counseling, receive testing for anemia and routine anthropometric monitoring, and obtain referrals to other health care resources.

Community health care nurses can refer clients to local WIC programs for assistance. Contacting the city, county, or state health department can identify the closest WIC clinic.

BOX 10-2   Sample Menu for Pregnant Women

Breakfast

Orange juice	½ cup
Whole-grain toast	1 slice
Banana	½ medium
Oatmeal	1 cup
Skim milk	1 cup

Midmorning Snack*

Some examples are:

- Cereal (ready to eat, ¾ cup) with skim milk (½ cup)
- Fresh or frozen berries (½ cup) with nonfat yogurt (½ cup)
- Apple/pear with cheese (1 oz) or peanut butter (1 Tbsp)
- Fruit and yogurt shake
- Open-face peanut butter and apple sandwich

Lunch

Roast beef (2 oz lean) sandwich on whole-grain bread with lettuce and tomato	
Green salad	1-1½ cups leafy greens, 1 Tbsp balsamic vinegar dressing
Orange wedges	1 cup
Skim milk[†]	1 cup

Midafternoon Snack*

See list at Midmorning Snack.

Dinner

Sesame chicken (or fish)	4 oz
Broccoli	1½ cup
Sweet potato	1 medium
Mixed salad (carrots, tomato, 1½ cups spinach, romaine lettuce)	
Olive oil	2 tsp
Fresh lime juice or vinegar	2 tsp
Whole-grain bread	1 slice
Butter	1 tsp
Fresh fruit salad	½ cup
Skim milk	1 cup

Snack (Evening if Needed) *

See list at Midmorning Snack.

*Snacks are all interchangeable.
[†]Assumes water is consumed throughout the day as a beverage in addition to skim milk.

The increase in protein intake over the nonpregnant state is necessary to build and maintain the variety of new tissues of pregnancy. A woman experiencing nausea and vomiting in the first trimester of pregnancy may find it difficult to increase sources of protein in her diet, particularly if meats (which have a strong cooking odor) aggravate the nausea. If this is the case, she should consume small amounts of high-quality protein as tolerated.

Vitamin and Mineral Supplementation

The DRIs are increased during pregnancy for most vitamins and minerals. Vitamins of concern are vitamins A and D.

Although the RDA for vitamin A is 750 to 770 µg RAE (Retinol Activity Equivalents) preformed vitamin A, the Tolerable Upper Intake Level (UL) is set at 2800 to 3000 µg RAE of preformed vitamin A per day because of the potential for birth defects from excessive intake (National Research Council [NRC], 2006). Similarly, excessive vitamin D during pregnancy may cause birth defects, so that the Adequate Intake (AI) (5 µg per day) and UL (50 µg per day) are the same for women regardless of physiologic state (NRC, 2006). Micronutrient needs may be met through a balanced diet, with a few notable exceptions, including folate and iron. All supplementation during pregnancy should be in the form of prenatal-type multivitamin-mineral supplements as recommended by primary health care providers or dietitians.

Folate. Substantial research has demonstrated that folate is important for the prevention of neural tube defects (NTDs) such as spina bifida and anencephaly, one of the most common congenital malformations in the United States. Approximately 2500 to 3000 infants are born with NTDs each year in this country, with an equal number likely lost to pregnancy termination and additional unknown numbers of spontaneous abortions. The U.S. Public Health Service and the American Academy of Pediatrics (AAP) now recommend that all women of childbearing age who are capable of becoming pregnant receive a daily intake of 400 µg of synthetic folic acid (from vitamin supplements, fortified grains, and other foods). Although fortification has been implemented, education continues to be needed to encourage awareness of folic acid intake by women of childbearing age. During pregnancy, the DRI increases to 600 µg DFE per day (NRC, 2006).

Iron. The RDA for iron during pregnancy is 27 mg per day. This level may be difficult to achieve with a normal diet that maintains recommended fat and kcal guidelines. Therefore, all women should take a supplement with 30 mg ferrous iron daily beginning in the second trimester to prevent iron-deficiency anemia in pregnancy (Turner, 2014).

Iron-deficiency anemia is one of the most common complications of pregnancy. The iron requirement increases secondary to the expansion of the maternal red cell volume. Iron-deficiency anemia can impair oxygen delivery to the fetus, which may have severe consequences. In addition, during the last trimester, the fetus stores iron in its liver to use during the first 4 months of life.

As discussed in Chapter 8, an unusual behavior associated with iron deficiency is pica. *Pica* is characterized by a hunger and appetite for nonfood substances, including ice, cornstarch, clay, and even dirt. These substances contain no iron, and their ingestion may lead to loss of additional minerals, particularly when clay and dirt are consumed. Intestinal blockages caused by consumption of these substances may be life-threatening. Of particular concern is the practice of pica during pregnancy, when the risk and implications of iron deficiency anemia are most severe. Although more common among African American women, pica has been diagnosed among all ethnic groups within all socioeconomic levels. A challenge to obstetric nurses is to elicit information about this type of dietary behavior when assessing clients.

Calcium. The AI for calcium is 1000 mg per day for women and 1300 mg per day for adolescents, neither of which is an increase over the nonpregnant state. Although calcium needs are great during pregnancy, particularly for mineralization of the fetal skeleton, changes occur in maternal calcium homeostasis, which result in an increase in intestinal calcium absorption. Many women, particularly adolescents, may not consume the AI for calcium before pregnancy. Women who are unable to consume rich sources of calcium may need to seek advice from a dietitian/nutrition specialist to determine whether supplements are necessary.

Nutrition-Related Concerns

Some pregnant women require particular attention through the course of pregnancy because of exposure to potential nonnutritive substances that may act as teratogens, problematic lifestyle behaviors, or development of medical conditions unique to pregnancy. Box 10-3 lists special needs populations of pregnant women.

Other concerns affecting the course and outcome of pregnancy are maternal age and medical conditions requiring nutrition intervention, such as hypertension, diabetes, phenylketonuria, and human immunodeficiency virus (HIV) infection.

Alcohol

The use of alcohol during pregnancy may produce fetal alcohol syndrome (FAS) or fetal alcohol spectrum disorder (FASD) in the infant. Symptoms include central nervous systems defects and specific anatomic defects such as a low nasal bridge, short nose, flat midface, and short palpebral fissures (separation between the upper and lower eyelids) (Figure 10-2).

There is no safe level of alcohol intake during pregnancy. FAS is not confined to heavy drinkers; anyone who uses alcohol during pregnancy puts her infant at risk of this preventable syndrome. Therefore, *all* pregnant women should be urged to cease consumption of *all* alcoholic beverages. Because alcohol use by pregnant women has been increasing, health care providers should screen women for alcohol use and counsel clients appropriately.

FIG 10-2 A young child with fetal alcohol syndrome features. (From Streissguth AP, et al: Teratogenic effects of alcohol in humans and laboratory animals, *Science* 209[4454]. 353-361, 1980.)

Foodborne Illness

Foodborne illness is a concern during pregnancy. Pathogens such as *Listeria monocytogenes, Salmonella* species, and *Toxoplasma gondii* are high risks for a pregnant woman and her fetus. In addition, commonly consumed foods may contain pathogens, not usually viewed as high risk, that can be problematic during pregnancy. Food safety strategies take on greater importance when a woman's body has reduced immunity or protections against pathogens. Box 10-4 highlights these concerns.

Maternal Age

Adolescents and women older than 35 years are at higher risk for poor pregnancy outcome. In any assessment of the nutritional status of the pregnant teen, there are several important factors to consider. These include the growth pattern of the mother, the psychologic maturity of the mother, possible lack of economic resources to provide for the infant, and potential delay in seeking medical care. Dietary factors to assess are the poor dietary habits typical of many teens, the frequency with which meals are eaten away from home each day, and the possible preoccupation with weight gain during pregnancy. This is still a major public health problem in the United States, affecting medical and nutritional status. Nutritional counseling targeted specifically to this age group is beneficial in reducing the risk of adverse outcomes commonly seen among pregnant adolescents (American College of Obstetrics and Gynecology [ACOG], 2002) (Figure 10-3).

Women who become pregnant after age 35 years have distinct nutritional needs, reflecting their longer medical

BOX 10-4 Food Safety Risks for Pregnant Women and Newborns

During pregnancy, women and their unborn children are more likely to become very ill from food poisoning. Newborns and infants also are at risk because their immune systems are not fully developed. Infections from foodborne illness can be difficult to treat and can recur in these groups.

In addition to keeping good food safety habits, there are certain foods that pregnant women should not eat:

- Rare, raw, or undercooked meats and poultry (rare hamburgers, carpaccio, and beef or steak tartare)
- Raw fish (including sushi, sashimi, ceviche, and carpaccio)
- Undercooked and raw shellfish (clams, oysters, mussels, and scallops)
- Fish containing high levels of mercury (swordfish, tilefish, king mackerel, and shark)
- Refrigerated smoked seafood
- Unpasteurized dairy products ("raw" milk and cheeses)
- Some fresh soft cheeses (Brie, Camembert, blue-veined varieties, and Mexican-style queso fresco) unless made with pasteurized milk
- Raw or undercooked eggs (soft-cooked, runny, or poached)
- Food items that contain undercooked eggs (unpasteurized eggnog, Monte Cristo sandwiches, French toast, homemade Caesar salad dressing, Hollandaise sauce, some puddings and custards, chocolate mousse, tiramisu, and raw cookie dough or cake batter)
- Raw sprouts (alfalfa, clover, and radish)
- Deli salads
- Unpasteurized fruit and vegetable juices
- Refrigerated paté or meat spreads

Some ready-to-eat foods require reheating before use. They include hot dogs, luncheon and deli meats, and fermented and dry sausages. Packaged items should be thrown away once their "use-by" dates have passed. If you think you have contracted a foodborne illness, contact your health care provider immediately.

Modified from the American Dietetic Association: *Food safety risks for pregnant women and newborns,* 2012. Accessed on March 10, 2014, from www.eatright.org/Public/content.aspx?id=5984&terms=foodborne+illness+pregnancy.

history, potential long-term use of oral contraceptives (which may affect folate levels), and the possibility of a longer history of poor eating habits. In addition, older women are at risk for nutrition-related complications such as gestational diabetes. Careful nutritional evaluation of these patients can be useful in providing guidance to reduce the risk of nutritional imbalances that cause pregnancy complications.

Preeclampsia

Preeclampsia, also known as pregnancy-induced hypertension, is considered hypertension with proteinuria (excess protein in urine) after 20 weeks' gestation (Turner, 2014). Clinically, the mother experiences a sudden and severe rise in arterial blood pressure, rapid weight gain, and marked edema, often necessitating immediate delivery of the fetus to save the lives of both mother and infant.

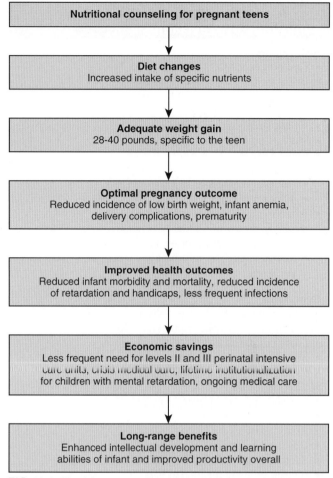

FIG 10-3 Nutrition counseling during teen pregnancy. (From Mahan KL, Escott-Stump S: *Krause's food & nutrition therapy,* ed 12, Philadelphia, 2008, Saunders.)

Preeclampsia may occur in as many as 3% to 5% of pregnancies and is one of the leading causes of prematurity and maternal and fetal death. Risk factors for and symptoms of preeclampsia are listed in Box 10-5.

Preeclampsia may progress to eclampsia. This disorder may result in seizures that can be fatal to the mother and the infant. The cause of eclampsia is unknown, and no screening test is available for it (Turner, 2014).

Nutritional support during preeclampsia includes provision of a well-balanced diet with generous sources of protein to replace losses in proteinuria and with adequate vitamins and minerals. It should supply a sufficient amount of energy. Energy intake should not be limited in an attempt to restrict maternal weight gain.

Currently, low vitamin D status is being studied as an associative factor of preeclampsia. Lower levels have been reported in women with preeclampsia, particularly dark-skinned women from northern latitudes whose levels are lower than those of white women in the same area. Nonetheless, any women with preeclampsia may be experiencing hypovitaminosis D, and testing should be conducted. For those with low levels, dietary changes and/or supplementation may be appropriate (Erick, 2012).

BOX 10-5 Risk Factors for and Symptoms of Preeclampsia

Risk Factors
- First pregnancies
- Diabetes mellitus (type 1; type 2)
- Hypertension (for at least 4 years)
- Advanced maternal age
- African American heritage
- Multiple pregnancies
- Renal disease
- Age at conception:
  - 19 years or younger
  - 40 years or older
- Preeclampsia in earlier pregnancies:
  - Family history of mother or sister having preeclampsia
  - Family history of hypertension, vascular disease
  - Being researched: Inflammatory response, insulin resistance, and oxidative stress

Symptoms
- Headaches (continuous and severe)
- Hypertension (change from usual level)
- Edema of hands and face
- Sudden weight gain
- Excessive nausea and vomiting
- Vomiting blood
- Smaller amounts of urine or no urine
- Blood in urine
- Rapid heartbeat
- Dizziness and blurred or double vision
- Sudden blindness
- Ringing or buzzing sound in ears
- Drowsiness
- Fever
- Pain in the abdomen
- Slowed fetal growth
- Protein in urine (proteinuria)

Diabetes Mellitus

Women with preexisting diabetes mellitus (DM) (type 1 and type 2) require specialized care during pregnancy. Pregnancy significantly affects insulin requirements. Control of glucose levels and avoidance of ketosis by adjustment of nutrient intake and insulin dosage lend support for healthy birth outcomes. There is an increased risk of birth defects, especially of the heart and central nervous system (Turner, 2014). Other complications include macrosomia (larger body size), hypoglycemia, erythremia (abnormal increase of red blood cells), and hyperbilirubinemia. Hyperbilirubinemia is a neonatal condition in which excessively high levels of bilirubin (red bile pigment) lead to jaundice, in which bile is deposited in tissues throughout the body.

These infants may experience hypoglycemia after birth. The maternal source of glucose is no longer available, and because glucose readily crosses the placenta, levels of glucose in utero tend to be high, especially if the diabetes has been poorly controlled. Infants born to mothers with diabetes require immediate monitoring in the neonatal intensive care unit (NICU).

Fortunately, there may be a decreased prevalence of many of the maternal and fetal complications associated with DM when normal blood glucose level (normoglycemia) is achieved before conception and maintained throughout pregnancy. The current recommendation is for women to achieve tight glucose control *before* conception to maximize the likelihood of a healthy mother and infant while avoiding perinatal risks. Control involves prudent blood glucose monitoring, adherence to diet, moderate exercise, and strict adherence to the prescribed insulin regimen. Total energy intake and energy distribution will likely need modification during pregnancy because of the increased energy needs of pregnancy. Insulin dosages will require adjustment because many of the hormones of pregnancy, such as estrogen, progesterone, human chorionic gonadotropin (HCG), somatotropin, and maternal cortisol, act in an antagonistic fashion with insulin. All women with diabetes should discuss drug treatment options with their physicians before conception.

Gestational diabetes mellitus (GDM) is a form of diabetes occurring during pregnancy, most commonly after the twentieth week of gestation. Pregnancy affects glucose control and insulin needs. For nondiabetic women, insulin sensitivity is decreased by placental and ovarian hormones. In response, more insulin is secreted to ensure appropriate glucose levels. The pancreatic reserves of approximately 5% to 10% of women are unable to compensate and do not secrete adequate insulin, and gestational diabetes develops. Patients experience abnormal carbohydrate metabolism much like other persons with diabetes. Of all forms of diabetes during pregnancy, GDM is the most common, affecting 4% of all pregnancies (Turner, 2014). All women should undergo screening for GDM during the second trimester, with repeat testing for women whose results are borderline.

Treatment of GDM consists primarily of dietary control combined with moderate exercise leading to an appropriate weight gain. Insulin may be required if glycemic control is not achieved through dietary control and exercise. Risk factors for GDM include delivery of a previous large infant, prepregnancy weight, family history of diabetes, ethnicity, a prior perinatal death, glycosuria, and maternal age greater than 30 years (Box 10-6). The majority of women with GDM have normal glucose tolerance following delivery, but they may remain at risk for type 2 diabetes mellitus later in life.

Maternal Phenylketonuria

Phenylketonuria (PKU) is an inborn error of metabolism characterized by extremely low levels of the enzyme phenylalanine hydroxylase, which catalyzes the conversion of phenylalanine to tyrosine. Absence of this crucial enzyme causes a failure in the metabolism of the amino acid phenylalanine and low levels of tyrosine. Successful treatment of this disorder occurs through adherence to a strict diet low in phenylalanine and supplemented with tyrosine beginning in the first

BOX 10-6   Risk Factors for and Symptoms of Gestational Diabetes Mellitus

Risk Factors
- Obesity
- Advanced maternal age
- African or Hispanic heritage
- Recurrent infections
- Gestational diabetes in previous pregnancy
- In a previous pregnancy, child having a congenital malformation or birth defect and/or unexplained death of fetus or newborn
- Previous newborn weighing more than 9 pounds

Symptoms
Often there are no symptoms, but the following may occur:
- Increased thirst
- Increased urination
- Weight loss with increased appetite
- Fatigue
- Blurred vision
- Frequent infections, including those of the bladder, vagina, and skin
- Nausea and vomiting

week of life. Failure to detect the disease or a lack of compliance with the dietary therapy results in irreversible mental retardation.

Forty years ago most patients with PKU did not conceive and bear children. Most likely, they were disabled before they were diagnosed or able to properly adjust their diets. However, with the advent of neonatal PKU testing in all 50 states, diagnosis and treatment of the disorder allow many young women to lead normal, productive lives, including having children. Women with PKU require specialized nutrition care during pregnancy. Maternal PKU, particularly if not well controlled at the time of conception, poses a great risk to the unborn offspring. Mothers with untreated PKU have a high likelihood of experiencing spontaneous abortion or having an infant born with microcephaly, mental retardation, congenital heart defects, or intrauterine growth retardation, even if the infant does not have the genetic defect. Conscientious adherence to a low-phenylalanine diet may lessen, but not completely eliminate, the risk of an adverse pregnancy outcome (Elsas and Acosta, 2014). Total nutrient intake and maternal weight gain should be monitored throughout pregnancy.

All young women with PKU should continue their low-phenylalanine diets throughout the childbearing years. Family planning is strongly encouraged to establish safe phenylalanine levels before conception and to educate women regarding the high risk of poor pregnancy outcome, even with good dietary control.

Human Immunodeficiency Virus Infection

In the United States, most of the female cases of HIV infection are among women of childbearing age. Pregnancy may put an additional strain on the already fragile immune system of a woman with HIV, because the hormones and proteins of pregnancy (including estrogen, progesterone, HCG, alpha fetoprotein, corticosteroids, prolactin, and α-globulin) have immunosuppressive effects.

The HIV-infected woman experiencing an opportunistic infection during pregnancy has increased needs for kcal, protein, vitamins, and minerals. Weight gain must be strictly monitored, although there are no specialized weight gain recommendations for this population. Other issues pertaining to HIV are presented in Chapter 20.

Common Nutrition-Related Discomforts of Pregnancy

The following sections discuss the common discomforts of pregnancy and methods of relief.

Nausea and vomiting. Nausea and vomiting, often referred to as "morning sickness," during the first trimester of pregnancy can be annoying, but they generally begin to subside by the beginning of the second trimester. Symptoms of morning sickness may actually occur at any time throughout the day, although vomiting tends to be more common between 6 AM and noon. Although the etiology of nausea and vomiting during pregnancy is unknown, it may be caused by hormonal factors such as a rise in estrogen or the placental hormone HCG. Stress or fatigue may exacerbate the condition. There is no cause for alarm unless the mother begins to lose weight or becomes severely dehydrated. If she cannot retain either foods or fluid for 6 hours or longer, a physician should be contacted.

If nausea or vomiting persists into the second trimester or severely interferes with the mother's life, it may be a more serious condition. Hyperemesis gravidarum is severe and unrelenting vomiting and usually requires intravenous replacement of nutrients and fluids. If the mother receives total parenteral nutrition or nasogastric tube feedings for the treatment of hyperemesis gravidarum, appropriate levels of vitamins and minerals should be included, with careful monitoring and follow-up.

There are no specific foods to avoid, but many women find it is helpful to eat small, frequent meals, to drink liquids between rather than with meals, and to avoid fried and greasy foods. Some women find it helpful to reduce coffee intake and to prepare meals near an open window to avoid cooking odors. If nausea upon getting out of bed in the morning is a problem, dry toast or crackers eaten before getting out of bed may provide relief. Snacks to keep handy while working or traveling include dried fruit, crackers, and small cans of juice.

Heartburn. In late pregnancy, when the fetus rapidly grows in size, the uterus pushes up against the stomach, possibly causing a feeling of fullness in the mother. Additionally, because of the action of progesterone (which can cause relaxation of smooth muscles), a relaxation of the gastroesophageal sphincter may occur, resulting in some reflux of gastric contents into the lower esophagus. This is the cause of the heartburn so common during the final weeks of pregnancy. The best dietary remedies are eating small, frequent meals, avoiding foods high in fat, drinking fluids between rather than with meals, limiting spicy foods, and avoiding lying down for 1 to 2 hours after eating. Many women find relief by wearing clothing that is loose-fitting around the abdomen. Expectant mothers should not take antacids without approval of a primary care provider. Heartburn generally disappears after delivery of the infant.

Constipation. Constipation is common during the first and third trimesters of pregnancy. During the first trimester, progesterone (which slows GI motility) may be responsible. In the third trimester, the growing fetus crowds the other internal organs, again possibly slowing GI motility. Although bothersome, constipation responds well to dietary treatment. A generous intake of fiber, such as whole-grain cereals, fresh fruit, and raw vegetables, as well as inclusion of plenty of fluids should alleviate constipation. Moderate exercise such as a daily walk may also help. The recommendations for alleviating constipation also help prevent hemorrhoids. Over-the-counter laxatives or enemas should not be used by a pregnant woman unless prescribed by a physician.

NUTRITION DURING LACTATION

All sexually mature female mammals possess milk-producing mammary glands and are able to produce milk specifically formulated to provide optimum growth and development for their offspring. Although there are historical accounts of wet nurses and even artificial feeding implements dating back to Greek and Roman times, breastfeeding (lactation) was the primary mode of infant feeding until the previous century in the United States and around the world.

Since World War II there has been a dramatic decline in the incidence and duration of breastfeeding worldwide. Currently 76% of mothers in the United States initiate breastfeeding at hospital discharge, but by 6 months after birth, only about 42% of American infants are breastfed (Ran and Zhou, 2006). In many developed countries, such as Sweden, all women initiate breastfeeding and continue for most of the infant's first year of life. Although there is not one isolated cause for lower breastfeeding rates in the United States, it can be attributed to a multitude of causes. These include the advertising of breast milk substitutes, lack of support for the breastfeeding mother, lack of health care professional knowledge about lactation, short postpartum hospital stays, and the rise in maternal employment without appropriate facilities to nurse infants or pump and store breast milk (James, et al, 2009).

The American Dietetic Association and the AAP have policy statements advocating exclusive use of human milk as the preferred feeding choice for infants for at least the first 6 months of life (AAP, 2012; James, et al, 2009). Ideally, breastfeeding should occur for the entire first 12 months accompanied by appropriate weaning foods. Although primary nourishment is provided by breast milk for the first 6 months, introduction of complementary foods may first occur from 4 to 8 months of age, depending on individual feeding behaviors and needs. Breastfeeding offers advantages for both infant and mother (Box 10-7).

Anatomy and Physiology of Lactation

The human breast begins development in utero and goes through two further stages of change after birth: at puberty and during pregnancy. The mature human breast consists of a system of alveoli and ducts. Myoepithelial cells surround the milk-producing glands, located in the alveoli. The ductules emerge from the alveoli to carry the milk to the lactiferous ducts, which eventually empty into the lactiferous sinuses. The lactiferous sinuses are located behind the areola, or the darkened area of the nipple where the infant latches on during nursing (Figure 10-4).

Throughout the course of pregnancy, the breast tissue undergoes considerable development. Under the influence of

---

> **BOX 10-7** **Benefits of Breastfeeding**
>
> - Provides immunologic protection to the infant against many infections and diseases (especially respiratory and gastrointestinal)
> - Offers uniquely suited nutrient composition with high bioavailability
> - Reduces risk of food allergy in the infant
> - Promotes infant oral motor development
> - Offers convenience: always fresh, available, and at the right temperature
> - Is generally less expensive than formula feeding
> - May protect infant against some chronic diseases such as type 1 diabetes and childhood leukemia
> - Promotes mother-infant bonding
> - Facilitates uterine contractions and controls postpartum bleeding
> - Promotes return to prepregnancy weight

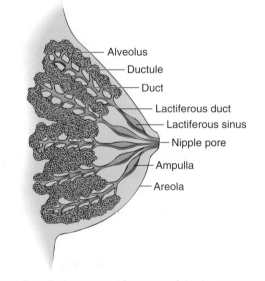

FIG 10-4 Detailed structural features of the human mammary gland. (From Rolin Graphics.)

progesterone, the lobules or alveoli increase in size and number, and estrogen stimulates proliferation of the ductal system. Together, these changes render the breast completely capable of milk production after delivery. An uncommon occurrence is a failure of the breasts to undergo development during pregnancy. A woman who does not notice any changes in her breasts during pregnancy, particularly if she is pregnant for the first time, should receive postnatal assistance to determine her ability to fully lactate. Most women are able to fully lactate with no problems. Actual size of breast has no bearing on the ability to breastfeed.

Lactation is a normal process beginning when various hormones interact following delivery of the infant. Before the onset of labor, there is a rise in serum levels of oxytocin. This hormone is instrumental in initiating the uterine contractions of labor that bring about birth. Oxytocin and another hormone, prolactin, set off the lactation process. Prolactin is primarily responsible for milk synthesis; oxytocin is involved with milk ejection from the breast.

When an infant is allowed to suckle after birth, a nerve impulse is sent to the mother's hypothalamus. This stimulates the anterior pituitary to secrete prolactin, which then stimulates milk production in the alveolar cells (Figure 10-5). The infant sucking stimulus initiates the release of oxytocin from the posterior pituitary. The flood of oxytocin into the breast tissue causes the myoepithelial cells around the glands to contract, thereby ejecting the milk into the infant's mouth. This is called the *let-down reflex,* or the *milk-ejection reflex.* Many women report feeling a tingling sensation in their breasts when the let-down occurs. Additionally, if a mother hears her infant's cry or sees another infant, she may experience a let-down accompanied by a rush of milk ejecting from her breasts. Deterrents to the let-down reflex include fatigue, stress, alcohol, smoking, and some prescription medications.

An important point to note is that milk production is a supply-and-demand mechanism. The more an infant is allowed to nurse, the more nerve stimulation there will be, resulting in a rise in prolactin levels followed by increased milk production. No restrictions should be placed on the number of times an infant, particularly a newborn, nurses per day (James, et al, 2009).

Of particular value is colostrum, the fluid secreted from the breast during late pregnancy and the first few days postpartum. When consumed by a newborn, colostrum provides immunologically active substances (maternal antibodies) and essential nutrients.

Promoting Breastfeeding

To increase the incidence and duration of breastfeeding in the United States and around the world, health care professionals can take measures ensuring that appropriate breastfeeding policies are adopted and practiced in hospitals providing maternity care. In 1991, the World Health Organization and UNICEF (United Nations International Children's Emergency Fund) launched the Baby Friendly Hospital Initiative (Ebrahim, 1993). The initiative includes "Ten Steps to Successful Breastfeeding" that the hospital must be willing to take to become infant friendly. Among the steps is breastfeeding education for all mothers, no separation of mother and infant following birth except for medical reasons, and no supplemental feedings unless medically indicated. Nurses play a key role in prenatal counseling and in postpartum support to help mothers successfully establish and maintain lactation. Obstetric nurses should consult a lactation specialist if an infant or mother has difficulties initiating breastfeeding.

Another influence on successful lactation is acceptability of lactation within the cultural and ethnic communities of which the mother is a part. Cultures in which breastfeeding is common are Chinese, Finnish, Indian, Saudi Arabian, Muslim, South African, and Swedish. In the following cultures, breastfeeding is common, but infants are not given colostrum because it is considered bad or unclean: Cambodian, Filipino, Haitian, Japanese, Korean, Laotian, Mexican, and Vietnamese. Socioeconomic and education levels are influences that help or hinder a mother's attempt at lactation. Organizations such as La Leche League and community-based mothers' groups may provide invaluable support to nursing mothers, particularly those nursing for the first time.

Energy and Nutrient Needs During Lactation

A large proportion of the energy stores laid down as adipose tissue during pregnancy are mobilized in lactation. Both BMR and maternal activity return to their prepregnant levels. The energy cost of milk production is approximately 500 to 800 kcal per day, depending on the volume of milk production. The RDA recommends increases for protein (71 g per

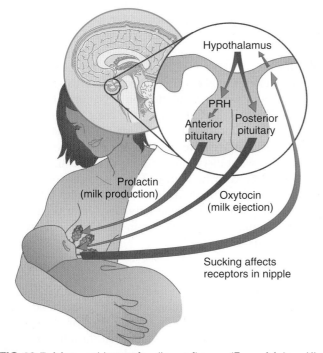

FIG 10-5 Maternal breastfeeding reflexes. (From Mahan KL, Escott-Stump S: *Krause's food & nutrition therapy,* ed 12, Philadelphia, 2008, Saunders.)

day) and for most of the vitamins and minerals over the normal adult levels. The mother can meet most of these increases by consuming a well-balanced diet (see Table 10-2).

A woman need not avoid certain foods while breastfeeding unless a problem occurs. For example, some infants are fussy following the mother's consumption of gas-producing vegetables such as cabbage, onions, and broccoli.

Adequate fluid intake is important during lactation. The average woman produces 750 to 1000 mL of milk per day. She can replace this fluid through consumption of water or juice. Coffee or cola drinks should be avoided or used on a minimal basis. They may act as diuretics in the mother's body, and caffeine, a stimulant, passes into breast milk in small amounts. The old myth stating that alcohol helps a mother relax and enhances milk production should not be followed. Alcohol not only passes into milk, thus becoming available to the infant, but also may inhibit oxytocin, consequently reducing the let-down reflex.

Despite the desire of most women to return to their pre-pregnancy weight quickly, rapid weight loss should not be encouraged during breastfeeding; reduction in milk production may result. Research shows that women may achieve weight loss without compromising their nutritional intake or the infant's if they breastfeed without the use of supplementary formula for at least 6 months. Sufficient milk may be provided with a modest caloric reduction for healthy lactating women with a 1-lb per week loss. An energy intake of at least 1800 kcal per day should be maintained for adequate lactation regardless of maternal fat stores (Erick, 2012).

Nutrition-Related Concerns

Common colds, the flu, and even most illnesses requiring short-term antibiotic therapy do not require cessation of breastfeeding. A number of maternal illnesses or conditions, however, are contraindications to breastfeeding:

- Active tuberculosis
- Human immunodeficiency virus/acquired immunodeficiency syndrome (HIV/AIDS)
- Herpes simplex lesions on the maternal breast
- Maternal alcoholism
- Maternal drug addiction
- Malaria
- Maternal chicken pox (first 3 weeks postpartum only)
- Maternal breast cancer requiring treatment

Most medications for mild illnesses are safe for the mother to take while breastfeeding. If the need for a medication arises, the mother should always remind her health care provider that she is nursing an infant. The American Academy of Pediatrics has classified medications into five categories based on safety considerations. For mild illnesses, as well as for chronic diseases, a medication compatible with breastfeeding can usually be found and substituted for one that is contraindicated. The amount of the maternal dose of drug actually secreted into the milk depends on the route of administration, the size of the molecule, ionization, the pH of the medication, solubility, and protein binding (AAP, 2012). Health care providers might keep this information in mind as they consider prescription medications for nursing mothers.

The Centers for Disease Control and Prevention (CDC) recommend that all women in the United States infected with HIV not breastfeed their infants (CDC, 2006). In developing countries where the risk of death from diarrhea due to inappropriate bottle feeding is far greater than the risk of transmission of HIV via human milk, the World Health Organization recommends that breastfeeding by HIV-infected mothers continue (Coutsoudis, et al, 2008). The woman with active AIDS and opportunistic infections is unlikely to have the physical strength to successfully lactate.

Because of the advent of hepatitis B vaccinations given at birth, hepatitis B is no longer a contraindication to breastfeeding. However, there is mother-to-infant transmission of hepatitis C, and therefore, mothers with hepatitis C should not breastfeed.

NUTRITION DURING INFANCY

Energy and Nutrient Needs During Infancy

Dramatic changes in growth and development occur during the first 12 months of life. In the first year, a human infant is expected to triple his or her birth weight and increase its length by 50%. In addition, after birth, organs such as the kidney and brain continue to develop and mature. In no other period of life do growth and development occur so rapidly. To support this rapid growth and development, the appropriate balance of all nutrients is essential. At the same time, parents, caregivers, and health care professionals must realize that infants have specialized nutrient needs. Advice that is appropriate for adults, and even older children, is inappropriate for infants, particularly with regard to fat and fiber intake and weight gain patterns.

Energy

Adequate energy intake will be reflected in satisfactory gains in length and weight as plotted on a National Center for Health Statistics (NCHS) growth chart (www.cdc.gov/growthcharts/clinical_charts.htm). Infants' fat intake should not be restricted. Well-meaning parents should not put their infants on low-fat diets. Human milk, in fact, is high in cholesterol and fat content. Omega-3 fatty acids are plentiful in human milk, particularly if the mother includes fish in her diet on a regular basis. These fatty acids have been found to be essential for proper brain and nervous system development.

Protein

Protein needs of infants have been hard to determine because of the difficulty of performing nitrogen balance studies on this population. Requirements are estimated on the basis of the intake and growth rates of normal, healthy breastfed infants. Protein requirement is highest during the first 4 months of life, when growth is the most rapid. It is suggested that infants receive 9 g per day from birth to 6 months of age

TABLE 10-3 Recommended Supplementation of Infant Diets

TYPE OF FEEDING	IRON	VITAMIN D	FLUORIDE	VITAMIN K
Human milk	1 mg/kg/day*	10 µg/day	0.25 mg/day	Single intramuscular dose of 0.5 to 1 mg or oral dose of 1 to 2 mg
Formula	Iron-fortified formula	—	0.25 mg/day†	Single intramuscular dose of 0.5 to 1 mg or oral dose of 1 to 2 mg

*May be provided through iron-containing foods after 6 months of age.
†If fluoride content of water is less than 0.3 part per million.
Adapted from Committee on Nutrition, American Academy of Pediatrics: *Handbook of pediatric nutrition,* ed 6, Elk Grove Village, IL, 2009, American Academy of Pediatrics.

and 11 g per day for the second half of the first year. An excess of protein in an infant's diet can be problematic. Protein has a significant influence on renal solute load. The infant kidney is immature and unable to handle the large renal solute loads of an adult's. Therefore, increasing a normal infant's protein intake above the recommended amount should be avoided.

Vitamins and Mineral Supplementation

The DRIs may be consulted for appropriate levels of vitamins and minerals for infants. Breast milk or commercial formula should provide infants with all the vitamins and minerals needed for proper growth and development (Table 10-3).

During the third trimester of pregnancy, the fetus stores iron in its liver to be used during the postnatal period. By 4 months of age, this supply of iron is usually depleted. The iron in breast milk, although lower in absolute amounts, is more bioavailable than iron from commercial formula. Many breastfed infants do not need an iron supplement. However, their iron levels should be assessed periodically. Infants who consume commercial formula should be given the iron-fortified variety to prevent iron-deficiency anemia.

Humans are able to manufacture vitamin D through exposure to the sun; many young infants may not receive enough sun exposure for adequate synthesis. Breast milk contains vitamin D, but it may not be present in levels sufficient to prevent vitamin D–related rickets. In the United States, there have been several documented cases of vitamin D–related rickets, particularly among fully breastfed infants who receive little or no sunlight exposure. Therefore, it is recommended that all breastfed infants receive a daily oral supplement of vitamin D, unless they receive substantial sunlight exposure. Vitamin D can be toxic, so the recommended dosage should not be exceeded. Because vitamin D is present in commercial infant formula, formula-fed infants need not receive a supplement. Use of milk alternatives such as "milks" made from rice, soybeans, almonds, or coconut have also resulted in rickets. These alternatives, which are low in protein, calcium, and vitamin D, are not nutrient dense in comparison with breast milk, formula, or cow's milk. Health care providers need to emphasize to caregivers that although the term "milk" is used in reference to these beverages, they are not nutritionally equal to milk produced by humans or animals.

The water supply of most major cities in the United States contains fluoride as a preventive measure against tooth decay. The availability of fluoride may be particularly important for infants and young children whose teeth are developing. Routine fluoride supplementation is not recommended for infants younger than 6 months. Older infants may need to receive fluoride if their local water supply is not fluoridated, but an assessment of total exposure to fluoride (via water, or juice prepared from local water source) should be made before systemic fluoride is prescribed. For example, many rural families who rely on well water should have their water supplies assessed for fluoride content. Excess fluoride can result in fluorosis, or mottling of tooth enamel, so precise dosing of this mineral is critical.

Newborns are vulnerable to vitamin K deficiency (and thus hemorrhaging) in part because they lack intestinal bacteria to synthesize the vitamin. As a preventive measure, U.S. hospitals routinely give infants 0.5 to 1 mg of vitamin K by injection, or 1 to 2 mg orally, once shortly after birth.

Food for Infants

The ideal food for the first 4 to 6 months of life is exclusive use of breast milk, which has the correct balance of all the essential nutrients as well as immunologic factors that protect the infant from acute and chronic diseases. The breast should be offered at least 10 to 12 times per 24 hours in the first several weeks. As the infant develops a stronger suck, more milk will be extracted with each nursing session, and the frequency of feeding may decline. Although there is no specified time the infant should stay on the breast, between 10 and 15 minutes per breast (offering both breasts per session) is a good recommendation. It is important to realize this is a *general* guideline because all infants have different nursing styles. It may in fact be more appropriate to watch the *infant*—not the *clock*—in an effort to allow the infant to dictate when satiety is reached. The *Teaching Tool* box Guidelines for Successful Breastfeeding offers some suggestions to facilitate breastfeeding.

If a mother chooses not to breastfeed or if she has a medical condition contraindicating breastfeeding, a variety of formulas made from either cow's milk or soy are available. In addition, a number of specialty formulas, such as protein hydrolysate formulas, are available for infants with medical problems. The parents should consult their primary health care provider or nutrition care specialist to identify the most appropriate formula for their infant.

Formulas are supplied either as ready-to-feed, with no mixing required, or as a powder or liquid concentrate to be

BOX 10-8   Formula Preparation

1. Clean all necessary equipment and wash hands before preparing formula.
2. Read formula label and dilute formula exactly as recommended by the manufacturer.
3. Use cold tap water for preparation of concentrated or powdered formula, unless directed otherwise by physician or nurse.
4. Never heat formula in a microwave oven.
5. Discard unused prepared formula after 2 hours.

✱ TEACHING TOOL

Guidelines for Successful Breastfeeding

Although breastfeeding is the most natural and easiest way to feed infants, mothers who decide to breastfeed will welcome the following suggestions:

- Offer both breasts at each nursing session.
- Open infant's mouth wide to latch on correctly.
- Place at least ½ to ¾ inch of the areola in the infant's mouth, not just the nipple.
- Check that the infant's lips make a tight seal around the breast.
- Sore nipples are usually caused by incorrect positioning; position the infant correctly in a tummy-to-tummy fashion or in a "football hold." Support the newborn's head and back with extra pillows on your lap or with your arm cradling infant.
- Do not limit nursing time in the first several days. Doing so does not prevent sore nipples and may hinder milk production.
- Remember that milk is produced by supply and demand— the more often the infant nurses, the more milk produced.
- Expect growth spurts at approximately 10 days, 2 weeks, 6 weeks, and 3 months. At these times, expect a fussy infant who wants to nurse frequently.
- Offer no bottles of formula or water while the milk supply is being established. The artificial nipple may confuse the infant, and substitute feedings that replace breast stimulation may diminish milk production.
- Once milk supply is established, breast milk may be expressed manually or by a pump and saved in a bottle in the refrigerator (up to 48 hours) or in the freezer (several months).
- Learn your infant's cues for satiety.

---

mixed with water (Box 10-8). In older homes and buildings, old pipes, joints, or faucets may contain lead. To reduce the chance of lead leaching into water, tap water should be run for 15 to 30 seconds before using for drinking, cooking, or formula preparation. Only cold water should be used for formula preparation. The formula should be mixed exactly as stated on the package unless otherwise directed by a primary health care provider. Adding insufficient water can result in a high renal solute load, putting strain on the immature infant kidneys; overdiluting will precipitate undernutrition.

For parents or caregivers who may be non–English speaking or may have low literacy skills, pictorial mixing instructions may be useful. Alternatively, asking the caregiver to demonstrate appropriate formula mixing may be suitable. Formula should never be heated in a microwave oven because microwaves heat food unevenly. Contents of a bottle appearing to be cool on testing may actually have portions that could scald an infant. All unused formula at the end of a feeding should be discarded if not used within 2 hours because of contamination by enzymes and bacteria in the infant's saliva. Home-prepared formulas made from evaporated milk, popular in some cultures, are likely to be low in iron, vitamin C, and other essential nutrients and should be avoided.

Before 1 year of age, cow's milk, regardless of fat content or form (evaporated, liquid, or dried), should not be fed to infants. The fat in cow's milk is less digestible than the fat in breast milk or formula and contains less iron and more sodium and protein. These higher levels of solutes may lead to dehydration caused by the increase in urine volume that occurs to reduce solute levels in the body. Deficiencies of other nutrients, such as vitamin C, essential fatty acids, zinc, and possibly other trace minerals, develop because cow's milk is a poor source of these nutrients.

Cow's milk may be introduced after 1 year of age, when at least two-thirds of energy needs are fulfilled by foods other than milk. The delay in cow's milk consumption reduces the risk for development of a milk allergy. Reduced-fat milk and nonfat milk are not recommended until age 2 years.

Introduction of Solid Foods

Solid foods may be added to the infant's diet between the ages of 4 and 6 months. Infants who are introduced to solid foods before this time may be prone to excessive kcal intake, food allergies, and GI upset. Many parents and even some health care professionals believe that offering an infant cereal in the evening will promote sleeping through the night. This belief, however, is not supported by research.

Two basic issues when one is considering the introduction of solid foods to the infant's diet are how to introduce them and what foods to introduce.

How to introduce solid foods. Parents and other caregivers may be anxious to introduce foods other than breast milk or formula to their infant's diet. Health professionals can assure them that it's best for the infant to be developmentally ready for solid foods. The infant should be able to sit with some support; move the jaw, lips, and tongue independently; be able to roll the tongue to the back of the mouth to facilitate a food bolus entering the esophagus; and show interest in what the rest of the family is eating. For example, the infant may try to reach and grab an item off of a family member's plate at mealtime. Likewise, parents should become familiar with satiety cues so as not to overfeed the infant. To indicate fullness, the infant may turn the head to the side, refuse to open the mouth, or grimace when the spoon comes close to the mouth. The caregiver should respect these cues. The infant should never be force-fed. If the infant is overtired or

TABLE 10-4 Solid Foods During the First Year of Life

AGE	FOOD	FOODS TO AVOID IN THE FIRST YEAR OF LIFE
4-5 months	Iron-fortified infant cereal	Honey (may cause infantile *Clostridium botulinum* poisoning); hot dogs, grapes, hard candies, raw carrots, popcorn, nuts, peanut butter (choking hazards); skim milk (insufficient calories); cow's milk (potential allergen, may replace breast milk or formula); egg whites (potential allergen)
5-6 months	Strained fruits and vegetables	
6-8 months	Mashed or chopped fruits and vegetables Juice from a cup	
9-12 months	Crackers, toast, cottage cheese, plain meats, egg yolk, finger foods	

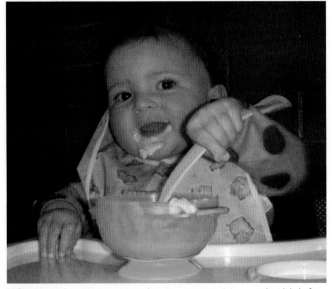

FIG 10-6 A messy experience as an 11-month-old infant strives to feed herself with a spoon.

is not interested in food, he or she ought to be removed from the high chair, and the foods offered again later.

At age 9 to 12 months, an infant may enjoy self-feeding. Although this may be a messy process, caregivers should encourage the development of these skills through food exploration (Figure 10-6).

Appropriate solid foods during the first year of life. The second half of the first year of life should be thought of as a transitional period; breast milk or formula is still the primary food, and the solid foods are complementary. Solid foods should be introduced gradually and one at a time with a 4- to 5-day interval between new foods. This timing is suggested because if the infant has any type of allergic reaction, such as GI upset, upper respiratory distress, or skin reactions (e.g., eczema, hives), the offending food can be easily identified. Families with a documented history of allergies should delay introduction of solid foods until the infant is about 6 months old. If solid foods are introduced too early, the large protein molecules of the offending food may cross the intestinal barrier and elicit an immunologic response in the infant. As the gut matures, it is less likely to allow large unhydrolyzed proteins to cross the mucosa.

Solid foods offered to the infant need not be commercial. Home-prepared foods are good, practical alternatives. Strict

attention should be paid to sanitary food preparation procedures. Although infants should not be offered excessive sweets, naturally sweet fruits such as peaches offer them a taste satisfaction. Although salt should not be added to an infant's food, complete elimination of sodium from foods in the diet is neither practical nor recommended.

A variety of textures, colors, and tastes is important for infants, whether they receive home-prepared or commercial infant foods. The *Personal Perspectives* box Developing "Nutrition Intelligence" provides strategies for introducing infants and older children to a diverse selection of foods. General guidelines for infant feeding are listed in Table 10-4.

Beverages During the First Year of Life

Fruit juice, particularly apple juice, is offered to many infants. Fruit juice can make an important contribution to the diet as a source of vitamin C, water, and possibly calcium (if fortified). Its use, though, needs to be monitored. From age 6 to 12 months, no more than 4 to 6 fluid ounces per day should be offered. Excess fruit juice (more than 12 fluid ounces per day) may lead to diarrhea from carbohydrate malabsorption, growth failure, or, in some children, obesity caused by excess calories. Juices can be diluted with water, providing a beverage with less sweetness. All fruit juices given to infants (and children) should be pasteurized. As discussed earlier in the chapter, it is important to note that beverages made from soy, rice, almond, or coconut do not contain the level of nutrients found in breast milk or infant formula unless they are specifically fortified as infant formulas.

An additional issue is the dental health effects when infants fall asleep with fluids in their mouths. See Box 10-9.

Nutrition-Related Concerns

The nutrition requirements of children with congenital or acquired health problems deserve special attention. These infants often have higher nutrient requirements, increased losses, or malabsorption. Significant drug-nutrient interaction often takes place as well. Although it is beyond the scope of this chapter to describe all of such children's special needs one might encounter in practice, a few of the major disorders are outlined. In all of these cases, a registered dietitian/nutritionist should be a part of the medical team.

The Premature Infant and the Low-Birth-Weight Infant

An infant is considered premature if born before 37 weeks' gestation. Low-birth-weight infants may be full term

👤 PERSONAL PERSPECTIVES

Developing "Nutrition Intelligence"

Alan Greene, MD, is a practicing physician who also teaches at Stanford University School of Medicine, but he is most known for advocating the green baby movement. The movement entails raising our young in a natural manner that is most supportive of their well-being and sustaining for our communities and world. He has coined the phrase "nutrition intelligence" to represent having a full understanding and experience of eating and enjoying great wholesome food. This excerpt is from his book Feeding Baby Green: The Earth-Friendly Program for Healthy, Safe Nutrition.

The Eight Essential Steps for Teaching Nutritional Intelligence

These eight simple steps to teaching nutritional intelligence will help you lay a strong foundation for building a healthy and delicious future for your child.

1. ***Take Charge!*** You are your child's first teacher and the primary agent of change in the way she approaches what she eats. It's not an overstatement to say that unless you take steps to prevent it, your child's food style will likely become a blend of the way you eat and the predominant American kids' food culture—weighted strongly toward the latter. The prevailing current is strong, but by making conscious choices now, you can make a lasting difference in your child's health and his enjoyment of food.

2. ***Use Windows of Opportunity.*** Every child has his or her own unique developmental process. Yet the stages of early development—from birth through about the end of the second year—provide special opportunities for you to make a deeper impact on future choices more easily than it will be later on. Learn to advance your child's food development in coordination with other unique stages of development that you see happening in your baby. Being out of sync often leads to food battles or refusing healthy food. Working together is one of life's joys.

3. ***Engage All the Senses.*** Use your baby's senses, even before birth, to help teach her to love great food, to create a deep sense of familiarity and joy about these healthy foods, and to help forge the comfort foods of her future. Enlist food's many flavors, aromas, and textures, and even its appearance and the language you use to talk about food....

4. ***Choose the Right Amount.*** The amount of food your child eats—before birth and after—not only affects growth now but can change hunger, metabolism, and health far into the future. Learn how to tell how much and what to feed your child at every age, and how to help her learn how much is just right for her.

5. ***Choose the Right Variety.*** Repetition is critical to acquiring tastes for new flavors, but so is novelty. A balanced diet is just that: a wide variety of colors and types of foods that meet all of your child's nutritional needs....

6. ***Customize Needs for Every Body.*** Learn to use foods to help address your family's specific health issues, including ADHD, allergies, asthma, cancer, diabetes, ear infections, and eczema. Learn to adapt the Feeding Baby Green program if you or your child has the "bitter taste" gene and to fit your food preferences, schedule, beliefs, or culture.

7. ***Exercise!*** Exercise really is good for every body—yours and your child's. It's closely linked to how a body desires and uses food every day. Working in tandem with good nutrition, it's the best start you can give your baby. ...

8. ***Reap the Benefits of Green***. Making connections—with where food comes from, with how it is prepared, and with others who share the food—is a powerful way to instill love for real food. The basics are simple: Eat seasonally. Eat locally. Grow something together. And choose organic. Avoiding extra hormones and toxic synthetic chemicals in our food and food containers is good for the environment and great for your baby.

From Greene A: *Feeding baby green: The earth-friendly program for healthy, safe nutrition,* San Francisco, CA, 2009, Jossey-Bass.

BOX 10-9 Baby Bottle Tooth Decay

Baby bottle tooth decay (BBTD), also known as early childhood caries (ecc), *nursing bottle caries, nursing bottle mouth,* and *nursing bottle syndrome,* is a distinctive pattern of tooth decay in infants and young children. It most commonly affects the maxillary incisors, although other teeth may be affected as well. For BBTD to develop, the mouth requires the presence of fermentable carbohydrate and a pathogenic organism.

BBTD commonly occurs in infants who are allowed to sleep with a bottle of milk, juice, or other sweetened liquid. As the infant falls asleep, the vigorous suck-swallow pattern that normally occurs during feeding diminishes. Moreover, saliva production decreases, resulting in a loss of saliva's buffering action in the mouth. Liquid pools in the infant's mouth, particularly behind the central incisors, becoming a ready source of fermentable carbohydrate for the bacteria colonizing the oral cavity. The acid produced by bacterial metabolism then destroys tooth enamel and initiates caries.

Prevention of BBTD is important for long-term dental health. Infants should never be put to bed with a bottle of milk, formula, juice, or other sweetened liquid. If a bottle is needed at bedtime, it should be plain water only. Oral hygiene may begin as soon as teeth erupt, as a daily gentle cleaning of the tooth surfaces with gauze or a washcloth. Finally, sharing of food and utensils between adults and infants should be discouraged because of transmission of bacteria from the adult to the infant. Weaning from the bottle should occur as soon as the child can drink from a cup.

or premature but weigh 2500 g or less at birth. As medical technology becomes increasingly sophisticated, infants are surviving at younger ages and lower weights. However, their developmental outlook may still be tenuous. Nutrition support of these infants plays a crucial role in successful long-term outcome. The major issues of concern in the premature infant are low birth weight, immature lung development, poor immune function, immature GI and neurologic function, insufficient production of digestive enzymes, inadequate bone mineralization, and minimal energy and mineral reserves.

Because the coordinated suck-swallow reflex is not fully developed until an infant reaches 34 weeks' gestation, initial feeding of the premature infant may need to be via total parenteral nutrition, tube feeding, or gavage feeding. Many criteria influence the route of nutrient delivery, and thus, each infant should receive an individualized nutrition assessment by a registered dietitian who specializes in high-risk pediatric patients.

Premature infants have increased needs for protein, kcal, calcium, phosphorus, sodium, iron, zinc, vitamin E, and fluids. The best feeding choice for a premature infant is mother's milk with the addition of "human milk fortifier," which contains additional minerals and protein needed by the premature infant. Although the infant may not suckle well or may tire easily at the breast, the nurse can play a key role in helping the mother pump and store her milk in the neonatal nursery. The milk may then be given by gavage even when the mother is not present. If the mother chooses not to breastfeed, a variety of specialized infant formulas are available to meet the special nutritional requirements of the infant.

Research suggests these formulas should be fortified with long-chain fatty acids to mimic what would be delivered via the placenta. Long-chain fatty acids are essential for proper retinal and neurologic development. Premature and low-birth-weight infants require continual nutritional follow-up after discharge for at least the first year of life because they are at risk for feeding problems, developmental delays, and growth retardation.

Failure to Thrive

Failure to thrive (FTT) is defined as a drop of two standard deviations in weight gain over an interval of 2 months or longer for infants younger than 6 months of age or over an interval of 3 months or longer for infants older than 6 months of age. An alternative definition is a weight-for-length measurement less than the fifth percentile or weight for age below the third percentile.

FTT may have organic causes, such as an underlying metabolic disorder. Congenital heart disease or HIV infection may cause such an increased energy requirement that oral intake is not able to keep up with metabolic need.

Nonorganic FTT may be diagnosed when no medical reason for poor growth can be recognized. There may be psychosocial causes for FTT, such as either extreme of parental attention (neglect or excessive attentiveness). Neglect may include inadequate maternal-infant bonding, poverty, child abuse, or neglect. Treatment for nonorganic FTT must include nutrition intervention to promote weight gain and therapy to correct developmental delays and any psychosocial problems in the home environment (Krugman and Dubowitz, 2003).

Inborn Errors of Metabolism

Phenylketonuria and galactosemia are described below. Other inborn errors of metabolism that require nutrition therapy that are not discussed further include urea cycle disorders, maple syrup urine disease, and homocystinuria.

Phenylketonuria. All 50 states have newborn screening programs to detect PKU. When it is discovered early, dietary therapy can begin immediately, and long-term prognosis is good. Without treatment, phenylalanine and its metabolites reach toxic levels in the blood, resulting in damage to the central nervous system, including mental retardation. Likewise, because phenylalanine cannot be converted to tyrosine, low levels or absence of tyrosine may contribute to the mental retardation.

Treatment consists of a low-phenylalanine diet to be followed throughout the individual's life. In infancy the use of a special formula such as Lofenalac is recommended. Partial breastfeeding is permitted, but phenylalanine levels in the infant's blood must be monitored carefully (Elsas and Acosta, 2014). As children with PKU are introduced to solid foods and make the transition to table foods, meals require careful planning. The use of low-protein breads and pastas is advised. This condition requires close monitoring of dietary intake by specialized dietitians.

Galactosemia. Galactosemia is another rare, autosomal recessive disorder caused by an enzyme deficiency and is part of the newborn screening panel. Absence of the enzyme galactose-1-phosphate uridylyltransferase results in an inability to metabolize galactose. Because the milk sugar lactose is a disaccharide of glucose and galactose, infants without this enzyme are unable to tolerate any milk products containing lactose. Manifestations include diarrhea, growth retardation, and mental retardation. Treatment is dietary therapy that excludes all milk products, including human milk. Soy formulas and casein hydrolysate formulas are acceptable. Even with lifelong diet therapy, there may be long-term health consequences such as nervous system or ovarian dysfunction (Elsas and Acosta, 2014). Specialized pediatric dietitians closely monitor the diet of infants and children who have this disorder.

NUTRITION HEALTH PROMOTION: PREGNANCY, LACTATION, AND INFANCY

Knowledge

The metabolic, hormonal, anatomic, psychologic, and physiologic changes that occur during pregnancy can be bewildering for the mother and for those around her. Having an understanding of the process can ease adaptation to these changes. Focusing on the nutrient needs of the mother assures appropriate weight gain to support the growth of the fetus. Knowledge of the anatomic and physiologic changes that occur after childbirth prepares the mother's body for lactation. Nutrient requirements of the mother remain elevated during lactation to produce nourishment for the infant. Recommendations for the specific nutrient needs of the first year of life are important for parents and caregivers to provide.

Techniques

There are numerous resources to assist with pregnancy, lactation, and infancy. Whether in printed form or on the Internet, strategies for dealing with challenges abound. Care needs to be taken to assess the credibility of the source of information. Government sites (.gov) are trustworthy, and applicable sites are available for each of the areas of concern. For example, the MyPlate site (MyPlate.gov) includes specific categories for pregnancy and lactation. In addition, sites from professional medical associations also provide potential solutions to the challenges of this life-span category.

Community Supports

Community supports may be government sponsored, such as the WIC program discussed in the *Social Issues* box Providing the Essentials. Health care providers can be familiar with such programs and recommend patients to take advantage of such services. In addition, interest groups have a strong presence either locally or through the Internet. Most notable is the La Leche League (www.llli.org/), which provides mother-to-mother support of breastfeeding women, ranging from local chapter meetings through a larger mission as an international nonprofit organization. Within individual communities, mothers (and fathers) may organize to assist one another with the trials and tribulations of pregnancy and the first year of life issues of their babies. This interaction may occur through a group blog or on a dedicated website.

NUTRITION DURING CHILDHOOD

Once we pass the specific nutrition and health necessities of pregnancy and infancy, the rest of the life span categories share more similarities than differences regarding nutrient intake and dietary patterns.

Stages of Development

The life span stages reflect psychologic and physiologic maturation. Approaches to health promotion take into account these stages and their impact on nutrient requirements, eating styles, and food choices.

Childhood (1 to 12 Years)

The accelerated growth of infancy slows down by about age 1 year, marking the transition to childhood. Growth then occurs unevenly until puberty heralds the onset of adolescence. This growth deceleration during childhood results in varying hunger levels, reflecting physiologic need. Parent and caregiver awareness of these fluctuations allows children to stay in tune with their internal hunger cues.

Nurses sensitive to normal growth patterns as affected by genetics and environmental influences can help families to understand the growth curves of their children. Height, weight, and head circumferences are used with the standard growth charts from the National Center for Health Statistics to monitor growth (available at www.cdc.gov/growthcharts). See Chapter 11 for a detailed description of clinical nutrition assessment procedures.

Childhood categories are based on a combination of psychosocial and physiologic developmental stages. Physiologic requirements are the basis of the age and gender divisions of the DRIs. This discussion highlights the nutrients of concern—protein, iron, calcium, and zinc. For other specific age-related nutrient recommendations, refer to the DRI tables inside the front cover of this book.

Children depend on adults for the provision of food. A discussion of the nutrient needs of the growing body is not complete without a consideration of the role of adults in nourishing children. Children are influenced by adults and model the behaviors of adults. Adults control the quantity and quality of foods prepared as well as the environment within which foods are presented for consumption. Serving sizes should represent appropriate quantities for the ages of the children. The children themselves, however, control the actual amount consumed. Easily distracted children may need gentle coaxing to try new foods or to ingest sufficient amounts to meet energy and nutrient needs.

Adults are responsible for not only what meals are offered but also *when* meals are offered. Regularity of mealtimes at home—breakfast and dinner—helps support success at school. Breakfast supplies energy in the morning for school learning (see the *Teaching Tool* box What's the Best Breakfast?); dinner supports the ability to complete homework, study, and relax before bedtime. Most children eat lunch away from home and either bring a prepared lunch from home or purchase meals through a school lunch program. (School lunches are discussed later in this chapter, under the heading "Community Supports.")

Snacks boost daily nutrient intake; for children whose energy and general dietary intake are adequate, snacks may sometimes include sweets such as cookies and even an occasional candy bar. A common myth is that sugar makes children hyperactive; studies have shown no convincing evidence that consumption of sugar causes attention- deficit/hyperactivity disorder. High-sugar-containing foods, however, can displace more nutritious foods and contribute to nutrient deficiencies (such as of calcium and dietary fiber) or excessive caloric and dietary fat intake. Of significant concern is childhood excess adiposity or overweight bodies. No food should be forbidden; frequency and quantity should be the guides.

Children too young for school may attend daycare programs if their parents work. The impact on their nutrition may be positive or negative, depending on the quality and attitude of the programs to nutrition and mealtimes. Most young children, regardless of parental employment, attend some form of preschool; for many, the food and social

What's the Best Breakfast?

Foods considered best for breakfast have changed. Although traditional breakfasts consist of eggs, bacon, white toast, and whole milk, this combination is now recognized as being too high in fat and protein. In addition, in the rush of morning preparation, few of us have the time to prepare this type of meal. Nonetheless, breakfast, which breaks our fast, is an important contributor of nutrients and energy.

As we teach clients and their families about nutrition and optimum dietary intake patterns, we can assure them that breakfast can be simple yet still provide appropriate levels of nutrients. Following are some ideas for parents to use to ignite their children's breakfast appetites:

- For children (and adults) who eat and run, have quick foods available such as fruit, granola bars (low fat/low sugar), muffins (low fat/low sugar), and raisins/nuts.
- For older children, offer to prepare a simple breakfast. Although they are able to prepare their own meal, the extra nurturing—and time saved—will be appreciated.
- To create appetite, toast bread while family members are dressing. The enticing scent will spark their taste buds.
- For picky eaters, create small smorgasbord plates with several choices such as a small container of yogurt, crackers with cheese, and some pear slices.
- Be a role model by also eating breakfast yourself.

experiences broaden acceptance of a variety of foods and eating styles.

Although adults may have predominant influence over the eating behaviors of children, another primary influence for some children is television. The influence of TV commercials has been studied extensively and is most often condemned as negatively influencing children's food choices. In addition, watching television while family meals are eaten appears to affect the types of foods served, resulting in consumption of foods higher in fat and lower in fiber—possibly reflecting the categories of foods most often advertised on television. Parents and caregivers can watch television with their children to assess the type of products advertised and then discuss their nutritional value. As more healthful products are marketed, even if targeted at adults, acceptance by children may increase. Occasional treats of advertised products may lessen their appeal if children are accustomed to high-quality snacks and meals.

The *Acceptable Macronutrient Distribution Range* (AMDR) for daily dietary fat intake recommends about 30% kcal intake. This level of dietary fat intake may also assist with obesity prevention and emphasizes fruits, vegetables, and complex carbohydrates. It is easier to enjoy whole foods that are naturally low in fat throughout childhood than to convert one's eating style as an adult. Other AMDRs include for carbohydrates 45% to 65% kcal; for protein 5% to 20% kcal for young children and 10% to 30% kcal for older children; added sugars not exceeding 25% of total calories; and adequate intake dietary fiber of 19 g/day for children 1 to 3 years,

25 g/day for those 4 to 8 years, 31 g/day for boys 9 to 13 years, and 26 g/day for girls 9 to 13 years (Nicklas, et al, 2008).

Despite national dietary recommendations, trends in children's total energy intake have shown an increase. Although calories increased, total intake of milk, vegetable, soups, breads, grains, and eggs decreased, and intake of fruits, fruit juices, sweetened beverages, poultry, and cheese increased. When food groups were considered, about 16% of U.S. children did not meet any food group recommendations, whereas only 1% consumed recommended amounts for all food groups. Approximately two thirds of U.S. children do not consume suggested servings of fruits and vegetables. Consumption of whole grains is extremely low, with consumption of two or more servings of whole grains daily by less than 13% of children. Those who did meet dietary recommendations had intakes that were high in fat (Krebs-Smith, 2010). Consider that for some children the principal vegetable is French fries. These findings indicate that nutrition education is still needed for parents and their children. (The *Cultural Considerations* box Child Health Education for Foreign-Born Parents offers suggestions for educating foreign-born parents about their child's health.)

Child Health Education for Foreign-Born Parents

Providing child health education for foreign-born parents presents special concerns related to language and culture. An innovative, culturally relevant approach should be used to present basic child health information in English, with translators present as facilitators. Foreign-born parents who need a partial or complete language interpretation then have readily available access to translation support. Parents can ask questions, provide comments and suggestions, and evaluate the presentation through the translator. Because participants can be grouped with an appropriate translator, each presentation can accommodate more than one language.

The presentation, conducted in English, is paced to allow for discussions. Child care is provided in a nearby setting, allowing parents to focus on the presentation without the concern of child care. Vocabulary relative to health care is developed from English into the parents' primary language with the support of the translator.

Application to nursing. This is an example of one cultural-specific strategy used to meet minority and ethnic health needs. Nurses are also encouraged to provide translated health education materials for the populations with whom they teach.

Data from Baker R: Child health education for the foreign-born parent, *Issues Compr Pediatr Nurs* 24:45-55, 2001.

Stage I: Children 1 to 3 Years Old

Usually referred to as "toddlerhood," the age span of 1 to 3 years old is a busy time for young children. They are dealing with issues of autonomy. Often food and eating create an arena for asserting newly discovered independence. The eating relationship between parent (or caregiver) and child is forming, and adult reaction to autonomy sets the stage for future encounters. Consistency of mealtimes is important. Meals are best accepted when hunger, tiredness, and emotions are still controllable; an overly tired child just cannot eat. Equally important is fostering self-reliance by allowing young children to feed themselves in a manner most appropriate for their psychomotor abilities. Regardless of the messy results, children's attempts to self-feed provide the roots of self-empowerment crucial to overall physical and psychologic development.

Hunger, rather than adult meal schedules, guides the child's perception of time to eat. Meals for toddlers are based on the same design and food selections as adults, only in smaller portions. (Of course, overly spicy foods may not be acceptable to young taste buds.) Snacks are a necessity in addition to meals. Toddlers are able to eat only small amounts at each meal or food encounter. Planned snacks provide required additional nourishment between meals to ensure an adequate dietary intake.

Nutrition requirements. Growth, BMR, and endless activity require an energy supply of 1300 kcal/day for children ages 1 to 3. Protein needs increase to 16 g to meet the demands of growing muscles. For children aged 1 through 6 years, a general guideline is one fruit or vegetable serving equals one level-measuring tablespoon of fruit or vegetable per year of age. A serving of bread or cereal is equal to about one-fourth of an adult's serving. Up to age 3, children should consume two or three 8-ounce cups of milk per day or about 16 to 24 ounces per day, and meats or meat substitutes can be offered at least twice per day (Heird, 2014). Caregivers should be advised that alternative milk products such as rice milk and soymilk, unless sufficiently fortified, may not provide the same quality of nutrients as animal-derived foods.

When children are between 1 and 3 years old, they should be introduced to lower-fat versions of commonly eaten foods. Fat-containing foods should not be obsessively restricted; however, high-fat foods are often filling and may displace other nutrient-containing foods.

This is also a prime time to introduce toddlers to a variety of foods. (See the *Personal Perspectives* box Developing "Nutrition Intelligence.") Toddlers imitate the adults around them; therefore, adults can model behavior by eating a variety of foods themselves. Clever introductions to foods are always helpful to catch the attention and appetite of toddlers. Broccoli is more than just a vegetable; cut up, it looks like little trees. Peas steamed in their pods are not just peas but green pearls waiting to be discovered.

Although breast milk or formula is the milk of choice until age 1, toddlers should drink breast milk, whole milk, or formula until age 2, after which low-fat or skim milk is best. Sometimes toddlers consume too much milk or juice, particularly if they are given an unlimited number of servings. Perhaps drinking from feeding bottles throughout the day simply becomes a habit. Unfortunately, the child fills up on milk or juice, both low sources of iron, and then does not have an appetite for iron-containing foods such as meat,

fish, poultry, eggs, or legumes. Iron-deficiency anemia may develop. Additionally, apple juice is sweet tasting and has few nutrients beyond carbohydrate kcal. Its frequent consumption may habituate young children to sweet drinks. Later, apple juice may be replaced with sugar-laden sodas or beverages, which displace more nutrient-dense beverages. One possible solution is to dilute juices with water. Milk can be served with meals and diluted juices drunk between meals. Parents and caregivers can view bottles as cups or glassware. Few of us drink from a cup continually while watching television, reading, or playing games. Similarly, once past infancy, young children's use of feeding bottles and/or lidded cups or "sippy" cups should be viewed as beverages that are part of a meal or snack. Healthful snacks can provide energy for playing.

Stage II: Children 4 to 6 Years Old

Stage II is characterized by independent eating styles, although modeling of adults still occurs. Children of this age clearly understand the time frame of meals and can save their appetite for meals. Snacks are still an integral part of the children's nutrient intake. Far from the messy eating styles of toddlers, these children accept foods more easily if presented separately, not mixed in a casserole style. Variations in hunger and appetite levels may confuse parents and caregivers. The most practical approach is to be respectful of these variations of hunger; this approach diffuses power plays over food consumption.

New foods can continue to be introduced. Children may require repeated exposures, as many as 8 to 10 attempts, before they accept a food. For some families, backup meal plans can encourage trying new foods. For instance, if a child does not accept a new dish after a reasonable attempt, the child may be allowed to prepare a peanut butter sandwich or cereal and fruit. By establishing backup meals in advance, parents avoid becoming short-order cooks preparing three or more individualized meals for dinner.

Another approach is to have at least one meal (eaten at home) include new foods along with favorite foods. In addition to the new foods, the child will recognize some familiar foods on his or her plate. A meal can consist of a sampling of food items; several will probably be acceptable.

At this stage, children can develop a sense of responsibility for healthful food selections. They can understand that although all foods are okay, some foods, such as fruits, vegetables, and low-fat foods, can be eaten more often than others.

Sometimes a child develops a food jag, wanting to eat only a narrow range of foods. Parents and teachers can educate the child that each food contains a different assortment of nutrients and offer substitute choices that contain additional nutrients, with the child making the final selections. Eventually food jags diminish, and the child consumes a broader selection of foods.

Nutrition requirements. Energy requirements jump to 1800 kcal/day at 4 to 6 years of age, reflecting continued growth and activity levels. Protein intake needs increase to 24 g.

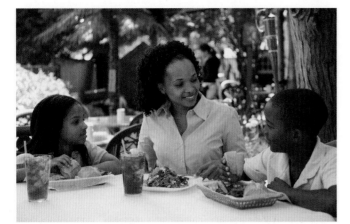

FIG 10-7 A child can be reminded to "stop eating when you are full."

Stage III: Children 7 to 12 Years Old

The years from 7 to 12 are tumultuous. Although actual growth may slow down, the body is preparing and seemingly storing up for the puberty growth spurt. Puberty may begin for girls from around age 9; boys may reach puberty in the early teen years. This prepuberty time may be reflected by weight buildup; an increase in chubbiness is not alarming if moderate eating and physical activities are maintained. Adults must be careful not to overreact, or they may plant the seeds of eating disorders. To rule out overeating, children can be asked whether they are really hungry for food or only tired or thirsty. These are different sensations. A child can be reminded to "stop eating when you are full" (Figure 10-7). If hunger returns, a snack of fruit can be provided. By taking time to consider these sensations, children can stay in touch with internal cues of true hunger.

Exposure to other dietary patterns takes place as children spend more time away from home at school and in socializing with friends. Peer influence at school lunchtime increases; having the right kind of lunch may be as important as wearing the right kind of clothes. Adults need to be sensitive to these issues. As long as a basic lunch of some protein, complex carbohydrates, and a beverage (preferably milk, juice, or water) is consumed, missing nutrients can be adjusted for later in the day, especially through after-school snacks.

It is at this age—when midmorning school snacks disappear and school lunch scheduling has more to do with numbers of students than with actual lunchtime appetites—that after-school hunger may intensify. This is the time to provide healthful snacks or at least stock the kitchen shelves with an assortment of nutrient-dense treats (see Box 10-10). If children purchase snacks away from home, adults can develop guidelines with children this age to maintain positive eating styles.

The intent is to supplement the nutrients received during meals with nutrient-dense snacks so the total caloric and nutrient intake is adequate to meet the needs of growth at each childhood stage. Snacking, though, seems to have changed in definition and frequency. A study of 31,337 children and adolescents assessed snacking and meal intake trends from 1977 to 2006 (Piernas and Popkin, 2010). On average, the numbers of both calories and eating events (a total of snacks and meals) increased substantially over time. In comparison with the 1970s, about half of American children in the twenty-first century average 4 snacks a day, whereas others consume snacks and meals as many as 10 times a day, or basically eat nonstop. This means that an excessive number of calories, most likely less nutrient-dense snack foods, are being consumed and that the consumption of nutrient-dense meal time foods is decreasing. Although the increase in snack calories is only 168 kcal, this number represents an average, signaling that for many children the excess intake is higher. With increased eating episodes, there can be a concern that eating is due not to physiologic hunger but to a habit from needing a constant state of satiation.

Nutrition requirements. Energy needs for 7- to 12-year-olds increase to 2000 to 2200 kcal/day. Protein requirements rise to between 28 and 46 g, depending on sexual maturity. Sexual maturity leads to an increase in lean body mass, particularly for boys, which requires more dietary protein for growth and maintenance.

BOX 10-10   Healthy Snacks

Snacks are a way to bridge energy levels between meals. They are not meant to be so energy dense that intakes during meals are compromised or that daily total caloric intakes are significantly increased. Frequent snacking (or nonstop eating) throughout the day has been associated with increased body weight in children (and adults!).

Here are some suggestions for healthy snacks:

- Ready-to-eat cereals: reserve presweetened cereals as special snack treats or mix a sweet cereal with a less sweet cereal—the best of both worlds
- Snack smorgasbord: cut-up apples and oranges, popcorn, cheese, crackers, and cookies
- Fruit juice pack
- Low-fat chocolate milk pack
- Open-face peanut butter sandwich (child-made) with cut fruit, jelly, coconut, and raisins
- Sliced apple or pear with thin spread of nut butter (peanut, almond, or cashew)
- Fresh or canned fruit (in fruit juice) with cottage cheese (in 4-ounce size)
- English muffin (oat bran, raisin, or sourdough) with a small amount of fruit spread
- Healthier Danish: a slice of toasted bread with low-fat ricotta cheese and preserves
- Bagel with a spread of whipped cream cheese, margarine/butter, or nut butter (peanut, almond, or cashew); freeze a variety of bagels
- Smoothie or fruit shakes made with skim milk or fruit juice, plain or fruit-flavored yogurt, fresh or frozen fruit—just mix in a blender
- Leftovers from lunch or dinner; a bowl of soup with bread for dipping instead of a prepackaged snack

Mineral needs rise as well. Because of greater bone growth and mineralization, calcium AI recommendations jump from 800 mg/day at age 8 to 1300 mg/day throughout adolescence. Iron and zinc allowances increase as well. Well-chosen dietary intakes will provide sufficient amounts of these nutrients. Marginal intakes of zinc have been noted among schoolchildren who are finicky eaters; low zinc intakes can affect growth rates (Cole and Lifshitz, 2008).

NUTRITION HEALTH PROMOTION: CHILDHOOD (1 TO 12 YEARS)

Knowledge

The growth cycle of this age span is important for both parents and children to understand. Attention to issues related to weight, appropriate appetite, and meal patterning is crucial for positive eating relationships and may prevent the development of eating disorders. By understanding the relationship of nutrients and kcal to their growth needs, children possess sufficient information to take responsibility for certain aspects of their food choices and dietary patterns. Children with special needs who are challenged by physical and/or mental limitations may require additional support to achieve nutritional adequacy (Box 10-11). Ultimately, however, adults must provide nourishment for children and guidance as to positive health behaviors.

Techniques

Several techniques can be used with children this age. MyPlate for Kids is similar to the adult version but presents games and other creative approaches for children to visualize and understand the serving sizes and types of foods that result in a balanced nutrient intake. It can be found at myplate.gov. Another source for appropriate techniques is the Fruits & Veggies—More Matters website, which offers resources for parents and children (www.fruitsandveggiesmorematters.org).

Community Supports

Community supports for children are currently divided into two categories based on location and services or education offered: (1) school food service and (2) classroom nutrition education.

School food service. National School Lunch Program (NSLP) was established to protect the health and wellness of American children. Formalized in 1946, the program provides lunches at varying cost, depending on family income, to all schoolchildren at public and nonprofit private schools and residential child care institutions. At the federal level, the program is administered by the Food and Nutrition Service (FNS) of the USDA, at the state level by various agencies, and locally by school boards. As an entitlement program, the NSLP provides funds to all schools that apply and meet the criteria of eligibility. Currently, about 95% of all school districts participate in this program. Every school district is required to implement a local school wellness policy to focus on obesity prevention and, through modification of school

---

BOX 10-11   Nutrition Requirements of Children with Special Needs

Although the basic nutrition needs of all children are the same, some children may be challenged by the limitations of physical and mental differences and the physical and pharmacologic consequences of chronic disease treatment. The ability to self-feed may be highly related to life expectancy. Enhancing feeding skills to the greatest extent possible is an involved procedure. Nutrition education has valuable skills and experiences to offer. Keep the following issues in mind:

- All children can enjoy working together to prepare foods. The process of measuring, mixing, arranging, and eating food that they helped to prepare enhances self-esteem and provides the acquisition of other skill competencies such as math and science, and the interpersonal skills of cooperation.
- Positioning of children with physical handicaps may require adaptive equipment and alternative eating strategies for special conditions. Oral stimulation before eating may be required for children with low muscle tone, and certain textures of foods may be better received than others. If chewing and swallowing are problematic, textures of foods may need adjustment. Low muscle tone may also affect functioning of the large intestine and require adequate fiber and water to reduce the risk of constipation.
- Medications may increase or decrease appetite. Caregivers and teachers should be aware of these effects, and meals and snacks should be offered when hunger is the strongest.
- Children with sensory integration difficulties may be sensitive to textures, temperature, and even colors of foods. Preferences should be accommodated when possible to ensure adequate nutrition and to provide the children a sense of control over food choices.
- Children experiencing growth retardation or malnutrition should be reassessed by a registered dietitian/nutritionist (RDN) to determine whether alternative feeding strategies can improve their nutritional status. Parents should regularly receive assessments of nutritional status to fully understand their children's conditions.
- Periodic nutritional assessments of children with special needs should be conducted by RDNs who have the expertise to evaluate nutritional status and offer practical strategies for everyday eating situations.

Data from Fung EB, et al: Feeding dysfunction is associated with poor growth and health status in children with cerebral palsy, *J Am Diet Assoc* 102(3):361, 373, 2002; and correspondence on Society for Nutrition Education (SNE) list/serv February 19, 1998, from Susan Piscopo, associate professor, University of Malta; Sharon Davis, education director, Home Baking Association; Collette Janson-Sand, associate professor, University of New Hampshire; and others.

---

environments, to support healthy eating habits and physical activity (Food Research & Action Center [FRAC], *National School Lunch Program,* n.d.).

At participating schools, there are two types of eligibility to qualify for free or reduced price meals; both usually require the family to complete and return application forms. Categorical eligibility is based on the child's household receiving the Supplemental Nutrition Assistance Program (SNAP) or

Temporary Assistance for Needy Families (TANF) or participating in the Food District Program on Indian Reservations (FDPIR), and free meals for the homeless, runaways, and children of migrant workers. Income-based eligibility offers reduced-price meals to children whose household income is below 185% of the federal poverty level; free meals are available to those with incomes below 130% of the poverty level. Through the process of direct certification, school districts qualify children without requiring submission of family applications. School districts work with state or local SNAP, TANF, and FDPIR agencies to certify children in households.

During the 2011-2012 school year, NSLP served meals daily to 29 million children in about 98,000 schools and residential child care institutions. More than 65% of these children received free or reduced-price lunches (FRAC, *National School Lunch Program*, n.d.).

New standards were issued by USDA in January 2012 as required by the Healthy, Hunger-Free Kids Act to provide school meal nutrition standards that implement the U.S. Department of Health and Human Services *Dietary Guidelines for Americans*. The new standards include increasing the amount of fruits and vegetables served with a focus on whole grain–rich foods. Only lower-fat or nonfat milk is to be served, and other reductions in saturated fat, sodium, and calories are required. Also included are increasing cultural food options to meet the needs of local communities.

Basically, lunch must provide approximately one third or more of the recommended levels for key nutrients, providing no more than 30% kcal from fat and less than 10% of kcal from saturated fat. For low-income children participating in the program, this lunch provides one third to one half of their daily intake.

The School Breakfast Program, created in 1966, has reduced tardiness and improved school attendance. During the 2011-2012 school year, more than almost 90,000 schools and institutions participated in the School Breakfast Program, serving 12.5 million children. About 84% of the participants qualify for free or reduced-priced meals. More than 47% of the children from low-income families receive both school lunch and school breakfast (FRAC, *National School Breakfast Program*, n.d.).

The breakfast can comprise an assortment of foods, but the program requires milk (either as a beverage or with cereal), a serving of fruit (either whole or as juice), and two servings of a bread/cereal product or meat/meat alternative or a combination of bread and meat servings. The breakfast is designed to provide one fourth or more of the daily recommended level for key nutrients and limits fat to no more than 30% kcal with less than 10% kcal of saturated fat.

During summer, the Summer Food Service Program for Children (SFSP) functions through a range of eligible organizations including schools, summer camps, and community agencies, as well as various federal, state, and local government departments. The purpose is to serve meals to school-age children when schools are not in session in communities where children depend on school meals as an essential component of their daily nourishment.

School nurses and community health nurses should be aware of these programs as valuable sources of nutrition. Sometimes children do not participate because school payment policies create a stigma associated with participation. Intervention by a health professional may be required to ensure that children's health needs are met in a socially sensitive manner. As health advocates, nurses may be able to highlight the importance of school lunch and breakfast programs to educational administrators and the community at large.

Classroom nutrition education. Health has been taught for many years in most school systems. What vary are the depth of school health curricula and the qualifications of the instructors. Both may affect the quality of the nutrition education. Although basic nutrition facts can be taught within a short-term health course, lifestyle changes that affect dietary patterns take longer to achieve. Unless they have special preparation, instructors may not feel comfortable teaching the intricate and ever-changing discipline of nutrition. This may lead to either poor-quality teaching or the imparting of negative attitudes to nutrition and food selections.

NUTRITION DURING ADOLESCENCE

The adolescent years (13 to 19 years) are marked by change. Not only does puberty initiate growth acceleration, but emotional and social developmental struggles also occur as academic and personal responsibilities escalate. Adults often assume that teenagers can take care of themselves. Although teens need to take responsibility for their behavior and overall health status, they still need the guidance and nurturing of caring adults. There is a fine line between allowing adolescents to be responsible and neglecting their needs. Adult involvement is still necessary to provide physical and emotional support during the stressful years of adolescence.

Part of the physical and emotional support includes creating guidelines for dietary patterns and providing food for consumption. Creating guidelines means maintaining a household in which meals are available, even if family members may not be able to eat together. Knowing that dinner just needs to be reheated means someone was thinking of the welfare of all family members. Of course, shared responsibility for meal preparation may be an appropriate component of family duties. A kitchen stocked with nourishing snack foods and ingredients for simple meals helps to make stressful, chaotic teenage schedules more manageable.

Older teens may be adjusting to the new demands of the college environment, including adapting to dining hall meals. Some campuses provide flexible meal plans with several locations for meal acquisition around campus. Others offer salad bars and food "stations" to provide a variety of selections. Individuals requiring special dietary requirements such as kosher meals or lactose-reduced meals should discuss these issues with food service staff or with student service personnel.

As their sense of social awareness develops, some teens may adopt a vegetarian dietary pattern. Creative planning on the part of the teen and the family meal planner results in meals that meet everyone's nutritional needs without compromising personal convictions.

Discussions of the eating habits of teens tend to be critical of their fast-food consumption. Fortunately, most teens can afford the extra kcal that typically higher-fat foods such as hamburgers, fries, and pizza may contain. If teens have grown up accustomed to well-balanced meals, they will more than likely still prefer those meals to high-fat delights. Eating in fast-food restaurants, where prices tend to be low, may have more to do with socializing among peers than with nutrient values.

When fast foods become the mainstay of an individual's diet, regardless of age, some nutrients, such as vitamin A and C, may be lacking, and overconsumption of dietary fats and kcal may occur. Although teens may be seen at such restaurants, most other customers are families with young children as well as older adults. Fast foods affect the nutrient intake of all ages.

Nutrition Requirements

Because of the natural physiologic differences between adolescent males and females, nutrient requirements from age 9 and older are divided by gender. Females need about 2200 kcal and 45 g of protein daily. Recommendations for males are 2500 to 2900 kcal and 45 to 59 g of protein daily. These values for kcal and protein reflect the greater lean body mass developing in males. They do, however, only represent suggested amounts; physical activity, either work or athletic endeavors, affects the actual nutrient needs for both males and females.

Calcium AI recommendations are the same for the two genders, 1300 mg per day, to allow for skeletal growth (particularly for boys) and for bone mineralization, a prime physiologic function during adolescence. Bone mineralization for girls is a concern because teenage girls often don't consume enough calcium-rich foods.

Teenage girls and sometimes teenage boys are at risk for dieting-related disorders and eating disorders. By regularly under-consuming nutrients during a time when the human body is completing maturation, girls are at risk for various deficiencies as they progress to adulthood and the nutrient requirements of potential pregnancies. In addition to calcium, iron allowances are important to fulfill, particularly for girls who begin menstruation; iron is also needed by boys, whose accelerated growth necessitates an increased blood volume and lean body mass.

NUTRITION HEALTH PROMOTION: ADOLESCENCE

Knowledge

The adolescent body benefits from a dietary intake most similar to an adult's; however, some nutrient needs are greater. Energy requirements are higher than at any other time of life, especially for adolescents involved in competitive athletics. Calcium recommendations increase to ensure adequate mineralization of bones. Parental tolerance for alternative food styles enhances overall dietary intake and allows for the acceptance of dietary suggestions to maintain appropriate nutrient consumption.

Teenagers can comprehend the body's physiology and nutrient needs. Ideally, this information should be taught within family life, health, or science curricula in schools. This knowledge provides a rationale for consumption of nutrient-dense foods, especially as preparation for sports activities. Although adults may supply provisions for meals and snacks, especially those that can be reheated, ultimately, most adolescents take responsibility for their own nutrient intake. Teens can help shop for and plan meals that meet the family's nutritional needs while incorporating alternative food styles.

Awareness of the risk factors for and symptoms of disordered eating and drug/alcohol abuse can be provided through health classes or interactions with health and educational professionals and parents. Even mild substance abuse in the face of the increased nutritional needs of adolescence can compromise nutritional status. For example, alcohol adversely affects absorption of folate and zinc, two nutrients required for normal growth. Nurses need to be aware of the indicators of substance abuse so they can guide adolescents into treatment. Nutrition assessment, intervention, and support are part of comprehensive physical and psychologic rehabilitation of all substance abusers.

Techniques

As they do for children, the concepts found at the MyPlate and "Fruits & Veggies—More Matters" websites provide a basis for adolescent food choices (adolescents use MyPlate for adults). Often the forces overriding good food choices are lack of time and scheduling demands. One strategy accommodating both is to ensure the availability of simple meals that are easily eaten and reheatable. Scheduling of meals in a home or institutional setting (e.g., school cafeterias, dining halls) can take into account school, sports, work, and recreational agendas. To improve the quality of food choices, adolescents should be included in meal planning and food preparation.

Community Supports

Except for federal government programs serving children and adults, no food programs are specifically targeted at adolescents. At a time when teens are developmentally ready to be empowered to take care of themselves, society provides few supports. In fact, school, sports, and work schedules often hinder adolescents from taking responsibility for their health behaviors. Television, radio, the Internet, and print messages rarely promote healthy behaviors. Although the increased interest in physical pursuits of basketball, soccer, biking, skateboarding, weight lifting, and other recreational sports enhances fitness, the nutrition component is often overlooked or cloaked in misinformation. This is an area to which all health professionals should be sensitive.

One of the few community supports is a comprehensive school health program. The depth of health issues covered varies and may not include sufficient nutrition guidance, but at the least, these programs highlight basic concerns of nutrition and health.

NUTRITION-RELATED CONCERNS OF CHILDHOOD AND ADOLESCENCE

Food Asphyxiation

Asphyxiation from food is possible at any point in the life span, but toddlers and older adults tend to be more at risk. (Older adults are discussed in the next section of this chapter.) As toddlers first become accustomed to a variety of food textures and substances, they sometimes misjudge the size of food being chewed or may be too active while eating and accidentally swallow before sufficiently chewing. Some foods that are potential problems are peanut butter (large clumps can stick in the throat), peanuts, popcorn, hot dogs, potato chips, hard candies, gum, grapes, and foods containing bones (e.g., beef, poultry, fish). Efforts by parents and caregivers to serve appropriate foods to young children can prevent choking incidents (Box 10-12); adults with responsibility for caring for children should know how to perform the Heimlich maneuver. Children can be reminded to chew food well and sit quietly while eating.

Lead Poisoning

Lead poisoning can be an invisible health hazard. Found in old paint dust or chips, enameled porcelain fixtures (bathtubs), and soil or air from industrial and transportation pollution, lead can be absorbed into the body in excessive amounts. Children are most at risk; they naturally absorb greater amounts of minerals than adults. Nutritional deficiencies of iron, calcium, and zinc tend to increase the absorption of lead. Lead poisoning and iron-deficiency anemia are sometimes diagnosed concurrently. Excessive exposure to lead can permanently affect cognitive and perceptual abilities. These reduced functions affect learning ability (Wessling-Resnick, 2014).

Role of Nurses

School and community nurses in higher-risk areas should be sensitive to this risk to both physical and intellectual health. Higher-risk areas for children include lower socioeconomic areas with poor housing conditions. Once lead poisoning is determined through blood testing, local health departments work with families to ascertain the sources of contamination in the home or school environment while physicians implement lead-reduction therapy.

Overall levels of lead in the environment are lower than in the past because of standards established and enforced by the Environmental Protection Agency. Levels of lead in some communities, however, are still high enough by Centers for Disease Control and Prevention standards that primary prevention activities to further reduce lead poisoning should remain a community-wide goal.

Obesity

During childhood and adolescence, weight and height continually change. This affects the standard measurements used to assess body composition of fat and lean mass. Therefore, direct application of standards used to evaluate obesity in adults to children is inappropriate. Gender and age also affect body composition during growth. For example, during adolescence, fat redistributes differently for males and females. Males gather body fat centrally around the waist, whereas females tend to collect body fat, gluteally on the lower body. Overweight may be determined as a BMI of 30 or greater and/or through skinfold measurements.

The prevalence of obesity or excessive body fat composition among American children and adolescents has grown substantially over the past 30 years. Among children aged 6 to 18 years, the proportions who were obese rose from 6% in 1980 to 17% by 2010 (Polsky, et al, 2014). Racial, ethnic, and gender differences reveal that black non-Hispanic girls and Mexican American boys have been at greater risk of being overweight than other American children. Severe overweight or obesity has increased more quickly than even the increases of moderate overweight.

The etiology of these changes is not obvious but may be considered multifactorial. Eating more food as snacks and meals away from home may be a subtle factor for children and adults. These food portions are larger and higher in calories and dietary fat than those eaten at home. Another factor may be the increase in sedentary lifestyles. Physical activity has decreased with a related decline of fitness. Although TV watching has not increased substantially over the years, children may be more sedentary than in the past because they play video and computer games and "surf" the Internet. Physical and behavioral environmental influences also affect the level of physical activity. If facilities are not available or not safe to use, physical activity is limited. Concerns over increasing numbers of latchkey children (grade-school children arriving home without adult supervision until the evening) focus on the use of food for emotional comfort and security. All of these factors affect the influence of genetics, which may predispose children to heavier weights and should be considered as interventions are being contemplated.

Clinical assessment of childhood overweight consists of completing a health history, including the pattern of weight gain, emotional health status, and physical activity patterns. If BMI is greater than 30, a further discussion of weight issues may be appropriate, but first a consultation with parents or guardians may be preferable to determine whether intervention is warranted.

As with adults, intervention regarding weight with a child or adolescent should be initiated only when the patient is motivated or is experiencing weight-associative disorders. Conducting a 24-hour food intake recall provides an opportunity to engage in a discussion of dietary intake patterns such as excessive or imbalanced intake of non–nutrient-dense foods such as sodas, sweets, and fast foods. (This type of discussion may be appropriate regardless of the child's weight.) Physical examinations need to be sensitive to the

BOX 10-12   Choking Prevention

Choking prevention for young children can be approached through the following measures:

1. Appropriate selection of foods based on size, shape, and texture
2. Application of prevention strategies.
3. Knowledge of the Heimlich maneuver procedures for use with children

Food Selection for Choking Prevention

Size

Both small and large pieces of food can cause choking. Small, hard pieces of food may get caught in the airway if they are swallowed before being chewed well. Larger pieces, those that are more difficult to chew, are more likely to completely block the throat. Examples are:

- Nuts
- Raw carrots, broccoli, and cauliflower
- Hard fruit, especially with peels, such as crisp apples

Shape

Food items shaped like a tube may cause choking because they are more likely than other shapes to completely block the throat. Examples are:

- Hot dogs
- Link sausage
- Whole carrots
- Grapes
- Frozen banana pieces

Texture

Foods that are firm, smooth, or slick may slide down the throat into the airway. Examples are:

- Hard candy
- Whole-kernel corn
- Peanuts, especially Spanish peanuts

Dry, hard foods may be hard to chew but easy to swallow whole. Examples are:

- Hard pretzels
- Tortilla chips
- Popcorn

Sticky foods can stick to the back or roof of the mouth and block the throat and are difficult to remove. Examples are:

- Nut butters alone
- Processed cheese chunks or slices
- Gummy bears
- Marshmallows
- Fruit roll-ups

Hard-to-chew foods that are fibrous and tough can present hazards. Examples are:

- Bagels
- Steak, roast, or other fibrous meats
- Meat jerky
- Toddler biter biscuits

Applying Prevention Strategies

Always supervise eating: Children do best when sitting to eat. It lets them concentrate on chewing and swallowing. Join the children at the table. Eating or drinking while running or playing is a distraction and can cause choking problems.

Decrease outside distractions: Reduce activities such as television, games, pets, and so on, during meals and at snack times.

Cut food into bite-sized pieces or thin slices: Grind or mash tough food.

Cook food until soft, especially beans, pasta, and rice: These foods are favorites but need to be soft enough to chew easily.

Steam vegetables, such as carrots and broccoli.

Eating in cars/buses may also cause problems: It is hard for the driver to safely pull over fast enough if a child is choking.

Serve small amounts of food at a time: Keep portion sizes small. With babies, be sure the mouth is clear before giving the child another spoonful of food.

Heimlich Maneuver

Choking is fairly common. Choking deaths occur most commonly in children younger than 3 years old and in senior citizens, but they can occur at any age. The Heimlich maneuver has been valuable in saving lives and can be administered by anyone who has learned the technique.

Modified from Child Care Health Program, Public Health—Seattle & King County: *Preventing choking on food by children: Safe practice guidelines for child care facilities,* Seattle, 2005, updated October 2008, Author. Accessed March 10, 2014, from www.kingcounty.gov/healthservices/health/child/childcare/education/choking.aspx.

child regarding his or her weight and body issues. If weight is excessive, the assessment can determine whether the weight is causing physical symptoms such as sleep apnea. Morbidly obese adolescents may require a more comprehensive physical examination and intervention approaches.

Type 2 Diabetes Mellitus

Obesity during childhood, when combined with lack of physical activity, is of significant concern as a risk factor for type 2 diabetes mellitus (T2DM). Until recently, T2DM was a concern just of older adults, but with the significant increase in childhood overweight combined with lack of physical activity and poor-quality dietary intakes, the age of risk has gotten progressively younger. Risk is multidimensional because genetics and race also predispose individuals to T2DM. Asians experience diabetes at lower body weights than people of other races; Hispanics and African Americans appear to have diabetes in greater numbers than other ethnic groups. Increased risk is also tied to the everyday lifestyle habits often set in childhood; such habits as sedentary activities (video games/TV) and excessive fat/sweet snacking have a lasting impact on diabetes risk. As the incidence of T2DM rises among the American adult population, the behaviors that put these adults at risk are being adopted by their children (Nestle, 2005).

T2DM is almost completely preventable by a balance of energy intake with energy output. This may sound like a simple solution, but as the rates of obesity and T2DM increase among children, particularly Hispanic and African American children, societal changes seem to fuel the risk factors, creating much more complex situations. Societal changes affect family structures, educational system, communities, consumer demands, food production, and business practices, all of which affect behaviors associated with overweight and diabetes risk for all ages (Nestle, 2005). Table 10-5 lists the consequences of these changes.

Current prevention efforts focus on the responsibility of the individual to reduce his or her risk factors for overweight and diabetes. Instead, a public health approach would be more effective. A public health approach provides community supports to ease the transition to positive health-promoting behaviors. For example, local governments could create and provide funds for after-school programs for different types of physical activities suitable for children of varying ages.

Treatment

Treatment of obesity, if warranted, must include the family. The goal is to maintain the current weight of the child while growth continues. Children should not be "dieting," but guidance can be provided to the child and caregivers as to healthier eating patterns. Education about dietary patterns such as those on the MyPlate site and food choices to restructure dietary intake patterns may be sufficient and should be conducted by a dietitian who has the expertise to work with children and their families. The goal of treatment should not be to reach an "ideal weight" but to develop and maintain a healthy lifestyle that includes acceptance of diverse body sizes. Additional T2DM treatment concerns are discussed in Chapter 15.

Role of Nurses

Nurses support the goals of health promotion for overweight children by being sensitive to the emotional, social, and physical dimensions associated with weight and body composition. As allies, nurses create an affirming medical environment for large children through awareness of their own behavior when they conduct physical examinations, such as quietly recording weight rather than announcing weight aloud in a medical office or school setting. Pediatric offices should also have examining gowns large enough for larger pediatric patients.

TABLE 10-5   Recent Societal Changes That Affect Children's Diet and Activity Patterns

CHANGE	CONSEQUENCES
More families with working parents	Parents unable to supervise children's meals and active play
Neighborhoods and parks perceived as increasingly unsafe	Children unable to play outside without supervision
Reduced tax revenues for schools	Introduction of soft drink contracts, vending machines, fast food, and food advertising in schools
Limits on school physical education	Less play during and after school
Increased agricultural production	Increased competition for market share; promotion of more junk food directly to children
Increased demands for convenience foods	More eating occasions; more calories consumed
Greater consumption of food prepared outside the home	Larger portions; more calories consumed
Business deregulation	Unrestricted marketing to children
Television deregulation	More commercials for junk foods during children's programming
Increased use of computers	Food marketing on the Internet; more sedentary behavior
Increased media consolidation	Alliances with food companies to market to children
Increased Wall Street expectations for corporate growth	Expansion of fast-food chains, food products, and marketing to children

From Nestle M: Preventing childhood diabetes: The need for public health intervention, *Am J Public Health* 95(9):1497-1499, 2005.

Iron Deficiency Anemia

For children, poverty is a significant risk factor for iron-deficiency anemia. Economically deprived children of inner cities are most at risk because of the dual risks of lead poisoning, which reduces the amount of iron absorbed by the body, and of chronic hunger, which limits the intake of adequate nutrients. Lead poisoning and iron deficiency each contribute to learning failure. The ability to learn is decreased because cognitive and motor abilities are altered, limiting the ability to explore, focus on, and benefit from the education environment. Poor Americans of any group are at risk, but African American, Hispanic American, and Native American children are most likely to have inadequate intakes of iron.

Malnourished children may be developmentally delayed and unable to benefit from educational experiences. The effects of iron-deficiency anemia may begin in childhood and carry through adolescence and into adulthood, limiting the productivity and potential accomplishments of individuals.

Although iron deficiency has been recognized as a public health issue for many years, it is still a concern. It is possible that federal government programs to improve nutrition status among poor Americans may actually work against decreasing iron deficiency. For example, the U.S. Federal Commodity Food Program releases cheese and butter to the poor. Not only are these foods high in fat, but they also are particularly poor sources of iron and may contribute to the continuing prevalence of iron deficiencies. Another contributing factor may be that in 1997, the USDA began to allow the School Lunch Program to substitute yogurt for meat/protein requirements. For the general population, the effect on iron intake may be minimal, but for economically disadvantaged children, the amount of iron consumed through school lunch servings of meat, poultry, fish, and beans is significant. The effects of chronic poverty and malnutrition are so intertwined that simple nutritional intervention will not overcome the deficits of social deprivation (Perez-Escamilla, 2014).

Role of Nurses

Nurses, particularly school nurses, can educate teaching staff about the relationship between iron deficiency and learning ability. Children may be labeled as slow learners and "behavior problems" in whom iron deficiency may be the true cause of learning difficulties.

NUTRITION DURING ADULTHOOD

Aging is a gradual process that reflects the influence of genetics, lifestyle, and environment over the course of the life span. The purpose of cell creation begins changing around age 30. No longer supplying new cells for growth and development, cell metabolism slows down and instead creates new cells to replace old cells. At older ages, this process of cell replication slows even more, and the effects of aging on body organs begin to appear. Some body systems are more affected than others, and the changes may begin to affect nutritional status. Other organ functions that may be altered include taste and smell, saliva secretions, swallowing difficulties, liver function, and intestinal function. For example, the gastrointestinal tract functions are diminished by reduced production of gastric juices such as hydrochloric acid, which results in decreased absorption of nutrients. The systems and the effects of aging are listed in Table 10-6.

How an individual body responds to these changes reflects health status across the life span. Consequently, everyone ages differently. The role of nutrition during the life span categories of adolescence through the middle years (40s and 50s) provides a foundation to adequately support body processes to effectively deal with the effects of lifestyle and environmental factors. Nutrient intake and dietary patterns directly influence the risk of developing the chronic disorders of osteoporosis, coronary artery disease (CAD), diabetes, hypertension, and obesity. The effect of nutrient intake, though, is mediated by lifestyle behaviors, including physical activity, stress, smoking, alcohol consumption, and exposure to

TABLE 10-6 Effects of Aging

EFFECT ON NUTRITIONAL STATUS	CAUSE	ORGAN(S) INVOLVED
↓Ability to taste salt and sweets	↓Taste buds	Tongue and nose
↓Palatability of food	↓Taste and olfactory nerve endings	
↓Food intake		
↓Taste and smell		
↓Sense of thirst/dry mouth	↓Saliva production	Salivary glands
Minor effects on swallowing (but may progress to dysphagia)	Muscle contractions may malfunction	Esophagus (and swallowing process)
↓Bioavailability of vitamins, minerals, proteins	↓Hydrochloric acid (HCl) secretion and intrinsic factor	Stomach
↓Absorption of vitamin B$_{12}$ and folate	↓Pepsin	Stomach
↓Drug doses (adjustments possible to prevent overdosing)	↓Production of drug-metabolizing enzymes	Liver

↓, Reduction in.
Data from Rosenberg IH, et al: Aging and the digestive system. In Munro HN, Danford E, editors: *Nutrition, aging, and the elderly*, New York, 1989, Plenum Press.

environmental factors. For example, how a young woman eats and the amount of exercise she performs affects the density of her bones and the level of lean body mass of her body. If her nutrient intake is adequate and the exercise is weight bearing, she may reduce her risk of osteoporosis (as well as the risk of the other chronic disorders) decades later when she is in her 60s or 70s.

Stages of Adulthood

The Early Years (20s and 30s)

Students tend to imagine that once they finish high school or college and enter the working world, they will then be able to eat better, sleep more, and generally take better care of themselves than they do during their hectic school years. Unfortunately, that is rarely the experience of young adults. Many find that their lifestyles may be even more time restricted, and positive health behaviors such as regular meal patterns and exercise may fall by the wayside.

These years mark a transition from one stage of the life span to another; young adults separate from their family of origin, focus on personal and career goals, and often face reproductive decisions (Figure 10-8). As such, it is a prime time to either refine or establish an eating style that promotes health, possibly preventing future development of diet-related diseases. National surveys, though, continue to report that few adults consume the health-promoting recommended intakes of fruits and vegetables. A self-review or assessment by a nutrition professional can assist in creating a personal schedule that allows time for planning and preparation of simple yet high-quality meals.

Many women bear children during these years. The nutrition and health requirements of pregnancy are detailed in earlier in this chapter. Layered on these needs during this life span stage are often employment and other family commitments, all of which affect nutritional and health behaviors. Physically caring for young children, although eminently rewarding, may be exhausting. Throughout the mother's pregnancy and during childbearing, the father's role in terms of health issues is often ignored. Although the woman's body is nourishing fetal development, the father is under stress as he prepares to support additional responsibilities. Fathers also need to be at optimum health, especially during the first few years of childrearing when physical stamina is put to the test.

Nutrition requirements. Growth tends to be completed by the late teens for women and early 20s for men, as reflected by the DRI. For women, the Recommended Dietary Allowance (RDA) for energy is 2200 kcal daily; for men, it is 2900 kcal. This reflects the typical differences in body weight and lean body mass of men and women. When this stage includes a departure from high school or college sports training, energy intake should be reduced to meet actual need, or weight gain could occur. A teenage boy's serious athletic training may require as much as 5000 to 6000 kcal a day to maintain weight. Switching to a desk job and exercising for 1 hour per day does not equal previous energy requirements.

The RDA for protein increases for women from 46 to 50 g and for men from 58 to 63 g daily; these ranges reflect lean body mass growth that may occur in both men and women through about age 24. Vitamin and mineral needs do not significantly change. Calcium and phosphorus needs for men and women decline after age 18 because skeletal growth is almost complete. Daily Adequate Intake (AI) recommended calcium levels up to age 18 are 1300 mg, dropping to 1000 mg from 19 years on. For phosphorus, RDA levels up to age 18 are 1250 mg a day, dropping to 700 mg from 19 years on. Maintaining calcium and iron intake continues to be a concern for women because of their often-restricted intake of food during dieting. (See also Box 7-1 or Box 8-3 regarding nutrients and their functions.)

The Middle Years (40s and 50s)

The years from 40 to 50 are marked by a continuation of family demands and career involvement. Some middle-year adults may be faced with caring for aging parents; this increased stress and responsibility may be offset by the seemingly reduced parenting of their own children. As older children leave for college or move into their own residences, the resultant "empty nest" necessitates rediscovering preparation of dinners for two or, for single parents, dinners for one. With family meals no longer a requirement, many middle-year adults often have the finances and time for restaurant dining. However, making the transition to food preparation styles and dietary patterns that maintain healthful dietary patterns is crucial.

The impact of continued positive dietary patterns coupled with regular exercise provides continued prevention or delay of diet-related diseases such as type 2 diabetes mellitus (T2DM) and CAD. Increased stamina is an additional benefit of such behaviors.

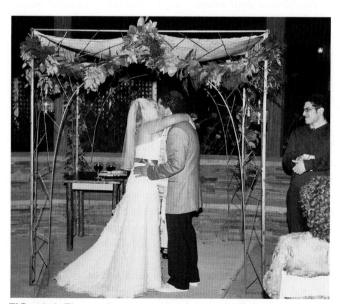

FIG 10-8 The early years of adulthood often include the forming of long-term relationships. (Copyright Jean Kallina, 2005.)

Nutrition requirements. During the middle years, cell loss rather than replication occurs. Kcal needs decline as lean body mass is lost and replaced by body fat, which is less metabolically active. Women in particular experience an increase in body fat composition. Body fat increases can be slowed by exercise and strength training to continue maintenance of lean body mass. After age 50, daily energy needs drop from 2200 to 1920 kcal for women and from 2900 to 2300 kcal for men. It is a challenge to meet the same nutrient needs with reduced kcal intake. Protein needs remain constant for both genders. Iron requirements for women drop from 18 to 8 mg, which reflects reduced iron loss because of menopause. (See also Box 7-1 or Box 8-3 regarding nutrients and their functions.)

Overall, dietary patterns that are nutrient dense and feature lower-fat protein foods coupled with fiber-containing fruits, vegetables, and grains best meet the nutrient needs of middle-year adults.

The Older Years (60s, 70s, and 80s)

The United States has never had a population with as high a percentage of older adults as it has. As our life span increases in years, senescence (older adulthood) is for many people a time of life for continued professional or career advancement and recreational enjoyment. Others are in transition, adjusting to retirement and settling into new patterns of activities. Gerontology, the study of aging, has provided insights into the emotional, physical, and social aspects of the later years of life. Preparation for the social and physical transitions of aging actually begins many years earlier, as individual approaches to lifestyle health behaviors, career fulfillment, and leisurely pursuits evolve.

Overall, quality of life for older adults depends on factors that influence daily experiences. These factors include health status; nutritional well-being; spirituality; living arrangements; physical activity; social interactions; physical, mental, and emotional functioning; disease management; and level of financial and physical independence. The level of wellness experienced during this stage of life often reflects the quality of life resulting from health behaviors through the several life span stages.

Physical activity. A lifetime of physical fitness and good nutrition allows an individual to enter these years with more stamina, cardiovascular conditioning, and solid health-promoting habits that enable him or her to overcome the inevitable slowing down or physical limitation of the later years. Even those who were not always active have been shown to benefit from regular exercise. Strength training has improved the muscle tone and stamina of older men and women.

Physical, mental, and emotional functioning. During these later years, individuals may struggle with the deaths of family members and friends and adjustment to retirement. Although some delight in retirement, others view it as a loss of social status. This combination of death and loss of status may lead to isolation and depression, resulting in loss of appetite (anorexia) or other forms of malnutrition. The

economic realities of retirement without a solid financial base may thrust some older adults into unexpected poverty, because Social Security and Medicare payments may not be sufficient to cover living and medical expenses. Resources for food purchases may be limited and may negatively affect nutritional status. Unless social networking and family supports are strong, these conditions may persist. Older adults may abuse alcohol as a way to deal with these perceived difficult events.

Disorientation or senility often associated with aging may be caused by improper use of medications, marginal nutrient deficiencies (e.g., vitamin B_{12}), or simple dehydration. Older clients may intentionally restrict fluid intake because of incontinence, nocturia (excessive urination at night), or the inability to get to the toilet on their own. Some older adults lose their sense of thirst and forget to consume enough fluids. Fluid requirements in older adults remain the same as in younger adults (about 8 cups daily is sufficient) unless a medical condition or medication prescribes otherwise. The signs of dehydration are listed in Box 10-13. Medical diagnosis should be sought to determine the specific etiology of these signs.

Nutritional well-being. Nutritional status of older adults may be affected by restrictions in access to food and ability to prepare meals. Shopping may be difficult without transportation, and mobility to walk through stores may be limited. Funds for food may be constrained, and often, food quantities available are beyond the amounts that can be used by individuals living alone. (See Figure 10-9.) Once foods are purchased, preparation may be affected by physical limitations caused by progressive chronic illnesses such as arthritis. Some older adults may no longer have an interest in cooking. Others have become so frightened about foods containing too much fat or cholesterol that they become malnourished. For individuals in this age bracket, there is not sufficient evidence to warrant restrictive dietary intake; in actuality, malnutrition and underweight are more detrimental than excess dietary fat and cholesterol intake. Box 10-14 lists risks factors for malnutrition in older adults.

Dietary management for older adults may be more complicated than for other stages of adulthood. For younger adults, reducing BMI decreases health risks. For older adults, decreased BMI may be associated with increased risk of strokes. Having an average BMI provides healthful weight

BOX 10-13   Signs of Dehydration in Older Adults
Confusion
Weakness
A hot, dry body
Furrowed tongue
Decreased skin turgor (may not be valid finding in older adults)
Rapid pulse
Elevated urinary sodium

BOX 10-14 Risk Factors for Malnutrition in Older Adults

Alcoholism
Anorexia
Chewing and swallowing problems (dysphagia)
Consuming only one meal a day
Dental difficulties
Depression or dementia
Diabetes
Diminished physical functioning
Feeding problems
Food purchasing/preparation difficulties
Impaired acuity of taste and smell
Living in long-term care institution
Loss of spouse
Taking multiple medications
Nerve disorders
Poverty
Pulmonary disease
Surgery

Data from Chernoff R: Nutrition and health promotion in older adults, *J Gerontol A Biol Sci Med Sci* 56(Spec 2[2]):47-53, 2001; copyright the Gerontological Society of America.

FIG 10-9 Socializing around food preparation assists with the adjustments of the older years.

reserves during times of illness (Chapman, 2010). Studies of weight reduction strategies seldom include older participants, so their complex physiologic, behavioral, and social needs are not considered. Additionally, such strategies may overly limit intake of essential nutrients, further worsening malnutrition.

Another aspect of older adult dietary management is protein adequacy. Total body protein decreases as aging progresses. Although the loss of skeletal muscle is the most noticeable body protein lost, organ tissue, blood components, and immune bodies are also affected, leading to compromised wound healing, loss of skin elasticity, reduced ability to battle infection, and longer recuperation from illness and surgeries (Chernoff, 2004). Dietary intake may be further altered when these physical factors combine with social factors, leading to reduced protein intake. Consumption of micronutrients found in protein foods also may be limited, leading to deficiencies of vitamins B_{12}, A, C, and D, calcium, iron, zinc, and others. Frail elderly women are most at risk for these micronutrient deficiencies. This need, combined with the greater turnover of whole-body protein in aging bodies, results in a need for greater dietary protein intake in older adults. Protein consumption may be improved by consumption of 30 g of protein per meal (Paddon-Jones and Leidy, 2014).

Living arrangements. Living arrangements also affect nutritional status. A variety of living arrangements exists for older adults. Although many continue to live in their own homes or with family members, some opt for retirement communities, and others, because of health conditions, may reside in long-term care facilities or nursing homes. Living in one's own home provides the freedom to prepare and eat foods whenever desired; illness, however, may make shopping

for and preparing food difficult. Retirement communities may provide transportation to food stores and more social events involving meals (Figure 10-9), although residents may still be responsible for their own food preparation. Long-term care facilities usually provide prepared meals, but the style of cooking may not be as appealing or comforting as home-prepared meals.

A challenge for meeting the nutritional needs of institutionalized older adults is that the DRIs used to guide nutrient levels are intended to meet the needs of healthy older adults. Adjustments are necessary for individual circumstances of acute or chronic illness to achieve rehabilitation, recuperation, or maintenance to reduce the risk of further complications. Consequently, it is now recommended that diets in long-term care facilities be liberalized to improve dietary intake of this age group (Kuczmarski, et al, 2005).

Dietary patterns and preferences of older adults are the result of long-established habits. When they are ill, lonely, or under stress, older adults may strongly prefer foods they associate with pleasant memories. Ethnic favorites may provide security and comfort. The psychologic and social meanings of foods can play an important part in helping an older client recover from illness or adjust to changed circumstances.

Demographic and lifestyle characteristics may, as noted, put older adults at nutritional risk. Factors may include gender, smoking, alcohol abuse, dietary patterns, educational level, dental health, chronic illnesses, and living situations. Interventions to assist older adults must account for these influences and should view support services through a continuum of care. Continuum of care provides continuity of care while the older individual moves through different living situations, and services such as health, medical, and supportive services are provided in suitable care environments. Care settings may range from acute medical settings to community and daycare, from assisted-living retirement housing to traditional nursing home facilities and hospices.

Nutrition requirements. The DRIs remain constant from age 51 years and older for men and women, except for vitamin D. What does change is the ability of the body to either process or synthesize certain nutrients. Synthesis of vitamin D is reduced; the AI for vitamin D for individuals older than age 70 increases to 20 μg a day, up from 15 μg a day for those aged 51 to 70 years. Older adults either need more exposure to sunlight to produce required amounts of vitamin D or require a supplement if so diagnosed by a physician, qualified nutritionist, or dietitian. Because of decreased production of gastric juices and intestinal enzymes, digestion and absorption may be reduced, further highlighting the need for optimum nutrient intake. The production of the intrinsic factor required for vitamin B_{12} absorption also may be reduced, increasing the risk of pernicious anemia. New recommendations suggest the use of vitamin B_{12} supplements or consumption of foods fortified with vitamin B_{12} to meet the RDA of 2.4 μg/day (see also Box 7-1 or Box 8-3 regarding the functions of nutrients).

Other factors may affect nutritional status. A marginal deficiency of zinc can alter the sensitivity of taste receptors. This deficiency heightens the ability to taste bitter and sour flavors and reduces sweet and salty sensations; excessive use of sugars and salt to make foods taste appealing may result.

Overconsumption of simple sugars and sodium may exacerbate other diet-related disorders, such as diabetes and hypertension. As the muscularity of the digestive system weakens, constipation may be a problem, especially after a lifetime of low-fiber foods. Constipation may be alleviated by slowly increasing consumption of whole-wheat products, fruits, vegetables, and fluids as well as increasing exercise.

Dental health may also affect the ability of older adults to be well nourished. Loss of teeth caused by periodontal disease limits the ability to chew foods such as meats, a prime source of zinc. For some, chewing ability may still be compromised after dentures have been fitted to replace missing teeth. Dentures may need to be periodically refitted. When dentures do not fit properly, some people do not use them. Instead, they tend to eat foods that can be gummed rather than chewed.

The Oldest Years (80s and 90s)

As life expectancy increases in years, the number of those in the most golden years rises. Although nutrient needs remain basically stable after age 80, the effects of aging may continue to reduce the ability of the body to absorb and synthesize nutrients. Optimum nutrition continues to be critical. The healthiest of the oldest develop individual patterns of dietary intake that most meet their physical and social needs.

Nutrition requirements. Malnutrition and being underweight become a concern during this stage (see Box 10-14). As food preparation becomes more physically difficult to

---

BOX 10-15   Strategies for Overcoming Barriers to Good Nutrition

Counteract Decreased Senses of Taste and Smell
Recommend that smokers refrain from smoking at least 1 hour before meals.
Suggest sipping water before and during the meal to moisten a dry mouth.
Amplify flavors with the use of seasonings other than salt.
Recommend chewing food thoroughly to fully release flavor and aroma.
Vary food textures and flavors.

Encourage Social Interaction
Find others who are willing to share food preparation and mealtimes.
Investigate congregate meal programs available through senior citizen centers, religious organizations, and hospital community outreach programs.
Avoid noisy dining areas for people with hearing aids.

Present Food Attractively
Use colorful foods and table settings.
Provide enough lighting to see food clearly.

Provide Outside Support
Arrange for Meals-on-Wheels for homebound adults.
Refer eligible clients to the Supplemental Nutrition Assistance Program (SNAP), Emergency Food Assistance Program, Child and Adult Care Program, or community food banks or soup kitchens.
Locate grocery stores with delivery service.
Refer to the Expanded Food and Nutrition Education Program (EFNEP) of the Cooperative Extension Service for recipes, meal suggestions, and budgeting assistance.
Refer clients to home health nurse for routine nutrition screening and appropriate interventions.

---

accomplish, kcal intake may diminish. Illness and accompanying medications may reduce appetite; malnutrition is associated with increased complications. Relatives, friends, and health care professionals can assist in ensuring that adequate meals are available and consumed (Box 10-15). Those in the oldest years may be most at risk for dehydration. Particularly at risk are African Americans and men. Risk rises because of decreased ability of the kidneys to concentrate urine, limited movement, drug interactions, and malfunctioning thirst sensation. Limited ability to move may increase fears of incontinence that lead to decreased fluid intake. Nearly half of older adults hospitalized as Medicare patients experience dehydration (Kuczmarski, et al, 2005) (see also Box 7-1 or Box 8-3 regarding functions of nutrients).

Older adults may be at risk for asphyxiation of food because of reduced chewing ability from loss of teeth or poorly fitting dentures. Neurologic conditions such as Parkinson's disease and effects of stroke may result in chewing and swallowing difficulties (dysphagia) that may cause asphyxiation (see Chapter 19). Counseling older adults about problematic foods may avert asphyxiation. Referrals to a registered dietitian/nutritionist with expertise in these disorders should be considered.

Although assessment is the responsibility of all health care professionals, home health nurses are particularly able to conduct routine nutrition screening and implement appropriate interventions to prevent or halt malnutrition among this population. Government and community meal programs help fill this need and are discussed later in the section on community supports.

NUTRITION HEALTH PROMOTION: ADULTHOOD

Knowledge

Health promotion integrates nutrition education and focuses on three areas of knowledge: (1) adequate intake of nutrients found in foods (rather than supplements), (2) the relationship between diet and disease, and (3) moderate kcal intake coupled with regular exercise for physical fitness and obesity prevention.

Techniques

Many strategies can be used for adult health promotion:

1. *To reduce risk of diet-related disorders such as coronary heart disease, some cancers, T2DM and obesity, consider:*
   - Scheduling routine food shopping so staples such as fruits, vegetables, and grains are available for meal preparation.
   - When shopping, occasionally comparing fat content of commonly purchased foods with that of similar products and purchasing the lower-fat product.
   - Aiming to limit foods that contain visible fat.
   - Reorganizing work and personal priorities if necessary to allow time for meal preparation and consumption; for example, get up earlier for breakfast, pack a lunch or afternoon snack, preplan easy-to-prepare dinner menus.
   - Keeping track of dietary intake using MyPlate or the Fruits & Veggies—More Matters plan. Review Chapter 5 for other dietary fat–lowering techniques and Chapter 4 for approaches that increase the use of complex carbohydrates and fiber-containing foods.
2. *To reduce osteoporosis risk and strengthen bone health, consider:*
   - Focusing on routine dietary habits—for example, drink a glass of milk at lunch each day. A food pattern assessment can assist in creating a practical calcium consumption plan.
   - Reviewing Chapter 8 for other approaches to increasing calcium consumption.
3. *To decrease the risk of sodium-sensitive hypertension and CAD, consider:*
   - Adopting the DASH (Dietary Approach to Stop Hypertension) eating plan, which focuses on increasing intake of fruits and vegetables. See Chapter 17 for more details.
   - Learning the food categories that are generally salty, and either consume them only occasionally or, if available, purchase low-sodium versions. See Chapter 17 for other sodium-reducing strategies.
   - Reducing overall intake of fat, particularly saturated fat.
4. *To achieve a healthy body weight and decrease the possibility of diet- and lifestyle-related obesity, consider:*
   - Responding to actual hunger with low-fat, high-fiber foods (with occasional splurges) rather than focusing on dietary restrictions.
   - Exercising regularly to increase stamina, strength, and a sense of wellness. Depending on conditioning, incorporate exercise gradually. A 10-minute walk may be comfortable for some, but others can begin with more strenuous endeavors.
   - Consulting Chapter 9 for related strategies (see also the *Cultural Considerations* box Live Long and Prosper … the Okinawa Way!)

Community Supports

Government, corporate, and social institutions create the environments and structures that can support lifestyle health promotion behaviors. Although the actions of these institutions affect particular groups of the public, employees, or communities, it is the individual who can choose to reap the rewards.

Government agencies such as the U.S. Food and Drug Administration (FDA) create regulations that either provide consumer information for decision making (e.g., nutrition labeling) or control the quality of foods, which in turn affects the nutrient viability of manufactured products.

In New York City, an ordinance was passed that requires restaurants and food chains with 10 or more locations to post the nutrient content of foods served. This information may be posted on signs, as in fast-food restaurants, or on menus in traditional restaurants. Whether this requirement will influence consumer choices is yet to be determined, but at least it makes the possibility of informed decision making available. Ordinances banning the use of artificial *trans* fats in the preparation of foods for direct consumption by consumers in restaurants and other food outlets have been implemented in several cities in the United States. The FDA has recently proposed removing artificial *trans* fat from the Generally Recognized As Safe (GRAS) list of ingredients because of its effect on blood cholesterol levels. Any use of *trans* fat would then be as a food additive requiring specific regulations to allow for its use.

Corporations can support health promotion activities by offering comprehensive employee health promotion programs to their employees. This can be accomplished through wellness centers providing programs about healthy lifestyles. Although most corporations may not be able to provide on-site gyms or similar facilities, some have arranged for corporate discounts at local gym facilities.

Government agencies and community groups provide socioeconomic support within the community. Government programs include the Supplemental Nutrition Assistance

Program (SNAP), The Emergency Food Assistance Program (TEFAP), and community food banks and meals. Boosting people's food purchasing power improves their overall nutrient intake. SNAP is administered nationally by the USDA and on the state and local levels by welfare or human services agencies. The federal government pays the actual food assistance costs; administration costs are divided among the other agencies.

As an entitlement program, SNAP is available to all who are eligible without restriction of age or family size. Financial and nonfinancial factors of households are considered to determine eligibility. Financial factors include income and economic resources, such as savings and vehicles; nonfinancial considerations consist of a variety of factors, such as social security eligibility, citizenship, and work requirements. Gross incomes must meet certain percentages of the poverty level on the basis of overall factors; the level of support varies according to family membership and net income (USDA, 2014).

The Food and Nutrition Service of the USDA administers TEFAP. Various local agencies may administer the program. State agencies determine their own criteria for eligibility based on household income. The program serves two functions: to reduce government-held surplus dairy commodities and to supplement the dietary intake of low-income households through the distribution of basic commodities. The types of foods distributed vary between actual surplus foods and foods purchased especially for this program. In addition to dairy products such as nonfat dry milk and cheese, TEFAP has distributed canned meat, peanut butter, citrus juices, legumes, dried potatoes, and canned and dried fruit. Some of this program's funds are used by states to fund emergency feeding programs such as soup kitchens and food banks (USDA, 2014).

Community food banks and emergency feeding programs may be partially funded by TEFAP in addition to support from foundations and other charitable organizations (Figure 10-10). Some programs also collect food from the surrounding community and surplus donations from supermarkets and restaurants. Personnel at these facilities are usually volunteers from youth groups, religious organizations, and civic associations. Food banks often provide a bag of food staples to help bridge the gap that may occur when food stamps and monthly welfare support are exhausted before the beginning of the next month. Emergency feeding programs such as soup kitchens may provide hot meals as a safety net to help individuals of lower socioeconomic populations avoid malnutrition.

Other USDA supports specifically for older adults are the Child and Adult Care Food Program and the Senior Nutrition Program. Community groups may sponsor some of the government programs or may develop their own local programs.

The Child and Adult Care Food Program provides meals and snacks for children up to age 12 and to senior citizens and specific categories of handicapped people participating in daycare programs that are nonprofit, licensed, or receive agency approval. Reimbursement rates differ for programs that serve children and adults. Family income of the participants may be considered. Like other programs, it is administered on the federal level by the Food and Nutrition Service of the USDA and on the state level by human services or education departments. Adult daycare programs may be administered locally by a variety of community sponsors. For children, eligible programs include Head Start, after-school programs, and family daycare (USDA, 2014).

The Senior Nutrition Program serves only older adults and was created to offer inexpensive meals, education, and socialization. The Congregate Meals Program and Home-Delivered Meals Program are both part of the Senior Nutrition Program. This program provides for those in financial need as well as those in social need. Eligibility is open to everyone 60 years or older; spouses of participants may also be served regardless of their age. To participate in the Home-Delivered Meals Program, individuals must reside in the program service area and be unable to prepare their own meals. Meals are generally provided Monday through Friday. Those receiving meals at home may also be given frozen meals for weekend consumption (USDA, 2014). Distribution of meals varies among programs.

TOWARD A POSITIVE NUTRITION LIFESTYLE: RATIONALIZING

Rationalization is one of the psychologic defense mechanisms used to protect our sense of self when we are under stress. When our behaviors, feelings, or perceptions are irrational or unreasonable, we may use rationalization to assign reasonable explanations to ourselves as to why we behaved as we did.

For example, from adolescence on through the older years, some individuals rationalize their poor eating habits. The list of reasonable explanations may include not enough time to prepare better meals, lack of knowledge about nutrition, and lack of cooking skills. Although these may be reasonable explanations, they do not help improve nutritional status.

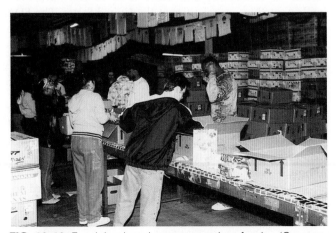

FIG 10-10 Food bank volunteers sorting foods. (Courtesy Community Food Bank of New Jersey, Hillside, NJ.)

Often these types of rationalizations make it harder to change unproductive behaviors.

Consider the same explanations in a more positive way:

- Not enough time to prepare better meals but can reorganize schedule to create time.

- Lack of knowledge about nutrition or of cooking skills but can take a nutrition or cooking course or read books on nutrition and use simple cookbooks to learn basic skills.

- Instead of continuing negative rationalization, positive rationalization may provide the means to change.

SUMMARY

- The importance of nutrition during pregnancy, the benefits of breastfeeding, and the establishment and maintenance of positive eating styles during infancy are crucial to overall health goals.
- Lactation is a natural, physiologic process beginning shortly after delivery and completing the cycle of the female body from pregnancy through motherhood.
  - Human milk is the best health promoter for the neonate.
  - Breastfeeding should begin immediately after birth and continue every 2 to 3 hours during the initial postpartum weeks.
  - Lactating women should continue to consume a diet with adequate sources of protein, energy, vitamins, and minerals.
- Sound nutrition practices during the first year of life lay the foundation for good health.
  - The ideal food for the first 4 to 6 months of life is breast milk.
  - Supplemental foods may be introduced one at a time at 4 to 6 months of age.
  - Feeding of breast milk (or formula) should continue until the infant reaches 1 year of age.
- Children with medical problems may require specialized nutrition support.
- Psychologic and physiologic maturation reflect life span stages: childhood (ages 1 through 12), adolescence (ages 13 through 19), and adulthood.
- Health promotion depends on knowledge, techniques, and community supports.
  - Approaches to health promotion take into account these stages and their effect on nutrient requirements,

eating styles, food choices, and supports from the larger community.
- Barriers to health promotion during childhood and adolescence may include food asphyxiation, lead poisoning, overweight/diabetes, and iron-deficiency anemia.
- The role of nutrition in each of the adult life span categories reflects the value of adequate nutrient intake to reduce the risk of chronic disorders of such as osteoporosis, CAD, DM, hypertension, and obesity.
- During the early years (20s and 30s), establishment of positive health behaviors is desirable because these years are the childbearing and child-rearing years, with health implications for both women and men.
- The middle years (40s and 50s) are years of career and family demands. Chronic diet-related diseases, such as type 2 diabetes mellitus and CVD, may occur during these years. Positive dietary and exercise behaviors may provide protection. Nutrient needs for women change as menopause occurs. In particular, adequate calcium consumption is recommended to offset loss of bone density.
- The older years (60s, 70s, and 80s) are most reflective of lifestyle behaviors practiced over many years, although psychosocial issues may affect adequacy of nutrient intake.
- During the oldest years (80s and 90s), malnutrition and underweight bodies are of concern.

◎ THE NURSING APPROACH

Case Study: Breastfeeding

Rebecca, age 24, delivered her first child 2 days before meeting with the nurse practitioner. She said she and the baby boy, Bobby, were doing well, but she had some questions about breastfeeding.

Assessment
Subjective (from Patient Statements)
- "He nurses OK and seems happy, though he wants to eat every 2 hours."
- "My nipples are not sore, but I feel really tired."
- "I plan to keep breastfeeding until Bobby is about 6 months old. I like the closeness I feel to him."

- "I'm wondering what to do about feeding when I need to leave the baby with my husband for a few hours."
- "How do I know if Bobby is getting enough to eat?"

Objective (from Physical Examination)
- Birth weight 7 pounds 10 ounces and length 19.7 inches
- Newborn at fiftieth percentile for weight and length
- Loose yellow stool and light yellow urine in diaper

Diagnoses (Nursing)
1. Effective breastfeeding as evidenced by the mother's statement that the newborn infant "nurses OK and seems

Continued

◎ THE NURSING APPROACH—cont'd

happy," the mother likes the closeness, the newborn is at fiftieth percentile for weight and height, and the loose yellow stool and light yellow urine in infant's diaper

2. Readiness for enhanced knowledge as evidenced by questions about saving milk and evaluating adequacy of milk intake

Planning
Patient Outcomes
Short term (at the end of this visit):
- Rebecca will state how to determine whether the infant is eating enough.
- She will demonstrate how to express milk and state how to save milk for the infant for times when she cannot breastfeed.
- She will identify resources for continued success with breastfeeding.

Long term (follow-up visit after 4 weeks):
- The infant will continue to gain weight to stay in the fiftieth percentile for weight and length.
- Rebecca will say she is satisfied with breastfeeding.

Nursing Interventions
1. Assess Rebecca's feelings about breastfeeding.
2. Discuss nutrition requirements for breastfeeding and promote a healthy lifestyle.
3. Educate Rebecca on the benefits of breastfeeding, how to express and store breast milk, and how to determine whether the infant is getting enough milk.
4. Provide resources for Rebecca.

Implementation
1. Assessed Rebecca's feelings and attitudes about breastfeeding.
   The nurse can accept and support a woman's decision to breastfeed or bottle feed. If the mother is not successful with breastfeeding, the nurse can try to help her. If the mother is not happy with breastfeeding, the nurse should present her with the alternate choice of using formula in bottles.
2. Encouraged drinking at least 3000 mL of water, milk, and juices per day, and eating a well-balanced diet per recommendations from ChooseMyPlate.gov.
   Adequate hydration, adequate nutrients, and extra kcal (about 500 kcal more than usual) are needed to support lactation and the health of the mother. Alcohol and caffeine should be avoided because they can be secreted in the breast milk.
3. Reviewed benefits of breastfeeding.
   It is rewarding for the mother to know that the infant may have fewer infections, fewer allergies, and easier digestion with breast milk. In addition, it is usually more convenient and economical to breastfeed rather than bottle feed.

4. Discussed how to express breast milk and save it in a bottle.
   Milk may be expressed manually or with a pump. It needs to be saved in a bottle in the refrigerator (up to 48 hours) or in the freezer (several months). Cleanliness and good hand washing are essential.
5. Discussed how to determine whether the infant is getting enough milk.
   Breastfeeding should be done on a demand schedule, and the infant should generally be content after eating. At least six wet diapers and one bowel movement per day indicate adequate hydration and milk. Weight gain should follow a standard growth chart.
6. Provided literature about breastfeeding and La Leche League support groups, and wrote down a contact number for the clinic.
   Written materials reinforce learning. Contacts and support personnel are helpful when questions arise about breastfeeding.

Evaluation
Short term (at the end of the first visit):
- Rebecca identified how to determine whether the infant is getting enough milk.
- She demonstrated how to express milk and stated how she can save milk.
- She said she might contact someone from La Leche support group.

Goals met.
- Long term (in 1 month):
- Infant gained weight and remained in fiftieth percentile for height and weight.
- Rebecca reported her satisfaction and infant's contentment after breastfeeding.
- She reported that infant has a bowel movement with each feeding and urinates several times a day.
- Rebecca said she rented a breast pump and was able to save enough milk to go on a date with her husband while the grandmother cared for the infant.

Goals met.

Discussion Questions
At the follow-up visit, Rebecca said she was drinking a lot of diet cola to increase her fluid intake and production of breast milk. She was restricting her calorie intake so that she could quickly lose the 25 pounds she needed to lose to get back to prepregnancy weight. She would like to begin introducing solid foods into the infant's diet but is not sure what foods to start with or whether Bobby is ready.

1. Role-play a conversation the nurse could have with Rebecca about her fluid intake and her restriction of calories.
2. How soon should Rebecca add solid food to the infant's diet? What food may be tolerated best?

APPLYING CONTENT KNOWLEDGE

Elena, age 18, is a client at the city Special Supplemental Nutrition Program for Women, Infants, and Children (WIC); she is beginning her third trimester of pregnancy. She attended nutrition education classes taught by the WIC nutritionist. The nutritionist, though, is concerned because Elena has not been gaining sufficient weight to support her pregnancy although she is otherwise healthy. The nutritionist suspects that Elena does not understand the relationship between her dietary intake and the health of her fetus. The nutritionist asks you as a WIC nurse to reinforce these concepts when Elena comes in for her monthly checkups. What will you discuss with Elena?

WEBSITES OF INTEREST

La Leche League

www.lalecheleague.org

Advocates breastfeeding through education, information, and support via publications, conferences, and local chapter meetings.

KidsHealth

www.kidshealth.org

Provides information for children, teens, and parents on health, food, and fitness, including games and colorful animations.

Office of Minority Health and Health Disparities (OMHD)

www.cdc.gov/omhd

Aims to eradicate health disparities for vulnerable and at-risk populations and to maximize the health impact of the Centers for Disease Control and Prevention (CDC) on the U.S. population.

National Women's Health Information Center

www.womenshealth.gov/

Functions as a single point of entry for federal and private sector sources on women's health issues; created by the Office on Women's Health, U.S. Department of Health and Human Services.

REFERENCES

American Academy of Pediatrics (AAP): Policy statement on breastfeeding and the use of human milk, *Pediatrics* 129(3):e827–e841, 2012.

American College of Obstetrics and Gynecology (ACOG), Committee on Obstetric Practice: ACOG committee opinion: Exercise during pregnancy and the postpartum period, *ACOG Committee Opinion* 267:171–173, 2002.

Bitler PM, Currie J: Does WIC work? The effects of WIC on pregnancy and birth outcomes, *J Policy Anal Manage* 24(1):73–91, 2005.

Centers for Disease Control and Prevention (CDC): Achievements in public health: Reduction in perinatal transmission of *HIV* infection—United States, 1985-2005, MMWR, *MMWR Morb Mortal Wkly Rep* 55(21):592–597, 2006.

Chapman IM: Obesity paradox during aging, *Interdiscip Top Gerontol* 37:20–36, 2010.

Chernoff R: Protein and older adults, *J Am Coll Nutr* 23(6 Suppl): 627S–630S, 2004.

Cole CR, Lifshitz F: Zinc nutrition and growth retardation, *Pediatr Endocrinol Rev* 5(4):889–896, 2008.

Coutsoudis A, et al: HIV, infant feeding and more perils for poor people: New WHO guidelines encourage review of formula milk policies, *Bull World Health Organ* 86(3):210–214, 2008.

Ebrahim GJ: The baby-friendly hospital initiative, *J Trop Pediatr* 39:2, 1993.

Elsas LJ II, Acosta PB: Inherited metabolic diseases: Amino acids, organic acids, and galactose. In Ross AC, et al, editors: *Modern nutrition in health and disease*, ed 11, Philadelphia, 2014, Lippincott Williams & Wilkins.

Erick M: Nutrition during pregnancy and lactation. In Mahan LK, et al, editors: *Krause's food & the nutrition care process*, ed 13, Philadelphia, 2012, Saunders.

Food Research & Action Center (FRAC): *National school lunch program*, n.d. From: http://frac.org/federal-foodnutrition-programs/national-school-lunch-program. Accessed January 14, 2014.

Food Research & Action Center (FRAC): *School breakfast program*, n.d. From: http://frac.org/federal-foodnutrition-programs/school-breakfast-program. Accessed January 14, 2014.

Heird WC: Nutritional requirements of infants and children. In Ross AC, et al, editors: *Modern nutrition in health and disease*, ed 11, Philadelphia, 2014, Lippincott Williams & Wilkins.

James DC, et al: Position of the American Dietetic Association: Promoting and supporting breastfeeding, *J Am Diet Assoc* 109:1926–1942, 2009.

Krebs-Smith SM, et al: Americans do not meet federal dietary recommendations, *J Nutr* 140:1832–1838, 2010.

Krugman SD, Dubowitz H: Failure to thrive, *Am Fam Physician* 68(5):879–884, 2003.

Kuczmarski MF, et al: Position paper of the American Dietetic Association: Nutrition across the spectrum of aging, *J Am Diet Assoc* 105(4):616–633, 2005.

Mathews TJ, MacDorman MF: Infant mortality statistics from the 2009 period linked birth/infant death data set, *Natl Vital Stat Rep* 61(8):1–27, 2013.

National Research Council (NRC): *Dietary reference intakes: The essential guide to nutrient requirements*, Washington, DC, 2006, The National Academies Press.

Nestle M: Preventing childhood diabetes: The need for public health intervention, *Am J Public Health* 95(9):1497–1499, 2005.

Nicklas TA, et al: Position of the American Dietetic Association: Nutrition guidance for healthy children ages 2 to 11 years, *J Am Diet Assoc* 108(6):1038–1047, 2008.

Paddon-Jones D, Leidy H: Dietary protein and muscle in older persons, *Curr Opin Clin Nutr Metab Care* 17(1):5–11, 2014.

Perez-Escamilla R: Food insecurity in children: Impact on physical, psychoemotional, and social development. In Ross AC, et al, editors: *Modern nutrition in health and disease*, ed 11, Philadelphia, 2014, Lippincott Williams & Wilkins.

Piernas C, Popkin BM: Trends in snacking among U.S. children, *Health Aff* 29(3):398–404, 2010.

Polsky S, et al: Obesity: Epidemiology, etiology, and prevention. In Ross AC, et al, editors: *Modern nutrition in health and disease*, ed 11, Philadelphia, 2014, Lippincott Williams & Wilkins.

Ran AS, Zhou W: Lower breastfeeding rates persist among the Special Supplemental Nutrition Program for Women, Infants, and Children participants, 1978-2003, *Pediatrics* 117:1136–1146, 2006.

Smith C: The effect of wartime starvation in Holland upon pregnancy and its product, *Am J Obstet Gynecol* 53:599–608, 1947.

Turner RE: Nutrition during pregnancy. In Ross AC, et al, editors: *Modern nutrition in health and disease*, ed 11, Philadelphia, 2014, Lippincott Williams & Wilkins.

U.S. Department of Agriculture (USDA): *Programs and services*, 2014. From: www.fns.usda.gov/programs-and-services. Accessed on January 15, 2014.

Wessling-Resnick M: Iron. In Ross AC, et al, editors: *Modern nutrition in health and disease*, ed 11, Philadelphia, 2014, Lippincott Williams & Wilkins.

CHAPTER 11

Nutrition Assessment and Patient Care

Hippocrates made the link between nutrition and disease almost 3000 years ago, but the modern medical community has just rediscovered its importance. The tremendous advances of medical technology are meaningless if the individual is at nutritional risk or already malnourished.

ⓔ http://evolve.elsevier.com/GRODNER/FOUNDATIONS

LEARNING OBJECTIVES

- Discuss the basic nutrition status assessment performed by nurses.
- Explain how the nutrition status of patients may be compromised by illness and the impact of nutrition status on recovery.
- Describe the role of the registered dietitian (RD/RDN).

- Outline the process and data collection of a comprehensive nutrition assessment conducted by a dietitian.
- Compare and contrast the Nutrition Care Process (NCP) and the Nursing Process.
- Summarize the types of potential interactions between food or nutrients and drugs.

NUTRITION IN DISEASE MANAGEMENT

The first half of this text discusses nutrition as it relates to health and wellness. The second half provides information for nursing professionals on how nutrition pertains to the physiologic stresses of disease states. The Quality and Safety Education (QSEN) nursing competencies (patient-centered care, teamwork and collaboration, quality improvement, safety, and informatics) are basic and serve as the underlying theme.

Role of Genetics on Disease Onset

Knowing how genes affect nutrient metabolism and how nutrients affect gene expression affirms the old adage "We are what we eat." In fact, a woman's prenatal diet affects the long-term health of her children (referred to as the *fetal origins of adult disease*). Placental insufficiency, maternal malnutrition, and intrauterine growth restriction (IUGR) can impair infant growth and eventually lead to hypertension, cardiovascular disease, and type 2 diabetes in adults (Hallows, et al, 2012). Not only is it important to eat well during pregnancy, but we now realize that the life-long adequacy of a person's diet affects the onset and severity of acute and chronic illnesses. Accumulation of errors in the genome and damage to biomolecules cause functional tissue changes, even aging. With

exciting research in field of Nutritional Genomics, more will become known about the role of specific nutrients and genes in health and wellness. A DNA assessment may become part of the routine nursing assessment!

THE NUTRITION TEAM

Doctors are generally responsible for writing admission orders, including diet. However, nurses are often the first health professionals with whom the hospitalized patient comes into contact. By using information gathered during assessments, they are in a good position to identify patients in need of nutrition services. Furthermore, nursing staff often perform basic nutrition screening and provide nutrition education.

On admission, key issues include decreased appetite and unintentional weight loss, which are red flags for nutritional decline. A patient's age, medical history, hydration status, and illness severity are also important to share with the nutrition team. When more in-depth nutrition assessment is needed, care is provided by registered dietitians-nutritionists (RDNs). This text will refer to the "RD" or "RDN" for simplification, but both credentials require the minimum Bachelor of Science degree from an accredited university, 1200 hours of supervised practice (often a dietetic internship), and passing a national examination. Most states also require licensure.

The RD is specially qualified to conduct the Nutrition Care Process (NCP) and serve as a valuable partner with the nursing team. The NCP encompasses detailed nutrition assessments, establishment of a nutrition diagnosis, provision of nutrition therapies, monitoring, and evaluation of outcomes. Nutrition therapy is often needed to treat an illness, injury, or related condition. Dietetic technicians, registered (DTRs) can assist the RD by taking diet histories, collecting information for nutrition screening and assessment, and working directly with patients who are having problems with their meals. A DTR may provide basic nutrition education but should not be asked to counsel patients about complex disease modifications.

Medical nutrition therapy (MNT) is a legal term that applies to patients with prerenal failure and diabetes who receive nutrition treatments under Medicare. To avoid confusion, this text will use the term "nutrition therapy" to discuss the provision of food and nutrients, nutrition education, nutrition counseling, and coordination of care.

NUTRITION RISK AND MALNUTRITION

An important relationship exists between dietary intake and a healthy population. The capacity for recovery from illness or disease depends on good nutrition status. Poor nutrition status delays recovery and decreases quality of life (QoL). It is important, therefore, to determine the current nutrition status of those undergoing medical treatment or cure. A return to wellness is the goal.

Nutrition Risk from Hunger

Many people have inadequate access to food. Hunger and food insecurity are prevalent in both developed and developing countries. More than 2 billion people in the world are micronutrient deficient; 1.5 billion people are overweight or obese; 870 million people have inadequate food energy intake; and 783 million people lack potable drinking water (Nordin, et al, 2013). In the United States, "food deserts" are urban or rural locations where individuals lack access to healthy, affordable food (U.S. Department of Agriculture [USDA], 2013).

Undernutrition and chronic micronutrient deficiencies are a form of "hidden hunger" (Burchi, et al, 2011). In the United Kingdom, for example, malnutrition affects more than 3 million people; 93% of them are living in their own homes (Blaikley, 2012). When they are admitted to hospitals or nursing homes, they are already "at nutritional risk" and may experience poor wound healing, longer lengths of stay, and a decline in overall health. In addition, both frail elderly and sick people may experience loss of appetite, depression, or alterations of taste and smell perception. Nurses and registered dietitians have a responsibility to help patients achieve their optimal nutrition status (Shepherd, 2012). Adequate nutrient intake is the concern, independent of weight status (Nordin, et al, 2013).

Nutrition Risk Assessment

Nutrition risk assessment focuses on the potential to become malnourished because of primary (inadequate intake of nutrients) or secondary (caused by disease or iatrogenic affects) factors. The Academy of Nutrition and Dietetics (Academy) and the American Society for Parenteral and Enteral Nutrition (ASPEN) recommend that a standardized set of diagnostic characteristics be used to identify and document adult malnutrition in routine clinical practice (White, et al, 2012; Mueller, et al, 2011).

Stays in acute care hospitals play havoc with patients' nutritional intake. During hospitalization, patients admitted in good nutrition status encounter psychologic and physiologic factors that put them at nutrition risk. Tests, surgical procedures, interruptions, medications, and illness can all cause a decline in nutrition status. If patients are admitted in compromised nutrition status, as nearly half are, risks are even greater and of more consequence. Moderate to severe nutritional depletion is associated with higher readmission and death rates than low or no nutrition risk (Aziz, et al, 2011).

Nursing personnel can help prevent malnutrition by paying particular attention to inadequate diet orders. Risk is high when patients have had nothing but clear-liquid or full-liquid diets for more than 24 hours, or intravenous feedings that contain only glucose and saline. Those are the times to contact the RD for a more complete evaluation of the patient's nutrition status.

Challenges of the Hospital Setting

Imagine you have been taken to a place where, after answering a multitude of questions about your condition, insurance, financial status, and durable power of attorney (a legal document in which a competent adult authorizes another competent adult to make decisions for him/her in the event of incapacitation), you are whisked off to a sterile-looking room that you must share with a stranger. In this room your clothes are replaced with a thin, flimsy gown that won't close in the back. You answer more questions about your medical history from the nurse who admits you. Once he or she finishes, a resident/intern comes into your room to ask many of the same questions and conduct a physical examination (Figure 11-1).

During a stay in the hospital, your eating habits are open to scrutiny and change. You're away from your own kitchen, and meals are served on a schedule that may or may not coincide with your personal preferences. Depending on your diagnosis, the food is likely to be modified in texture, consistency, nutrients, or energy. While you're in the hospital, different staff routinely enter your room to ask questions, ranging from what you ate yesterday to your elimination habits, to draw blood, and to take you elsewhere in the hospital for tests that may or may not be invasive. Although no harm is intended, little privacy is afforded while you undergo tests and examinations that may provide critical information about your prognosis. During these trying times, food becomes very important, physiologically and psychologically.

FIG 11-1 Patients are interviewed by many members of the health care team.

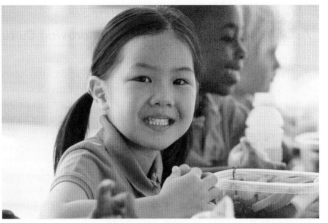

FIG 11-2 Food provides emotional comfort as well as nutrition, especially for children.

Food is one of the few familiar experiences encountered in a hospital setting (see *the Personal Perspectives* box Sharing an Orange).

👤 PERSONAL PERSPECTIVES

Sharing an Orange

Machines were whirling as I entered the cardiac intensive care unit to visit my husband Lenny's grandmother. I didn't know what to expect. Grandma Ethel was the most energetic older adult I ever knew. Eighty-six years old, still running her own gift shop, and always ready to go out with Lenny and me, until she had this heart attack.

Grandma Ethel was sitting upright in a chair with all kinds of wires attached to her body. She was pale but immediately her radiant smile spread across her face. She said, "Come and sit, have lunch with me," as she invited me to share the hospital lunch that was on a tray in front of her. Now I certainly wasn't going to eat any of her lunch, especially hospital food. But I was definitely needed. She wanted the soup, but with the wires and being somewhat weak, couldn't get the lid off the Styrofoam cup. So I came to the rescue. Uncover the lid from the plate of soft chicken and mashed potatoes? Again I was handy. Open the juice container and decaffeinated coffee cup? Who knew I was so competent?

"Michele, here have the orange." The orange was in a bowl surrounded by plastic wrap. I gently suggested she should have it because it was good for her. "No, I'm too full. Take it home … take it home for the boys [my sons; her great-grandsons] and take the brownie too!" I then realized that the real issue was not to feed Grandma Ethel's body, but to let her soul feed us. Her soul needed to nourish us with her gift of a sweet orange and a rich brownie. And we were nourished.

Michele Grodner
Montclair, NJ

Particularly for hospitalized toddlers and adolescents, food can become a battleground because of its emotional connotations (Figure 11-2). The same is true for elderly patients when they receive meals that contain unfamiliar or disliked foods. A temper tantrum is possible—at any age!

Food or an alternative method of nourishment can mean the difference between a good and a poor prognosis. Part of the initial assessment should include questions related to cultural, ethnic, or religious food preferences (see the *Cultural Considerations* box Asking the Right Questions and Improving Cultural Competency).

Effects of Bed Rest on Nutrition

Occasionally, complete bed rest is prescribed as part of patients' medical care. Some patients may be unable to ambulate because of the severity of their illnesses or because they are "hooked up" to a multitude of necessary life-saving equipment at bedside. Although it is often necessary or unavoidable, complete immobilization because of bed rest can have injurious effects on a patient's body. Inactivity leads to measurable changes in muscle and bone, reduces exercise capacity, impairs the immune system, and decreases the sensitivity to insulin (Loenneke, et al, 2012). Low-intensity and resistance exercises can be quite beneficial (Loenneke, et al, 2012).

Skin integrity may be compromised after just 24 hours of immobilization, and after 3 days of lying supine in bed, muscle tone, bone calcium, plasma volume, and gastric secretions diminish. In addition, glucose intolerance and shifts in body fluids and electrolytes may also occur. Nursing personnel can prevent or delay some injurious effects by frequently turning and repositioning patients. Good skin care is essential.

Malnutrition

Nearly 40% of patients admitted to hospitals are malnourished upon admission or demonstrate malnutrition during their hospitalization (Barker, et al, 2011; Jensen, et al, 2010). Patients may experience physiologic stress from injury or illness, which increases nutritional demands. Nutrition needs may be further compromised because of periodic fasting needed before laboratory testing or diagnostic procedures. Highly restricted, nutritionally inadequate diets, meals missed because of procedures and tests, and unmonitored dietary intakes can lead to malnutrition; see Chapter 12 for details on managing diet orders.

🌐 CULTURAL CONSIDERATIONS

Asking the Right Questions and Improving Cultural Competency

Health care professionals serve patients from a variety of diverse backgrounds in hospitals, nursing homes, the community, and sometimes patients' homes. When providing care, nurses must be sensitive to the cultural needs and expectations of their patients and family members. To be culturally competent, nurses need to understand the knowledge and attitudes of each cultural group in relation to food, especially those with symbolic or religious connotations.

It is impossible to know all of the specific cultural food practices of diverse groups around the world, so asking the right questions is important. Andrews and Boyle's (2002) Cultural Nutritional Assessment Guide, presented here in slightly modified form, helps obtain information that forms an important part of a patient's health history. Information obtained from the patient or family member can improve the patient's satisfaction, the nurse's cultural competency, and the patient's nutrition outcome.

Cultural Nursing Assessment Guide: Nutrition

- What nutritional factors are influenced by the client's cultural background? What is the meaning of food and eating to the client?
- With whom does the client usually eat? What types of foods are eaten? What is the usual timing and sequencing of meals?

- What does the client define as food? What does the client believe comprises a "healthy" versus an "unhealthy" diet?
- Who shops for food? Where are groceries purchased (e.g., special markets or ethnic grocery stores)? Who prepares the client's meals?
- How are foods prepared at home—preparation methods, cooking oils used, length of time foods are cooked (especially vegetables), amount and type of seasonings added to various foods during preparation?
- Has the client chosen a particular practice such as vegetarianism or abstinence from alcohol or fermented beverages?
- Describe how the client's religious beliefs and practices influence the type, amount, preparation, or delineation of acceptable food combinations (e.g., kosher diets). Does the client fast or abstain from certain foods at regular intervals, on specific days of the week, or on certain dates determined by the religious calendar?
- If the client's religion mandates or encourages fasting, what does the term *fast* mean (e.g., refraining from certain types or quantities of foods, eating only during certain times of the day)? For what length of time is the client expected to fast?
- During fasting, does the client refrain from liquids/beverages? Does the religion allow exemption from fasting during illness? If so, does the client believe that an exemption applies to him or her?

Adapted from Andrews M, Boyle J: *Transcultural concepts in nursing care,* ed 4, Philadelphia, 2002, Lippincott Williams & Wilkins.

Adult forms of malnutrition have been defined as "starvation-related malnutrition" when there is chronic starvation without inflammation, "chronic disease-related malnutrition" when inflammation is chronic and of mild to moderate degree, and "acute disease or injury-related malnutrition" when inflammation is acute and of severe degree (Jensen, et al, 2010). The indicators are used to assess individuals. Examples include starvation-related malnutrition in a patient with anorexia nervosa, chronic malnutrition in a patient with cancer, or acute disease-related malnutrition for the febrile patient with burns.

NUTRITION CARE PROCESS

Most patients entering the health care system have special nutrition needs, depending on their injury or illness. Patients at nutrition risk need to be identified so high-quality nutrition care can be provided. Poor nutrition status may lead to complications such as increased morbidity and mortality, longer lengths of stay, and higher cost of care (The Writing Group, 2008).

For nutrition intervention to be efficacious and successful, a systematic, logical strategy is necessary. The Nutrition Care Process was designed to serve this purpose (Box 11-1).

Screening

The Joint Commission (TJC) requires that all patients admitted to a hospital be screened for nutritional concerns within 48 hours of admission (TJC, 2012). Nutrition screening identifies characteristics known to be associated with nutrition problems, such as unintended weight loss (Lee and Nieman, 2010). It is not possible, or necessary, to complete a full nutrition assessment on every patient. It is necessary, however, to have a system in place to quickly identify patients at risk for nutrition problems such as malnutrition (TJC, 2012; Lee and Nieman, 2010). In long-term care facilities, screening and assessments must be completed on all residents within 14 days of admission.

Nutrition screening can be executed by nurses, RDs, DTRs, dietary managers, physicians, or other trained personnel. Whether or not the RDs directly perform the nutrition screening, they are responsible for the identification of suitable screening parameters. The nutrition screening process facilitates completion of early intervention goals, includes collection and interpretation of relevant data, helps determine the need for a nutrition assessment, is cost effective, and may be completed in any setting.

A referral to an RD is necessary when a patient shows signs of nutrition risk, especially unintended weight loss or poor appetite. The RD is responsible for conducting the nutrition assessment, selecting relevant nutrition diagnoses, and providing appropriate nutrition care.

Nutrition Assessment

The first step of the NCP is a comprehensive nutritional assessment conducted by the RD. Data are collected from

BOX 11-1   Academy of Nutrition and Dietetics: Nutrition Care Process

Definition of Nutrition Care Process (NCP)

Providing nutrition care starts when a patient is recognized as being at nutritional risk and requiring additional support to attain or maintain positive nutritional status. The NCP is defined "as a systematic problem-solving method that dietetics professionals use to critically think and make decisions to address nutrition-related problems and provide safe and effective quality nutrition care." It is composed of the following four separate but interrelated and associated steps:

1. Nutrition assessment
2. Nutrition diagnosis
3. Nutrition intervention
4. Nutrition monitoring and evaluation

Each stage builds upon the preceding one, but the process is not necessarily linear. Figure 11-3 provides a visual illustration of the model.

Step 1: Nutrition Assessment

Techniques such as those outlined previously in the chapter are used to systematically obtain information necessary to determine or reassess whether a nutrition problem (or diagnosis) exists. If so, the problem is diagnosed using the PES (problem, etiology, signs/symptoms) statement described in Step 2.

Step 2: Nutrition Diagnosis

Before nutrition intervention can take place, the nutrition problem(s) must be identified. This identification is accomplished with the nutrition diagnosis. Standardized language has been developed to make the nutrition diagnosis clear to other nutrition and health care professionals. When the nutrition problem has been identified, it is labeled with a specific, standardized diagnostic term. The nutrition diagnosis statement, or PES statement, is organized in three distinct parts: the problem (P), etiology of the problem (E), and signs and symptoms associated with the problem (S). Typically, nutrition diagnoses fall into one of three categories or domains: intake, clinical, and behavioral-environmental.

Here is an example of how a nutrition diagnosis is written:

"Disordered eating pattern related to harmful belief about food and nutrition as evidenced by reported use of laxatives

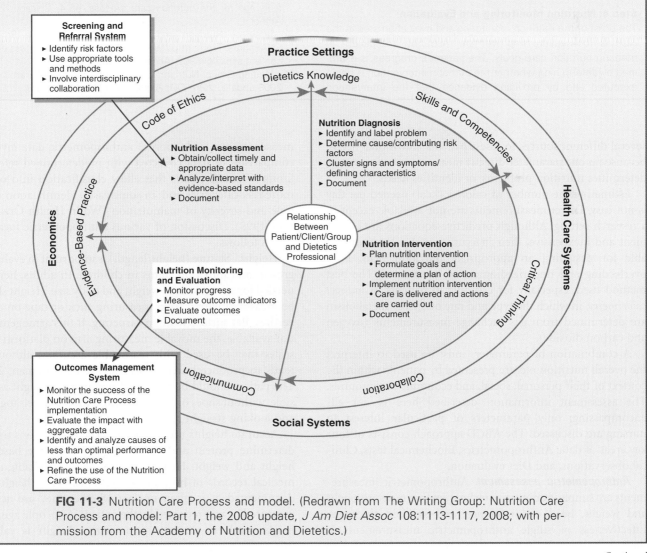

FIG 11-3 Nutrition Care Process and model. (Redrawn from The Writing Group: Nutrition Care Process and model: Part 1, the 2008 update, *J Am Diet Assoc* 108:1113-1117, 2008; with permission from the Academy of Nutrition and Dietetics.)

Continued

after meals and statements that calories are not absorbed when laxatives are used."

Step 3: Nutrition Intervention

Intervention begins once the nutritional diagnosis is identified. It is generally aimed at the etiology (E) of the nutrition diagnosis and is directed at reducing or eradicating the effects of the signs and symptoms (S). Nutrition interventions are intended to modify a nutrition-related problem and comprise two interconnected components: planning and implementation. Nutrition diagnoses are prioritized in the planning component, whereby implementation is the "action phase." The plan is communicated and carried out, data continue to be collected, and the nutrition intervention is revised as necessary. Four categories or domains of nutrition intervention have been identified:

- Food and/or nutrient delivery
- Nutrition education
- Nutrition counseling
- Coordination of care

Step 4: Nutrition Monitoring and Evaluation

The point of the nutrition monitoring and evaluation step in the NCP is to measure improvement made by the patient in meeting nutrition care goals. The patient's progress is examined by determining whether the nutrition intervention is being executed and by providing evidence that the intervention

is or is not altering the patients' nutrition status. Nutrition monitoring and evaluation terms are organized into four categories or domains:

- Food/nutrition-related history
- Biochemical data, medical tests, and procedures
- Anthropometric measurements
- Nutrition-focused physical findings

Summary

The Nutrition Care Process allows for continuous monitoring and evaluation of the patient. As the condition of the patient changes, plans or interventions change, as do diagnoses and/or interventions. If the patient shows no response to interventions, new interventions can be developed. Additionally, any or all nutrition interventions should be planned along with patients and/or their caregivers or significant others.

References

Academy of Nutrition and Dietetics: *International dietetics and nutrition terminology (IDNT) reference manual: Standardized language for the nutrition care process*, ed 4, Chicago, 2012, Author.

Academy of Nutrition and Dietetics: Nutrition Care Process SNAPshots. From: http://www.eatright.org/HealthProfessionals/content.aspx?id=5902. Accessed August 8, 2013.

The Writing Group: Nutrition Care Process and model: Part 1: The 2008 update, *J Am Diet Assoc* 108:1113–1117, 2008.

several different sources to assess patients' nutritional needs, because no one parameter directly measures nutrition status, determines nutrition problems, or identifies needs.

Estimating the number of calories (kcal) needed per day is not easy. Direct measurements are not available except in a research setting. Although predictive equations are convenient and inexpensive, their inaccuracy makes them unreliable for designing an appropriate nutrition plan. Both overfeeding and underfeeding are to be avoided. The best method used, especially for critically ill patients, is *indirect calorimetry,* in which the type and rate of energy metabolism are determined from gas exchange measurements (oxygen and carbon dioxide).

A combination of parameters must be used to interpret the overall nutrition picture presented by patients within the context of their personal, social, and economic backgrounds. The assessment information described here is not all-encompassing; only parameters of particular interest to nursing are discussed. The ABCD approach consists of four key areas of data: **A**nthropometrics, **B**iochemical tests, **C**linical observations, and **D**iet evaluation.

Anthropometric assessment. Anthropometric measurements are simple, noninvasive techniques that measure height and weight, head circumference, and skinfold thickness. Effectiveness of single anthropometric measurements is limited, but certain serial measurements can be useful to assess body composition changes or growth over time. Standardized techniques must be used to obtain valid and reliable

measurements. Evaluation of anthropometric data involve a comparison of data collected with predetermined reference limits or cutoff points that allow classification into one or more risk categories and, in some cases, identification of the type and severity of malnutrition (World Health Organization, 1995). Discussion of various anthropometric measurements follows.

Height. Stature (height/length) is important in evaluating growth and nutrition status in children. In adults, height is needed for assessment of weight and body size. Height should be measured with a fixed measuring stick or tape on a true vertical, flat surface with no carpeting. If this arrangement is not available, the movable measuring arm on platform clinic scales may be used with reasonable accuracy, although it tends to produce lower measures (Lee and Nieman, 2010). The patient should be measured standing as straight as possible, without shoes or head coverings, with the heels together, and looking straight ahead (Box 11-2).

Accurate heights are important. The calculations used to determine protein and energy requirements are based on height and weight. Heights are not always available in the medical records of hospitalized patients. When heights are documented, it is often unclear whether they are actually measured or just reported by the patient. As people age, their height tends to decline, so a current height is valuable information.

Asking patients about their height does not usually produce accurate information. On average when asked,

BOX 11-2   Measuring Height

1. Have patient stand erect with weight equally distributed on both feet.
   a. If the legs are of unequal length, place boards under the short limb to make the pelvis level.
   b. When possible, make sure the head, shoulder blades, buttocks, and heels all touch a vertical surface.
   c. Instruct patient to let arms hang free at the sides with palms facing the thighs.
2. Have patient look straight ahead (so the line of vision is perpendicular to the body), take a deep breath, and hold that position while the horizontal headboard is brought down firmly on top of the head. (Measurer's eyes should be level with the headboard to read the measurement.)
3. Read the measurement to the nearest 0.1 cm or ⅛ inch.

From Lee RD, Nieman DC: *Nutritional assessment,* ed 5, New York, 2010, McGraw-Hill.

FIG 11-4 A recumbent length board used to take height measurements horizontally. (From Mahan LK, Escott-Stump S, Raymond JL: *Krause's food & nutrition therapy,* ed 13, St. Louis, 2012, Elsevier.)

people report being slightly taller than they actually are. Men overstate height more often than women, and the extent of overstating height increases as people age (Lee and Nieman, 2010). If the height of a patient recorded in the medical record is not a measured height, it should be documented as a stated height.

When measuring an infant or child (younger than 2 to 3 years) who cannot stand or another patient unable to stand erect without assistance, a recumbent measure can be taken while the subject is lying down or reclining. A recumbent length table can be used. A recumbent length table or board has a fixed headboard, a movable footboard, and a permanent measuring scale along the side (Figure 11-4). To measure a patient, he or she should be placed supine on the board or table with shoulders and legs flat against the measuring board (table) and arms at the sides. The head should firmly touch the headboard while the line of vision is perpendicular to the board or table. Soles of the feet should be vertical, and the footboard should touch the bottoms of the feet so that the soft tissue is compressed. Length can be recorded from the measure at the footboard. Two people are often needed to take an accurate measurement (Merrill and Richardson, 2009).

When the patient is comatose, critically ill, or unable to be moved for other reasons, taking a recumbent bed height may

BOX 11-3   Measuring Recumbent Bed Height

1. Remove pillows and make the bed level.
2. Straighten the patient out in the bed but with the feet flexed.
3. With a clipboard or ruler, extend perpendicular lines from the top of the head and the bottom of the feet out to the side of the bed.
4. Mark the two positions on the bed sheet, and measure the distance between them to the nearest 1/2 inch.

Data from Gray D: Accuracy of recumbent height measurement, *JPEN J Parenter Enteral Nutr* 9:712-715, 1985.

FIG 11-5 If a patient is nonambulatory, a bed scale can be used to measure patient weight.

be possible (Box 11-3). Note that in comparison with standing height, bed height is significantly greater by at least 2% (Gray, 1985). A more accurate measurement for patients who cannot stand is *knee height,* which is minimally affected by aging but requires the use of special calipers. Other possible measurements are *forearm length* (useful for patients with contractures) and *demi-span* (useful for patients with lower limb dysfunction); details on measuring heights in bedridden patients can be found at the following website: http://www.rxkinetics.com/height_estimate.html.

Weight. When accurately measured, body weight is a simple, gross estimate of body composition. In fact, body weight is one of the most important measurements in assessing nutrition status and is used to predict energy expenditure (Blackburn and Thornton, 1977). Beam scales with movable but nondetachable weights or accurate electronic scales are recommended to obtain accurate results. Spring scales are not recommended. If the patient is not ambulatory, wheelchair or bed scales should be used (Figure 11-5).

Scales should be checked for accuracy periodically and recalibrated when necessary. Like heights, actual measured

TABLE 11-1 Weight Change as an Indicator of Nutrition Status

% WEIGHT CHANGE	TIME	NUTRITION STATUS
1-2	1 week	Moderate weight loss
>2	1 week	Severe weight loss
5	1 month	Moderate weight loss
>5	1 month	Severe weight loss

weights are more accurate than patients' estimated weights because men slightly over-report their weights and women report slightly lower weights (Merrill and Richardson, 2009).

For accurate weights, the patients should be clothed in underwear or a hospital gown. Weight should be measured at the same time of day and after voiding. The patient should stand still with the weight evenly distributed on both feet while weight is recorded to the nearest 0.1 kg, or 0.25 pound (Lee and Nieman, 2010).

As a nutrition screening tool, weights can be used to detect changes that may represent or suggest serious health problems. Magnitude and direction of weight change are more meaningful when dealing with sick or debilitated patients than standardized desirable weight references (see Table 11-1). Percent weight change is a useful nutrition index and may be computed as follows:

$$\% \text{ Weight change} = (\text{Usual weight} - \text{Actual weight}) \div \text{Usual weight} \times 100$$

Example 11-1

Mrs. Welch is admitted to your unit. Her weight on admission is 120 pounds. During the admissions interview, she indicates that 3 months ago she weighed 135 pounds. Her percent weight change from usual weight is calculated with the formula:

$$\% \text{ Weight change from admission weight} = (\text{Usual weight} - \text{Actual weight}) \div \text{Admission weight} \times 100$$

as follows:

$$(135 - 120) \div 135 \times 100 = 15 \div 135 \times 100$$
$$= 0.11 \times 100, \text{ or } 11\% \text{ Weight change}$$

Mrs. Welch's (actual) weight is 11% less than her usual weight.

Example 11-2

Mr. Tucker is a patient in the long-term care facility where you work. When he was admitted more than a year ago, he weighed 180 pounds. He has weighed 170 pounds for the past 6 months, but today you weigh Mr. Tucker and he weighs 165 pounds. His percent weight change from admission weight is calculated as follows:

$$(170 - 165) \div 180 \times 100 = 5 \div 180 \times 100 = 0.0278 \times 100$$
$$= 2.78\%, \text{ or } 3\% \text{ Weight change}$$

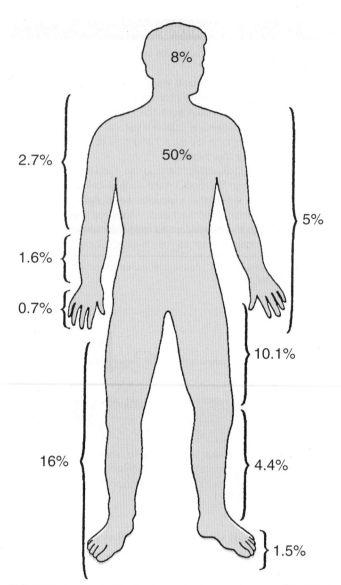

FIG 11-6 Approximate body weight percentages. (Modified from Brunnstrom S: *Clinical kinesiology,* Philadelphia, 1962, FA Davis.)

Mr. Tucker's (actual) weight is 3% less than his admission weight. His % weight change since a nutrition intervention is as follows:

$$(\text{Usual weight} - \text{Actual weight}) \div \text{Preintervention weight} \times 100$$

Example 11-3

Mrs. Bussard was started on a feeding tube because her weight has decreased from her usual weight of 130 pounds to 115 pounds. She has been on the feeding tube for 1 week, and when you weigh her today, she weighs 122 pounds. Her percent weight change since nutrition intervention is calculated as follows:

$$(130 - 122) \div 115 \times 100 = 8 \div 115 \times 100 = 0.067 \times 100$$
$$= 6.96\%, \text{ or } 7\% \text{ Weight change}$$

Mrs. Bussard's weight has increased 7% since the tube feedings were initiated.

TABLE 11-2 Classifications of Overweight And Obesity by Body Mass Index (BMI)

	BMI (kg/m²)
Underweight	<18.5
Normal	18.5-24.9
Overweight	25.0-29.9
Obesity	≥30

Special care should be taken to identify patients with ascites, edema, or dehydration. Their weight changes may be more reflections of fluid shifts than actual changes in body composition. A gain of more than 1 pound in a day's time may signify excess fluid. It is also important to examine any unplanned weight loss the patient might experience; see Table 11-2. Reported or measured percent weight losses of these magnitudes could be cause for alarm.

For older adult patients who cannot be weighed because of the severity of their medical condition, or if bed or chair scales are not available, Chumlea et al (1988) developed gender-specific equations to predict body weight in people 60 to 90 years of age. The estimated weights are based on recumbent measures of arm circumference (AC), calf circumference (CC), subscapular skinfold (SSF), and knee height (KH).

The equation for women is as follows:

$$Weight (cm) = [0.98 \times AC (in\ cm)] + [1.27 \times CC (in\ cm)] \\ + [0.4 \times SSF (in\ mm)] + [0.87 \times \times KH (in\ cm)] \\ 62.35$$

The equation for men is as follows:

$$Weight (cm) = [1.73 \times AC (in\ cm)] + [0.98 \times CC (in\ cm)] \\ + [0.37 \times SSF (in\ mm)] + [1.16 \times KH (in\ cm)] \\ 81.69$$

Another challenge in obtaining weights occurs in patients who have missing body parts because of accidents or amputation. Figure 11-6 shows the approximate percentages of body weight contributed by individual body segments; using this information allows a patient's desirable weight to be calculated.

Body mass index. Body mass index (BMI) is a ratio of weight to height and has been associated with overall mortality and nutrition risk (Lefton and Malone, 2009). BMI does not determine body composition (lean body mass or adipose tissue) but is a dependable gauge of total body fat, which is interrelated with risk of disease (National Heart, Lung, and Blood Institute [NHLBI], 2013). Although BMI measurements are valid for men and women, they do have limits (Lefton and Malone, 2009; NHLBI, 2013):

- BMI has not been validated in acutely ill patients.
- BMI may underestimate body fat in the elderly and others who have lost muscle mass.
- BMI may overestimate body fat in individuals who have a muscular build.

You can determine BMI by dividing weight in kilograms by height in squared meters—[BMI = Weight (kg) ÷ Height (m)²]—using the following three steps:
1. Divide weight in pounds by 2.2 to convert it into kilograms.
2. Multiply height in inches by 2.54, and divide the result by 100 to convert height to meters; then multiply height in meters by itself (that is, square it).
3. Divide weight in kilograms (result of step 1) by the square of height in meters (result of step 2). The result is BMI.

The desired BMI range for healthy adults is 18.5 to 24.9 kg/m², which reflects a healthy weight for height; see Table 11-2. Although at low risk for health problems, people with BMI values between 25 and 29.9 kg/m² are approximately 20% above desirable levels. A patient with a BMI less than 18.5 kg/m² is classified as underweight; this status is associated with risk factors such as respiratory disease, tuberculosis, digestive disease, and some cancers (NHLBI, 1998).

Waist measurements. Waist circumference (WC) is an economical and straightforward measure that can be used to assess abdominal (visceral) fat content. BMI and waist circumference can be used classify overweight/obesity (Moore, 2009). A circumference greater than 40 inches in men and 35 inches in women indicates risk for disease. It should be noted that visceral adiposity may vary among racial and ethnic groups (Moore, 2009).

Waist-to-hip ratio (WHR) is sometimes used for patients with human immunodeficiency virus–acquired immunodeficiency syndrome (HIV-AIDS). For WHR, measure waist circumference and divide by hip circumference. A third calculation, Waist-to-height ratio (WHtR), has been shown to have greater predictive capacity than either BMI or WC for diabetes, hypertension, cardiovascular risks and outcomes in both men and women (Ashwell, et al, 2012). For WHtR, measure waist circumference and divide by height (Browning, et al, 2010). A simple message here is to keep waist circumference to less than half of height (<0.5).

Nutrition-Focused Physical Examination and Functional Assessments

A nutrition-focused physical examination includes but is not limited to fluid assessment, functional status, wound status, and clinical signs of malnutrition, overnutrition, and/or nutrient deficiencies (Academy of Nutrition and Dietetics [ADA], 2013). Involuntary weight loss should be addressed, as previously noted; note the pathway shown in Figure 11-7.

Poor muscle quality is often a predictor of mortality, especially in the elderly. Manual muscle testing (MMT) and hand-grip strength (HGS) dynamometry assessments have been used to evaluate muscle weakness in patients. Further study is needed to verify whether these tests are valid as part of a nutrition screening or assessment.

Biochemical assessment. Many routine blood and urine laboratory test results recorded in patient charts are useful for objective assessment of nutrition status. However, care should be taken in interpreting test results for a number of reasons. First, no single test is available for evaluating short-term

Nutrition411 *Interdisciplinary Nutrition Care Plan*

Involuntary Weight Loss

Patient Name: _____ Pt #:_____ Initiated by:_____ Date:_____

Goals (check any/all):

❏ Prevent nutritional decline/adverse events in _____ (goal time)

❏ Encourage improvement as evidenced by: wt gain/increased strength in _____ (goal time)

❏ Correct causes of involuntary weight loss where possible in _____ (goal time)

Screening
Nutrition Screen indicates Involuntary Weight Loss
Signed_____date_____

Assess Acuity (Check any/all)
❏ Poor oral intake
❏ Complex diet order
❏ BMI < 20 (high risk)
❏ Wt loss: > 3 lbs/wk or > 5%/mo or > 10%/6 mo
❏ Nausea / diarrhea / vomiting
❏ Infection (eg, pneumonia, UTI, URI)
❏ Pressure ulcers, wounds
❏ Poor strength
Signed_____date_____

Moderate Risk Interventions
(Check any/all)
❏ "Food Record" provided and reviewed
❏ RD chart consult
❏ Weight monitoring q:_____
❏ BID/TID supplements
❏ Other:_____
   See notes for documentation

Signed_____date_____

Key
❏ **Recommended intervention for best practice:**
   • Patient Education Materials provided and assessed for comprehension
❏ **Optional intervention:**
   • Nutrition support initiated (oral/enteral)
   • Referrals
   • Monitoring

High Risk Interventions (Check any/all)
❏ "Food Record" provided and reviewed
Obtain Dr. orders as needed:
   ❏ Weight monitoring q:_____
   ❏ RD referral for home visits
   ❏ BID/TID supplements
❏ Other:_____
   See notes for documentation

Signed_____date_____

Assess Response (Check any/all)
❏ Further wt loss
❏ Wt gain < goal
❏ New onset infection
❏ Declining strength
❏ Other:_____
See notes for documentation
Signed_____date_____

Outcomes Achieved
Document improved:
❏ Strength
❏ Weight
❏ Other:_____
❏ Repeat nutrition screen in _____ days.
See notes for documentation
Goals met
Signed_____date_____

Assess Response (Check any/all)
❏ Further wt loss
❏ Wt gain < goal
❏ New onset infection
❏ Declining strength
❏ Other:_____
See notes for documentation
Signed_____date_____

Outcomes Achieved
Document improved:
❏ Strength
❏ Weight
❏ Other:_____
❏ Repeat nutrition screen in _____ days.
See notes for documentation
Goals met
Signed_____date_____

Outcome Not Achieved
Reassess acuity/evaluate need for EN/PN (refer to Tube Feeding Nutrition Care Plan)
Document on variance reporting form

Review Date 12/12 • G-1436

FIG 11-7 Interdisciplinary care plan for involuntary weight loss. (From www.nutrition411.com/ clinical-nutrition/care-algorithms/item/648-interdisciplinary-nutrition-care-plan-involuntary -weight-loss/)

response to nutrition therapy. Laboratory values should be used in conjunction with anthropometric data, clinical data, and results of dietary intake assessments. Second, some tests may be inappropriate for certain patients; for example, serum albumin might not be useful in the evaluation of protein status in patients with liver failure because this test assumes normal liver function. Third, laboratory tests conducted serially will give more accurate information than a single test.

Although serial measures can be obtained in long-term care settings, patients in acute care facilities are rarely hospitalized long enough for serial measures to be obtained. Therefore, it might be more appropriate to compare test results with known standards. Biochemical parameters can be used to evaluate visceral proteins and immune function, which may reflect nutrition status.

Visceral proteins are proteins found in internal organs and blood rather than those found in muscle. Visceral protein status is estimated through tests of serum albumin and prealbumin. Interpretation of albumin values must be cautious, however, because inflammation, infection, hydration, and illness affect these values; low values do not necessarily indicate poor dietary intake.

Normal serum albumin values are within 3.5 to 5 g/dL. For nutritional analysis, values between 2.8 and 3.5 g/dL indicate compromised protein status; values less than 2.4 g/dL may precede pressure ulcer development. This measurement is most useful when used to monitor long-term nutrition changes because the half-life of albumin is 14-20 days. In addition, if patients are experiencing dehydration or have received infusions of albumin, fresh frozen plasma, or whole-blood serum albumin, serum levels may appear normal. Abnormally low values may be caused by infection, burns, trauma, congestive heart failure, fluid overload, chronically low protein intake, and severe hepatic insufficiency (Heimburger and Ard, 2006).

Prealbumin (transthyretin) also can provide a measure of visceral protein status assessment. Normal values range from 16 to 40 mg/dL. This test is useful in monitoring short-term changes in visceral protein status because of its short half-life, 2 days. Compromised protein status is indicated when levels are between 10 and 15 g/dL. Factors that result in abnormally low levels of prealbumin include chronic kidney disease, surgical trauma, stress, inflammation, infection, and liver dysfunction (Heimburger and Ard, 2006).

Serum hemoglobin measurement is another useful test. This oxygen-carrying protein molecule is especially important for children; iron-deficiency anemia impacts their health, their cognition, and subsequently their educational achievement (Best, et al, 2010). In adults, iron-deficiency anemia leads to fatigue, pale skin, weakness, and cold extremities. Indeed, many biochemical assessments provide useful information to determine the effects of nutrition or of medical conditions on the health status of patients. Table 11-3 provides more content.

Immune function may be evaluated nutritionally, on the basis of vitamin D levels. Vitamin D affects hundreds of genes in the body (Christakos, et al, 2013; NIH, 2013). Vitamin D receptors (VDRs) have been found in bone, skin, placenta, and cancer cells. Adequate serum levels may help with immunity, pregnancy, and aging as well as may prevent autoimmune diseases, cancer, obesity, cardiovascular and respiratory disorders, erythropoiesis, diabetes, and muscle dysfunction (Christakos, et al, 2013; National Institutes of Health [NIH], 2013).

Vitamin D is produced by the body when sunlight strikes the skin; then two metabolic steps are required in the liver and the kidney to convert to the active form, vitamin D_3 (calcitriol). Dietary sources of this vitamin are few, and the rate of conversion to the active form is lower with aging. Thus, individuals who avoid the sun, have darker skin, are older, consume no vitamin D–rich foods, or habitually use sunscreens with high sun-protective factors may not acquire sufficient amounts. Serum vitamin D levels should be 50 to 125 nmol/L; a level between 30 and 50 nmol/L is mildly inadequate, and levels below 30 nmol/L are detrimental for bone and health.

Clinical assessment. Clinical assessment incorporates data from several sources: medical history, social history, and physical examination. Environmental, social or family, and past and present medical factors can affect nutrition status. This information can be found by reviewing the patient's medical record or through direct interview. Many physical signs and symptoms associated with malnutrition are also sought as an integral part of assessing nutrition status.

Features associated with nutrition deficiency may be identified through histories and clinical categories. Historical data includes alcohol abuse, poverty, avoidance of specific food groups (e.g., fruits or vegetables), weight loss, drug use (or abuse), family history of inborn errors, and cigarette smoking (Heimburger and Ard, 2006). Clinical features are recent surgery or wounds, blood loss, skin and hair changes, and many other indicators. Findings may be organized according to symptoms of the eyes, face, skin, muscles, tongue, and central nervous system; see Table 11-4. Although these signs are typically taught thoroughly to dietitians, nurses may overlook them. For example, in a patient with spoon-shaped nails, an assessment for iron-deficiency anemia may be an appropriate request for the physician to consider.

Dietary intake assessment. There are several methods for collecting information regarding actual and habitual dietary intake. Most commonly, data are collected using dietary recall methods (historical/retrospective) or documented food records (current/prospective). Each method has its pros and cons, so it is important to choose a method suitable for the type of information needed. These data provide information regarding intake of calories (kcal), protein, carbohydrate, fat, vitamins, minerals, and fluid. Results can be calculated manually with food composition tables or analyzed by computer software. More than 100 computer programs are available to analyze dietary intake.

24-Hour diet recall. In 24-hour diet recall, the patient is asked by a trained interviewer to report all foods and beverages consumed during the past 24 hours. Detailed descriptions of all foods, beverages, cooking methods, brand names, condiments, and supplements, along with portion sizes in common household measures, are included. Food models,

TABLE 11-3 Serum Biochemical Parameters*

SERUM ANALYTE NORMAL VALUE/RANGE)	FUNCTION	COMMENTS

Albumin:
  Normal: 3.5-5.0 g/dL
  Depletion:
    Mild: 3.0-3.4 g/dL
    Moderate: 2.4-2.9 g/dL
    Severe: <2.4 g/dL
  Half-life ~ 14-20 days
	Maintains plasma oncotic pressure; carrier for small molecules	Not sensitive or specific for acute protein malnutrition or response to nutrition therapy; affected by hydration status, disease state, clinical condition
		Often low because of inflammation
		Can be used as prognostic indicator of morbidity, mortality, and severity of illness

Prealbumin (transthyretin, thyroxin-binding prealbumin):
  Normal: 16-40 mg/dL
  Depletion:
    Mild: 10-15 mg/dL
    Moderate: 5-9 mg/dL
    Severe: <5 mg/dL
  Half-life ~ 2-3 days
	Carrier protein for thyroxin
	Combined with retinol-binding protein, transports vitamin A
		Influenced less than albumin by intravascular fluid volume
		Not affected as early or as significantly with liver disease (compared with albumin)
		More likely to be a reflection of recent dietary intake than an accurate indicator of nutrition status

Hemoglobin:
  Normal:
    Males: 13.8-17.2 g/dL
    Females: 12.1-15.1 g/dL
  Depletion:
    Males: <13.5 g/dL
    Females: <12 g/dL
  In general:
    Mild anemia = 10-12 g/dL
    Moderate anemia = 8-10 g/dL
    Severe anemia = <8 g/dL
	Carries oxygen to cells; gives blood cells red color	Hemoglobin estimation is a useful index of the overall state of nutrition; in addition to anemia, it also suggests protein and trace element status
		High levels may be indicative of dehydration but not necessarily a high dietary iron intake
		The hemoglobin finding interpretation must be made in concert with that of other values before iron-deficiency anemia can be diagnosed
		Low serum levels may occur from blood loss, hidden gastrointestinal bleeding, or absorption problems (celiac disease, inflammatory bowel disease, etc.)
		Patients may exhibit shortness of breath, pale skin and gums, fast heartbeat, and extreme fatigue

Glucose (70-99 mg/dL [fasting])	Used for monitoring diabetes mellitus (DM) and other conditions such as hypoglycemia and ketoacidosis	Fasting glucose > 125 mg/dL indicates DM (oral glucose tolerance tests are not needed for diagnosis); fasting glucose > 100 mg/dL is indicator of insulin resistance

Creatinine
  (Males: 0.6-1.2 mg/dL; 53-106 μmol/L
  Females: 0.5-1.1 mg/dL; 44-97 μmol/L)
	Muscle breakdown molecule	Increased in renal disease and decreased in malnutrition (i.e., blood urea nitrogen/creatinine ratio >15:1)

Blood urea nitrogen (BUN) (5-20 mg urea nitrogen/dL; 1.8-7 mmol/L)	Protein in the bloodstream	Increased in renal disease and excessive protein catabolism Decreased in liver failure, negative nitrogen balance, and pregnancy
Total bilirubin (0.3-1.0 mg/dL; 5.1-17.0 μmol/L)	Important value in liver disorders	Increased in gallstones, biliary duct diseases, hepatic immaturity

Serum electrolytes:
  Na^+ (135-145 mEq/L)†
  K^+ (3.6-5 mEq/L)†
  Cl^{2-} (101-111 mEq/L)†
	Used to monitor most patients, especially those with cardiac, pulmonary, renal, or liver problems	Sodium levels are altered by hydration status
		Hypokalemia is seen in diarrhea, vomiting, and licorice ingestion, and with diuretics and some other drugs
		Hyperkalemia in renal diseases, crush injuries, and infection
		Chloride levels may be low with prolonged episodes of vomiting

Total calcium (8.5-10.5 mg/dL)	Transported bound to albumin; level may be altered by albumin level Important in bone and blood health	Hypercalcemia associated with endocrine disorders, malignancy, and hypervitaminosis D Hypocalcemia associated with vitamin D deficiency and inadequate hepatic or renal activation of vitamin D, hypoparathyroidism, magnesium deficiency, renal failure, and nephrotic syndrome

TABLE 11-3 Serum Biochemical Parameters—cont'd

SERUM ANALYTE NORMAL VALUE/RANGE)	FUNCTION	COMMENTS
Phosphorous (phosphate) (3-4.5 mg/dL)	Important part of energy metabolism (forms adenosine triphosphate molecules)	Hyperphosphatemia associated with hypoparathyroidism and decreased intake Hypophosphatemia associated with hyperparathyroidism, chronic antacid ingestion, and renal failure
Total cholesterol (<200 mg/dL)	Cholesterol is an important precursor of steroid hormones and vitamin D	Decreased in patients with some forms of malnutrition, liver diseases, and hyperthyroidism
Triglycerides (40-160 mg/dL)	Levels vary by age and sex	Increased in patients with glucose intolerance and in some alcoholics

*Biochemical assessment for nutrition starts from a general overview but will then be targeted according to medical diagnosis. Reference ranges may vary slightly among laboratories.

†mEq/L = 1 mmol/L.

Adapted from Lab Tests on Line. Accessed from http://labtestsonline.org/map/sindex/; Lee RD, Nieman DC: *Nutritional assessment*, ed 5, Boston, 2010, McGraw-Hill; and Thompson CW: Laboratory assessment. In Charney P, Malone AM, editors: *ADA pocket guide to nutrition assessment*, ed 2, Chicago, 2009, American Dietetic Association.

TABLE 11-4 Physical Signs That Suggest Nutrient Imbalance

AREA OF CONCERN	POSSIBLE DEFICIENCY	POSSIBLE EXCESS
Hair		
Dull, dry, brittle	Pro	
Easily plucked (with no pain)	Pro	
Hair loss	Pro, Zn, biotin	Vit A
Flag sign (loss of hair pigment in strips around head)	Pro, Cu	
Head and Neck		
Bulging fontanel (infants)		Vit A
Headache		Vit A, D
Epistaxis (nosebleed)	Vit K	
Thyroid enlargement	Iodine	
Eyes		
Conjunctival and corneal xerosis (dryness)	Vit A	
Pale conjunctiva	Fe	
Blue sclerae	Fe	
Corneal vascularization	Vit B_2	
Mouth		
Cheilosis or angular stomatitis (lesions at corners of mouth)	Vit B_2	
Glossitis (red, sore tongue)	Niacin, folate, vit B_{12}, and other B vit	
Gingivitis (inflamed gums)	Vit C	
Hypogeusia, dysgeusia (poor sense of taste, distorted taste)	Zn	
Dental caries	Fluoride	
Mottling of teeth		Fluoride
Atrophy of papillae on tongue	Fe, B vit	
Skin		
Dry, scaly	Vit A, Zn, EFAs	Vit A
Follicular hyperkeratosis (resembles gooseflesh)	Vit A, EFAs, B vit	
Eczematous lesions	Zn	
Petechiae, ecchymoses	Vit C, K	
Nasolabial seborrhea (greasy, scaly areas between nose and lip)	Niacin, vit B_{12}, B_6	
Darkening and peeling of skin in areas exposed to sun	Niacin	
Poor wound healing	Pro, Zn, vit C	

Continued

TABLE 11-4 Physical Signs That Suggest Nutrient Imbalance—cont'd

AREA OF CONCERN	POSSIBLE DEFICIENCY	POSSIBLE EXCESS
Nails		
Spoon-shaped nails	Fe	
Brittle, fragile	Pro	
Heart		
Enlargement, tachycardia, failure	Vit B$_1$	
Small heart	Energy	
Sudden failure, death	Se	
Arrhythmia	Mg, K, Se	
Hypertension	Ca, K	
Abdomen		
Hepatomegaly	Pro	Vit A
Ascites	Pro	
Musculoskeletal and Extremities		
Muscle wasting (especially temporal area)	Energy	
Edema	Pro, vit B$_1$	
Calf tenderness	Vit B$_1$ or C, biotin, Se	
Beading of ribs, or "rachitic rosary" (child)	Vit C, D	
Bone and joint tenderness	Vit C, D, Ca, P	
Knock knee, bowed legs, fragile bones	Vit D, Ca, P, Cu	
Neurologic		
Paresthesias (pain and tingling or altered sensation in the extremities)	Vit B$_1$, B$_6$, B$_{12}$, biotin	
Weakness	Vit C, B$_1$, B$_6$, B$_{12}$, energy	
Ataxia, decreased position and vibratory senses	Vit B$_1$, B$_{12}$	
Tremor	Mg	
Decreased tendon reflexes	Vit B$_1$	
Confabulation, disorientation	Vit B$_1$, B$_{12}$	
Drowsiness, lethargy	Vit B$_1$	Vit A, D
Depression	Vit B$_1$, biotin, B$_{12}$	

Ca, Calcium; *Cu*, copper; *EFAs*, essential fatty acids; *Fe*, iron; *K*, potassium; *Mg*, magnesium; *Na*, sodium; *P*, phosphorus; *Pro*, protein; *Se*, selenium; *Vit*, vitamin(s); *Zn*, zinc.

measuring cups, life-size pictures, or abstract shapes (squares, circles, and rectangles) are used to assist the patient in estimating correct portion sizes of foods consumed. This method is useful in screening or during follow-up to evaluate adaptation of or compliance with dietary recommendations. The advantages of this method are that it is quick (only 15 to 20 minutes is needed) and that it can be used with most age groups. Because it is retrospective, the patient does not modify his or her actual intake. The information can be obtained by face-to-face interview, telephone interview, or patient self-reporting. Some of the drawbacks of this method are that it relies on the memory, motivation, and awareness of the patient. Also, because it records only a single day's intake, the results may not be representative of the patient's actual diet.

Food records. Estimated or measured food records can provide a more realistic picture of a patient's usual intake. For this method of dietary data collection, the patient must be literate, numerate, and well-motivated (Lee and Nieman,

2010). All foods, beverages, snacks, and supplements are recorded by the patient, usually over 1 to 7 days using household measures. The patient must be trained with food models, measuring cups, or other measuring devices that will help ensure recording of proper or actual portion sizes. Cooking methods, recipe ingredients, and descriptions must be recorded as completely and accurately as possible. If information is needed to identify behavioral as well as nutritional patterns, the recorder is also asked to record locations, times, events, and feelings in addition to foods eaten. A 7-day food record is considered optimal for gathering this kind of information, but it does tend to be tedious. Shorter periods are less representative of usual intake, but a 3-day record (2 weekdays and 1 weekend day) is most common.

Calorie counts. In an acute or a long-term care setting, one of the most common forms of food records is a calorie (kcal) count. In actual practice, all nutrients can be assessed, but energy and protein intakes are most often quantified. Information gathered in this manner is used to determine the adequacy of patients' daily oral intake or to document need for nutrition support (any nutrition intervention used to minimize patient morbidity, mortality, and complications).

Nursing observations are essential for early identification of malnutrition and prevention of weight loss during the hospital stay. Staff responsible for recording calorie intake must be accurate in their recordings. It is important to record foods and beverages consumed in measurable amounts (e.g., cups, ounces, teaspoons, tablespoons, mL) or in percentage of amount eaten (50% baked chicken, 75% bread, 25% green beans). Subjective terms such as "two bites, ate well," and "three swallows" are not useful and cannot provide objective information needed to calculate protein and kcal intake. See box Teaching Tool *Conducting an Effective Calorie Count*.

Managing Nutrition Risk

The nutrition care process involves assessing patients' nutritional status, estimating nutrition needs, determining whether there is a nutrition diagnosis (problem) to treat, and planning nutrition intervention. If done appropriately, early intervention works as treatment of established malnutrition and prevention of malnutrition among those at high nutrition risk. Areas to consider regarding nutrition risk are age, weight, laboratory test results, body systems, and feeding modalities (Table 11-5), as follows (Heimburger and Ard, 2006):

Age: Age-related high risk is possible for patients aged 75 years or older; for children, high risk most often occurs for those younger than 5 years. Moderate nutrition risk occurs among adults between ages 65 and 75 years and for children older than 5 years.

Weight: Weight loss is a potential nutrition risk factor, depending on its cause. The percentage of body weight lost combined with the evaluation or cause of the loss determines the possible level of risk.

Laboratory test results: As noted previously, biochemical tests of albumin, prealbumin, vitamin D levels provide a cursory assessment of nutrition risk.

Body systems: Conditions affecting various body systems can pose either moderate or high nutrition risk. Moderate nutrition risk may be experienced when a patient undergoes chemotherapy because of its effects on dietary intake. High risk is incurred among individuals with eating disorders or pregnant women with diabetes.

Feeding modalities: Moderate nutrition risk is associated with transition from restrictive intervention to a regular diet. Risk is also high with modified diets that have the potential to cause nutrient deficiencies. Patients may be at high risk if they receive parenteral feeding or tube feeding, are on NPO (i.e., nothing by mouth) status, or are consuming only clear liquids for more than 3 days.

Nutrition assessment involves examination of anthropometric data, biochemical data, clinical data, and dietary data. It is important to remember that there is no one absolute index for measuring nutrition status. Accurate and meaningful assessment can be made only by incorporating data from several sources.

Screening and Assessment Tools

A variety of tools have been established to evaluate nutrition screening and assessment factors, especially in relation to

---

✳ TEACHING TOOL

Conducting an Effective Calorie Count

Policy

Residents/patients will receive a Calorie Count/Nutrient Intake Analysis, as ordered by the physician.

Procedure

A Calorie Count/Nutrient Intake Analysis is the calculation of a resident's food and beverage intake for calories and protein for 72 hours. In addition, the analysis of other nutrients sometimes is ordered.

1. A physician's order is obtained for a calorie count, which is conducted for 72 hours (3 days). Extensions sometimes are ordered.
2. Nutrient intake analysis begins with the first breakfast meal after the order is written and received by the Nutrition Department.
3. Nursing staff must contact the nutrition professional and give the name, room number, and current diet order. The diet sheet must indicate that a calorie count has been ordered.
4. Nursing staff will initiate the 72-hour (3-day) calorie count.

5. Nursing staff will record the resident's food and beverage intake for each meal on the actual menu and attach it to the calorie count form (shown here). It is also necessary to record all between-meal snacks, nourishments or nutrition supplements on the calorie count form.
6. The nutrition designee picks up the completed calorie count form
7. The nutrition professional records a summary of analysis in the resident's medical record.
8. The nutrition professional makes recommendations in the medical record and communicates these recommendations to the physician, as per policy, if findings indicate a need for further assessment and/or interventions.
9. References to help calculate nutrient intake may include:
   - Nutrient analysis of menu items
   - *Food values of portions commonly used*, ed 19, 2009, Lippincott Williams & Wilkins.
   - *USDA agriculture handbook 8: Composition of foods—raw, processed, prepared*, and its revisions, and/or supplements
   - Exchange lists

Continued

✳ **TEACHING TOOL—cont'd**

CALORIE COUNT FORM

Please record all foods and beverages consumed by patient including the amounts consumed. Please note if patient did not eat at a meal.
Attach menus to show foods chosen when possible.

Day 1 Date: _____	Breakfast/Morning	Lunch/Noon	Supper/Evening	Snacks/am-pm-bedtime	Dietitian's Calculations
Day 2 Date: _____	**Breakfast**	**Lunch**	**Supper**	**Snacks**	
Day 3 Date: _____	**Breakfast**	**Lunch**	**Supper**	**Snacks**	

Adapted with permission from http://www.nutrition411.com/nutrition-management/clinical-policies-and-procedures/item/286-nutrient-intake-analysis-calorie-count

TABLE 11-5 Nutrition Risk Categories

DATA SOURCE	MODERATE RISK	HIGH RISK
Age	65-75 years Children > 5 years of age	≥75 years Children < 5 years of age
Weight	Evaluation of loss (i.e., self-induced)	5% weight loss in 1 month 10% loss in 6 months Length/height for age <5th percentile Weight/height <5th percentile or <80th percentile of standard
Laboratory	Albumin 3-3.5 g/dL*	Albumin ≤3 g/dL
Systems (risk depends on the individual population)	Heart, antepartum, pain, orthopedics, selected oncology, short hospital stay, chemotherapy	Renal, pancreas, gastrointestinal, liver, diabetes with pregnancy, eating disorders, oncology, transplants, any condition in children associated with development of protein-calorie malnutrition
Feeding modalities	Transitional (stable) Some selected modified diets with education component	Parenteral nutrition, tube feeding, nothing per mouth (NPO), or clear liquids >3 days

Data from Grant A, DeHoog S: *Nutritional assessment and support,* ed 5, Seattle, 1999, Anne Grant/Susan DeHoog.
*A *Nutrition Risk Score* (NRI) developed originally for populations with acquired immunodeficiency syndrome) AIDS or cancer was derived from the serum albumin concentration and the ratio of actual to usual weight, as follows: NRI = (1.519 × serum albumin, g/dL) + [41.7 × present weight (kg)/ideal body weight(kg)] (Aziz, et al, 2011).

length of hospital stay and other morbidity factors (Kyle, et al, 2010). It is important to determine how the tools were validated and for which population and care setting they were developed (Anthony, 2008). Of the many tools, six are mentioned here: Nutrition Risk Screening 2002, the Malnutrition Universal Screening Tool, Mini Nutritional Assessment, Short Nutritional Assessment Questionnaire, the Subjective Global Assessment, and the Malnutrition Screening Tool.

Nutrition Risk Screening–2002 (NRS-2002) can be used in the community, in the hospital, or for the elderly. Some tools have been designed by groups, such as the Malnutrition Universal Screening Tool (MUST) from the British Association of Parenteral and Enteral Nutrition. Some were designed specifically for the elderly, such as the Mini Nutrition Assessment (MNA) from the Nestle Institute or the Short Nutritional Assessment Questionnaire (SNAQ65+). Finally, some were designed for specific conditions; the Subjective Global Assessment (SGA) was developed in the 1980s for patients with liver disease or cancer. However, only one has been found to be both reliable and valid for identifying undernutrition in a variety of patients and settings: the Malnutrition Screening Tool (MST) from Abbott (Skipper, et al, 2012) (Figure 11-8).

For malnourished adults with chronic starvation: Order meals and snacks according to appetite and preferences ; encourage a small snack approximately every 2 to 3 hours. Some individuals may need feeding assistance.

For recent acute illness or injury with inflammation: Offer balanced, nutritious meals in small amounts. Use oral supplements between meals if intake is poor at mealtime and for patients who are frail or have infections, impaired wound healing, or pressure ulcers.

For sarcopenia: Oral diet is best, but enteral or parenteral routes may also be needed. Extra dietary protein or amino acids may be useful; whey protein powder is a good source. Some individuals may need feeding assistance.

Drug Interactions with Food and Nutrients

One of the key aspects of nutrition assessment and patient care includes ongoing review of potential or actual food-drug and drug-nutrient interactions. All drugs have physiologic effects, some of which are unintended side effects and constitute the risks of medication use. The amount and rate of drug absorption can be affected by the composition and timing of food intake. Conversely, food intake, absorption, and metabolism can be altered by medication. Drug-nutrient interactions may reduce drug efficacy, interfere with disease control, and foster nutritional deficiencies. Key interventions may involve a change in foods or nutrient administration, patient education or counseling, and coordination of care with the dietitian.

The Joint Commission strongly recommends evaluation of drug and diet combinations. Documentation of these interactions, which may be done by the registered dietitian or nurse, is essential in complying with TJC standards. In addition to medications, use of alcohol and street drugs affects nutrition status and nutrient requirements.

Risk Factors for Drug-Nutrient Interactions

Determination of risk for drug-nutrient reactions depends on characteristics of the individual, including age, physiologic status, multiple-drug intake, hepatic and renal function, and typical dietary intake.

Age. Older adults are more at risk for drug-nutrient reactions because of the greater variety of medications used and the reduced physiologic functioning, which affects drug absorption and efficacy. Older patients often experience several different disorders simultaneously, each with complications and medications that may interact. Young children

Malnutrition Screening Tool (MST)

STEP 1: Screen with the MST

❶ Have you recently lost weight without trying?

No	0
Unsure	2

If yes, how much weight have you lost?

2-13 lb	1
14-23 lb	2
24-33 lb	3
34 lb or more	4
Unsure	2

Weight loss score:

❷ Have you been eating poorly because of a decreased appetite?

No	0
Yes	1

Appetite score:

Add weight loss and appetite scores

MST SCORE:

STEP 2: Score to determine risk

MST = 0 OR 1
NOT AT RISK
Eating well with little or no weight loss

If length of stay exceeds 7 days, then rescreen, repeating weekly as needed.

MST = 2 OR MORE
AT RISK
Eating poorly and/or recent weight loss

Rapidly implement nutrition interventions. Perform nutrition consult within 24-72 hrs, depending on risk.

STEP 3: Intervene with nutritional support for your patients at risk of malnutrition.

Notes: _____

_____

_____

_____

_____

_____

Ferguson, M et al. *Nutrition* 1999 15:458-464

FIG 11-8 The MST Screening Tool. (Reprinted from Ferguson, et al: Development of a valid and reliable malnutrition screening tool for adult acute hospital patients, *Nutrition* 15:458-464, 1999.)

also can be affected by drug-nutrient interactions. Use in children of vitamins/minerals, dietary supplements, and over-the-counter (OTC) medications intended for adults can result in drug-nutrient reactions because the substances will be metabolized differently.

Physiologic status. Impaired ability to absorb, metabolize, or excrete nutrients and medications because of disorders of the gastrointestinal (GI) tract and reduction in hepatic and renal functioning increases the risk of drug-nutrient reactions. Postoperative trauma or injury may also trigger atypical physiologic responses to drug-nutrient interactions. Age alters physiologic status as the body matures. Drug doses can vary according to a person's weight and metabolic function as an aspect of age-related physiologic status. Use of medications during pregnancy requires caution because of the multiple effects on the fetus and on the nutritional status of the mother.

Polypharmacy (multiple-drug intake). Certain types of illness or disease groups tend to require combinations of therapeutic drugs plus other medications, including OTC drugs, for relief of symptoms. The resulting drug-nutrient reactions may be related to the disease itself or be a reaction to medications. For example, intestinal bleeding often causes iron deficiency anemia among patients with arthritis. This intestinal bleeding is a common side effect of long-term use of nonsteroidal anti-inflammatory drugs (NSAIDs), either prescribed or OTC, taken to reduce the symptoms of arthritis.

Influence of typical dietary intake. The basis of a person's nutritional status depends on foods regularly consumed; the nutritional content of these foods affects body functions. A well-nourished individual is better able to withstand a medical regimen that may affect nutrient functioning. In contrast, individuals who are malnourished or marginally deficient in nutrient intake are more at risk for complications of drug-nutrient reactions as the body's stores of nutrients are diminished. For example, individuals who excessively consume alcohol tend to be marginally deficient in a number of nutrients either because of inadequate food intake (alcohol is an appetite suppressant) or because of drug (alcohol)–nutrient interactions.

Prescription and Over-the-Counter Medications

Television, radio, and print media present numerous advertisements about prescription drugs. Patients now approach primary health care providers requesting prescriptions for drugs that treat conditions for which they have not yet been diagnosed. Although the public has become more educated about prescription drugs, OTC medications may be viewed as harmless because prescriptions are not required, but harmless they are not. Interactions of OTC drugs with other medications, foods, nutrients, and supplements such as herbs may occur.

Effects of Drugs on Food and Nutrients

Most drug absorption occurs through the GI mucosa, predominantly in the small intestine. Before a drug can be absorbed, it must first be metabolized and dissolved in gastric juices of the stomach. The speed with which the drug leaves the stomach depends on the gastric emptying time, which affects the rate of drug absorption. This rate may either increase or decrease according to the amount of food in the GI tract. In the fasting state, the medication leaves the empty stomach quickly and is absorbed from the small intestine. For some drugs that is too quick, because time is needed for their disintegration into absorbable particles. For those drugs, it is better to take the medication in the fed state, in which the stomach, containing food, empties more slowly, especially after the consumption of large meals, heated food, and meals with fat, all of which slow emptying time.

Drugs can alter food intake, nutrient absorption, metabolism, and excretion. These drugs include prescription medications, OTC drugs, and even alcohol. Drugs used to lower serum cholesterol levels bind with fat-soluble vitamins and bile salts. As a result, both the bile salts and vitamins are excreted. Some drugs can decrease the amount of digestive enzymes available and thereby decrease nutrient absorption. The tables in this chapter provide information on selected drug-nutrient interactions.

Mineral status can be affected by drugs. Depletion may occur from the simultaneous use of several medications that have the side effect of mineral depletion. Potassium-depleting diuretics along with laxatives may cause significant loss. Older adults often use these products; their dietary intake may be marginal in mineral content as well. Potassium overload may occur in instances in which renal function is compromised and potassium-sparing diuretics (e.g., spironolactone) and potassium supplements are used. Patient education is vital regarding the use of potassium supplements. Clear information is essential. Patients should be taught about the kind of diuretic they are taking and its potential side effects to reduce inappropriate supplementation.

Medications can alter food intake by acting as appetite suppressants or stimulants (Box 11-4), altering taste sensations (Box 11-5), or producing nausea and vomiting, which further decrease appetite. The *Teaching Tool* box Minimizing Drug Side Effects provides a number of specific suggestions.

Drugs may cause additional nutrition problems by affecting GI tract motility (which can change nutrient absorption) or GI tract pH. Drugs also may cause injury of GI mucosa, development of drug-nutrient compounds, decreased bile acid function, and depressed nutrient transport mechanisms. The metabolic and excretion rates of the drug itself may also interfere with nutrient metabolism and excretion. Oral contraceptives may cause marginal deficiencies of B vitamins and vitamin C by increasing the body's use of these vitamins. Table 11-6 presents information on how various drug classes affect food intake, nutrient absorption, metabolism, and excretion.

Effects of Food and Nutrients on Drugs

Foods and nutrients may also affect drug action, producing uncomfortable side effects. Most noteworthy are the adverse side effects associated with monoamine oxidase inhibitors

BOX 11-4 Selected Drugs That Affect Appetite

Appetite Stimulants

Antidepressants
Amitriptyline (Elavil, Endep)
Clomipramine HCl (Anafranil)
Monoamine oxidase inhibitor (MAOIs)
Tranylcypromine sulfate (Parnate)

Antihistamines
Astemizole (Hismanal)
Cyproheptadine HCl (Periactin)

Bronchodilator
Albuterol sulfate (Proventil, Ventolin)

Steroids
Anabolic steroids
Oxandrolone (Anavar)
Corticosteroids
Hydrocortisone (Cortef)
Glucocorticoids
Dexamethasone (Decadron)
Methylprednisolone (Medrol)

Tranquilizers
Lithium carbonate (Lithane)
Benzodiazepines
Chlordiazepoxide HCl (Librium)
Diazepam (Valium)
Prazepam (Centrax)
Phenothiazines
Chlorpromazine HCl (Thorazine)
Promethazine HCl (Phenergan)

Appetite Suppressants

Amphetamines
Benzphetamine HCl (Didrex)
Fenfluramine HCl (Pondimin)
Phenylpropanolamine (Dexatrim, Dimetapp, Triaminic)

Antidysrhythmics
Digitalis
Digitoxin (Crystodigin, Digitoxin)
Digoxin (Digoxin, Lanoxin)

Antibiotics
Amphotericin B (Fungizone)
Gentamicin (Garamycin)
Metronidazole (Flagyl)
Zidovudine (AZT)

Antidepressant
Fluoxetine HCl (Prozac)

Antihistamine
Azatadine maleate (Optimine)

Antihypertensives
Amiloride and hydrochlorothiazide (Moduretic)
Captopril (Capoten)
Chlorthalidone (Hygroton)

Muscle Relaxant
Dantrolene sodium (Dantrium)

Stimulant/Anti–Attention Deficit Disorder Agent
Methylphenidate HCl (Ritalin)

Data from Pronsky ZM: *Food-medication interactions,* ed 17, Birchrunville, PA, 2012, Food-Medication Interactions.

BOX 11-5 Selected Drugs That Alter Taste

Antidysrhythmics
Amiodarone (Cordarone)
Antiarthritic/Chelating agent
Penicillamine (Cuprimine, Depen)

Antibiotics
Ampicillin
Clarithromycin (Biaxin)

Anticonvulsant
Phenytoin (Dilantin)

Antidepressants
Clomipramine HCl (Anafranil)
Fluoxetine HCl (Prozac)

Antifungal
Griseofulvin (Fulvicin, Grifulvin V, Grisacrin)

Antigout Agent
Allopurinol (Zyloprim)

Antihypertensives
Captopril (Capoten)
Labetalol HCl (Normodyne, Trandate)

Antimanics
Lithium carbonate (Eskalith, Lithane, Lithobid)
Lithium citrate (Cibalith-S)

Antiparkinsonian
Levodopa (Dopar, Larodopa)

Antiviral/Anti–Human Immunodeficiency Virus Agent
Didanosine (Videx)

Muscle Relaxant
Dantrolene sodium (Dantrium)

Muscle Relaxant/Antispasmodic
Baclofen (Lioresal)

Stimulant/Amphetamine
Dextroamphetamine sulfate (Dexedrine)

Data from Pronsky ZM: *Food-medication interactions,* ed 17, Birchrunville, PA, 2012, Food-Medication Interactions.

✳ TEACHING TOOL

Minimizing Drug Side Effects

A number of drugs have side effects—symptoms that are not caused by the illness for which the drugs have been prescribed but are physiologic responses of the body to the drugs themselves. The side effects may be mild or quite bothersome. Some may be serious enough to warrant a change in medication. Before using these strategies as education tools, consult the client's primary health care provider to ascertain whether additional medical intervention is required.

Side Effect: Diminished Appetite

- Consider eating several small meals or snacks throughout the day.
- Describe a setting and atmosphere for mealtimes that enhances appetite. Assist the client in exploring approaches to encourage an optimum eating environment.
- Discuss client's favorite foods. Brainstorm about how recipes can be adapted to comply with dietary therapeutic plans.

Side Effect: Modified Taste Sensations

- Visit a dentist regularly to maintain oral hygiene.
- Mask the taste of medications, if needed, with fruit sauces such as applesauce, crushed pineapple, or milk products. First determine whether combinations are acceptable and not contraindicated.

Side Effect: Increased Appetite

- Alert client to the appetite stimulant effect of certain medications.

- Evaluate client's typical dietary intake. Suggest high-fiber foods to provide a quick sense of feeling full.
- Advise limiting availability of high kcal foods and drinks to minimize excess kcal intake.
- Increase activity.

Side Effect: Gastrointestinal Tract Irritation and Discomfort

- Advise client to sit up or stand after taking medications that have the potential to cause heartburn or indigestion.
- Reduce intake of fat, greasy, and/or highly acidic foods, including citrus juices and tomato products.
- Limit food intake in the evening to prevent reflux.
- Control consumption of spicy foods, peppermint, colas, chocolate, alcohol, pepper, decaffeinated coffee, and caffeine if they produce gastric discomfort.

Side Effect: Nausea

- Control liquid intake by serving after meals, or drink only small quantities with meals.
- Sustain adequate fluid volume; cold, carbonated, or clear liquids are easier to tolerate.

Side Effect: Dry or Sore Mouth

- Consume softer, moist foods such as applesauce, puddings, pureed foods, and mashed potatoes.
- Include iced and cold foods throughout the day; consider ice pops, frozen yogurt, ice cream, sorbets, and cooled melons.
- Encourage oral hygiene before and after eating.
- Avoid mouthwashes, which can further dry the oral mucosa.

Data from Pronsky ZM: *Food-medication interactions*, ed 17, Birchrunville, PA, 2012, Food-Medication Interactions.

TABLE 11-6 Medications That Affect Food and/or Nutrients

DRUG OR CLASS	EXAMPLES	ACTION	NUTRIENTS AFFECTED	HOW TO AVOID
Alcohol, particularly excessive use	Beer, wine, spirits	Increases turnover of some vitamins; substitution of alcohol for food	Vitamin B_{12}, folate, and magnesium	Limit alcohol consumption to 2 drinks per day for men or 1 drink per day for women
Analgesics, nonsteroidal anti-inflammatory drugs	Salicylates (aspirin), ibuprofen (Motrin, Advil), naproxen (Anaprox, Aleve, Naprosyn), acetaminophen (Tylenol)	Increase loss of vitamin C and compete with folate and vitamin K	Vitamin C, folate, vitamin K	Increase intake of foods high in vitamin C, folate, and vitamin K; take with 8 oz of water
Antacids	Aluminum antacids, histamine H_2 blockers	Inactivates thiamin; decreased absorption of some nutrients	Thiamin (vitamin B_1)	Foods containing thiamin (B_1) should be consumed at a different time- Take antacid after meals; take iron, magnesium, or folate supplements separately 2 hours before or after; take antacid separately 3 hours before or after citrus fruit or juices or calcium citrate

Continued

TABLE 11-6 Medications That Affect Food and/or Nutrients—cont'd

DRUG OR CLASS	EXAMPLES	ACTION	NUTRIENTS AFFECTED	HOW TO AVOID
Antiulcer agents (histamine blockers)	Ranitidine (Zantac), Cimetidine (Tagamet), famotidine (Pepcid)	Decreases vitamin absorption	Vitamin B_{12}	Consult physician or registered dietitian regarding vitamin B_{12} supplementation
Antibiotics	Tetracycline, Ciprofloxacin (Cipro)	Chelation of minerals; ingestion with caffeine may increase excitability and nervousness	Calcium, magnesium, iron, and zinc; caffeine	Take tetracycline at least 1 hr before or 2 hr after a meal; do not take with caffeine-containing products
Antineoplastic drugs	Methotrexate	Cause mucosal damage, which may lead to decreased nutrient absorption	Folate and vitamin B_{12}; also see *Antibiotics*	Consult physician or registered dietitian regarding supplementation
Anticholinergics	Amitriptyline (Elavil), chlorpromazine (Thorazine)	Thicken saliva, which loses its ability to prevent tooth decay	Fluids	Increase intake of fluids
Anticonvulsants	Phenobarbital, phenytoin (Dilantin)	Increase metabolism of folate (possibly leading to megaloblastic anemia), vitamin D (especially in children), and vitamin K	Folate, vitamin D, and vitamin K	Increase folate, vitamins D and K intake
Antidepressants	Lithium carbonate (Lithane, Lithobid, Lithonate, Lithotabs, Eskalith)	May cause metallic taste, nausea, vomiting, dry mouth, anorexia, weight gain, and increased thirst	Fluids	Drink 2-3 L of water per day and take with food; have a consistent sodium intake
Antihyperlipidemics	Cholestyramine (Questran), colestipol (Colestid)	Bind bile salts and nutrients	Fat-soluble vitamins (A, D, E, K), folate, vitamin B_{12}, and iron	Include rich sources of these vitamins and minerals in diet
Antituberculosis	Isoniazid (INH)	Inhibits conversion of vitamin B_6 to active form	Vitamin B_6	Vitamin B_6 supplementation is necessary to prevent deficiency and peripheral neuropathy
Corticosteroids	Prednisone, Solu-Medrol, hydrocortisone	Increase excretion	Protein, potassium, calcium, magnesium, zinc, vitamin C, and vitamin B_6	Increase intake of foods high in protein, potassium, calcium, magnesium, zinc, vitamin C, and vitamin B_6
Loop diuretics	Furosemide (Lasix)	Increase mineral excretion in urine	Potassium, calcium, magnesium, zinc, sodium, and chloride	Include fresh fruits and vegetables in diet
Thiazide diuretics	Hydrochlorothiazide (HCTZ)	Increase excretion of most electrolytes but enhances reabsorption of calcium	Potassium, calcium, magnesium, zinc, sodium, chloride, and calcium	Increase intake of foods high in potassium, calcium, magnesium, zinc, sodium, chloride, and calcium
Potassium-sparing diuretics	Triamterene (Dyrenium)	Hyperkalemia	Potassium	Avoid potassium-based salt substitutes
Laxatives	Fibercon, Mitrolan	Decreases nutrient absorption	Vitamins and minerals	Consult physician or registered dietitian regarding supplementation
Sedatives	Barbiturates	Increases metabolism of vitamins	Folate, vitamin D, vitamin B_{12}, thiamine, and vitamin C	Increase intake of foods high in folate, vitamin D, vitamin B_{12}, thiamine, and vitamin C

TABLE 11-6 Medications That Affect Food and/or Nutrients—cont'd

DRUG OR CLASS	EXAMPLES	ACTION	NUTRIENTS AFFECTED	HOW TO AVOID
Mineral oil	Agoral Plain	Decreases absorption	Fat-soluble vitamins (A, D, E, K), beta carotene, calcium, phosphorus, and potassium	Take 2 hours before or after food and fat-soluble vitamins
Oral contraceptives	Estrogen/progestin	May cause selective malabsorption or increased metabolism and turnover	Vitamin B_6 and folate	Increase foods high in B_6 and folate

From Long S: Drug-nutrient interactions. In Schlenker ED, Long S, editors: *Williams' essentials of nutrition & diet therapy,* ed 10, St. Louis, 2010, Mosby.

TABLE 11-7 Drugs That May Cause Nutrition Problems

NUTRITION PROBLEM	DRUGS	USE
Depression that results in weight fluctuation	Carbidopa/levodopa	Antiparkinsonian
	Beta blockers	Antihypertensive
	Clonidine	Antihypertensive
	Benzodiazepines	Antianxiety
	Barbiturates	Antianxiety
	Anticonvulsants	Antiepileptic
	Histamine H_2 blockers	Peptic ulcer disease
	Calcium channel blockers	Antihypertensive
	Thiazide diuretics	Antihypertensive
	Digoxin	Antidysrhythmic
Delayed gastric emptying time	Anesthetic agents	Anesthesia
	Opiates	Narcotic
	Tricyclic antidepressant	Antidepressant
	Clonidine	Antihypertensive
	Calcium channel blockers	Antihypertensive
	Nitrates	Antianginal
	Meperidine	Analgesic
	Theophylline	Bronchodilator
	Caffeine	Stimulant
Increased gastric emptying time	Metoclopramide	Antiemetic
	Cisapride	Cholinergic enhancer
	Bethanechol	Cholinergic
	Erythromycin	Antibacterial
Folate deficiency	Phenytoin	Seizures
	Methotrexate	Antimetabolite
	Trimethoprim	Antibacterial

Continued

(MAOIs). MAOIs, such as phenelzine (Nardil) and tranylcypromine (Parnate), may be prescribed to treat depression. These drugs inhibit the enzyme monoamine oxidase, the function of which is to inactivate tyramine found in some foods. Without monoamine oxidase, the level of tyramine increases the release of norepinephrine. Elevations of norepinephrine may cause headache, pallor, heart palpitations, and life-threatening severe hypertension. Patients who take MAOIs should avoid foods and drugs that contain tyramine, such as Chianti wine, aged cheese, and several fermented foods. Locate the list in your facility's diet manual and discuss any concerns with the dietitian.

Medications must be absorbed to have a therapeutic effect. Food intake and composition of the food may affect drug absorption. Table 11-7 lists some common drug classes in which absorption is affected by food. A specific food example is grapefruit juice. Grapefruit juice, which patients sometimes use to take medications, can affect the bioavailability of certain drugs (Box 11-6). Table 11-8 lists foods and nutrients that affect medications.

Timing of Medication Administration

The timing of drug administration and meals also has clinical significance. If its absorption is increased by the presence of

TABLE 11-7 Drugs That May Cause Nutrition Problems—cont'd

NUTRITION PROBLEM	DRUGS	USE
Drowsiness and, possibly, missed meals	Antihistamines	Allergies
	Beta blockers	Antihypertensive
	Skeletal muscle relaxants	Relieve stiffness, pain, discomfort
	Antiemetics	Nausea and vomiting
	Benzodiazepines	Antianxiety
	Antipsychotics	Psychotic disorders
	Antidepressants	Depression
Nausea and vomiting	Selective serotonin reuptake inhibitors (SSRIs)	Antidepressant
	Antibiotics	Antibacterial
	Antineoplastic agents	Chemotherapy
	Digitalis	Antidysrhythmic
	General anesthetics	Anesthesia
	Theophylline	Bronchodilator
	Opioid derivatives	Narcotic

Data from Losben N: Dietitians and consultant pharmacists: A team approach to improved quality care (in *The Consultant Pharmacist*), Alexandria, VA, 1997, American Society of Consultant Pharmacists. Accessed February 21, 2010, from www.ascp.com/public/pubs/tcp/1997/dec/dietitians.html; and MedlinePlus: *Drugs & supplements*, Bethesda, MD (updated January 2006), U.S. National Library of Medicine and National Institutes of Health. Accessed February 21, 2010, from http://medlineplus.gov.

BOX 11-6 Grapefruit "Juices Up" Certain Medications

Almost all oral drugs (including alcohol) go through the liver via hepatic portal circulation, which removes some of the active substance from the blood before entering the general circulation. This means that a fraction of the original dose of the drug will not be "available" because bioavailability of the drug has been lowered. One mechanism responsible for this effect is an enzyme system found in the intestinal wall and liver called the cytochrome P450 3A4 system. Most medications are lipid soluble and readily absorbed. To eliminate toxins (i.e., drugs) from the body, however, the cytochrome P450 system either breaks them down in the gut or changes them into more water-soluble versions in the liver, allowing them to be eliminated via urine.

Grapefruit juice blocks the CYP3A4 enzyme in the wall of the small intestine, thus increasing bioavailability of the drugs. The serum drug level is then higher, which may have unpleasant consequences or even cause toxicity. It is believed that more than one component present in grapefruit juice may contribute to this effect. A single glass (8 oz) of grapefruit juice has the potential to increase bioavailability and enhance beneficial or adverse effects for up to 72 hours after consumption. The following table indicates drugs that are influenced by grapefruit juice:

Interactions between Grapefruit Juice and Medications

CATEGORY	GENERIC NAME	BRAND NAME	EFFECT(S) OF GRAPEFRUIT JUICE
Antihypertensive (calcium channel blockers)	Felodipine	Plendil	Flushing, headache, tachycardia, decreased blood pressure
	Nifedipine	Procardia, Adalat	
	Nimodipine	Nimotop	
	Nisoldipine	Sular	
	Nicardipine	Cardene	
	Isradipine	DynaCirc	
	Verapamil	Calan, Isoptin	Same as above plus bradycardia and atrioventricular (AV) block
Immunosuppressant	Cyclosporine	Neoral, Sandimmune, SangCya	Kidney toxicity, increased susceptibility to infections
	Tacrolimus	Prograf	
Statin (HMG-CoA reductase inhibitors)	Atorvastatin	Lipitor	Headache, gastrointestinal complaints, muscle pain, increased risk of myopathy
	Lovastatin	Mevacor	
	Simvastatin	Zocor	Nervousness, overstimulation

BOX 11-6 Grapefruit "Juices Up" Certain Medications—cont'd

CATEGORY	GENERIC NAME	BRAND NAME	EFFECT(S) OF GRAPEFRUIT JUICE
Antianxiety, insomnia, or depression	Buspirone	BuSpar	Increased sedation
	Diazepam	Valium	
	Alprazolam	Xanax	
	Midazolam	Versed	
	Triazolam	Halcion	
	Zaleplon	Sonata	
	Carbamazepine	Tegretol	
	Clomipramine	Anafranil	
	Trazodone	Desyrel	
Protease inhibitors	Saquinavir	Fortovase, Invirase	Doubles bioavailability, resulting in increased efficacy or toxicity depending on dose and patient variability
Sexual dysfunction	Sildenafil	Viagra	Delayed absorption (takes longer to become effective)

Medications Considered Safe for Use with Grapefruit

Cetirizine	Zyrtec, Reactine	Loratadine	Claritin
Fexofenadine	Allegra	Pravastatin	Pravachol
Fluvastatin	Lescol		

From Long S: Drug-nutrient interactions. In Schlenker ED, Long S, editors: *Williams' essentials of nutrition & diet therapy*, ed 10, St. Louis, 2010, Mosby.

TABLE 11-8 Foods and/or Nutrients That Affect Medications

DRUG CLASS	EXAMPLES	USE	FOOD(S)/ NUTRIENT(S)	ACTION(S) OR EFFECT(S)	HOW TO AVOID
Alcohol, particularly excessive use	Beer, wine, spirits	Lowers inhibitions; central nervous system (CNS) depressant	Food	Slowing of absorption	Consume alcohol with food or meals
Analgesics and nonsteroidal anti-inflammatory drugs	Salicylates (aspirin), Ibuprofen (Motrin, Advil), naproxen (Anaprox, Aleve, Naprosyn), Acetaminophen (Tylenol)	Pain and fever	Alcohol	Increase in hepatotoxicity, liver damage, or stomach bleeding	Limit alcohol intake to 2 drinks per day for men, 1 drink per day for women
Antiulcer agents (histamine blockers)	Cimetidine (Tagamet)	Ulcers	Alcohol	Increased blood alcohol levels	Limit alcohol intake to 2 drinks per day for men, 1 drink per day for women
			Caffeine-containing foods and beverages	Reduced caffeine clearance	Limit caffeine intake
Antibiotics	Ciprofloxacin (Cipro)	Infection	Dairy products	Decrease absorption	Avoid dairy products
Anticoagulant	Warfarin (Coumadin)	Blood clots	Vitamins K and E (supplements)	May reduce efficacy	Limit foods high in vitamin K: broccoli, spinach, kale, turnip greens, cauliflower, Brussels sprouts; avoid high dose of vitamin E (400 IU or more)
			Alcohol and garlic	May increase anticoagulation	Avoid alcohol and garlic

Continued

TABLE 11-8 Foods and/or Nutrients That Affect Medications—cont'd

DRUG CLASS	EXAMPLES	USE	FOOD(S)/ NUTRIENT(S)	ACTION(S) OR EFFECT(S)	HOW TO AVOID
Antineoplastic drugs	Methotrexate	Cancer	Alcohol	Increased hepatotoxicity with chronic alcohol use	Avoid alcohol
Antiemetic	Amitriptyline HCl (Elavil), chlorpromazine HCl (Thorazine)	Antidepressant; antipsychotic/ antiemetic	Alcohol	Increased sedation	Avoid alcohol
Anticonvulsants	Phenobarbital	Seizures, epilepsy	Alcohol	Increased sedation	Avoid alcohol
Antidepressants: monoamine oxidase inhibitors (MAOIs)	Phenelzine (Nardil), tranylcypromine (Parnate)	Depression, anxiety	Foods or alcoholic beverages containing tyramine	Rapid, potentially fatal increase in blood pressure	Avoid beer; red wine; Camembert and aged blue cheeses; aged Cheddar, bleu, Brie, mozzarella, and Parmesan cheeses; yogurt; sour cream; beef or chicken liver; cured meats such as sausage and salami; game meats; caviar; dried fish; yeast extracts; sauerkraut; kimchee; fish or shrimp sauce; soy sauce; miso soup; broad (fava) beans
Antihistamine	Fexofenadine (Allegra), loratadine (Claritin), cetirizine (Zyrtec), astemizole (Hismanal)	Allergies	Alcohol	Increases drowsiness and slows mental and motor performance	Use caution when operating machinery or driving
Antihypertensives	Angiotensin-converting enzyme inhibitors, angiotensin II receptor antagonists, beta blockers, verapamil HCl	Hypertension	Natural licorice (Glycyrrhiza glabra) and tyramine-rich foods	Reduced effectiveness	Avoid natural licorice and tyramine-containing foods (see previous list for Antidepressants)
Antihyperlipidemics such as statins	Atorvastatin (Lipitor), lovastatin (Mevacor), pravastatin (Pravachol), simvastatin (Zocor)	High serum cholesterol	Food/meals	Altered absorption	Lovastatin should be taken with evening meal to enhance absorption
			Alcohol	Increased risk of liver damage	Avoid large amounts of alcohol
Antiparkinsonian	Levodopa (Dopar, Larodopa)	Parkinson's disease	High-protein foods (eggs, meat, protein supplements); vitamin B_6	Decreased absorption	Spread protein intake equally in 3-6 meals per day to minimize reaction; avoid B_6 supplements and multivitamin supplements
Antituberculosis agent	Isoniazid (INH)	Tuberculosis	Food	Reduced absorption	Take on empty stomach

TABLE 11-8 Foods and/or Nutrients That Affect Medications—cont'd

DRUG CLASS	EXAMPLES	USE	FOOD(S)/ NUTRIENT(S)	ACTION(S) OR EFFECT(S)	HOW TO AVOID
			Alcohol	Increased hepatotoxicity and reduced INH levels	Avoid alcohol
Bronchodilators	Theophylline (Slo-bid, Theo-Dur)	Asthma, chronic bronchitis, and emphysema	Caffeine	Increased stimulation of CNS	Limit caffeine-containing foods/beverages (chocolate, colas, teas, coffee)
			Alcohol	Can increase nausea, vomiting, headache, and irritability	Avoid alcohol
Corticosteroids	Prednisolone (Pediapred, Prelone), methylprednisolone (Solu-Medrol); hydrocortisone	Inflammation and itching	Food	Stomach irritation	Take with food or milk to decrease stomach upset
Hypoglycemic agents	Chlorpropamide (Diabinese) metformin (Glucophage)	Diabetes	Alcohol	Severe nausea and vomiting	Avoid alcohol

From Long S: Drug-nutrient interactions. In Schlenker ED, Long S, editors: *Williams' essentials of nutrition & diet therapy,* ed 10, St. Louis, 2010, Mosby.

food, the medication should be taken with a meal or a snack. If the drug's absorption is depressed by the presence of food in the stomach, optimum absorption occurs if the medication is taken at least 1 hour before or 2 hours after eating or tube feeding.

The established drug administration schedules in health care facilities often conflict with the optimal bioavailability of a prescribed drug. As a general guideline, drugs should be given at least 1 hour before or 2 hours after a meal unless the medication causes GI distress when taken on an empty stomach. Such timing should enhance drug absorption and decrease hindrance of nutrient absorption. Tube feedings present other issues of drug-nutrient interactions (Box 11-7).

Effects of Herbs on Food, Nutrients, and Drugs

Herbs are not innocuous; they can have significant effects on the bioavailability of foods, nutrients, and drugs. Of particular concern are the effects of certain commonly used herbs on a body undergoing surgery. Ginkgo, feverfew, garlic, ginger, ginseng, dong quai, and danshen affect blood clotting. Other herbs, such as valerian, kava kava (which may also cause liver damage), and St. John's wort, can prolong the effects of narcotic and anesthesia drugs.

Nurses should ask detailed questions about a patient's supplement intake, such as the following:

- Do you use any dietary supplements? (Direct patient to include in the answer vitamins, minerals, botanicals, amino acids, concentrates, and extracts.)
  - If so, what dosage do you take? What other directions do you follow, such as taking with meals or at bedtime?
- What is the purpose of taking the dietary supplement? (Avoid questions like "What is that supposed to do?" because such implied skepticism can embarrass the patient and discourage honest reporting of supplement use.)
- Have you experienced any side effects?
- Do you take an herbal product, herbal supplement, or other "natural remedy"?
  - If so, do you take any prescription or nonprescription medications for the same purpose as the herbal product?
- Have you used this herbal product before?
- Are you allergic to any plant products?
- Are you pregnant or breastfeeding?
- Are you seeing an herbalist, naturopathic practitioner, nutritionist, or natural healer?
- Is your physician or primary health care provider aware that you take these supplements (in addition to any prescribed medications)?

It is useful to keep an open mind and remain current in this quickly changing area. Table 11-9 lists herbs and the potential drug interactions that are of concern.

Text continued on p. 259

BOX 11-7 Tube Feedings and Drug-Nutrient Interactions

Drug-nutrient interactions can compromise pharmacologic and nutritional objectives of safety, efficacy, and quality of care. Moreover, these interactions can affect cost effectiveness of health care. Before administering an oral drug through a gastric or nasogastric feeding tube, ask yourself the following questions:

1. Is the feeding tube placed correctly?
2. Can the medication be crushed and delivered through a feeding tube?
3. Will there be an interaction between the medication and the feeding solution?
   - If so, will the interaction degrade the nutritional components of the feeding solution?
   - Or alter the medication's availability?
   - Or clog the tube?

4. Will the medication change the osmolality or pH in the feeding system?
   - Or cause nausea, vomiting, cramping, or diarrhea?

Pharmacists have valuable expertise in optimizing prescriptions. The number of potential drug–feeding formula interactions is nearly endless, and new medications and feeding formulas are marketed almost daily. Consultation with pharmacy services is recommended to detect possible incompatibilities and recommendations for appropriate alternative forms of medications if necessary. Questions regarding specific feeding formulas and adverse drug reactions can be directed to the dietitian. The following chart offers solutions to potential problems that may occur.

POTENTIAL PROBLEM	SOLUTION
Should I administer the tablet or liquid form of the medication?	Whenever possible, use the liquid form of a drug because it bypasses the dissolution process. But be aware that many liquid medications are formulated for pediatric patients; therefore, large volumes must be dispensed to meet the required dose for adults. This often leads to diarrhea as a result of excessive amounts of sorbitol in the adjusted dose.
Okay, I checked and the only form of the medication available is a tablet. What should I do?	If a tablet is the only preparation available, consultation with the pharmacist is mandatory. Some tablets can be crushed if they are simple, compressed tablets designed to dissolve immediately in the gastrointestinal (GI) tract. Keep in mind that crushing the tablet allows it to enter the bloodstream faster. The difference may or may not be clinically significant. Always confirm the type of coating on the tablet with the pharmacy.
I've checked with the pharmacy and was told the tablet could be crushed. How do I do that?	Ideally, medication(s) should be crushed in the pharmacy. But if you must do it yourself, the best technique is to position a unit-dose tablet in a mortar without removing it from the package. Then crush the tablet by tapping it through the package with a pestle (to avoid tearing the package, don't grind). If the medication isn't packaged as a unit-dose, place it between two paper medicine cups and pulverize the tablet with the mortar and pestle. Mix the crushed tablet thoroughly with 15-30 mL water (5-10 mL for children), and administer through the feeding tube. Tubing must be flushed with a minimum of 30 mL of room temperature sterile water before and after administration of each medication.
It seems like it would be easier to add the medication to the feeding formula.	Never add medications directly to the feeding formula. This can alter the medication's therapeutic effect and disrupt the integrity of the feeding formula, causing it to resemble curdled milk.
The pharmacy has the prescribed medications in liquid form. Is there anything special I need to do?	Check whether dilution of the medication formulation before administration is required. Hypertonic, irritating, or viscous medications should be diluted in at least 30 mL of water immediately before infusion to avoid gastric irritation and diarrhea. In some cases, 90 mL of water may be necessary for dilution. Adjust water amounts appropriately for pediatric patients and patients on fluid restrictions. Document the amount of water used on the patient's intake and output records.
If sugar-coated tablets can be crushed, are there tablets that cannot be crushed?	Some types of tablets must not be crushed. These include: *Buccal or sublingual tablets* (e.g., nitroglycerin or isosorbide) are intended to be absorbed by veins under the tongue or in the cheek, thus bypassing the liver (avoiding first-pass effect) and protecting the medication from contact with other drugs, foods, and GI secretions that could affect the medication's potency or bioavailability. *Enteric-coated tablets* (e.g., bisacodyl [Dulcolax] and ferrous sulfate [Feosol]) are formulated to inhibit release of the active drug until after the tablet has passed from the stomach into the small intestine. Moreover, the tablet's coating protects the stomach from irritation from the medication. Crushing the tablet would put an end to the protective coating. *Uncoated gastric irritants* (including aspirin) remain effective following crushing, but they are more apt to trigger undesirable GI reactions such as cramping and bleeding. Ask for an alternative form or different medication. *Sustained-release or effervescent tablets* (e.g., Slow-L, Procan SR, Theolair-SR, Inderal LA) were designed to dissolve and release medication gradually (they contain 2 or 3 doses of the medication). As a result, if such a tablet were crushed, the patient would receive an overdose. In addition, the planned beneficial effects would not be maintained throughout the dosing interval.

BOX 11-7 Tube Feedings and Drug-Nutrient Interactions—cont'd

POTENTIAL PROBLEM	SOLUTION
The prescribed medication is in the form of a capsule. Can't I just place it in the tube and flush it down with some water?	Capsules should not be crushed, but you can open some and mix the contents with water: *Hard gelatin capsules* (e.g., ampicillin and doxycycline) contain a medication in a powdered form. The capsule can be opened (it's designed to separate in the middle), and the powder mixed thoroughly with water. *Sustained-release capsules* (e.g., Slo-bid and Feosol Spansules) release the active medication slowly, over time, through coated beads or pellets inside the capsules. They are designed to dissolve in the GI tract at different rates, lengthening the medication's duration of action. Obviously, crushing capsules or their contents would damage the timed-release coatings. A better alternative would be a liquid form or a simple compressed tablet that can be crushed (ascertain that dosage frequency is increased appropriately). *Soft gel capsules* (e.g., chloral hydrate, some vitamin preparations) can be dispensed through a feeding tube by poking a pinhole in one end and squeezing out the liquid contents. The liquid contents can also be drawn up in a syringe. Neither method should be used if delivering an exact dose is important. Some of the drug will always remain inside the capsule. Dissolve the capsule in 15-30 mL of warm water (5-10 mL for pediatric patients), then administer. The drug-water mixture will also work if you plan ahead—dissolving the capsule can take as long as 1 hour.

Data from Lehmann S, Barber JR: Giving medications by feeding tube, *Nursing* 91:58-61, 1991; Lourenco R: Enteral feedings: Drug/nutrient interaction, *Clin Nutr* 20(2):187-193, 2001; and Belknap DC, et al: Administration of medications through enteral feeding catheters, *Am J Crit Care* 6(5):382-392, 1997.

TABLE 11-9 Commonly Used Herbal Products and Nutraceuticals That May Be Used to Treat Selected Conditions*

CONDITION/HERB	USE OR ACTION	ASSOCIATED ADVERSE EFFECTS; COMMENTS
Asthma		
Tylophora indica, T. asthmatica	Inhibits histamine release	Sore mouth, loss of taste for salt, morning nausea and vomiting
Adhatoda vasica	Bronchodilator	Vomiting and diarrhea; lack of conclusive efficacy data
Picrorhiza kurroa	Bronchodilator	Vomiting, cutaneous rash, anorexia, diarrhea, itching, giddiness, headache, abdominal pain, increased dyspnea
Khellin	Bronchodilator	Avoid taking with prescription bronchodilators
Onion extract *(Allium cepa)*	May inhibit leukotriene and thromboxane	Delirium, tachycardia, nausea, high incidence of gastrointestinal (GI) side effects
Ginkgo *(Ginkgo biloba)*	Smooth muscle relaxant	Clinical efficacy unproven
Anxiety and Depression		
Chamomile *(Chamaemelum nobile, Matricaria chamomilla, M. recutita)*	GI spasm or irritation, sedative	Therapeutic amounts may vary depending on effect chamomile has on an individual; side effects infrequent
Valerian *(Valeriana officinalis)*	Insomnia, mild to moderate anxiety, stress and tension, premenstrual tension, hyperactivity, depression, insomnia, migraine headaches	Side effects not reported, but if used in too large a dose initially, it may cause excitability
Passion flower *(Passiflora incarnate)*	Relaxation and sleep	Not recommended for children <2 years; use of decreased initial dose recommended for those >65 years
Kava *(Piper methysticum)*	Sedative, anticonvulsive, antispasmodic, central muscular relaxant	Prolonged use causes a temporary yellow coloring of skin, hair, and nails; may cause liver damage; not recommended for use with other central nervous system depressants, including alcohol
Hops *(Humulus lupulus)*	Insomnia, digestive aid, treatment of intestinal ailments	

Continued

TABLE 11-9 Commonly Used Herbal Products and Nutraceuticals That May Be Used to Treat Selected Conditions—cont'd

CONDITION/HERB	USE OR ACTION	ASSOCIATED ADVERSE EFFECTS; COMMENTS
Ginseng (Panax quinquefolius, P. ginseng, Eleutherococcus senticosus)	Increase energy, improve stamina, enhance memory	Typically mild and dose related; most commonly observed are nervousness, sleeplessness, nausea, and occasionally headache
St. John's wort (Hypericum perforatum)	Depression	Fatigue, pruritus, weight gain, emotional vulnerability; photosensitivity; decreased effectiveness of oral contraceptive therapy possible
Black cohosh (Cimicifuga racemosa)	Sedative, relaxant	Not for use in pregnancy
California poppy (Eschscholzia californica)	Hypnotic, tranquilizer	
Damask rose (Rosa damascene)	Antidepressant	Use only good-quality damask rose
Jamaican dogwood (Piscidia erythrina)	Insomnia, migraine	
Linden (Tifia europaea)	Reduces nervous tension	
Gotu kola (Centella asiatica)	Relaxant	Gotu kola may cause rash; avoid during pregnancy and breastfeeding
Pasque flower (Anemone pulsatilla)	Sedative action	Use only dried plant
Lavender (Lavandula species)	Sedative	Avoid high doses in pregnancy
Wild lettuce (Lactuca virosa)		Excess amounts can lead to insomnia
Wood betony (Stachys officinalis)		Large doses can cause vomiting; avoid high doses in pregnancy
Cancer Prevention and Treatment		
Shark cartilage	Antiangiogenic effect	Doubtful oral bioavailability of biologically active components
Aloe vera	May stimulate macrophage function (antitumor activity)	May have deleterious effects in patients with acquired immunodeficiency syndrome (AIDS)
Echinacea (Echinacea angustifolia, E. pallida)	Immunostimulatory activity	Unknown whether effective orally
Mistletoe (Phoradendron species and Viscum species)	Potent inducer of cytokines stimulating release of tumor necrosis factor-α and interleukin-1	
Antioxidant vitamins A and E	May reduce risk of lung cancer by reducing formation of free radicals	Vitamin A can be toxic
Garlic and onion (Allium sativum and A. cepa)	May decrease nitrosamine formation	
Green tea	Antioxidant properties, inhibits nucleoside transport	Contradictory epidemiologic studies regarding efficacy in cancer
Chaparral (Larrea tridentate, L. divaricata, L. mexicana)	Antioxidant properties	Hepatoxic; unproven and dangerous
Ginseng (Panax quinquefolius, P. ginseng, Eleutherococcus senticosus)	Antiestrogen properties	More data needed
Laetrile	May have tumor static activity	Unproven
Goldenseal (Hydrastis canadensis)	May prevent carcinogenesis	Use may be limited by toxicity
Pineapple	May cause tumor regression	More study needed
Sweet and red clover (Trifolium pretense)	Stimulates macrophage activity	
Cloud fungus	Immunostimulatory activity	
Colds and Flu		
Anise (Pimpinella anisum)	Expectorant action	May cause contact dermatitis; avoid use during pregnancy and breastfeeding
Boneset (Eupatorium perfoliatum)	Antipyretic; influenza	Individuals with hypersensitivity to the Asteraceae family (e.g., chamomile, feverfew) should avoid use
Coltsfoot (Tussilago farfara)	Antitussive	Possible hepatotoxicity; has abortifacient effects, should not be taken during pregnancy and breastfeeding

TABLE 11-9 Commonly Used Herbal Products and Nutraceuticals That May Be Used to Treat Selected Conditions—cont'd

CONDITION/HERB	USE OR ACTION	ASSOCIATED ADVERSE EFFECTS; COMMENTS
Echinacea (Echinacea angustifolia, E. pallida)	Prophylaxis and treatment of cold and flu symptoms	Continuous use (>6-8 weeks) may lead to immunosuppression; contraindicated in autoimmune diseases Purple coneflower (E. purpurea) is a different species with similar properties
Horehound (Marrubium vulgare)	Controversial use as expectorant, antitussive, cough suppressant, digestive aid, appetite stimulant	Large doses have produced cardiac irregularities
Slippery elm (Ulmus rubra)	Demulcent and emollient to treat sore throats	Pollen can be an allergen; may cause contact dermatitis
Zinc lozenges	Reduce duration and severity of cold symptoms	Possible nausea, unpleasant taste
Diabetes		
Karela (Momordica charantia)	Hypoglycemic	May sufficiently lower blood glucose to merit decrease in insulin or oral medications to avoid or minimize incidence of hypoglycemia; karela juice will cause greater decrease in blood glucose than when slices of karela are fried
Ginseng (Panax quinquefolius, P. ginseng, Eleutherococcus senticosus)	Hypoglycemic	Korean or Chinese ginseng may exert greater hypoglycemic effect than Japanese ginseng
Brewer's yeast	Hypoglycemic	May cause unfavorable variability in blood glucose control if medical staff is unaware of concomitant use with chromium
GS₄ (Gymnema sylvestre)	Hypoglycemic	May decrease insulin and glyburide requirements but should not be relied on for blood glucose control
Devil's claw (Harpagophytum procumbens)		May cause hyperglycemia
Ephedra or ma huang (Ephedra sinica)		
Dyslipidemia and Atherosclerosis		
Nicotine acid (niacin)	Reduces total serum cholesterol, low-density lipoprotein (LDL) cholesterol, and triglycerides; increases high-density lipoprotein (HDL) cholesterol	Should be used only under physician's supervision; may raise blood glucose levels; severe hepatotoxicity may occur, especially with sustained release nicotinic acid products
Soluble fiber products (oat bran, guar gum, psyllium, and other dietary sources)	Can lower total serum cholesterol and LDL cholesterol depending on product and amount consumed	Flatulence, cramping, bloating, nausea, diarrhea, indigestion, heartburn
Fish oils (omega-3 fatty acids)	Inhibit platelet aggregation, lower triglyceride levels when consumed in high doses (20-30 g/day)	Triglyceride-lowering effect may diminish with continued use; variable effects (decreases and increases) on blood cholesterol levels; may increase bleeding risk
Vitamin E	200 International Units or more per day *may* reduce risk of coronary heart disease	
Garlic (Allium sativum)	Standardized powdered garlic products may produce modest reduction in total cholesterol	
Nuts	Lower plasma lipoprotein levels	
Beta-sitosterol	May produce modest reductions in total and LDL cholesterol	
Alfalfa seed (Medicago sativa)	May produce modest reduction in cholesterol	Potential toxic effects outweigh any advantages that might be obtained

Continued

TABLE 11-9 Commonly Used Herbal Products and Nutraceuticals That May Be Used to Treat Selected Conditions—cont'd

CONDITION/HERB	USE OR ACTION	ASSOCIATED ADVERSE EFFECTS; COMMENTS
Chromium	May produce modest cholesterol reductions; administration as picolinate salt seems to increase bioavailability	
Gastrointestinal Problems		
Aloes (*Aloe barbadensis, Aloe ferox, Aloe africana, Aloe spicata*)	Orally a powerful cathartic and not generally recommended	A harsh purgative; less toxic laxatives are available Contraindicated in patients with hemorrhoids, kidney disease, intestinal obstruction, abdominal pain, nausea, or vomiting
Bilberry fruit (*Vaccinium myrtillus*)	Treatment of diarrhea	No known side effects or interactions
Cascara (*Rhamnus purshiana*)	Stimulant laxative	Avoid during pregnancy and breastfeeding Fresh bark may cause severe vomiting Electrolyte imbalance with misuse; potentiates toxicities of cardiac glycosides and thiazide diuretics
Ginger (*Zingiber officinale*)	Treatment of motion sickness and nausea	May cause prolonged bleeding times; should be used with caution by patients on anticoagulant therapy
Licorice (*Glycyrrhiza glabra; G. uralensis*)	Treatment of peptic ulcer, expectorant	Considered unsafe Contraindicated in patients taking cardiac glycosides or thiazide diuretics
Peppermint (*Mentha piperita*)	Decreases muscle spasms of the GI tract Treatment of abdominal pain Enteric-coated capsules used to treat irritable bowel syndrome	Should not be used by infants or small children; tea from leaves can cause laryngeal and bronchial spasms Overuse can lead to heartburn and relaxation of laryngoesophageal sphincter
Psyllium (*Plantago arenaria, P. psyllium, P. indica, P. ovata*)	Bulk-forming laxative for constipation, irritable bowel syndrome	Possibly interferes with absorption of other drugs Bezoars (fibrous masses in GI tract) may occur if liquid intake is inadequate
Senna (*Cassia acutifolia; C. angustifolia, Senna alexandrina*)	Cathartic; used to treat constipation	Long-term use can result in electrolyte imbalance and potassium loss May increase toxicity of cardiac glycosides and thiazide diuretics
Hypertension		
Garlic (*Allium sativum*)	Antihypertensive	Routine use not recommended Avoid use of garlic with nonstyeroidal anti-inflammatory drugs, anticoagulants, drugs that inhibit liver metabolism (e.g., cimetidine), and drugs that may be affected by liver inhibition (e.g., propranolol, diazepam)
Grapefruit juice		May cause significant decrease in blood pressure if taken with nifedipine
Licorice (*Glycyrrhiza glabra; G. uralensis*)		May induce hypertension accompanied by hypokalemia Patients taking oral contraceptives or thiazide diuretics may be predisposed to licorice toxicity if taken concomitantly
Yohimbine (*Pausinystalia yohimbe*)	May be used to treat impotence secondary to antihypertensive medications	May increase blood pressure Should not be co-administered with tricyclic antidepressants or clonidine

*This table does not provide information on how to use herbs, nor is it an exhaustive look at every herbal product that may be used. Rather, the intent is to provide information regarding herbal products that patients may use.

Data from Miller LG, Miller WJ, editors: *Herbal medicinals: A clinician's guide,* New York, 1998, Pharmaceutical Products Press; and Tyler VE: *The honest herbal,* ed 3, New York, 1993, Pharmaceutical Products Press.

SUMMARY

- The capacity for recovery from illness or disease depends heavily on nutrition status.
- Nurses often perform basic nutrition screening, nutrition education, and monitoring.
- Nutrition status of patients may be compromised by acute care hospital or nursing home stays; nurses must evaluate whether patients actually receive the nutrients they are served.
- Psychologic and physiologic alterations of illness, the effects of bed rest, risks of malnutrition, food-drug interactions, and the effects of poor intake on immunity and healing require nutrition screening and monitoring.
- It is important to refer patients at nutrition risk to the nutrition team members who can enhance meals or offer alternative methods of intake.
- The registered dietitian (RD/RDN) is best qualified to provide in-depth knowledge about nutrition care, to consult individually with patients, and to participate in team meetings.
- A comprehensive nutrition assessment is conducted by dietitians to determine appropriate nutrition therapy based on identified needs (nutrition diagnoses) of the patient.

- Data are collected from several sources to assess patients' nutrition needs using the ABCD approach: **A**nthropometrics, **B**iochemical tests, **C**linical observations, and **D**iet evaluation.
- The Nutrition Care Process (NCP) addresses the unique nutrition needs of each patient.
- The NCP is similar to the nursing process and involves four steps to identify and solve nutrition-related problems: Assessment, Nutrition Diagnosis, Nutrition Intervention, and Monitoring-Evaluation.
- The NCP process is repeated as often as needed until the nutrition diagnoses have been resolved.
- Specific food or nutrient alterations may be required, or a patient may need education on how to choose foods wisely.
- Drug-nutrient interactions are common.
- Nutrients and foods may interact with drug function; drugs may affect the use of food and nutrients.
- Timing of meals and medication administration are sometimes in conflict in health care facilities.
- Knowledge of all types of potential interactions between food, nutrients, and drugs helps nurses provide more comprehensive patient care.

◎ THE NURSING APPROACH

A Comparison of the Nursing Process and the Nutrition Care Process

The Nursing Process and the Nutrition Care Process (NCP) are both systematic problem-solving methods that utilize critical thinking skills to develop a framework for the plan of care. The following is a case study used to compare the Nursing Process and NCP.

James is a 37-year-old African American man with a history of hypertension. He has been noncompliant with his medications for the past 2 years because of the high cost of medications and their unpleasant side effects. He smokes one pack of cigarettes per day but does not drink alcohol. He presents to the clinic today because he has been feeling tired and has had a headache for the past few days.

	NURSING PROCESS		**NUTRITION CARE PROCESS**
Assessment	**Subjective**	Assessment	**Anthropometric Measurements**
	"I work a lot, so I usually eat fast food or frozen meals for breakfast and dinner."		Height 5'9", weight 205 pounds "I've gained about 10 pounds within the past 3 months."
	"I've been really tired lately, and I've had this headache that won't go away."		
	"I've gained about 10 pounds within the past 3 months."		**Biochemical, Medical Tests, and Procedures**
	"I don't like to exercise."		BP 178/94 mm Hg, pulse 92 Laboratory tests have not been order yet
	Objective		**Client History**
	Height 5'9", weight 205 pounds BP 178/94 mm Hg, pulse 92		Hypertension
			Food/Nutrition-Related History
			"I work a lot, so I usually eat fast food or frozen meals for breakfast and dinner."
			"I've been really tired lately, and I've had this headache that won't go away."
			"I don't like to exercise."
			Based on the patients 24-hour recall, he consumes approximately 3500kcal/day

Continued

◎ THE NURSING APPROACH—cont'd

NURSING PROCESS	NUTRITION CARE PROCESS
	Sodium intake of approximately 4000mg/day Consumes 1-2 servings of fruits and vegetables per day **Nutrition-Focused Physical Findings** Obese
Diagnosis 1. Ineffective self-health maintenance related to lack of knowledge, difficulty modifying personal habits, and insufficient financial resources 2. Imbalanced nutrition: more than body requirements related to excessive intake in relation to physical activity as evidence by body mass index (BMI) >30	**Diagnosis** 1. Excessive energy intake related to food- and nutrition-related knowledge deficit concerning energy intake, as evidenced by BMI > 30, 10-pound weight gain, and reports of high-calorie meals 2. Excessive sodium intake related to food- and nutrition-related knowledge deficit concerning sodium intake, as evidenced by hypertension 3. Physical inactivity related to time constraints, as evidenced by BMI >30 and reports of infrequent physical activity
Planning **Patient Outcomes** *Short term (at the end of this visit):* • James will verbalize his personal risk factors and the potential complications of having hypertension • He will commit to taking his blood pressure medication • He will select low-sodium, low-fat options from a menu *Long term (at follow-up visit in 1 month):* Weight 201 pounds; BP 140/85 • Reports taking medication as prescribed • Feels more energized and no longer has a headache • Has started to quit smoking **Nursing Interventions** 1. Measure blood pressure, pulse, and weight. 2. Review medication and teach him when to notify the doctor. 3. Teach him about general dietary measures to reduce sodium and fat intake. 4. Provide education and information on how to quit smoking.	**Intervention** **Short-Term Goal** • Verbalize understanding of Dietary Approaches to Stop Hypertension (DASH) diet • Demonstrate how to read food labels and choose low-sodium foods • Verbalize plan to begin exercise regimen • Will schedule follow-up appointment **Long-Term Goal** • Adhere to DASH diet • Reduce sodium intake to 1.5 g/day • Begin playing tennis 3 times per week **Nutrition Education** • Provide support written and verbal instruction on DASH diet • Will instruct patient to limit dietary sodium to 1.5 g/day • Will instruct patient to begin walking for at least 20 minutes 3 times per week **Coordination of Care** • Organize referral to cardiac rehab program through local American Heart Association
Implementation 1. Explain risk factors and possible complications of developing hypertension. 2. Provide information about medication and importance of taking it as prescribed. 3. Teach guidelines for following a heart-healthy diet and provide information on how to lose weight. 4. Provide education and information on how to quit smoking.	**Monitoring & Evaluation** • Follow-up with patient in 1 month to assess dietary and lifestyle changes: BMI, BP, dietary patterns, physical activity

◎ THE NURSING APPROACH—cont'd

NURSING PROCESS	NUTRITION CARE PROCESS

Evaluation *Short term (at the end of the visit):*
- Verbalized his risk factors and the possible complications of developing hypertension
- Committed to taking his medication as prescribed
- Verbalized intent to quit smoking
- Identified heart-healthy foods
- Made follow-up appointment for 1 month

Goals met

Discussion Questions

1. Because it is difficult to obtain a true intake record, which question might be more effective? a. Do you use salt? b. For a typical meal, how many times do you shake salt onto a food?

2. Will it be necessary to provide support to this patient for the changes he is facing? Discuss.

3. If he asks, "Which is more important, eating better or quitting cigarettes?" what would your response be? Why?

⍰ CRITICAL THINKING

Clinical Applications—Role Play

Malnutrition is important to prevent or correct. Select two of the screening or assessment tools from the websites listed here. Invite a friend to help you. Conduct the two screening interviews and time yourself; do not rush the process. When you are finished, identify the pros and cons of each tool and its ease of use.

- Nutrition Risk Screening-2002 (NRS-2002): *http://www.sciencedirect.com/science/article/pii/S0261561403000980*
- Malnutrition Universal Screening Tool (MUST): *http://www.bapen.org.uk/pdfs/must/must_full.pdf*
- Mini Nutrition Assessment (MNA): *http://www.mna-elderly.com/*
- Short Nutritional Assessment Questionnaire (SNAQ65+): *http://www.fightmalnutrition.eu/fileadmin/content/malnutrition/Screening_tools/Snaq_65__engels_final.pdf*
- Subjective Global Assessment (SGA): *http://subjectiveglobalassessment.com/*
- Malnutrition Screening Tool (MST): *http://static.abbottnutrition.com/cms-prod/abbottnutrition.com/img/Malnutrition%20Screening%20Tool_FINAL.pdf*

Follow-up: review the tools found at *http://www.fightmalnutrition.eu/home-care/toolkit/*.

What will you do differently the next time you conduct a nutrition screening?

List three reasons why it is important to identify and correct malnutrition.

▮ WEBSITES OF INTEREST

Academy of Nutrition and Dietetics—Evidence Analysis Library
www.andevidencelibrary.com.
European Union: Fight Malnutrition Food-Drug Interactions
http://www.fightmalnutrition.eu/home-care/toolkit/

Food and Drug Administration: Food-Drug Interactions
http://www.fda.gov/downloads/Drugs/ResourcesForYou/Consumers/BuyingUsingMedicineSafely/EnsuringSafeUseofMedicine/GeneralUseofMedicine/UCM229033.pdf
National Center for Health Statistics, Centers for Disease Prevention and Control
www.cdc.gov/nchs/
Collects statistical data on every aspect of health status and use of health services by socioeconomic status, region, race or ethnicity, and other population attributes.
NCMND Center of Excellence for Nutritional Genomics, University of California, Davis
http://nutrigenomics.ucdavis.edu/
Useful website that addresses the human genome and interactions with diet.

REFERENCES

Academy of Nutrition and Dietetics, Evidence Analysis Library: *Critical illness nutrition practice recommendations.* From: www.adaevidencelibrary.com/topic.cfm?cat=4800. Accessed August 10, 2013.

Anthony PS: Nutrition screening tools for hospitalized patients, *Nutr Clin Pract* 23:373, 2008.

Ashwell M, et al: Waist-to-height ratio is a better screening tool than waist circumference and BMI for adult cardiometabolic risk factors: Systematic review and meta-analysis, *Obes Rev* 13:275–286, 2012.

Aziz EF, et al: Malnutrition as assessed by nutritional risk index is associated with worse outcome in patients admitted with acute decompensated heart failure: An ACAP-HF data analysis, *Heart Int* 6:e2, 2011.

Barker LA, et al: Hospital malnutrition: Prevalence, identification and impact on patients and the healthcare system, *Int J Environ Res Public Health* 8:514–527, 2011.

Best C, et al: The nutritional status of school-aged children: Why should we care? *Food Nutr Bull* 31:400–417, 2010.

Blackburn GL, Thornton PA: Nutritional and metabolic assessment of the hospitalized patient, *JPEN J Parenter Enteral Nutr* 1:11–22, 1977.

Blaikley C: Mind the Hunger Gap: a review of malnutrition in the community, *Br J Community Nurs* 10:S12–S14, 2012.

Browning LM, et al: A systematic review of waist-to-height ratio as a screening tool for the prediction of cardiovascular disease and diabetes: 0·5 could be a suitable global boundary value, *Nutr Res Rev* 23:247–269, 2010.

Burchi F, et al: The role of food and nutrition system approaches in tackling hidden hunger, *Int J Environ Res Public Health* 8:358–373, 2011.

Christakos S, et al: Vitamin D: Beyond bone, *Ann N Y Acad Sci* 1287:45–58, 2013.

Chumlea WC, et al: Prediction of body weight for the nonambulatory elderly from anthropometry, *J Am Diet Assoc* 88:564–568, 1988.

Gray D: Accuracy of recumbent height measurement, *JPEN J Parenter Enteral Nutr* 9:712–715, 1985.

Hallows SE, et al: The long and short of it: The role of telomeres in fetal origins of adult disease, *J Pregnancy* 2012:638476, 2012.

Heimburger DC, Ard JD: *Handbook of clinical nutrition*, ed 4, St. Louis, 2006, Mosby.

Jensen GL, et al: Adult starvation and disease-related malnutrition: A proposal for etiology-based diagnosis in the clinical practice setting from the International Consensus Guideline Committee, *Clin Nutr* 29:151–153, 2010.

Kyle UG, et al: Nutritional assessment and length of hospital stay, *CMAJ* 182:1831–1832, 2010.

Lee RD, Nieman DC: *Nutritional assessment*, ed 5, Boston, 2010, McGraw Hill.

Lefton J, Malone AM: Anthropometric assessment. In Charney P, Malone AM, editors: *ADA pocket guide to nutrition assessment*, ed 2, Chicago, 2009, American Dietetic Association.

Loenneke JP, et al: Blood flow restriction: an evidence based progressive model (review), *Acta Physiol Hung* 99(3):235–250, 2012.

Merrill RM, Richardson JS: Validity of self-reported height, weight, and body mass index: Findings from the National Health and Nutrition Examination Survey, 2001–2006, *Prev Chronic Dis* 6(4):A121, 2009.

Moore MC: *Pocket guide to nutrition assessment and care*, ed 6, St. Louis, 2009, Mosby Elsevier.

Mueller C, et al: A.S.P.E.N. clinical guidelines: Nutrition screening, assessment, and intervention in adults, *JPEN J Parenter Enteral Nutr* 35:16–24, 2011.

National Heart, Lung, and Blood Institute: *Clinical guidelines on the identification, evaluation, and treatment of overweight and obesity in adults: The evidence report*, Bethesda, MD, 1998, Author. (Pub No 98-4083).

National Heart, Lung, and Blood Institute: *Obesity education initiative*, n.d. From: www.nhlbi.nih.gov/health/public/heart/obesity/lose_wt/risk.htm. Accessed August 8, 2013.

National Institutes of Health, Office of Dietary Supplements: *Vitamin D: Fact sheet for health professionals*. From: ods.od.nih.gov/factsheets/VitaminD-HealthProfessional. Accessed August 8, 2013.

Nordin SM, et al: Position of the Academy of Nutrition and Dietetics: Nutrition security in developing nations: sustainable food, water, and health, *J Acad Nutr Diet* 113:581–595, 2013.

Shepherd AA: Nutrition through the life-span. Part 2: Children, adolescents and adults, *Br J Nurs* 17:1332–1338, 2012.

Skipper A, et al: Nutrition screening tools: An analysis of the evidence, *JPEN J Parenter Enteral Nutr* 36:292–298, 2012.

The Joint Commission: *2012 Comprehensive accreditation manual for hospitals: the official handbook (CAMH)*, Oakbrook Terrace, IL, 2012, Author.

The Writing Group: Nutrition Care Process and Model: Part 1, the 2008 update, *J Am Diet Assoc* 108:1113–1117, 2008.

U.S. Department of Agriculture: *Food deserts*, n.d. From: apps.ams.usda.gov/fooddeserts/foodDeserts.aspx. Accessed August 21, 2013.

White JV, et al: Consensus statement of the Academy of Nutrition and Dietetics/American Society for Parenteral and Enteral Nutrition: Characteristics recommended for the identification and documentation of adult malnutrition (undernutrition), *J Acad Nutr Diet* 112:730–738, 2012.

World Health Organization: *Physical status: The use and interpretation of anthropometry*, Geneva, 1995, Author. (Technical Report Series 854).

CHAPTER 12

Food-Related Issues

During trying times, food becomes very important, both physiologically and psychologically. It may be one of the few pleasant experiences patients encounter in a hospital. Having a special problem, such as not being able to eat orally or having a food allergy, can make the hospital stay quite stressful. The sudden onset of food poisoning can be frightening or even life-threatening. In addition, herbs or dietary supplements may cause unexpected interactions that must be addressed. Through all of these food-related issues, teamwork between nurses and dietitians can ease the stress and promote recovery.

http://evolve.elsevier.com/GRODNER/FOUNDATIONS

LEARNING OBJECTIVES

- Describe the nutritional therapy rationale for modified diets, including qualitative and quantitative changes.
- Explain appropriate interventions to resolve food allergy or food poisoning incidents.
- List the risks and benefits of TCAM (traditional, complementary, and alternative medicine).
- Distinguish between alternative medical therapies and integrative medical therapies.

- Summarize potential interactions of herbal dietary supplements with bioavailability of foods, nutrients, and drugs
- Compare and contrast enteral nutrition (EN) and parenteral nutrition (PN).

DIMENSIONS OF HEALTH

Food affects each dimension of health. Careful nursing supervision can ensure adequate nutrient intake to maintain or improve *physical health*. Effects can be detrimental when dietary supplements interact with medications and inadvertently alter the effects of medications.

The *intellectual* dimension is tested when nurses and caregivers have to observe patient intake, determine whether problems are caused by illness or food availability, and choose when to alert the clinical dietitian. Critical thinking skills are also needed to evaluate appropriateness of herbs and therapies that have been used by patients. The effects of non-oral feeding modalities also requires astute thinking by the nurse; side effects are often insidious, but the reactions must be quick and accurate.

Emotional health is challenged by the stress of dietary modifications that may be long term or permanent. Complementary nutrition approaches are often chosen to reduce anxiety when a patient is coping with a chronic disorder. *Social health* can be altered when patients are served meals in their rooms; they often feel isolated and eat less as a result. The same is true when a patient is given a tube feeding or parenteral nutrition. Instead of being able to eat orally, the patient experiences the loss of a basic human right. Beyond

this, food is significant for *spiritual health.* Many foods have religious significance, such as bread and wine used for Communion or matzoh used during the Jewish holiday of Passover. When such foods are restricted because of medical problems, patients may need spiritual or religious advice and support. When sensitive to these issues, nurses can help patients adjust and establish new meanings related to bodily and spiritual nourishment. The *environmental health* dimension may depend on having access to refrigeration to keep foods at their proper temperatures so as to reduce the risk of food poisoning.

DIETARY MODIFICATIONS

Sometimes dietary modifications are required to allow the body to heal, adjust to physical disability, or prepare for diagnostic tests or surgical procedures. Therapy may require texture changes to liquefied or pureed foods. Nutrients may also be modified, as when a low-sodium diet is used to lower blood pressure or when carbohydrates are restricted for diabetes management. Liquid diets are no longer mandated before surgery, but a patient with a wired jaw will need to sip liquids from a straw. If someone cannot or will not eat for a week or longer, a enteral (tube) feeding or parenteral (intravenous) nourishment may be needed. In the extreme, a patient may never again be able to eat orally. This chapter discusses typical hospital diets, enteral formulas, and parenteral nutrition.

DIET ORDERS

Specific diseases or conditions require modifications of the normal (regular, general, house) diet. Each modified diet has a purpose and rationale, and its use is usually determined by the physician or registered dietitian (RD).

Generally, doctors must order diets, including modifications. The Centers of Medicare and Medicaid Services (CMS) announced a rule change in May 2014 that would allow "privileged" RDs to independently order patient diets without requiring the supervision or approval of a physician or other practitioner, and to order laboratory tests to monitor the effectiveness of dietary plans and orders (see http://www.eatright.org/dietorders/). The rule applies only to RDs who are granted privileges by the hospital in which they work (i.e., "privileged registered dietitians"). Implementation of this CMS rule will expedite the correction of diet orders that are not effective for the patient because the RD would not have to request a change through the physician.

To appreciate the modified diets described in the following chapters, it is helpful to have an understanding of the basis for the diet order called "regular," "general," or "house" diet. The regular diet is designed to attain or maintain optimal nutritional status in people who do not require dietary alterations. Individual requirements for specific nutrients vary and are adjusted according to gender, age, height, weight, and activity level. A healthful regular diet is used to reduce risks for chronic diet-related diseases such as cardiovascular diseases and certain cancers.

Depending on individual food choices, a regular diet can be adequate in all of the recommended daily allowances (RDAs) of nutrients. In fact, the dietitian or manager who plans nonselect menus must document for regulatory agencies that the house diet meets these minimum requirements for good health. Dietary modifications of the regular diet may then be designed in two ways: quantitative or qualitative. *Qualitative diets* contain modifications in consistency, texture, or nutrients. *Quantitative diets* involve modifications in number or size of meals served or amounts of specific nutrients, such as "six small feedings" or "2-gram sodium" diets.

Whatever kind of diet orders a patient receives, the patient's acceptance is definitely influenced by nursing personnel. For example, if a caregiver expresses criticism about the food or its service, the patient is likely to do the same. Acceptance of the modified diet is also influenced by patient perception about food and nutrition as a part of medical therapy. Thus, genuine concern and education can make a difference. By explaining the rationale of why some foods are allowed and others not, the staff may enhance patient adherence to the modified diet. It is important to remember that food provides the energy and nutrients to heal and recover from illness. Food left on the tray does not help the healing process.

Food Service Delivery Systems

Nursing personnel are often on the front line of meal distribution. So it is important for them to understand how meals are prepared and delivered in health care facilities. Food service in a health care setting is the responsibility of the director of the food and nutrition services department. This person may be either an administrative dietitian or a specially trained food service manager. He or she is responsible for hiring, terminating, and supervising staff; ordering and purchasing food and supplies; delivering food to patients and staff; and overseeing quality improvements.

Clinical dietitians work with the food service director to assess patients' nutritional status, plan appropriate diets and nutrition intervention, and provide nutrition education. Other personnel from the food and nutrition department are cooks, clerks, dishwashers, aides, and dietetic technicians. Clinical dietitians may be members of the food service department or may work for a nutrition department, especially in larger facilities. Their jobs involve direct patient care.

Typically, only RDs (management or clinical) have the appropriate education and training in clinical nutrition with all of its contextual applications. Other nutrition team members work under the direction of the RD when it comes to the implementation of diet orders, altering nutrients, and making recommendations. Dietetic technicians registered (DTRs) work most closely with the RD in direct patient care services.

A selective menu system affords patients the feeling of some control over their lives while hospitalized. Even if the most nutritious meals are planned, malnutrition is a risk when patients do not eat well. A standardized house diet is planned, and then options are modified according to special nutritional needs. Some institutions provide selective menus for modified as well as regular diets. The menu for a modified diet lists only foods that are appropriate for that diet order, allowing a choice of foods that the patient will actually eat. If a selective menu is not available, simple changes or substitutions are allowed. See Figure 12-1.

Many hospitals offer hotel-style *room service* instead of pre-plated meal service delivered by carts to nursing units.

FIG 12-1 Selective menu planning often requires nursing assistance.

With this service, patients can order from their menu when hungry, and not just when mealtimes are scheduled. Greater satisfaction occurs when patients can choose when and what they eat within the constraints of a diet order (Marcason, 2012). (See the *Teaching Tool* box Assisting Patients with Menu Selections for more suggestions.)

Nursing personnel, on behalf of their patients, often interact with the staff of the food service system at their facility. It is useful to access the following information in your facility:

- Phone number or pager for the clinical dietitian to request assessments or education.
- Time schedule of meal service so requests or changes can be made *before* meal delivery.
- Location of the diet manual on the nursing unit, required by the Medicare Conditions of Participation for Hospitals and by The Joint Commission (TJC). The diet manual is the reference (usually in a three-ring binder or online) that describes the rationale and indications for using a specific diet; it lists allowed and restricted foods, and sample menus.

Meals in Long-term Care

Most of this information also applies to long-term care facilities, but there are a few additional concerns. Food service supplied to residents in long-term care facilities frequently relies exclusively on the food service department for nutritious foods and meals. Repetition and monotony also influence patient acceptance of foods and meals as served. Therefore, it is important that these patients be given food they can and will eat because they are at high nutritional risk. (See the *Personal Perspectives* box How We Should Care for One Another.)

✴ TEACHING TOOL

Assisting Patients with Menu Selections

When we select food items from a restaurant menu while socializing with friends or family, the process is fun. However, choosing foods from the restricted hospital selections, often with little descriptive information, can be a difficult and sometimes intimidating chore. Some hospitals are going to paperless menus, using palmtop computers for patients to make their selections. We are familiar with forms and computers that require us to choose quickly. Our patients may not share that ability and may need our help. Following are potential menu selection problems and possible solutions.

PROBLEM	SOLUTION
Patient is illiterate or too ill to read and write, or has reduced visual abilities or a low literacy level.	Read menu items to patient and mark his or her selections.
Patient does not understand the terms used on menu (menu names are not always common knowledge).	Clarify for patient or ask for clarification from dietetic technician, dietitian, or food service personnel.
Patient often must select foods from menu a day in advance, often resulting in delivery of too much or too little food (particularly a concern when appetite may be diminished from drug-nutrient interactions or the effects of the illness).	Remind patients they are selecting food for the next day. If they have not selected enough food, offer them foods kept on the nursing unit for snacks or order additional foods from food service. If they have selected too much food, cover, date, and store appropriate foods for use later in the day; discard if not consumed within 24 hours.
Patient does not understand why some of his or her favorite foods are not included on the menu, why smaller amounts are served, or why textures are modified. (Note that when we are ill, familiar foods are most desired and comforting.)	Discuss dietary concerns of the patient's illness, explaining why specific foods are not included or only limited amounts allowed. Menus are a great teaching tool for modified diets. Contact the dietitian to provide more education or counseling for patient.

👤 PERSONAL PERSPECTIVES

How We Should Care for One Another

Working in long-term care facilities made me aware of how important food is to all people. Every day, three times a day, the residents would make their way to the Dining Room for meals. Seated next to favorite friends, or sometimes newly admitted strangers, the social event of a meal was the highlight of their day. Whenever possible, serving meals family-style would make it more like home. Holidays were extra special, and guests would be invited for the festivities. The biggest celebrations were Thanksgiving, Mother's Day, and Father's Day. The Activities staff would have special musicians and singers come for the events. The meals were always beautifully prepared and served, with an emphasis on memorable choices and exquisite flavors. Knowing that the residents were living in their final "home" made us feel like a family. Our goal of adding comfort to their lives made the work very rewarding.

These experiences also prepared me to care for my own mother for the last five years of her life. During that time, she experienced the limitations of Parkinson's disease, hearing loss, cataracts, and a broken hip. In spite of these frustrating events, she maintained a bright outlook and her spiritual faith. Having her live with us deepened the empathy and compassion of our children, showing them a good example of how an extended family works and how we should care for one another … in good times and in bad.

Sylvia Escott-Stump
Winterville, NC

Basic Hospital Diets

For the appropriate content of diets served in your facility, check the diet manual. Table 12-1 lists the types of diets available in hospitals, some indications for and contraindications

TABLE 12-1 Types of Diets

DIET	INDICATIONS	CONTRAINDICATIONS	SAMPLE FOODS ALLOWED
Liquid diet	Provide oral fluids; before/after surgery; prepare bowel for diagnostic tests (colonoscopic examination, barium enema, and other procedures); acute gastrointestinal (GI) disturbances	Should not be used more than 24 hours; inadequate GI function; nutrient needs requiring parenteral nutrition	Broths, bouillon, apple juice, grape juice, gelatin made without fruit, 7-Up, ginger ale, coffee, and tea without milk/cream
Full liquid	Provide oral fluids; after surgery; transition between clear liquids and solid food; oral or plastic surgery to the face and neck; mandibular fractures; patients who have chewing or swallowing difficulties; esophageal or GI strictures; diarrhea	Dysphagia, wired jaw	Same as clear liquids and add all other juices, milk, ice cream, cooked eggs, eggnog, oral supplements, or milkshakes
Pureed diet	Neurologic changes; inflammation or ulcerations of the oral cavity and/or esophagus; edentulous patients; fractured jaw; head and neck abnormalities; cerebrovascular accident	Situations in which ground or chopped foods are appropriate	Any foods that can be blended and served without particles or strands that might cause choking Sufficient but not excessive fluids should be used for the blending process
Mechanical soft diet	Poorly fitting dentures; edentulous patients; limited chewing or swallowing ability; dysphagia; strictures of intestinal tract; radiation treatment to oral cavity; progression from enteral tube feedings or parenteral nutrition to solid foods	Situations in which regular foods are appropriate	All foods that are easily cut with a fork, chopped or blended Hard, stringy, or tough foods such as celery, broccoli, nuts, popcorn, and meat strands should be omitted because they may cause choking Depending on the reason for the modification, more foods might be eliminated or added back to the diet as the patient progresses
Soft diet	Debilitated patients unable to consume a regular diet; mild GI problems	Situations in which regular foods are appropriate	All foods served on the general diet with the exception of highly fibrous fruits and vegetables Most cooked or canned foods are acceptable choices Omit chewy, stringy, and tough foods

to the diets, as well as sample lists of allowed foods for each -.

Clear liquid diets. Clear liquid diets are used in preparation for gastrointestinal (GI) surgery or colonoscopy. A clear liquid diet consists of foods that are clear and liquid at room or body temperature, such as popsicles, plain gelatin, ice chips, and apple and grape juices. This diet helps prevent dehydration and keeps colon residue to a minimum. This diet is inadequate in protein, fat, fiber, and energy, so its long-term use is discouraged. Use of a clear liquid diet longer than a day can lead to compromised nutritional status and possible nutrient deficiencies. Your facility should have a policy that diet orders for clear liquid diets are valid for only 24 hours (similar to time-restricted orders for antibiotics).

Full liquid diets. A full liquid diet is one that consists of foods that are liquid at room or body temperature. It is used to provide oral nourishment for patients with wired jaws and those who have difficulty chewing or swallowing solid foods. Unlike the clear liquid diet, the full liquid diet offers more variety, and commercial nutritional supplements and milk

can be used to supply adequate amounts of energy and nutrients to make it nutritionally complete. Full liquid diets can be nutritionally complete if they are well planned and include between-meal snacks. Amounts of the diet consumed by patients should be monitored daily to ensure adequate energy and nutrient consumption.

Full liquid diets are excluded in most diet manuals but may still be ordered (Academy of Nutrition and Dietetics, n.d.). Because lactose-containing (milk-based) foods are included, patients who are lactose intolerant may experience nausea, vomiting, distention, or diarrhea when given lactose-rich liquids. Raw eggs should not be used in the preparation of any food served to patients, and patients and their families should be educated about the possible dangers of food-borne illness. Another special concern is for patients with dysphagia who cannot swallow thin liquids.

Dysphagia diets. Many patients require dysphagia diets after a stroke or with any other conditions in which swallowing is impaired. Signs of dysphagia include drooling, pocketing of food, choking, gagging, and taking longer than 2 to 10 seconds to swallow food. The National Dysphagia Diets begin with the most restrictive diet (pureed, often with thinned or thickened liquids) and progress back to a general diet if dysphagia improves (Heiss, et al, 2010). Level 1 is the Dysphagia Pureed diet; no coarse textures are allowed and foods are totally blended without lumps. Liquids are ordered separately, usually at pudding consistency. Level 2 is Dysphagia Mechanically Altered; foods are to be moist, softened, and easily chewed. Meats are ground and served with a gravy or sauce, or soft salads may be used (tuna or chicken salad, for example). Level 3 is Dysphagia Advanced; hard, dry, sticky and crunchy foods are omitted. Level 4 is a return to the general diet. Nurses should check with their institution's diet manual for the list of specific foods that may be served for each level of the dysphagia progression.

Mechanically altered diets.   When a patient has problems chewing or swallowing, foods can be chopped, ground, mashed, and pureed. Consistency of food can be varied according to the patient's ability to chew and swallow. The nurse, dietitian, and patient should work together to evaluate the patient's needs for modifying consistency according to the food preferences.

Some foods, such as mashed potatoes and ice cream, are already a smooth consistency. For other foods, small amounts of liquids (e.g., broth, milk, gravies) can be added to reach the appropriate consistency needed. Any liquid added to pureed foods should complement the food and should not conceal the food's original flavor. Care should be taken to add only enough liquid to achieve desired consistency yet allow the nutritional quality of the food to be retained.

Butter, margarine, gravies, sugar, or honey may be added to foods to increase kcal density. To make pureed foods more attractive, component pureeing may be used. For example, a cake-decorating tool (icing bag and tips) can be used to make pureed peas look like regular peas. Molds are also used to shape foods. A pork chop can be pureed and then put into a pork chop–shaped mold and reheated in a microwave oven.

The exact composition and consistency of a mechanically altered diet will vary according to the patient's needs. These diets can be modified for additional needs, such as low sodium, kcal control, and low fat. Care should be taken in evaluating the patient's needs for consistency. If a patient needs only meats pureed, then only the meats should be pureed. If a patient needs only ground foods, then they shouldn't be pureed. Sometimes, foods just need to be chopped coarsely or finely. Edentulous patients can often chew solid or soft foods.

Soft diets.   Soft diets are often used during transition from liquid diets to regular or general diets. Whole foods, low in fiber and only lightly seasoned, are used. Food supplements or between-meals snacks may be used if needed to add kcal. Soft diets can contain "hard to chew" foods such as white toast. This diet is not appropriate for patients requiring mechanically altered diets.

"Diet as tolerated."   Occasionally when patients are admitted, the physician writes an order for "diet as tolerated."

It is also common for this diet to be ordered postoperatively. It permits the patient's preferences and situation to be taken into consideration and also allows for postoperative diet progression at the patient's tolerance. This diet order provides an excellent opportunity for collaboration by the nurse, dietitian, and patient to plan and provide food that is eaten, tolerated, and nourishing.

Vegetarian diets.   A vegetarian diet is a normal diet but does not include meat, poultry, fish or seafood, or products containing those foods, and it can be healthful and nutritionally adequate if planned well (Craig, et al, 2009). A "Vegan" diet omits dairy products and eggs as well. Important nutrients that must be planned include protein, vitamins B_{12} and D, iron, zinc, and calcium. For patients who wish to follow this type of plan, the RD should be consulted. Note that Hindus, Seventh Day Adventists, Buddhists, and some other religious groups suggest following a vegetarian lifestyle.

OTHER FOOD CONSIDERATIONS

Food Allergy or Intolerance

A true *food allergy* is caused by the release of histamine and serotonin that can be reproduced in a double-blind food challenge (Ho, et al, 2014). These responses usually occur quickly, every time the food is eaten. In a hospital or nursing home setting, an allergic reaction can be quickly addressed if staff members know the typical symptoms and how to respond. The most common symptoms of food allergies are diarrhea, nausea, vomiting, cramping, abdominal distention, and pain. Although nearly 200 different foods have been known to produce an allergy or intolerance, only 8 foods (eggs, milk, wheat, soy, fish, shellfish, peanuts, and tree nuts) are major triggers in adults. Infants may react to cow's milk and soy, but most of them outgrow this sensitivity by age 4 years.

It is important to assess true food allergies (documented by a physician) versus food dislikes or intolerances. *Food intolerance* is a nonallergic reaction; it may be caused by toxins, drugs, or conditions such as lactose and gluten intolerances. Intolerances are often dose-responsive, occurring after a large amount has been consumed. Often patients state "I am allergic to milk" but will say they can use it on cereal; thus, they do not have an allergy. Most patients who are lactose intolerant can use treated milk (Lact-Aid), cheeses, and yogurt. Ask the RD to evaluate such patients further, as it is important to find ways to include calcium for individuals who are lactose intolerant. See Figure 12-2 for some of the more common diet orders that include allergens and food sensitivities.

Food Safety

Food poisoning can occur in any setting. Personal hygiene and hand washing are the most important factors in prevention. Food temperatures should be maintained below 40° F or above 140° F for safe food handling, storage, and holding. Refrigerators on nursing units should be checked regularly,

WHEAT FREE

DAIRY FREE

NUT FREE

GLUTEN FREE

SHELLFISH FREE

SUGAR FREE

LACTOSE FREE

EGG FREE

FIG 12-2 Common diet orders that may include food allergens.

and hot foods should be served to patients as soon as possible after they have been cooked.

Any protein-rich food (milk, eggs, cheese, meat/poultry/fish) should be discarded if left at room temperature longer than 2 hours. Items that are not consumed should be labeled and dated, then refrigerated and used within 24 hours. To prevent cross-contamination, refrigerators on nursing units should not mix drugs, personal foods, and patient foods.

A foodborne outbreak occurs when two or more individuals have the same symptoms over the same period—such as nausea, vomiting, diarrhea, abdominal cramping, vision problems, fever, chills, dizziness, and headaches. When there is an outbreak, it must be reported (by the food service director or director of nursing) to the local health department authorities. Suspected foods should be tested for microbial contamination.

The top causes of food poisoning are the norovirus, *Salmonella*, *Clostridium perfringens*, *Campylobacter spp*, and *Staphylococcus aureus*. The FDA Food Safety Modernization Act (FSMA), a sweeping reform of food safety laws, aims to ensure that the U.S. food supply is safe by shifting the focus of federal regulator from responding to contamination to preventing it (U.S. Food and Drug Administration [FDA], 2013). Preventive controls will be initiated from farm to table. The Centers for Disease Control and Prevention (CDC) website offers a useful pictorial at www.cdc.gov/outbreaknet/investigations/figure_food_production.html.

At the institutional level, all food service employees are taught about *HACCP (hazard analysis and critical control points)*. In HACCP, biological, chemical, and physical hazards from raw material production, procurement, and handling to manufacturing, distribution, and consumption of the finished product are controlled. This training discusses receiving, cooking, serving, and handing of high-risk foods and how to prevent illness. In-service sessions can be given to nursing staff upon request.

Cultural and Religious Implications of Food

It is important to ask a patient about cultural, ethnic, and religious beliefs and preferences related to food. All of us grow up in families and communities in which certain patterns and rituals are considered "the norm." Asking questions and understanding these individual needs and expectations are basic and important parts of the nursing assessment.

Cultural food patterns. Understanding the common food preferences and patterns used by different cultures helps nurses identify better food choices and reduce meal refusals. With the diversity of food choices in grocery stores and restaurants, Americans have adopted many foods into their daily lives that would have been considered "foreign food" to past generations.

Many older adults prefer simple choices and "comfort foods" over exotic and unfamiliar options. At the same time, enhancement of meals with simple herbs and spices (dill, onion, garlic, parsley) often helps increase intake for those individuals who have lost their sense of smell or taste. It is important to remember, as well, that medications and treatments such as chemotherapy alter taste buds. The patient who complains that the food "tastes lousy" should be given the opportunity to select something else during mealtimes to avoid the potential for nutritional decline. To read more about foods popular in various cultures, the following websites are useful.

- African American: www.cdc.gov/omhd/Populations/BAA/BAA.htm
- Asian: www.asiasociety.org/style-living
- Culinary History Timeline (social history, manners, and menus) www.foodtimeline.org/food1.html
- Health Resources and Services Administration's Cultural Competence website: www.hrsa.gov/culturalcompetence/index.html
- Indian Health Service: www.ihs.gov
- Mexican, Puerto Rican, and Cuban countries and their cultures: www.everyculture.com
- Native American and Alaskan Native: www.cdc.gov/omhd/Populations/AIAN/AIAN.htm
- Racial and ethnic populations: www.cdc.gov/omhd/Populations/populations.htm
- Think Cultural Health: www.thinkculturalhealth.hhs.gov/
- World Food Habits (resources for the anthropology of food and nutrition): http://lilt.ilstu.edu/RTDIRKS/

Religious implications for dietary patterns. Beliefs of several major religions include practices that affect or prescribe specific dietary patterns or prohibit consumption of certain foods. Individuals practicing these religions may or may not adhere to all of the customs. A brief review of some of these practices is found here.

Western and Near-Eastern Religions

Christianity: Some sects may not eat meat on holy days; others prohibit alcohol and caffeine consumption; see www.faithandfood.com.

Seventh-day Adventist: General restrictions of pork and pork-related products, shellfish, alcohol, coffee, and tea are followed. Some followers are ovo-lacto vegetarians, whereas others are vegans. See www.health20-20.org.

Church of Latter-Day Saints/Mormon: Alcohol and caffeine are prohibited or strongly discouraged. See www .mormon.org.

Islam: Pork and pork-related products are not eaten. Meats that are consumed must be slaughtered by a prescribed ritual called *halal*; these procedures are similar to the Judaic kosher slaughtering of animals, so Muslims may eat kosher meats. Coffee, tea, and alcohol are not consumed. During the month of Ramadan, Muslims fast during the day from dawn to sunset. See www.ifanca.org/index.php.

Judaism: No pork or pork-related products or fish without scales and fins are eaten. Dairy foods are not consumed with meat or animal-related foods (excludes fish). If meat or dairy is eaten, 6 hours must pass for the other to be acceptable for consumption. Animals are slaughtered according to ritual, in which blood is drained and the carcass is salted and rinsed; meat prepared this way is *kosher*. Preparation of processed foods must adhere to guidelines. Because meat and dairy must not mix, two sets of dishes and utensils are used at home and in kosher restaurants. Foods that are neither meat nor dairy are called *pareve* and labeled by food manufacturers. Additional customs affect food consumption on Saturday, the Sabbath, during which no cooking occurs. Fasting (no water or food) for 24 hours occurs during Yom Kippur (Day of Atonement). During Passover, an 8-day holiday, no leavened bread is consumed—only matzoh (made from flour and water) and products made from matzoh flour. Other symbolic food restrictions may be observed; see www.jewishvirtuallibrary.org/jsource/Judaism/kashrut.html.

Eastern Religions

Hinduism and Buddhism: Animal foods of beef, pork, lamb, and poultry are not eaten. Monks participate in fasting, as may some followers. Followers are lacto-vegetarians or vegans; see www.faithandfood.com.

Complementary-Alternative Medicine: Herbs and Botanicals

Nurses need to understand the benefits and risks of *TCAM (traditional, complementary, and alternative medicine)*, including efficacy, safety, harm, drug-supplement interactions, and appropriate referral sources (Leiby and Vazirani, 2012). TCAM consists of a cluster of medical and health care approaches, methods, and items not associated with conventional medicine (National Center for Complementary and Alternative Medicine [NCCAM], 2014).

Medical doctors and doctors of osteopathy practice conventional medicine (*allopathy*) and Western medicine, as do registered nurses, nurse practitioners, registered dietitians, and physician assistants. Some conventional physicians may also incorporate TCAM in their practices, often called an *integrative medicine* approach (Institute of Medicine [IOM], 2009). Previously, the efficacy of these therapies tended to

be anecdotal—based on the self-reported experiences of individuals. Well-designed studies continue to identify the efficacy of particular modalities for specific disorders, especially the active ingredients in herbs and botanical products.

The Eastern, traditional cultures base their system on the forces of nature, understood through the fundamental concept of *yin* and *yang*. Illness is viewed as an imbalance of these two forces, which are opposites of each other. Yin is dark, night, feminine, and contracting; yang is light, day, masculine, and expanding. The imbalance of these two forces affects *Qi*, the life force.

Acupuncture, energy work, body work, and herbal medicine have been part of traditional medicine for thousands of years. Eastern medicine treats the person as a whole, whereas conventional western medicine treats organ systems. The mind-body, nutrition, and exercise components of health are applied for daily wellness in the Eastern protocols.

Western culture has produced naturopathic medicine (NCCAM, 2013). The approach of naturopathic medicine is based on noninvasive, natural healing to recover from disease and to achieve wellness. This system incorporates techniques from Eastern and Western traditions. Techniques include acupuncture, exercise, massage, and dietary alterations. Some of the treatments conflict with evidence-based medicine, so there are controversies about some practices.

Herbs, botanicals, and dietary supplements, a component of TCAM, have become an everyday part of life for many Americans. To address this increased interest, the National Institutes of Health created the National Center for Complementary and Alternative Medicine. In a *person-centered therapeutic process*, both Western and traditional medical treatments should be considered to help people take better care of their own physical psychological and spiritual health, always guided by deep respect for individual autonomy, personal culture, religion, and beliefs (di Sarsina, et al, 2012). Box 12-1 shows some herbs commonly used by many people these days.

Complementary medicine refers to non-Western healing approaches used at the same time as conventional medicine (NCCAM, 2013). For instance, the patient who attempts to lower hypertension takes prescription medications (conventional) but also attends yoga classes (complementary) for physical and psychologic benefits. Alternative medicine replaces conventional medical treatment (NCCAM, 2013). An example is the use of herbal supplements to treat cancer instead of surgical intervention or chemotherapy. Integrative medicine merges conventional medical therapies with TCAM modalities for which safety and efficacy have been demonstrated by scientific data (IOM, 2009; NCCAM, 2013). Integrative medical centers under the direction of physicians and other conventional health professionals are available in larger hospitals.

Advanced practice nurses with a Master of Science degree in holistic health are often at the forefront of the integrative care provided. For example, a patient recovering from heart bypass surgery can be referred to a center for integrative medicine. Once there, a board-certified nurse practitioner

BOX 12-1 Natural Does Not Equal Safe!

Herbal remedies and dietary supplements are not regulated by the U.S. Food and Drug Administration (FDA), so the purity, potency, and safety of these products can and do vary. Manufacturers' claims of efficacy and safety are not subject to the rigorous testing that is mandatory for medications. Herbs and dietary supplements are likely to be contaminated with other herbs, pesticides, herbicides, and other products during growth, harvesting, preparation, and storage. Moreover, active chemical components in the herb may not be standardized, leading to dissimilar potencies from lot to lot, or even from capsule to capsule within the same lot. Safety, toxicity, and the likelihood of adverse interactions with other medications or treatments frequently have not been tested, particularly in children. Patients contemplating use of herbs and dietary supplements should proceed with caution and should seek out products only from reliable manufacturers.

HERB	TRADITIONAL USE*	DRUG(S) THAT INTERACT WITH THE HERB	ADVERSE EFFECTS/DRUG INTERACTIONS
Chamomile (English) (*Chamaemelum nobile, Matricaria recutita*)	Indigestion, reduction of tension and inducement of sleep, eczema, irritation of mucous membranes following chemotherapy or radiation (for cancer)	Anticoagulants: heparin, warfarin (Coumadin)	May increase bleeding time
		Benzodiazepines: alprazolam (Xanax), chlordiazepoxide (Librium), diazepam (Valium), flurazepam (Dalmane), lorazepam (Ativan), temazepam (Restoril), triazolam (Halcion)	Binds to benzodiazepine receptors, possibly altering effect of drug
		Central nervous system (CNS) depressants: alcohol, anticonvulsants, antiemetics, antihistamines, antipsychotics, antivertigo drugs, barbiturates, hypnotics, opioids, tricyclic antidepressants, paraldehyde (Paral)	May add to sedative effect
Chasteberry (*Vitex agnus-castus*)	Premenstrual syndrome (PMS), menopausal symptoms, amenorrhea, and other menstrual irregularities, fibrocystic breasts	Hormone replacement therapy, oral contraceptives	Herb binds to estrogen receptor, so may counteract oral contraceptives
Dong quai (*Angelica sinensis*)	Menstrual irregularities and menopausal complaints	Anticoagulants	May increase bleeding time; if using concurrently, obtain measurements of prothrombin time and International Normalized Ratio (INR) to rule out interactions
Echinacea (*Echinacea angustifolia, E. pallida, E. purpurea*)	Decrease duration of colds	Immunosuppressants: azathioprine, basiliximab, cyclosporine, daclizumab, interferon, muromaonab-CD3, mycophenolate, sirolimus, tacrolimus, corticosteroids	May decrease immunosuppressant effect
Ma Huang, Ephedra (*Ephedra sinica, E. equisetina, E. intermedia*)	Bronchodilator, decongestant, CNS stimulant, diuretic	Amitriptyline (Elavil)	Drug may decrease hypertensive effect of ephedrine
		Anticonvulsants	Sympathomimetic effects, which may interfere with drug
		General anesthetics	Concurrent use may result in arrhythmias
		Caffeine and other xanthine alkaloids	Increased effects and potential toxicity
		Monoamine oxidase inhibitors (MAOIs)	Increased sympathomimetic effects

BOX 12-1 Natural Does Not Equal Safe!—cont'd

HERB	TRADITIONAL USE*	DRUG(S) THAT INTERACT WITH THE HERB	ADVERSE EFFECTS/DRUG INTERACTIONS
		Antihypertensives: angiotensin-converting enzyme (ACE) inhibitors, alpha blockers, angiotensin II receptor blockers, beta blockers, calcium channel blockers, diuretics	Stimulant effect may decrease effectiveness of drug
		Insulin/oral hypoglycemic agents	Possible hyperglycemia with concurrent use
		Methylphenidate (Ritalin)	May displace drug from adrenergic neurons, possibly decreasing effectiveness of drug
		Morphine	Increases analgesic effect
		Oxytocin (Pitocin)	Possible hypertension
Evening primrose oil (*Oenothera biennis* L)	PMS, eczema, diabetic neuropathy, fibrocystic breasts, rheumatoid arthritis	Phenothiazines: chlorpromazine (Thorazine), fluphenazine (Prolixin), prochlorperazine (Compazine), promethazine hydrochloride (Phenergan)	May increase risk of seizures
		Anticoagulants	May increase risk of bleeding
Ginkgo (*Ginkgo biloba*)	Improvement of blood flow, protection against free-radical damage, attention-deficit/hyperactivity disorder (ADHD), dementia, macular degeneration, mental performance	Aspirin or Coumadin	May increase risk of bleeding
Ginseng American (*Panax quinquefolius*) Panax or Asian (*Panax ginseng*)	ADHD, stress reduction, chronic fatigue syndrome, fibromyalgia, age-related memory loss, menopausal cloudy thinking	Insulin/oral hypoglycemic agents	May enhance hypoglycemic effect
		Oral contraceptives/hormone replacement therapy	May alter effectiveness of exogenous hormones
		General anesthetics	Herb should be discontinued 7 days before surgery because it increases risk of hypoglycemia and bleeding
		Caffeine and other stimulants	Red ginseng (steamed) may be additive to stimulant effect
		Immunosuppressants	Ginseng has immunostimulant activity and should not be used concurrently
		Monoamine oxidase inhibitors (MAOIs)	Potentiates phenelzine, causing manic symptoms
Kava (or kava kava) (*Piper methysticum*)	Sleep disorders, antianxiety, tension headaches, menopausal anxiety, fibromyalgia	Alprazolam (Xanax)	Synergistic CNS activity of alprazolam
		Alcohol, tranquilizers (barbiturates), and antidepressants	May potentiate action
		Antiparkinsonian drugs	May increase tremors and make medications less effective
Senna (*Cassia senna*)	Laxative, weight loss	Any drug	May reduce intestinal absorption
		Antiarrhythmics	May potentiate drug effect
		Corticosteroids	May cause hypokalemia
		Digoxin/cardiac glycosides	May increase effects
		Diuretics	May interfere with potassium-sparing effect
St. John's wort	Depression, seasonal affective disorder	Theophylline and β_2 agonists	Possibility of increased anxiety
		Selective serotonin reuptake inhibitors (SSRIs)	Serotonin syndrome (sweating, agitation, tremor)
Valerian (*Valeriana officinalis*)	Sleep disorders, ADHD, menstrual cramps	Sedatives, barbiturates, CNS depressants, general anesthetics, thiopental	May intensify effects

*Not an exhaustive listing.

From Long S: Drug-nutrient interactions. In Schlenker ED, Long S, editors: *Williams' essentials of nutrition & diet therapy*, ed 10, St. Louis, 2010, Mosby.

or physician evaluates the patient and may recommend therapeutic massage for stress reduction and yoga for exercise to assist recovery. All services are provided within the same health care facility. Insurance companies have gradually increased coverage for such treatments, recognizing the cost benefits of many of these approaches.

Biologically based therapies encompass materials found in nature. These materials include functional foods, botanicals, and herbs. This category incorporates dietary supplements, alternative dietary patterns, and other treatments, such as shark cartilage for cancer treatment (NCCAM, 2013).

Functional foods include physiologically active (bioactive) substances found in food products. Functional foods provide good health through their physiologically active food components. These foods may have been modified to increase nutrient density, through being fortified, enriched, or enhanced (Academy of Nutrition and Dietetics, 2013). Some functional food components are marketed as dietary supplements, such as herb-enriched beverages. Care must be taken, though, because the amounts and sources of herb and other phytochemical ingredients are not sufficiently regulated (Lenoir-Wijnkoop, et al, 2013). A fruit juice beverage may contain the herb St. John's wort. However, consuming a small amount in a juice beverage is ineffective for depression treatment and pointless for any other purpose. Nonetheless, the development of new functional foods will continue because of the aging population, the increasing cost of health care, the growth of self-care, and food regulations (Lenoir-Wijnkoop, et al, 2013).

Dietary supplements are substances consumed orally as an addition to dietary intake. The ingredients of dietary supplements may include one or more of the following: minerals, vitamins, amino acids, herbs, plant extracts, enzymes, metabolites, and organ tissues. Dietary supplements are processed into various forms, such as tablets, liquids, capsules, extracts, powders, concentrates, gel caps, liquids, and powders; see Figure 12-3.

There are special requirements for supplement labeling. Under the Dietary Supplement Health and Education Act of 1994 (DSHEA), dietary supplements are considered foods, not drugs. DSHEA establishes a definition of dietary supplements as products that supplement dietary intake and contain one or more of the following (Center for Food Safety and Applied Nutrition [CFSAN], 2013):

- A vitamin or a mineral
- An herb or other botanical
- An amino acid
- A dietary substance for use to supplement the diet by increasing the total dietary intake
- A concentrate, metabolite, constituent, extract, or a combination of the preceding ingredients

On the basis of this definition, dietary supplements are to be considered foods; they are not drugs or food additives. This distinction affects the way they are regulated and actually eases the approval process. Drugs require more strident testing for safety and efficacy, and food additives must also meet more stringent criteria. Consequently, dietary supplements can enter the marketplace much more quickly with fewer data confirming their function.

Physicians and dietitians strongly recommend that nutrients be consumed together, through food rather than supplements. Supplements may be recommended as a safety net for groups at high risk for nutritional insufficiency: infants, children, teens, pregnant women, and the elderly. As a safety net, vitamin/mineral supplements at 100% or less of the Dietary Reference Intake (DRI) are appropriate.

Labeling of dietary supplements must follow the format used for nutrition labels (see Chapter 2). This means that the label needs to identify the product as a dietary supplement and must include the name and amount of each item contained in the product. Labels may also include approved statements of health claims such as are allowable on food product labels. For example, a claim may be made that a diet containing soluble fiber from whole oats and psyllium may reduce the risk of coronary heart disease.

Other health-related claims may also be made about the effect of the supplement on the "structure or function" of the body as well as on "general well-being." Claims related to reducing the risk of nutrition deficiency diseases are also acceptable. In addition, if claims are made, the label must include the statement "This statement has not been evaluated by the Food and Drug Administration. This product is not intended to diagnose, treat, cure, or prevent any disease" (NCCAM, 2013).

Application to nursing. Familiarity with alternative therapies is valuable. Acceptance without judgment provides support for patients in their quest for health. On the other hand, the nurse may be the first person to document the patient's use of products that could interact with other medical therapies or medications. Drawing attention to concerns such as these may prevent an unexpected medical incident.

It is possible that patients may use supplements instead of conventional medications because of high prescription costs. If this is the case, patients can be referred to social services or pharmaceutical company programs for financial assistance.

FIG 12-3 Dietary supplements may be consumed as liquids, capsules, extracts, powders, concentrates, gel caps, and powders.

Referral to registered dietitians for nutrition therapy involving dietary supplements or for general nutrition counseling is always an option. Health professionals and the public can consult the Academy of Nutrition and Dietetics website (www.eatright.org) for guidance on meeting specific health promotion or nutrition therapy goals. Additional concerns are discussed in the *Cultural Considerations* box Complementary Medicine and Cultural Implications.

🌐 CULTURAL CONSIDERATIONS

Complementary Medicine and Cultural Implications

Global Strategies

The global plan of the World Health Organization (WHO) provides guidelines for countries to develop national policies to evaluate and regulate traditional/complementary/alternative medicine (TCAM) to ensure its availability to populations throughout the world. The global plan supports strategies to expand the availability and uniformity of traditional medicine. Supporting this goal has led to a sharing of successful endeavors that adapt traditional practice to self-help approaches.

Application to nursing. One concern is that TCAM may be inappropriately applied when the benefits are translated from one culture to another. Nurses working with diverse cultural groups should become aware of the TCAM practices of their patients' culture of origin. A prime example is the herb *ma huang* (ephedra). In China, ma huang is used for a short period to reduce respiratory congestion. In the United States ma huang was marketed as a dietary aid to reduce weight and to increase energy potential, causing strokes, heart attacks, or death when used long-term.

Non-Oral Feeding

Any time the GI tract is used to provide nourishment, the feeding is a form of enteral nutrition. This includes liquid diets, soft and solid food diets, and special nutritionally complete formulas administered orally or via tubes. When a patient is not able to eat orally for more than a few days, a non-oral method must be used. If medical personnel talk about "enteral nutrition (EN)," they are referring to tube feedings.

Tube Feeding

Frequently, patients are unable or unwilling to consume adequate nutrients and calories orally. When this is the case and the GI tract is functioning, nutrients can be provided via feeding tubes placed into the alimentary tract. See the *Teaching Tool* box Tube Feeding the Infant or Child.

When the GI tract is functional, accessible, and safe to use, enteral feedings are preferred over parenteral nutrition because they are physiologically beneficial in maintaining the integrity and function of the gut. Enteral tube feedings are much less costly than parenteral nutrition for both the patient and the health care institution.

Tube feeding can be part of routine care when a patient experiences inadequate or reduced oral intake over the

✳ TEACHING TOOL

Tube Feeding the Infant or Child

Parents and caregivers need special support when their infants and children are tube fed. Assure them that the children can still be cuddled and can play without interfering with the tube nourishment. Teach the adults how the process works; they can be allies in helping young children accept and understand these procedures. Be sure to explain the procedures to the children as well. Dolls or stuffed animals can be used to explain how tube feeding helps speed the healing process.

Every infant and child has individual nutritional requirements based on growth needs and medical conditions. Check with the nurse or dietitian for appropriate rate, concentration, and volume of feedings. The following are some specific techniques to ensure adequate nutrient intake:

- Wash your hands with soap and water for at least 20 seconds (the time it takes to sing the "Happy Birthday" song twice).
- Flush feeding tube with 1-5 mL of water before and after each feeding, and before and after giving medications, to prevent the feeding tube from clogging.
- Never add new formula to formula already in the feeding container.
- Change the entire feeding setup every 24 hours.
- Place only 8 hr of formula or 4 hr of breast milk in the feeding container at any given time.
- Make sure your infant or child has pleasant sensations during feedings: Hold your child during feedings, and allow him or her to suck on a pacifier, sit in a high chair, and be a part of family meals.
- Give medications only in liquid form.
- Elevate the head of the bed 30 to 45 degrees if the child cannot be held.

Data from Cincinnati Children's Hospital Medical Center, *Nasojejunal tube feeding with enteral pump*, 2011. Accessed August 8, 2013, from www.cincinnatichildrens.org/health/info/abdomen/home/nasojejunal-kangaroo.htm.

previous 7 to 10 days. Other conditions warranting tube feeding are severe dysphagia, major burns, short bowel syndrome after resection, and intestinal fistulas (abnormal passages between the intestines). Conditions under which tube feedings are helpful, but not routine, include major trauma, radiation therapy, chemotherapeutic regimens, acute or chronic liver failure, and severe renal dysfunction.

Tube feeding is of limited value if intensive chemotherapy leads to GI tract dysfunction or if adequate postoperative oral intake is expected to resume within 5 to 7 days. If EN is not contraindicated (e.g., by hemodynamic instability, bowel obstruction, high-output fistula, or severe ileus), then the RD should recommend that EN be started within 24 to 48 hours after injury or admission to the intensive care unit (Academy of Nutrition and Dietetics, Evidence Analysis Library [EAL], 2013). The benefits of starting EN early include less risk for malnutrition, fewer complications, faster wound healing, and shorter length of hospital stay.

Types of formulas. For years, enteral formulas were prepared with the use of foodstuffs, vitamin/mineral preparations, and a blender. Today an extensive variety of commercially prepared formulas are used. Some formulas are nutritionally complete, some are formulated for specific diseases or conditions, and others (modular) provide specific nutrients to supplement a diet or other formula. Commercial products are preferred over hospital or home-blended solutions because they provide a known nutrient composition, controlled *osmolality* and consistency, and bacteriologic safety. They are also much easier to prepare and store. Many are nutritionally complete if consumed in the volumes recommended by the manufacturers.

Standard formulas. Standard (*polymeric*) formulas are composed of intact nutrients that require a functioning GI tract for digestion and absorption of nutrients. There are several categories of polymeric formulas that provide 1 to 2 kcal/mL. Standard formulas can be categorized into blenderized food products, milk-based products, high-kcal lactose-free products, and normocaloric lactose-free products. Normocaloric (1 kcal/mL) lactose-free formulas have low osmolality, which generally makes them well tolerated. Fiber-containing products are low osmolality and are used for patients with abnormal bowel regulation. These formulas contain fiber from natural food sources or soy polysaccharide.

Hypercaloric (1.5 to 2 kcal/mL) formulas are designed to meet kcal and protein demands in a reduced volume and have moderate to high osmolality. High-nitrogen lactose-free formulas (1 to 2 kcal/mL) are designed to meet higher protein demands at usual or increased energy needs. They have low to moderate osmolality.

Elemental formulas (predigested or hydrolyzed formulas) (1 to 1.3 kcal/mL) are composed of partially or fully hydrolyzed nutrients that can be used for the patient with a partially functioning GI tract, impaired capacity to digest foods or absorb nutrients, pancreatic insufficiency, or bile salt deficiency. These products are lactose-free and are usually hyperosmolar. They are not palatable and are best suited only for administration by tube. These products are used less often because most patients can tolerate standard formulas.

Modular formulas (3.8 to 4 kcal/mL) are not nutritionally complete by themselves because they are single macronutrients, such as glucose polymers, protein, or lipids. They are added to foods or other enteral products to change composition when nutritional needs cannot otherwise be met.

Specialty formulas (1 to 2 kcal/mL) are designed to meet specialized nutrient demands for specific disease states, such as diabetes, renal failure, liver failure, pulmonary disease, and human immunodeficiency virus/acquired immunodeficiency syndrome (HIV/AIDS). For critically ill patients, immune-enhancing formulas may be considered (EAL, 2013). These products contain omega-3 fatty acids, borage oil, antioxidants, and other additives. Some specialty formulas require additional supplementation with vitamins, minerals, or trace elements. Some are unpalatable, and all are more expensive than standard formulas.

Formula selection. The numerous types and brands of enteral feeding products on the market can make product selection a complex process. Whether a patient can digest and absorb nutrients indicates whether an elemental or polymeric formula should be used. Individual nutrient requirements determine the type and amount of tube-feeding formula. The RD will assist the physician with ongoing assessment of nutritional status and formula tolerance.

Feeding routes. Like the choice of an appropriate tube-feeding formula, selection of the correct feeding tube and feeding route involves consideration of various factors. If the tube feeding will be used for short duration, a nonsurgical placement can be made. If the feeding tube will be in place long term or permanently, surgical placement is necessary. Routes for tube feeding include the following (Figure 12-4):
Nasogastric: Tube is passed through the nose to the stomach.
Nasoduodenal: Tube is passed from the nose to the duodenum (small intestine).
Nasojejunal: Tube is passed through the nose to the jejunum (small intestine).
Esophagostomy: Tube is surgically inserted into the neck and extends to the stomach.
Gastrostomy: Tube is surgically inserted into the stomach.
Jejunostomy: Tube is surgically inserted into the small intestine.

Placing the feeding tube into the stomach, duodenum, or jejunum through the nose is the simplest and most commonly used tube-feeding technique. This technique is preferred for patients who will resume oral feedings in the near future. Feeding through a tube placed in the stomach simulates normal GI function but should be reserved for patients who are alert with intact gag and cough reflexes. Tube placement into the small intestine has less risk of aspiration, but elemental formulas are often required for easier absorption, and continuous feedings are better tolerated.

Surgical placement of the feeding tube is preferred when long-term use is anticipated or when obstruction makes insertion through the nose impossible. These procedures require surgery with general anesthesia. Placement of a percutaneous endoscopic gastrostomy (PEG) tube can be performed with minimal sedation and has fewer complications than surgical placement. PEG involves placing a feeding tube into stomach via the esophagus and then drawing it through the abdominal skin using a stab incision. Table 12-2 describes the classifications, advantages, and disadvantages of feeding routes.

Positioning. Unless contraindicated, patients should be positioned with the head of the bed elevated 30 to 45 degrees for tube feedings; this practice decreases the incidence of aspiration pneumonia and reflux of gastric contents into the esophagus and pharynx (EAL, 2013).

Method of administration. Proper administration safeguards delivery of the desired nutrients, enhances patient tolerance, and provides optimal nutrition support. Factors affecting decisions about appropriate methods of formula infusion include the patient's medical status and GI function, and the feeding route. Tube feedings can be administered by

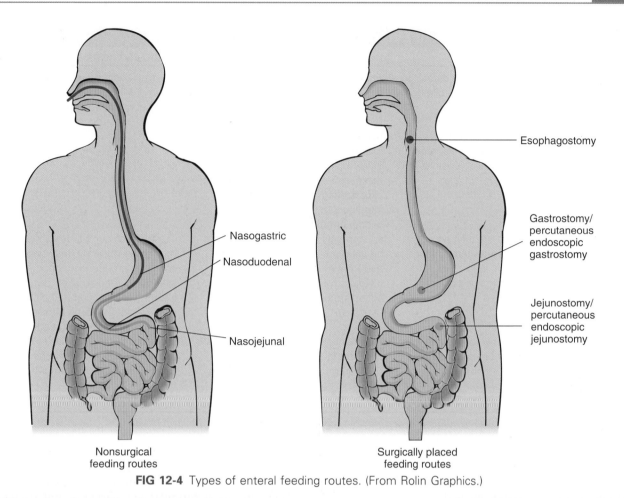

FIG 12-4 Types of enteral feeding routes. (From Rolin Graphics.)

TABLE 12-2 Advantages and Disadvantages of Enteral Feeding Routes

FEEDING ROUTE	CHARACTERISTICS	ADVANTAGES	DISADVANTAGES
Nasogastric	Tube extends from nose into stomach	Easy to place/easy to remove No surgery necessary Less expensive Medications can be administered	Greater risk of aspiration (compared with nasointestinal feeding) Gastric emptying must be monitored
Nasoduodenal or nasojejunal	*Nasoduodenal:* Tube extends from nose through pylorus into duodenum; tube must be advanced by peristalsis or videofluoroscopy *Nasojejunal:* Tube extends from nose through pylorus into jejunum and is usually placed by videofluoroscopy or endoscopy	Less aspiration (compared with nasogastric feedings) Helpful in patients with gastroparesis	Requires placement via endoscopy Gastric motility cannot be monitored
Gastrostomy or percutaneous endoscopic gastrostomy (PEG)	*Gastrostomy:* Tube placed through incision in abdominal wall into stomach *PEG:* Tube percutaneously placed in stomach under endoscopic guidance, secured by rubber "bumpers" or inflated balloon catheter	Intermediate/bolus feedings possible Patient comfort Size of tube allows medication administration and/or gastric decompression	Increased risk of aspiration in some individuals Stoma care required Potential for dislodgment of tube
Jejunostomy or percutaneous endoscopic jejunostomy (PEJ)	*Jejunostomy:* Types include needle catheter placement, direct tube placement, and creation of jejunal stoma that is catheterized intermittently *PEJ:* Weighted feeding tube (from PEG insertion) passed into duodenum; peristaltic action advances tube into jejunum	Early postoperative feeding possible Decreased aspiration risk	Smaller tube used, so tube may clog easily Stoma care required Intraperitoneal leakage possible Volvulus possible

Data from American Dietetic Association: *Manual of clinical dietetics,* ed 6, Chicago, 2000, Author.

TABLE 12-3 Administration of Enteral Tube Feedings

METHOD	INDICATIONS	ADVANTAGES	DISADVANTAGES
Continuous	Patients who have not eaten for a significant period; debilitated patients; patients with impaired gastrointestinal (GI) function; patients with uncontrolled type 1 diabetes mellitus; intestinal feedings	Feedings can be administered at constant rate over 24-hr period; feedings can be cycled (allows formula to be delivered over shorter period, allowing patients freedom of movement, and to promote oral intake if appropriate); gastric pooling minimized and fewer GI side effects experienced; continuous feeding into jejunum is similar to normal gastric emptying	Requires feeding pump if accuracy of volume delivered is required; continuous drip by gravity is possible, but less accurate
Intermittent	Feedings that are infused at specific intervals throughout the day (total volume of feeding divided and given 4-6 times/day)	Requires only simple equipment; can be used in home settings; may be more physiologic than continuous infusion; feedings can be administered by gravity over 30-90 minutes	In absence of pumps, feedings must be monitored vigilantly; may become time consuming depending on number of scheduled feedings per day; rate of intermittent infusion (rather than volume) seems to be a major reason for intolerance of tube feedings
Bolus	Appropriate *only* for feeding into the stomach; involves feeding large volumes of formula intermittently over short periods, usually by syringe	More manageable for the patient; rate of 30 mL/min or volume of 500-700 mL per feeding seems to be cutoff of physical tolerance	Associated with increased risk of aspiration, regurgitation, and GI side effects; not appropriate for postpyloric feedings

Data from Moore MC: *Pocket guide to nutrition assessment and care,* ed 6, St. Louis, 2009, Mosby/Elsevier.

three methods: continuous, intermittent, or bolus infusion. Table 12-3 summarizes indications for and advantages and disadvantages of each feeding method.

Continuous infusion is a common method of feeding. It provides controlled delivery of a prescribed volume of formula at a constant rate over a continuous period using an infusion pump. This method requires use of special equipment but is preferred when feeding into the small intestine; its effect is most similar to typical gastric emptying.

Intermittent infusion involves delivering the total quantity of formulas needed for a 24-hour period in three to six equal feedings. Each feeding is usually delivered by gravity over 30 to 60 minutes. This method represents a more normal feeding pattern, but patients often do not tolerate it if the rate is too rapid. Although equipment needs are minimal, this method is time consuming because feedings must be closely monitored to ensure proper delivery rate.

Bolus feedings involve infusing volumes of formula (250-500 mL) by gravity or syringe over short periods. This method requires minimal equipment and time but is associated with greater potential for aspiration, regurgitation, and GI side effects. It should not be used for intestinal feedings.

Starting the tube feeding. Before initiation of enteral tube feedings, placement of the feeding tube must be confirmed and documented. Tube placement is often confirmed radiologically after initial insertion. Thereafter, aspiration of gastric contents with a large syringe (60-mL) is used to reconfirm tube placement.

The high osmolality of a hypertonic formula can lead to GI distress such as intestinal distention and osmotic diarrhea. Diluting tube feedings will lengthen the amount of time necessary before nutritional requirements can be met. Therefore, most formulas are started at full strength but infused at a lower rate than goal. The rate of the feedings can be advanced to meet the desired volume, and then concentration can be gradually increased until kcal and protein needs are met.

Rate and concentration should never be advanced at the same time. If the feeding is not tolerated, rate or concentration can be reduced to the last level of tolerance, then gradually increased again. Other criteria to be considered to ensure optimal tolerance of the formula and safety of the feedings are solution temperature, prevention of bacterial contamination, prevention of aspiration, patency of tubing, administration of medications, and patient monitoring (Table 12-4).

Complications of tube feeding. Most problems in tube feeding can be prevented simply through the use of good hand washing techniques by the nursing staff administering the feeding. GI problems include diarrhea, nausea and vomiting, cramping, distention, and constipation. In past efforts to check for aspirated contents, blue dye was added to enteral formulas. However, the dye contributed to several deaths so should no longer be used to check for aspiration (EAL, 2013).

Mechanical complications consist of tube displacement or obstruction, pulmonary aspiration, and mucosal damage. Metabolic difficulties involve hyperosmolar dehydration or overhydration; abnormal (too high or too low) blood concentration levels of sodium, potassium, phosphorus, and magnesium; hyperglycemia; respiratory insufficiency; and

TABLE 12-4   Criteria for Safe Administration of Enteral Tube Feedings

CRITERION	CONSIDERATIONS
Temperature	Administer solutions infused by continuous drip chilled
	Administer intermittent and bolus feedings at room temperature to decrease incidence of gastrointestinal (GI) side effects
Prevention of bacterial contamination	Use closed feeding containers
	Prefilled, ready-to-feed closed systems are available for some products (less chance of contamination)
	Change extension tubing administration set and bag *daily*
	Never add new formula to old formula
	Do *not* hang feedings for longer than 4-8 hours
	Keep ice in pouch of bag at all times while formula is running
Prevention of aspiration	Check tube placement before administration
	Tubes placed into small bowel are associated with decreased risk for aspiration
	Head of bed (HOB) should be elevated 30-45 degrees
	Consider adding vegetable food coloring to formula to allow for detection of aspirated tube feeding from pulmonary secretions (*Remember:* This does not protect against aspiration)
Patency of tubing	Irrigate tubes every 6-8 hr with 40-50 mL of warm water (continuous feeds)
	For intermittent or bolus feedings, irrigate tubes after each feeding with 40-50 mL of warm water
	Flush tube with 40-50 mL of water each time feeding is stopped
	If tubing clogs, flush with 30-50 mL of warm water
	Systems are available that allow for self-flushing of the feeding tube (e.g., from Ross Laboratories)
Medications	Medications administered through the feeding tube should be in *liquid form*
	Flush tubing before and after giving the medication with 20 mL of water to prevent clogging
	If medication is not available in liquid form, consult the pharmacist *before* crushing or diluting the medication (some medications are pharmacologically altered by mechanical manipulation)
	Never crush time-released, liquid-filled capsules or enteric-coated medications
	Do *not* give sublingual medications through the tubing
	Because hyperosmolar liquid medications (KCl) may cause gastric irritation or diarrhea, dilute with water before administration
	Supplemental electrolyte preparations (KCl, NaCl, NaPO$_4$) increase the osmolality of the formula and may cause feeding tubes to clog
	Do not mix together multiple medications and deliver simultaneously unless the compatibility of the medications is known
	If feeding into the duodenum or jejunum instead of the stomach, check the effect of medication absorption
	Monitor patient response to medications given through the feeding tube, and make the changes needed
Monitoring	Confirm tube placement before initiating feeding and before each intermittent feeding
	Record urine glucose level every shift until final feeding rate and concentration are established
	Record gastric residuals every 4 hours (gastric feedings only)
	Record bowel movements and consistency
	Record tolerance to feedings
	Record daily:
	Weight
	Intake and output
	Record weekly:
	Serum electrolytes and blood counts
	Chemistry profile (including liver function tests, phosphorous, calcium, magnesium, total protein, and albumin)
	Nitrogen balance, if appropriate
	Reassess nutrition indexes weekly, adjusting energy and protein as needed

Data from Moore MC: *Pocket guide to nutrition assessment and care,* ed 6, St. Louis, 2009, Mosby/Elsevier.

rapid weight gain. Table 12-5 summarizes possible complications of tube feeding, probable causes, and suggested corrective actions.

Diarrhea, a common complication of enteral feedings, was once thought to be caused by the feeding solutions; however, other factors may contribute to this problem. Patients receiving tube feedings are frequently also started on liquid medications that contain sorbitol, which can cause diarrhea. Bacterial dysentery due to *Clostridium difficile* is also a common cause of diarrhea. Diarrhea should not be attributed to tube-feeding formulas until other causes have been ruled out.

Home enteral nutrition. The demand for home tube feeding has been growing steadily. Although it provides opportunity and convenience for patients, home enteral nutrition (HEN) imparts responsibility on the patient or home caregiver and involves risks that must be anticipated.

TABLE 12-5 **Complications of Tube-Feeding: Causes, and Corrective Actions**

PROBLEM	POSSIBLE CAUSE	CORRECTIVE ACTION
Gastrointestinal		
Diarrhea (defined as more than four bowel movements per day or liquid stools greater than 200 g)	Protein-energy malnutrition (PEM)	Switch to isotonic formula and feed at slow rate (will allow intestine to adapt to refeeding)
	Infection, microbial contamination of formula	Confirm with stool, blood, or formula cultures; limit hang time of formula to 8-12 hr, maintain ice in bag's pouch, change bag and tubing every 24 hr, and rinse after each bolus feeding or before filling bag for continuous feedings; use good hand washing technique
	Malabsorption	Check for pancreatic insufficiency, as pancreatic enzymes replacement may be necessary; change to low-fat, lactose-free, or elemental formula; change to continuous feeding
	Bolus feeding, volume overload, rapid administration, dumping syndrome	If infusion rate or concentration was advanced recently, return to previously tolerated rate/concentration; change to continuous feeding; decrease bolus volume and increase frequency of feedings
	Hyperosmolar formula	If started, reduce rate and increase gradually; dilute formula or change to isotonic product; if starting, rate should begin at 25 mL/hr, increasing every 12-24 hr
	Medications	Evaluate types of medications as primary cause (diarrhea has been related to administration of antibiotics and antacids, potassium supplements, cimetidine, and sorbitol-containing drops) and the possibility for change; stool samples should be taken for *Clostridium difficile* culture and toxin; change to fiber-containing formula
	Hypoalbuminemia	Albumin levels <2.5 g/dL result in decreased colloidal osmotic pressure* with accompanying peripheral edema (which may involve gastrointestinal [GI] tract); try peptide- based, low-fat formula with medium-chain triglycerides (MCTs)†
	Decreased bulk transit time and providing bulk	Fiber-containing formulas may help control diarrhea by normalizing GI
Nausea and vomiting, cramping, distention	High osmolality	Dilute formula to isotonic concentration if gastric residuals are consistently high; consider changing to isotonic formula
	Patient position	Reposition patient on right side to facilitate passage of gastric contents through pylorus
	Rapid increase in rate, volume, or concentration	Return to slower rate, and advance by smaller increments; advance only when current rate is tolerated
	Delayed gastric emptying	Stop feedings for 2 hr and check residuals; check residuals every 2-4 hr (continuous feedings) and before administration (bolus feedings); reduce fat content in tube feeding; consider transpyloric feeding; monitor for drugs or disease that may influence gastric or intestinal motility; ambulation may help
	Lactose intolerance	Change to lactose-free formula
	Cold formula	Warm formula to room temperature
	GI tract obstruction	Stop feeding immediately
	Excessive fat in formula	Change to low-fat formula
Constipation	Dehydration	Monitor intake and output; add free water if intake not greater than output by 500-1000 mL/day
	Decreased fiber	Use formula with fiber; make sure patient gets adequate water
	Medications	Evaluate medication side effects; suggest stool softener or bulk-forming laxative
	Inactivity	Increase patient activity if possible
	GI tract obstruction	Stop feedings
Mechanical		
Tube displacement	Coughing, vomiting	Replace tube and confirm placement before restarting feeding
	Dislodgement of by patient	Replace tube; restrain patient if necessary; use nasal bridle with small-bore tubes; consider alternate feeding route
	Inadequate taping of tube	Position tube; tape securely
Tube obstruction	Improperly crushed medication	Use liquid form of medication; medications should not be crushed without first checking with pharmacy; rinse tube with 20 mL warm water before and after giving medications

PROBLEM	POSSIBLE CAUSE	CORRECTIVE ACTION
	Medications mixed with incompatible formula	Review drug-nutrient interaction guidelines; flush tubing before and after adding medications
	Insufficient tube irrigation; failure to irrigate	Flush tubing with 20-50 mL warm water before and after bolus feeding, every 4-8 hr during continuous feedings, and whenever tube is disconnected or feeding is stopped
Pulmonary aspiration	Patient lying flat	Elevate head of bed 30-45 degrees during continuous feedings and for at least 30-60 minutes after bolus feedings
	Absence or weakness of gag reflexes	Feed into duodenum or jejunum
	Gastric reflux	May be caused by feeding tube, so change to smaller bore tube; feed into duodenum or jejunum
	Delayed gastric emptying	Monitor gastric residual; residual > 200 mL in patients with gastrostomy tubes and >100 mL in patients with gastrostomy tubes may indicate intolerance; hold feedings and recheck residual in 1-2 hr
	Improper tube placement	Confirm tube placement with radiology; reconfirm placement before each feeding and periodically during continuous feeding by injecting air into stomach and listening with a stethoscope
Mucosal damage	Extended use of large-bore tubes	Give conscientious mouth and nose care; consider changing to small-bore tubing or permanent gastrostomy or jejunostomy feeding tube
	Decreased salivary secretions caused by lack of chewing; mouth breathing	Moisten lips and mouth; let patient chew sugarless gum, gargle, or suck on anesthetic lozenges if appropriate
Metabolic		
Hyperosmolar dehydration	Hypertonic formula used without adequate water	Begin hypertonic feedings at slower rate; dilute with free water; or consider isotonic formula
Overhydration (fluid overload)	Refeeding patients with PEM; fluid overload	Restrict fluids; use concentrated formula
Hyponatremia	Congestive heart failure (CHF), cirrhosis; hypoalbuminemia; edema; ascites	Restrict fluids; administer diuretics; use concentrated formulas
	Excess GI losses	Monitor serum Na levels and hydration status, replacing Na as needed
Hypernatremia	Dehydration	Calculate patient's fluid needs: 35 mL/kg can be used unless patient's condition alters fluid needs, and <30 mL/kg for the elderly
Hypokalemia	Refeeding syndrome; insulin administration; diuretics; diarrhea	Monitor electrolytes daily, and replete with parenteral potassium
Hyperkalemia	Renal insufficiency; metabolic acidosis; anabolic metabolism	Reduce potassium intake; consider changing to a lower potassium tube-feeding formula; assess renal function
Hyperphosphatemia	Renal insufficiency	Use phosphate binder; consider changing formula
Hypophosphatemia	Refeeding syndrome; insulin administration	Replace phosphorus with parenteral supplement; monitor serum levels daily; once patient is repleted, monitor weekly
Hypomagnesemia	Refeeding syndrome; alcoholism	Replete with parenteral magnesium sulfate; monitor serum levels daily; once patient is repleted, monitor weekly
Hyperglycemia	Diabetes mellitus; temporary insulin resistance or insulin deficiency	Monitor blood glucose level frequently, and adjust insulin dose; reduce rate of tube feeding until blood glucose controlled; avoid formulas high in simple carbohydrates
Increased respiratory quotient; excess CO_2 production; respiratory insufficiency	Overfeeding (kcal), especially in form of carbohydrates	Balance kcal provided from fat, protein, and carbohydrates; consider using a higher-fat formula or adding modular fat
Rapid, excessive weight gain	Excess kcal, excess fluids, electrolyte balance	Decrease concentration or amount of formula; evaluate electrolyte status

*Pressure difference between the osmotic pressure of blood and that of tissue fluid or lymph; it is an important force in maintaining balance between blood and surrounding tissue and is usually caused by large particles such as protein molecules that will not pass through a membrane. This is also called oncotic pressure.

†Distinguished from other triglycerides by having 8 to 10 carbon atoms. MCTs are easily digested.

Data from Moore MC: *Pocket guide to nutrition assessment and care*, ed 6, St. Louis, 2009, Mosby/Elsevier; Mueller C, Bloch AS: Intervention: Enteral and parenteral nutrition support. In Mahan LK, Escott-Stump S, editors: *Krause's food & nutrition therapy*, ed 12, St. Louis, 2008, Saunders.

In addition to criteria already discussed, requirements that should be considered in the decision to send a patient home on EN include the following:

- Patient's nutritional needs cannot be met orally.
- Appropriate enteral access is in place and functioning, and patient is tolerating tube-feeding regimen.
- Patient and/or significant other are able and willing to perform HEN techniques safely and effectively.
- Underlying disease state is stable, and patient is ready for discharge and can be monitored in the home setting.
- Affordable HEN supplies are available.

Once a patient is considered an appropriate candidate for HEN, the nutrition care plan must be modified to an appropriate home plan that includes tailoring the enteral formula, route and method of administration, and feeding schedule.

The amount or type of formula may need to be adjusted to meet the patient's long-term nutritional requirements.

Homemade blenderized formulas are strongly discouraged because of reasons previously discussed. Feeding schedules may need to be arranged around family members' schedules or other daily routines. They should be planned to augment patient comfort and convenience and to maximize nutritional benefit.

The patient should be stabilized on the home feeding regimen while still hospitalized before patient education is initiated. Education should include oral instructions, written guidelines, staff demonstration, return demonstration by the patient and caregiver, and their assumption of full responsibility for tube feeding before the patients is discharged. Figure 12-5 shows an example of an HEN training checklist.

PURPOSE AND INSTRUCTIONS: This checklist will assist in identifying instructional responsibilities and aid in training patients in the skills needed for performing home enteral nutrition (HEN).

The nurse and dietitian will jointly instruct the patient on tube feeding administration and cares.

Date and initial section when instruction/demonstration is completed.

RNs: Document training in Nursing Notes.
RDs: Document training in Progress Notes.

STAGE I: INITIATION OF HEN PROGRAM

———— Patient assessment   (Dietitian-Nurse)
        Medical-social-nutritional history
———— Plan of care outlined   (Dietitian-Nurse)
———— Identification of dismissal date ———————————————— (Nurse)
———— Home enteral coordinator notified   (Dietitian)

STAGE II: IMPLEMENTATION OF HEN TRAINING   (Dietitian)

INTRODUCTION TO HEN PROGRAM   (Dietitian)

———— Discuss purpose
———— Introduce manual *Instructions for Tube Feeding at Home*

EQUIPMENT   (Dietitian-Nurse)
Discuss purpose, assembly, use, care, and cleaning of equipment.

	Discuss	Demonstrate	Patient Demonstrate
Feeding tube	————	————	————
Feeding bag	————	————	————
Gavage syringe	————	————	————
Enteral pump (if needed)	————	————	————

FORMULA—FLUIDS   (Dietitian)
————Show formula.
————Discuss purpose, type, amount, formula concentrations, fluid needs.
————Discuss preparation.
————Discuss administration schedule.
————Discuss weight expectations.

FIG 12-5 Home enteral training checklist. (From Nelson JK, Weckwerth JA: Home enteral nutrition. In Skipper A, editor: *Dietitian's handbook of enteral and parenteral nutrition*, Rockville, MD, 1989, Aspen.)

Patients should also be referred to a source for obtaining supplies such as formula and administration equipment before discharge. Some patients may need help in obtaining financial assistance for purchase of supplies. Most often, referral to home health agencies provides the necessary supplies, equipment, and staff for home follow-up visits, as well as assistance with third-party payers.

Parenteral Nutrition

Fortunately, there are alternatives for providing nutrients to patients when they can't or won't eat and tube feedings are contraindicated. Parenteral nutrition (PN) involves the provision of energy and nutrients intravenously. When nutrients are infused into a large-diameter vein, such as the superior vena cava or subclavian vein (Figure 12-6), the method is called central parenteral nutrition (CPN) or total parenteral nutrition (TPN). When a smaller, peripheral vein is used (usually in the forearm), parenteral nutrition is called peripheral parenteral nutrition (PPN).

CPN may mean the difference between life and death for patients who cannot be adequately nourished via the GI tract. Factors that should be considered before initiating CPN are the nature of the patient's GI dysfunction, severity of malnutrition, degree of hypercatabolism, medical prognosis, and wishes.

Components of Parenteral Nutrition Solutions

PN solutions contain the same nutrients and components found in any enteral nutrition source: water, amino acids, dextrose, electrolytes, vitamins, and trace elements. Fat is also included, often by means of piggyback administration or by adding it directly to the PN solution (usually called a three-in-one solution).

Carbohydrates. The most common carbohydrate used in PN is dextrose monohydrate. Used as an energy source, it yields 3.4 kcal/g because of its hydrated form. Dextrose solutions are available in initial concentrations of 5% through 70%. Higher glucose concentrations are useful when a patient's fluids need to be restricted; lower concentrations are often used to help control hyperglycemia. Concentrations greater than 10% (final concentration) are hypertonic and must be delivered via the larger central vein.

Amino acids. Protein is provided in PN solutions as a mixture of essential and nonessential crystalline amino acids that are available with or without added electrolytes. It is important that the amino acids be used for protein synthesis and not as an energy (kcal) source. Amino acid solutions are available in different concentrations as well as in various of amino acid compositions.

Fats. Intravenous (IV) lipid emulsions are used as concentrated energy sources and to prevent development of an essential fatty acid (EFA) deficiency. Commercial lipid emulsions are formulations of safflower oil, soybean oil, or a combination of the two, with glycerol added for isotonicity and egg phospholipid added as an emulsifying agent. The kcal density of lipid solutions is useful when volume restriction is necessary. A 10% fat emulsion yields 1.1 kcal/mL or 550 kcal per 500-mL bottle, and a 20% solution yields 2 kcal/mL or 1000 kcal per 500-mL bottle. Use of lipids increases calories without increasing osmolality as much.

Traditionally, lipid emulsions have been delivered peripherally with a piggyback system. Baseline serum triglyceride levels should be confirmed before administration of IV lipid emulsions and should be monitored according to institutional policy. If a lipid profile is ordered for a patient receiving lipids, the patient should not have received lipid emulsion for the 12 hours before the blood specimen is drawn.

Total nutrient admixtures. When lipid emulsions are added to dextrose and amino acid mixtures, the resulting solution is called a three-in-one mixture, or a total nutrient admixture (TNA) (Figure 12-7). Such solutions allow lipid infusion over 24 hours, decreasing carbon dioxide production and reducing hepatic accumulation of fat.

FIG 12-6 Placement of catheter for central parenteral nutrition, via the subclavian vein to the superior vena cava. (From Rolin Graphics.)

From IV feeder
Subclavian vein
Incision
Catheter inside superior vena cava

FIG 12-7 A three-in-one solution includes dextrose, amino acids, and lipids. (From Morgan SL, Weinsier RL: *Fundamentals of clinical nutrition*, ed 2, St. Louis, 1998, Mosby.)

Electrolytes. Electrolytes and minerals can be provided by the general amino acid solution or as a combined electrolyte concentrate, or they can be added separately as individual salts. Commercial electrolyte solutions are available. Magnesium, phosphate, and potassium requirements must be monitored carefully to prevent overfeeding and underfeeding of malnourished individuals.

Vitamins. Adult and pediatric multivitamin formulations for IV use are commercially available. In clear vitamin deficiency, multiples of daily doses can be given in accordance with clinical status. The FDA has amended its PN multivitamin requirements to increase amounts of thiamin, vitamins B_6 and C, and folic acid as well as adding 150 μg vitamin K (Shearer, 2009).

Trace elements. Trace element formulations contain zinc, copper, manganese, chromium, and selenium. Already combined commercial solutions may be used, or an institutional pharmacy may develop its own IV injectable formula.

Bioactive substances. Evidence suggests that additives such as prebiotics or probiotics, antioxidants, and glutamine may benefit certain patients. An individual assessment must be done.

Peripheral Parenteral Nutrition

PPN solutions composed of more than 10% (final concentration) dextrose and/or more than 5% (final concentration) amino acids are hypertonic and can be administered only into central veins. These solutions administered via peripheral veins must be isotonic to prevent damage to the veins. Isotonic PN solutions usually contain 5% to 10% dextrose (final concentration) and 3% to 5% amino acids, plus electrolytes, vitamins, minerals, and fat as needed. PPN is most often used when only short-term nutrition support is needed.

Monitoring Guidelines and Complications

Monitoring needs and protocols vary among institutions and patient populations. Frequency of monitoring ranges from every 6 hours to a one-time baseline reading, from biweekly to "as needed." Specific parameters and recommendations are listed in Box 12-2.

As with enteral tube feedings, complications can occur with PN. Most can be averted by following the recommendations for monitoring. Others can be circumvented by adhering to stringent technique. Technical complications are related to catheter placement; pneumothorax can be prevented by careful insertion of the central line using proper technique. Septic complications, like technical complications, are not unique to parenteral nutrition. Infections can be local or systemic, and they usually occur because of poor technique in aseptic catheter care. Metabolic complications are common because metabolic requirements (electrolytes and energy) differ from patient to patient. Hyperglycemia is common and can be treated by administering insulin or by adding it to the solution, reducing the dextrose load, or ensuring that the total calorie load is not excessive. Box 12-3 summarizes possible complications.

BOX 12-2   Monitoring Patients Receiving Central Parenteral Nutrition (CPN)

Every 8 Hours
Vital signs
Temperature
Urine fractionals

Daily
Weight
Fluid intake and output
Serum electrolytes, glucose, creatinine, blood urea nitrogen (BUN) until stable; then twice weekly

Weekly
Serum magnesium, calcium, phosphorus, albumin
Liver function tests
Complete blood count
Review of actual oral, enteral, and CPN intake

Fluid Disorders
Urine sodium or fractional sodium excretion
Serum osmolality
Urine specific gravity

Protein Status
Nitrogen balance, serum prealbumin

Lipid Disorders
Serum triglycerides or lipid clearance test
Respiratory quotient
Essential fatty acids (if fat-free CPN is necessary)

Hepatic Encephalopathy
Plasma amino acids

Gastrointestinal Losses
Serum trace elements
Stool electrolytes

Respiratory Compromise
$PaCO_2$
Indirect calorimetry, respiratory quotient

Acid-Base Disorders
Blood pH
Anion gap

Long-Term CPN
Body composition measures
Serum trace elements, vitamins

From Lenssen P: Management of total parenteral nutrition. In Skipper A, editor: *Dietitian's handbook of enteral and parenteral nutrition,* ed 2, Rockville, MD, 1998, Aspen.

Home Parenteral Nutrition

Home parenteral nutrition (HPN) enables selected patients who depend on PN to return to a reasonably normal lifestyle. A specialized catheter is used to reduce possibility of infection. The catheter is placed through a tunnel under the skin and exits the chest at a place where the patient or caretaker can care for it conveniently. As with HEN, HPN requires that

BOX 12-3 Complications of Parenteral Nutrition

Technical Complications
Pneumothorax
Malposition of catheter
Subclavian artery puncture
Carotid artery puncture
Catheter embolism
Air embolism
Catheter obstruction
Thrombosis

Septic Complications
Catheter-related sepsis
Septic thrombosis

Metabolic Complications
Hyperglycemia
Hyperglycemic hyperosmolar nonketotic dehydration
Hypoglycemia
Hyperkalemia
Hypophosphatemia
Hypocalcemia

Transitional Feedings

A period of adjustment, or weaning, is necessary before discontinuation of nutritional support or for conversion from one form of nutritional support to another. Transition to an adequate oral intake to maintain nutritional status differs from patient to patient. Although the GI tract responds quickly to enteral feeding, patients who have been receiving CPN usually have decreased appetites and it may take 1 to 2 weeks after complete cessation of CPN for them to feel hungry. This early satiety necessitates gradual weaning from PN as oral or tube feeding progresses to ensure continued adequate intake. Moreover, stopping CPN too quickly can result in hypoglycemia.

Parenteral Nutrition to Oral or Tube Feeding

Long periods of PN without enteral feedings result in atrophy of the GI tract. If not contraindicated, minimal enteral intake (sips of dilute fruit juice) helps maintain normal GI tract physiology and gut mucosal immunity. Before weaning from PN, judicious assessment of GI function is recommended to prevent problems with delayed gastric emptying, nausea, vomiting, or diarrhea. As PN is tapered and oral or tube-feeding intake increases, it is important to document actual enteral intake, including fluids, to facilitate nutrient sufficiency. If oral feedings or isotonic formulas are not well tolerated, an elemental formula may be needed.

Tube Feeding to Oral Feeding

In addition to documentation of intake per tube and orally, it will be important to assess the patient's swallowing ability before offering oral feedings. A full liquid diet is usually offered first, followed by pureed or soft foods. Tube feedings should be stopped at least 1 hour before and after mealtime to promote appetite. As oral intake increases, tube-feeding volume should be decreased. When oral intake consistently exceeds two thirds of energy requirements, the tube feedings can be discontinued.

both patient and caregiver are willing and able to perform daily procedures involved in administering the PN, which include monitoring laboratory values, temperature, weights, glucose measurements, and fluids. Home health care agencies may be used to provide equipment, supplies, and services.

Patients may be scheduled to receive HPN at night during sleep (cyclic CPN) to allow freedom to leave home or even work during the day. Sometimes, if the GI tract is functional, HPN is administered only on selected nights per week to supplement oral intake. Although expensive, HPN costs less than hospitalization, allows the patient to leave the hospital sooner, and in many cases allows the patient to resume a productive lifestyle.

SUMMARY

- All patient nutrition is provided through food service delivery systems of acute care hospitals and long-term care facilities.
- Staff includes a director of the food and nutrition services department, clinical dietitians, as well as cooks, clerks, dishwashers, aides, and dietetic technicians, registered.
- To provide nutritional therapy, regular or modified diets are developed to meet specific needs of patients as determined by the physician or registered dietitian.
- Qualitative diet changes include modifications in consistency, texture, or nutrients.
- Quantitative diet changes include modifications in size and number of meals served or amounts of specific nutrients.

- Incidents related to food allergy or food poisoning require appropriate interventions to address those incidents while promoting rapid recovery and a continuation of the healing process.
- TCAM is a significant component of health care in the United States.
- TCAM consists of a cluster of medical and health care approaches, methods, and items not associated with conventional medicine.
- Complementary medicine refers to non-Western healing approaches used at the same time as conventional medicine.
- Alternative medicine replaces conventional medical treatment.

- Integrative medicine merges conventional medical therapies with TCAM modalities for which safety and efficacy have been demonstrated by scientific data.
- Use of herbs as dietary supplements or as natural medications can interact with bioavailability of foods, nutrients, and drugs.
- Dietary supplements are substances consumed orally as an addition to dietary intake.
- The Dietary Supplement Health and Education Act of 1994 regulates supplement identity, potency, contents, and labeling under the supervision of the U.S. Food and Drug Administration.
- Supplement use has grown substantially and may interact with other medications and treatments.
- Oral and tube feedings are the preferred methods of nutritional intake.
- Feeding patients via the GI tract is safer, is easier to administer, aids in maintaining GI tract integrity, and is much less expensive than parenteral nutrition (PN).

- Commercial tube-feeding products supply intact nutrients and are readily available.
- When tube feedings are administered in the appropriate volume, 100% of the daily requirements for vitamins and minerals can be provided, as well as adequate amounts of energy and protein.
- When patients are unable to obtain nutrition by oral or tube feeding, parenteral nutrition can literally be lifesaving.
- Peripheral or central infusions of amino acids, dextrose, fat emulsions, vitamins, and minerals can provide the ordinary or extraordinary nutrient needs of patients.
- When managed through a team approach and routine monitoring, PN can provide a safe vehicle for meeting patients' nutritional goals.
- By working together, nurses and dietetic professionals can most efficiently meet the nutritional and medical needs of patients.

◎ THE NURSING APPROACH

Empathy and Dietary Teaching: Experiencing Modified Diets

An effective way for nursing students to learn about medical nutrition is to research modified dietary pattern guidelines and resources for specific disorders and conditions and then experience these diets personally. Following a modified diet even for 1 day provides students empathy with patients who need to change their regular eating habits and adhere to special dietary intakes. This dietary experience also supplies nursing students with strategies to reinforce teaching by dietitians.

Purposes of the Experience
- Experience a modified diet (for health promotion or nutrition therapy) for 1 day (24 hours).
- Identify components or principles of the diet and the specific foods allowed or restricted.
- Gain empathy for patients who are beginning nutrition therapy for disorders or conditions and need to adhere to modified dietary patterns.
- Reflect on teaching ideas for use with patients on the basis of this experience.

Choose One Diet and Follow It for a 24-Hour Period or Longer
- High fiber and adequate liquid (for diverticulosis)
- Gluten-free (for celiac disease)
- Carbohydrate counting (for diabetes)
- Dietary Approaches to Stop Hypertension (DASH) diet (for hypertension)

Answer These Questions
1. List three health problems that may make this diet modification necessary or desirable.
2. What general guidelines were followed?
   a. What types of food were consumed?
      (1) Food groups and temperature of foods; textures, such as solid, pureed, or liquid.
      (2) Examples of foods.

b. What amounts of food were consumed? Number of calories or specific measurements.
   c. At what time of day were foods consumed? Create a food diary. Include times and types of meals (e.g., breakfast, 7 AM).
      (1) What foods/beverages were avoided or restricted? List specific foods/beverages.
      (2) Rationale.
3. What resources besides this textbook were used to learn about the diet? Were any Internet sites especially useful?
4. What was your experience?
   a. How did you feel physically and/or emotionally?
   b. What did you learn by paying attention to food labels?
   c. What surprised you the most about this diet?
   d. What foods were challenging to include or eliminate?
   e. What were other personal barriers that made following this diet difficult?
5. Are there special dietary products that may help people with this diet?
   a. Are special products needed? Why?
   b. What products (helpful or not) are available?
   c. Which of these products would you buy if on this diet for a month?
6. What are the pros and cons of this diet?
   a. Benefits
   b. Disadvantages and/or risks
7. What aspect of this experience gave you empathy for a patient who is following this diet?
   a. What dietary guidelines would be especially difficult if you followed this diet for 1 month? Why (e.g., cost, not wanting to be different from peers)?
   b. Was it necessary to learn a large amount of new information? Explain the steps taken to gain this information.
   c. Would it be difficult to follow this diet indefinitely? Discuss.

◎ THE NURSING APPROACH—cont'd

8. How would you teach a patient about this diet?
   a. What would you do to promote understanding of this diet (which foods and why)?
   b. What patient education materials would assist a patient to make wise food choices?

   c. What would be a reasonable goal that a patient could successfully achieve by the end of the first week?
   d. What would you recommend as the first step a patient should take when beginning this dietary pattern?

？ CRITICAL THINKING #1*

Clinical Applications

Faye, a 20-year-old student from Germany, seeks medical attention at the urging of her roommates, who report that her mood has become increasingly depressed during the past two semesters. She has become withdrawn and moody—a significant change from her affect since first coming to the United States to attend college. She is otherwise healthy. Faye reports a 5-pound weight loss during the past 3 months. She takes oral contraceptives for regulation of menses. Her mother has been treated for depression with *Hypericum perforatum* (St. John's wort) by the family physician for the past 10 years. Faye reports smoking a pack of cigarettes per day. Plans are to treat her with 50 mg sertraline (Zoloft) per day and to provide counseling therapy. During the diet history, the dietitian asks Faye whether she uses any over-the-counter vitamins, minerals, or herbal supplements. She tells the dietitian that her mother suggested she try St. John's wort because in Germany it is prescribed to treat depression. Faye did as her mother suggested because it is available without prescription in the United States.

1. Faye's depression will be treated with sertraline, a selective serotonin reuptake inhibitor (SSRI). How do SSRIs work?
2. What is St. John's wort?
3. How is St. John's wort used in the United States? How is it regulated?
4. How does St. John's wort work as an antidepressant?
5. Does St. John's wort have any side effects?
6. How is St. John's wort used in Europe?
7. Why do you think people are interested in alternative medicine and herbal treatments?
8. What is your immediate concern regarding Faye's use of St. John's wort?

？ CRITICAL THINKING #2†

Clinical Applications

Advances in medical technology have provided mechanisms to feed or nourish patients who once could not otherwise be fed or nourished. However, like most medical advances, the advances also engender dilemmas and difficult decisions about patient care. Nutrition care dilemmas occur when this technology will keep the patient alive even though the patient has no hope of ever living a normal life. What happens if a person loses decision-making capacity? Who should decide? What should be decided? Who should the surrogate be? What should that person do?

In a perfect world, the person should be someone designated by the patient while the patient still has decision-making capacity (durable power of attorney for health care). In the world we actually live in, when a patient does not have the capacity to make decisions or has not made an advanced directive, some family member without legal authority has to make decisions about life and death matters, often in a time of crisis. And what happens if family members of the patient do not agree on what should be done? Often, the dilemma requires legal action for resolution.

Such was the situation in the case of 41-year-old Terri Schiavo. Schiavo collapsed at home and experienced several minutes of oxygen deprivation to the brain in 1990, leaving her in a persistent vegetative state (PVS). In 1993, her husband decided to withdraw artificial nutrition, hydration, and life support on the grounds that she would not want to be kept alive this way. Her mother and father, the Schindlers, disagreed, and a controversy began in 1993 that lasted more than 12 years, going back and forth to court. What made the Schiavo case different from its predecessors (those of Karen Ann Quinlan of New Jersey and Nancy Cruzan of Missouri) was the involvement of Jeb Bush, then governor of Florida; the Florida state legislature; U.S. Congress; and 19 judges in six courts, including the Florida Supreme Court and federal courts. The courts continually sided with Terri's husband, whereas Bush and the Florida legislature sided with the Schindlers. Her feeding tube was removed on March 18, 2005, and Terri Schiavo died 13 days later. What are your thoughts about the following circumstances?

- An 85-year-old man who suffers from many physical problems, but is not terminally ill, refuses to be tube fed.
- A 57-year-old woman is hospitalized as a result of a severe psychiatric disorder that prohibits her from speaking or eating. She is bedridden in a fetal position and has a gastrostomy tube. She repeatedly dislodges the feeding tube and is combative when it is replaced.
- A 75-year-old woman's husband has requested termination of her nasogastric feedings. She is brain dead and has no living will.

---

*Modified from Nelms MN, et al: *Medical nutrition therapy: A case study approach,* ed 3, Belmont, CA, 2009, Cengage/Wadsworth.
†Data from Edelstein S: *Ethical dilemmas and decisions,* San Marcos, CA, 1993, Nutrition Dimension; Jennings B: *Garrison colloquium: The long dying of Terri Schiavo—private tragedy, public danger,* Garrison, NY, 2005 (May 20), The Hastings Center.

WEBSITES OF INTEREST

Academy of Nutrition and Dietetics

www.eatright.org/HealthProfessionals/

Tips for managing diets, educating patients, working with dietitians.

American Botanical Council

www.herbalgram.org

Information and research findings to encourage appropriate use of phytomedicines and medicinal plants.

American Society of Parenteral and Enteral Nutrition (ASPEN)

www.nutritioncare.org

Dedicated to making sure patients receive the most appropriate nutritional therapy. Interactive features on the site allow users to post questions, register for conferences, and view links to other related organizations.

National Center for Complementary and Alternative Medicine (NCCAM)

www.nccam.nih.gov

Promotes scientific research on CAM and distributes information to the public and health professionals on the efficacy of CAM modalities.

National Dysphagia Diet

http://www.anfponline.org/Publications/ articles/2004_03_008Dysphagia.pdf

Tips and details for managing the dysphagia diet, which is designed in three stages.

Office of Dietary Supplements (ODS)

http://dietary-supplements.info.nih.gov

Supports research and distributes findings about dietary supplements to the public and acts as a resource for other federal agencies.

Office of Minority Health

http://minorityhealth.hhs.gov/

Great resource for addressing health disparities and cultural competency.

REFERENCES

Academy of Nutrition and Dietetics: *Nutrition care manual*, n.d. From: www.nutritioncaremanual.org. Accessed August 10, 2013.

Academy of Nutrition and Dietetics: Position on functional foods, *J Am Diet Assoc* 113:735–746, 2013.

Academy of Nutrition and Dietetics, Evidence Analysis Library: *Critical illness nutrition practice recommendations.* From: www.adaevidencelibrary.com. Accessed August 10, 2013.

Center for Food Safety and Applied Nutrition, Office of Nutritional Products, Labeling, and Dietary Supplements, Food and Drug Administration: *Dietary supplement labeling*, College Park, MD, 2013, Author. From: www.fda.gov/Food/DietarySupplements/default.htm. Accessed August 9, 2013.

Craig WJ, et al: Position of the American Dietetic Association: Vegetarian diets, *J Am Diet Assoc* 109:1266, 2009.

di Sarsina R, et al: Traditional, complementary and alternative medical systems and their contribution to personalization, prediction and prevention in medicine-person-centered medicine, *EPMA J* 3:15, 2012.

Heiss CJ, et al: Registered dietitians and speech-language pathologists: an important partnership in dysphagia management, *J Am Diet Assoc* 110:1290, 2010.

Ho MH, et al: Clinical spectrum of food allergies: A comprehensive review, *Clin Rev Allergy Immunol* 46(3):225–240, 2014.

Institute of Medicine: *Integrative medicine and the health of the public: A summary of the February 2009 summit*, Washington, DC, 2009, National Academies Press.

Leiby A, Vazirani M: Complementary, holistic, and integrative medicine: Crohn disease, *Pediatr Rev* 33:83–85, 2012.

Lenoir-Wijnkoop I, et al: Nutrition economics—food as an ally of public health, *Br J Nutr* 109:777–784, 2013.

Marcason W: What is the current direction for hospital room service? *J Acad Nutr Diet* 112:456, 2012.

National Center for Complementary and Alternative Medicine: *What's in a name?* (Publication No. D347) From: http://nccam.nih.gov/health/whatiscam. Accessed June 5, 2014.

Shearer MJ: Vitamin K in parenteral nutrition, *Gastroenterology* 137:S105–S118, 2009.

U.S. Food and Drug Administration: *FDA food safety modernization act (FSMA)*, n.d. At: http://www.fda.gov/Food/GuidanceRegulation/FSMA/default.htm. Accessed August 21, 2013.

CHAPTER 13

Nutrition for Disorders of the Gastrointestinal Tract

The ability to chew, swallow, digest, and absorb nutrients, while passing fiber and other substances on for elimination, may be compromised by disorders of the gastrointestinal (GI) tract. Almost everyone experiences intermittent GI complaints from time to time. Indigestion, gas, bloating, nausea, abdominal pain or cramping, diarrhea, and esophageal reflux are some of the symptoms occasionally experienced by healthy people.

http://evolve.elsevier.com/GRODNER/FOUNDATIONS

LEARNING OBJECTIVES

- List the organs affected by disorders of the GI tract.
- Describe how some disorders affect the flow of sustenance through the GI tract
- Identify how and why certain disorders cause site-specific tissue inflammation.
- Compare and contrast disorders caused by the inability to produce digestive enzymes and those caused by the inability to metabolize substances.

- Explain how inflammatory bowel disorders are autoimmune conditions.
- Discuss levels of individualized nutrition therapy for GI disorders.

DIMENSIONS OF GI HEALTH

Consider the six dimensions of health. *Physical health* is most affected when the GI disorder is chronic and intensive. Eventually, weight loss and nutrient deficiencies pose health risks in addition to the primary disorder. *Intellectual health* is tested as the patient tries to find food combinations and textures that are anesthetically pleasing. Some disorders require constant vigilance to restrict inadvertent consumption of problematic foods (e.g., gluten in celiac disease). *Emotional health* is taxed when patients struggle with acceptance of their dietary or physical limitations. Poorly managed symptoms diminish psychological well-being and overall quality of life. *Social health* strategies are needed to help patients handle the personal ramifications of colostomies, dumping syndrome, and other disorders. *Spiritual health* can be enhanced through yoga and meditation, which are tied to mind and body wellness. For those with GI disorders that may cause unexpected need for access to a bathroom, the *environmental health* dimension of facilities at home, at work, and/or during commuting or traveling may alter the sense of wellness.

COMMON DIGESTIVE DISORDERS

Many GI disorders have significant nutritional implications. In many situations, diet is the cornerstone of therapy for GI complaints. Evaluation of a patient's GI symptoms requires a team effort to separate GI symptoms associated with dietary practices from those associated with GI disease or dysfunction. The registered dietitian can identify unusual dietary practices, nutritional inadequacies, or food intolerances through an in-depth diet history assessment.

The simple act of eating an apple may no longer be easy for individuals with disorders of the GI tract. The ability to chew, swallow, digest, and absorb nutrients, while passing fiber and other substances on for elimination, may be compromised (Figure 13-1). GI disorders affect the availability of nutrients to all other organs and body systems, thereby influencing overall health.

We now know that gut health and integrity affect the immune system. Healthy interactions between gut microbiota and their host are needed to maintain homeostasis. Metabolic, signaling, and immune-inflammatory relationships connect the gut, liver, muscle, and brain (Nicholson, et al,

FIG 13-1 Major organs of the gastrointestinal tract.

2012). Microbiota function like a metabolic "organ," influencing nutrient acquisition, energy homeostasis, intestinal permeability, and a chronic low-grade inflammatory state (Frazier, et al, 2011). Research about the use of prebiotic and probiotic therapy shows great promise for many of the GI disorders described in this chapter.

ESOPHAGEAL DISORDERS

Dysphagia

Swallowing is often an involuntary activity that is not thought about, just like breathing or the beating of a heart. Swallowing takes place in three stages: oral preparation and transit, pharyngeal transit, and esophageal transit (Figure 13-2). A disorder affecting any of these stages may require specific nutrition interventions. For patients with chewing or swallowing difficulties, diets must meet individual nutritional needs while preventing aspiration. Box 13-1 lists some conditions that may cause dysphagia.

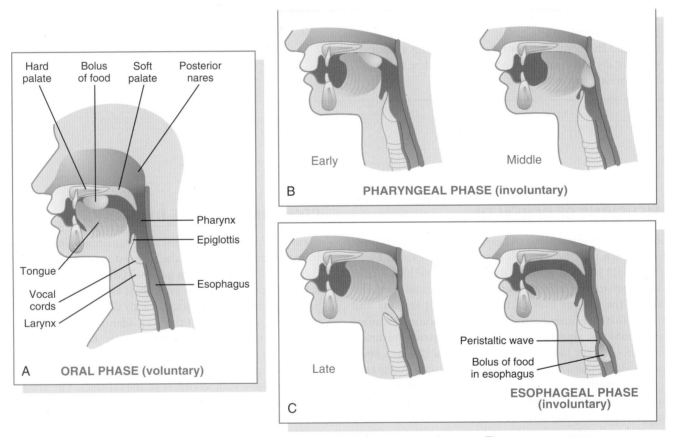

FIG 13-2 Swallowing occurs in three phases: **A**, Voluntary or oral phase. The tongue presses food against the hard palate, forcing it toward the pharynx. **B**, Involuntary, pharyngeal phase. Early: wave of peristalsis forces a bolus between the tonsillar pillars. Middle: soft palate draws upward to close posterior nares and respirations cease momentarily. Late: vocal cords approximate and the larynx pulls upward, covering the airway and stretching the esophagus open. **C**, Involuntary, esophageal phase. Relaxation of the upper esophageal (hypopharyngeal) sphincter allows the peristaltic wave to move the bolus down the esophagus. (From Mahan LK, Escott-Stump S, Raymond KL: *Krause's food & nutrition therapy,* ed 13, Philadelphia, 2012, Elsevier.)

BOX 13-1 Conditions That Cause Dysphagia

Achalasia
Acute cervical spinal cord injury
Alzheimer's disease/dementia
Amyloidosis
Amyotrophic lateral sclerosis (ALS, aka Lou Gehrig's disease)
Anoxia
Botulism
Cerebrovascular accident (CVA)/stroke
Chagas disease
Diabetes, type 1 (long-term)
Esophageal cancer
Esophageal varices
Gastroesophageal reflux (GERD)
Gastroparesis
Goiter
Guillain-Barré syndrome
Head and/or neck cancer, including brain stem tumors
Head injury
Human immunodeficiency virus (HIV) infection
Huntington's disease
Inflammatory masses
Intrinsic and extrinsic structural lesions
Lung inflammation, including chronic obstructive pulmonary disease (COPD), with excessive secretions
Multiple sclerosis (MS)
Multiple system atrophy (MSA)
Muscular dystrophies (MD)
Myasthenia gravis
Parkinson's disease
Poliomyelitis
Postintubation trauma
Presbyphagia (swallowing difficulty of old age)
Scleroderma
Stricture or inflammation of pharynx or esophagus
Tumor or obstruction of throat

Data from Academy of Nutrition and Dietetics: *Nutrition care manual*, Chicago, Author. Accessed August 14, 2013, from www.nutritioncaremanual.org.

PERSONAL PERSPECTIVES

The Pain of Parkinson's Disease

When Don Kaemmer met his soon-to-be second wife, Yetta, he was a physically active 70-year-old widower. A few years after they wed, he was diagnosed with a quickly advancing condition of Parkinson's disease that significantly affected his ability to speak and swallow. Here are some of Mrs. Kaemmer's reflections on her husband's dysphagia.

The doctor approached me and said, "I know what your husband had for dinner tonight." I just stared at him and thought how does he know? Hours after dinner that night, an ambulance brought Don to the hospital because of a kidney infection. While examining my husband, the doctor found partially chewed chicken in Don's mouth and throat. I thought Don swallowed his dinner but apparently not. An example of Parkinson's effect on daily activity became clear.

As the effects of the disorder progressed, my husband had trouble chewing and swallowing food and medications. I don't know if he was just too tired, too depressed, or didn't have an appetite to eat. He frequently looked as if he was wearing a mask with no emotion and said little. I often felt like a cheerleader trying to boost his spirits to get him to eat. How could he stay well if he didn't eat? I made soft foods like chicken soup with pieces of cut-up chicken and vegetables, split pea soup, puddings, and ice cream. During one hospital stay he had a supplement drink that he was willing to drink at home. It was expensive, so we would get a supply of it from the Veterans Administration because Don was entitled to benefits, having served in WWII. But toward the end, only small spoonfuls of ice cream or sherbet felt good. It took too much energy to drink. Instead of feeding with food, I nourished him by being there.

Yetta Kaemmer
Tamarac, Florida

Proper diagnosis and treatment of oral-pharyngeal dysphagia involve a multidisciplinary health care team effort; it starts with systematic screening of at-risk patients (Kaspar and Ekberg, 2012). The 10-item Eating Assessment Tool (EAT-10) is a useful tool (Nestle Nutrition Institute EAT-10 Questionnaire is available at http://www.nestlenutrition-institute.org/Documents/test1.pdf).

The onset of dysphagia can be frightening for patients and family members alike (Milazzo, et al, 1989). See the *Personal Perspectives* box The Pain of Parkinson's Disease.

Food and Nutrition Therapies

Systematic screening for dysphagia and resulting malnutrition among at-risk older adults is important (Kaspar and Ekberg, 2012). Patients sometimes give the following warning signs suggesting that they are at risk for swallowing problems (Academy of Nutrition and Dietetics [AND], 2013):

- Collecting food under the tongue, in the cheeks, or on the hard palate
- Tongue thrusting or spitting food out of the mouth
- Inability to control tongue
- Moving tongue excessively
- Altered oral transit time (fast or slow)
- Delay or absence of larynx elevation while swallowing
- Coughing before or after swallowing
- Choking
- Drooling
- Gargled voice after eating or drinking
- Regurgitating food or liquid through nose, mouth, or tracheostomy tube
- Inadequate intake of food and fluids, resulting in weight loss
- Increased time required to eat
- Resisting food, as by clenching the teeth, pushing food away, or clutching the throat.

A videofluoroscopy swallow study (VFSS) determines the level of bolus consistency the patient can tolerate. Solid foods and liquids should be evaluated separately, and needed modifications identified on the basis of texture, cohesiveness, density, viscosity, consistency, temperature, and taste. Different physiologic problems will dictate the necessity for different consistencies of food.

No two patients with dysphagia are alike. Therefore, diet must be individualized according to the swallowing ability and personal food preferences of the patient. Food must be served in a form that fits the specific anatomic and functional needs of the patient. Patients may need puréed foods to provide stimulation that provokes the reflex to swallow. For patients whose pharyngeal swallow is reduced (but not delayed or absent), liquids tend to be the most difficult consistency. Thickening agents can be used to acquire the appropriate consistency. For patients who have lost coordination of the upper esophageal sphincter (cricopharyngeal dysfunction), thin liquids are more appropriate.

Patients may require changes in food consistency during a hospital or nursing home stay. Thickening agents provide varying levels of consistency to accommodate individual needs. A nutritionally adequate diet for dysphagia considers these characteristics, along with careful planning to ensure nutritional adequacy. The three-stage dysphagia diet is outlined in Table 13-1.

Application to nursing. Enlisting the aid of a speech therapist is usually necessary to teach the patient various techniques to compensate for swallowing problems. The *supraglottic swallow* technique is appropriate for patients with reduced laryngeal function. This method involves teaching the patient to take a breath before swallowing, consciously hold the breath during the swallow, exhale forcefully or cough gently after the swallow, and swallow again to clear the mouth. The *Mendelsohn maneuver* is helpful for individuals with cricopharyngeal dysfunction. The patient is taught to elevate the larynx voluntarily to the maximum level during a swallow to allow food to pass.

In the care of patients with dysphagia at mealtime, several aspects are of concern: bolus consistency, feeding rate, specific swallowing techniques, and patient positioning. One of the safest eating positions for patients who have dysphagia is upright. If patients cannot sit up by themselves, the head of the bed should be raised to provide support, and pillows and wedges should be used to support arms, head, neck, or trunk when necessary.

The upright position allows gravity to assist with the passage of food along the esophagus and helps prevent choking and aspiration (AND, 2013). Aspiration of foreign materials (food, liquids) can lead to pneumonia and other upper respiratory infections. A patient who has aspirated may have a bluish tinge in the skin, wheeze, cough with foul sputum, rapid pulse, or excessive sweating or may experience chest pain.

Dehydration is another concern. Patients with dysphagia are usually not permitted to drink liquids on their own. Thus, attention must be paid to their total fluid intake throughout the day. Intake and output (I&O) records are very important for this population.

About one third of patients in long-term care facilities experience serious difficulties with swallowing solid oral

TABLE 13-1	**Three-Level Dysphagia Diet**	
LEVEL	**RATIONALE**	**DESCRIPTION**
Level 1: Puréed	Suitable for people with severely reduced oral preparatory–stage abilities, impaired lip and tongue control, delayed swallow reflex triggering, oral hypersensitivity, reduced pharyngeal peristalsis, and/or cricopharyngeal dysfunction.	Thick homogeneous textures are emphasized. Puréed foods should be "spoon-thick" or "pudding-like" consistency. No coarse textures, nuts, raw fruits, or raw vegetables are allowed. Liquid or crushed medications (refer to physician or pharmacist for pharmoefficacy of medications) are required and may be mixed with puréed fruits. Liquids and water are thickened with commercial thickening agent as needed to recommended consistency.
Level 2: Mechanically altered	Intended for patients who can tolerate a minimum amount of easily chewed foods. May be suitable for people with moderately impaired oral preparatory stage abilities, edentulous oral cavity, decreased pharyngeal peristalsis, and/or cricopharyngeal muscle dysfunction.	No coarse textures, nuts, raw fruits (except ripe or mashed bananas), or vegetables, except as noted. Puréed or slurried bread, if necessary. Liquid or crushed medications may still be required (refer to physician or pharmacist for pharmo-efficacy of medications). Liquids and water thickened as needed with commercial thickening agent to recommended consistency.
Level 3: Advanced	Designed for patients who chew soft textures. Based on a soft diet; may be appropriate for individuals with mild oral preparatory–stage deficits.	Textures are soft with no tough skins, no nuts or dry, crispy, raw, or stringy foods. Meats should be moist and tender or casseroles with small chunks of meat allowed. Fluid consistency ordered separately: may be thin, nectar-thick, honey-like, or spoon-thick. Moist potatoes, rice, and dressing allowed. All soups except those with tough meat or vegetables. Soft, peeled fruit without seeds. Moist breads and cereals allowed. All fats except those with chunky additives.

Data from Academy of Nutrition and Dietetics: *Nutrition care manual.* Accessed August 14, 2013, from www.nutritioncaremanual.org.

dosage forms (SODFs); manipulating the product can lead to medication errors and changes in efficacy (Stegemann, et al, 2012). The best way to administer medications to a patient with dysphagia should be discussed with the pharmacist.

When dry mouth is a problem, nursing personnel can use several techniques: Encourage the patient to think or talk about food before mealtime; this helps stimulate the flow of saliva for chewing and swallowing. Tart or sour foods can also stimulate saliva production. Have the patient practice oral swallowing exercises. Many exercises can be found at this resource: http://www.swallowingdisorderfoundation.com/oral-swallowing-exercises/ (National Foundation of Swallowing Disorders, 2013).

During meals, supervision is necessary to prevent or minimize swallowing problems. Patients should be reevaluated regularly to determine whether any changes need to be made in the consistency of fluids or food. Sometimes patients eat too quickly and then choke when trying to swallow. Staff can observe and supervise patients while they eat to remind them to complete the swallowing sequence before taking the next bite of food.

Evaluating and documenting the patient's food intake is prudent to ensure adequate nutritional intake and status. Make sure meals are as relaxing as possible; let patients eat at their own pace. Patience on the part of the feeding team is rewarded when patients eat with minimal difficulty while maintaining their nutritional status. Consider a tube feeding if intake is continuously less than 50% at meals.

✳ TEACHING TOOL

Recommendations for Feeding Patients with Dysphagia

1. Position patient upright, bent slightly forward, with the chin tucked and head tilted forward.
2. Eliminate distractions so the patient can focus all attention on the meal.
3. The person feeding should sit at or below patient's eye level while feeding.
4. Avoid asking patient to talk while eating.
5. Instruct the patient not to use liquids to clear the mouth of foods; in fact, they should be used only after the patient has cleared the food from the mouth. Encourage frequent dry swallows or coughing to help clear food from the mouth between bites.
6. Encourage small bites (½ to 1 teaspoon solid food or about 10 to 15 mL liquid), especially if patient's ability to manage food is impaired.
7. Allow adequate time to feed.
8. Use spoons rather than cups because patients have less difficulty taking food and liquid this way. A straw may be used by some patients to drink liquids and softened foods.
9. While patient eats, check for voice quality. A wet or gurgled voice indicates food may be resting on the vocal cords.

From Academy of Nutrition and Dietetics: *Nutrition care manual, 2013.* Accessed August 14, 2013, from www.nutritioncaremanual.org.

Heartburn and Gastroesophageal Reflux Disorder

Heartburn is a burning sensation felt in the esophagus when acid refluxes after food has already been passed to the stomach; it may pass back up through the cardiac sphincter into the esophagus. Some people consider it normal and never report the symptoms to their physicians.

Unlike the stomach, the esophagus is not lined with acid-resistant mucus, so the acidic mixture of food burns the walls of the esophagus and causes pain. Heartburn is also called gastroesophageal reflux. Depending on the frequency and severity of heartburn—including symptoms such as severe burning sensation under the sternum; asthma; chronic cough; and other ear, nose, and throat ailments—either gastroesophageal reflux disorder (GERD) or laryngopharyngeal reflux (LPR) (in which reflux affects the larynx or pharynx) may be diagnosed. The reflux usually takes place within 1 to 4 hours after a meal.

Food and Nutrition Therapies

It is important for patients with GERD to avoid high-fat meals. Slow emptying of the stomach from eating high-fat food increases sphincter relaxation, leading to potential reflux. Foods such as chocolate, alcohol, peppermint, spearmint, liqueurs, caffeine, and high-acid foods (tomatoes, vinegar-based foods, citrus fruits, and juices) may irritate the esophagus and cause heartburn. Patients should also avoid overeating, which slows emptying.

Application to nursing. Suggest prevention and treatment strategies to reduce pressure in the stomach so that the cardiac sphincter is not opened by excessive pressure from stomach contents. Straining to defecate affects the contents of the stomach by creating additional pressure; prevention and management of constipation are important.

✳ TEACHING TOOL

Recommendations for Managing Symptoms of Gastroesophageal Reflux Disorder

- Avoid lying down shortly after eating: Resting or sleeping with a full stomach may push contents against the cardiac sphincter. Wait several hours after a meal before lying flat or keep head and shoulders elevated when reclining.
- Avoid tight clothing: Wearing restrictive clothing around the waist and midriff affects the functioning of the stomach and may increase stomach pressure.
- Avoid eating "on the run": Eating meals while under stress or trying to do other activities at the same time may cause food to not be chewed enough. Big clumps of foods in the stomach force the stomach muscles to react strongly, which may cause reflux.
- Avoid some medications: Taking certain medications regularly may initiate heartburn. If heartburn often occurs when taking birth control pills, antihistamines, tranquilizers (e.g., diazepam [Valium]), or any drug taken often, check with the primary care provider.

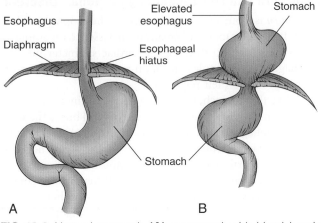

FIG 13-3 Normal stomach (**A**) compared with hiatal hernia (**B**). (From Rolin Graphics.)

HIATAL HERNIA AND ESOPHAGITIS

Normally, the lower esophageal sphincter (LES) prevents stomach contents from entering the esophagus. Factors that may decrease sphincter pressure include smoking, chocolate, alcohol, caffeine, and some medications; see Figure 13-3.

Unlike gastric mucosa, esophageal mucosa can be damaged when exposed to gastric contents. If not treated, chronic reflux can result in *esophagitis* (inflammation of the lower esophagus). Reflux is aggravated by reclining after eating, stress, and increased intra-abdominal pressure. Increased intra-abdominal pressure can occur with coughing, straining, bending, vomiting, obesity, pregnancy, trauma, ascites, clothing that fits tightly around the waist, lifting heavy objects, and strenuous exercise (AND, 2013).

Hiatal hernia is a condition in which part of the stomach bulges upward through the diaphragm. Older patients may experience respiratory symptoms, such as pneumonitis, chronic bronchitis, and asthma.

Food and Nutrition Therapies

Patients may be able to minimize symptoms of esophagitis or hiatal hernia by manipulating the way they eat and by avoiding certain foods, especially those high in fat. See the previous section on heartburn for more guidance.

Application to nursing. Esophagitis is treated medically by reducing intra-abdominal pressure and gastric acid production. Medical management can be divided into six stages (Box 13-2 and Figure 13-4). Table 13-2 summarizes medications that may be used. Attention to metabolism of these medications and their interaction with other prescribed and over-the-counter medications should be considered, particularly among members of different populations (see the *Cultural Considerations* box Biologic Variations of Medication Metabolism). If medical management does not work, surgical intervention may be necessary.

BOX 13-2 Management of Gastroesophageal Reflux Disease

Lifestyle Modifications
- Head of bed elevated 6 inches
- Decreased fat intake
- Smoking cessation
- Weight reduction for obese patients
- Avoidance of recumbent positions for 3 hours postprandially
- Small, frequent meals
- Avoidance of alcohol, chocolate, caffeine
- Avoidance of tight, waist-constricting clothing

Pharmacologic Therapy
- Antacid or antacid product
- Over-the-counter histamine H_2-receptor blocker
- With documented erosive esophagitis, a proton pump inhibitor may be used as first-line therapy
- Stool softeners

Surgery
- May be appropriate in patient with severe symptoms, erosive esophagitis, or disease complications
- Laparoscopic fundoplication procedure

FIG 13-4 Stretta procedure used to treat gastroesophageal reflux disease (GERD). **A,** Catheter positioned. **B,** Multiple sites treated with radiofrequency energy. **C,** Remodeling occurs with collagen formation. (Courtesy Curon Medical, Inc., Freemont, CA.)

🌐 CULTURAL CONSIDERATIONS

Biologic Variations of Medication Metabolism

Ethnic differences are affected by genetics and pharmacokinetics; clinical outcomes are affected accordingly (Phan, et al, 2011). Medications are metabolized differently by ethnic and racial groups. The result can be different therapeutic consequences from what is anticipated as well as unexpected side effects. Individuals are slow metabolizers when the drug-metabolizing enzyme functions are slowed or impaired by deoxyribonucleic acid (DNA) mutations (or differences). Others may be considered extensive metabolizers because they have normally functioning enzymes. Because significant disparities remain in health, health quality, and access to health care within the United States, more research on these biologic variations is needed. Demographic shifts because of a more diverse and aging population will require adaptation of existing programs and services to serve culturally diverse individuals and communities (Awosoqba, et al, 2013; Haughton and Stang, 2012.)

TABLE 13-2 Medications Used to Treat Gastroesophageal Reflux Disease

MEDICATION	ACTION	POTENTIAL ADVERSE EFFECTS AND COMMENTS
Antacids	Neutralize gastric acid	
Aluminum salts (AlternaGEL, Alu-Cap, Amphojel, Basaljel)		Constipation, hypophosphatemia, accumulation in patients with renal impairment
Calcium salts, Tums, Tums E-X, Titralac (Amitone)		Constipation, milk-alkali syndrome with high doses, rebound hyperacidity (depending on dosage)
Magnesium salts (Phillips' Milk of Magnesia, Mygel, Almacone)		Diarrhea
Sodium bicarbonate (Citrocarbonate)		Milk-alkali syndrome with high doses
Magnesium-aluminum combinations (Maalox, Maalox Plus, Mylanta, Mylanta Double Strength, Di-Gel, Gelusil)		Take iron or folic acid supplement separately by 2 hours; take separately from citrus fruit/juice or calcium citrate by 3 hours; minor changes in bowel function. Magnesium-containing products may accumulate in patients with renal impairment. Magnesium-containing products may cause diarrhea
Histamine H₂–Receptor Blockers	Inhibit histamine stimulation of gastric parietal cells, suppressing gastric acid secretion	
Nizatidine (Axid AR) Famotidine (Pepcid AD) Cimetidine (Tagamet HB) Ranitidine (Zantac)		Take at least 2 hours after iron supplement; take magnesium supplement or magnesium-aluminum antacids separately by at least 2 hours; limit caffeine/xanthine; avoid alcohol. Liquid cimetidine precipitates tube feeding
Prokinetic Agents	Increase gastric emptying and lower esophageal sphincter pressure	
Metoclopramide (Reglan) Bethanechol (Urecholine)		Most effective when used in combination with acid-suppression therapy; drowsiness, psychiatric symptoms, and extrapyramidal reactions may occur with long-term use
Proton Pump Inhibitors	Strongly inhibit gastric acid secretion by irreversibly inhibiting the H⁺-K⁺ adenosine triphosphatase pump of parietal cells	Uncommon; include diarrhea, nausea, dizziness, and headaches
Lansoprazole (Prevacid) Omeprazole (Prilosec) Pantoprazole (Protonix) Rabeprazole (Aciphex) Esomeprazole (Nexium)		Optimal: take 30-60 minutes before a meal; swallow whole, do not crush; omeprazole only—capsule may be opened and granules sprinkled on 1 Tbsp applesauce; avoid alcohol

Data from Pronsky ZM, Crowe JP: *Food-medication interactions,* ed 17, Birchrunville, PA, 2012, Food-Medication Interactions; and National Digestive Diseases Information Clearinghouse (NDDIC), National Institute of Diabetes & Digestive & Kidney Diseases (NIDDK): *Heartburn, gastroesophageal reflux (GER), and gastrointestinal reflux disease (GERD)* (NIH Pub. No 07-0882), Bethesda, MD, 2007, National Institutes of Health. Accessed August 14, 2013, from http://digestive.niddk.nih.gov/ddiseases/pubs/gerd/index.htm.

STOMACH DISORDERS

Vomiting

Vomiting is reverse peristalsis. Instead of food moving down the GI tract, the peristalsis muscles move the contents of the stomach back through the esophagus and forcefully out the mouth.

It is an involuntary muscular action that we cannot easily control. Often it is painful; the contents of the stomach already consist of a mixture of food and acidic gastric juices that burns the unprotected esophagus. A primary health care provider should be consulted to determine the cause of any chronic or persistent vomiting and to recommend treatment.

Vomiting is a way the body protects itself. When an intruding virus or toxin has entered the GI tract, vomiting removes the offending substance. Nausea and vomiting are found in GI diseases as well as in conditions unrelated to a GI disorder.

⁕ **TEACHING TOOL**

Recommendations for Living with a Hiatal Hernia

- Avoid large meals. If additional calories are needed for weight gain or maintenance, include midmorning and midafternoon snacks.
- Avoid eating meals and snacks for at least 2 hours before lying down.
- Avoid vigorous activity soon after eating.
- Avoid or limit foods and beverages that relax the lower esophageal sphincter (allowing stomach contents to back up), such as alcohol, carminatives (oil of peppermint or spearmint, garlic, onion), chocolate, and high-fat foods (fried foods, high-fat meats, cream sauces, gravies, margarine/butter, cream, oil, salad dressings).
- Avoid or limit foods and beverages that can irritate damaged esophageal mucosa. These will vary individually and may include carbonated beverages, citrus fruit and juices, coffee (regular and decaffeinated), herbs, pepper, spices, tomato products, and very hot or very cold foods.
- Increase intake of protein foods with low-fat content (lean meats, skim or 1% milk, cheeses, and yogurt made from skim milk) and carbohydrate foods with low-fat content (breads, cereals, crackers, fruit, noodles, potatoes, rice, and vegetables prepared without added fat).
- Achieve and maintain a desirable body weight.

Mixed messages regarding the body's sense of equilibrium during air or sea travel can result in motion sickness; nausea and vomiting may result. Pregnant women are often affected by vomiting with the hormonal shifts that occur, especially during the first trimester. In addition, some patients with cancer suffer from episodes of vomiting because of chemotherapy, radiation treatments, or use of medicines such as opioids.

Individuals who vomit as a way to control their weight and suffer from eating disorders such as anorexia nervosa and bulimia are at medical risk. Repetitive self-induced vomiting can injure the esophagus and wear away tooth enamel. Anyone practicing this self-destructive behavior should consult a primary care provider or mental health professional as soon as possible.

Food and Nutrition Therapies

Dehydration is a concern when vomiting is continual. Vomiting causes a loss of fluid and electrolytes, such as magnesium, potassium, and sodium, which stresses the functioning of the body. Infants are at particular risk for dehydration because their bodies consist mostly of fluids.

When patients are experiencing periods of nausea or vomiting, small cold meals may be better tolerated than large hot meals. For example, crackers and cheese, gelatin, fruit, or lemonade might be tolerated. Avoid mixing hot and cold foods, which may aggravate the problem. Hot, fried, spicy, and strong-smelling foods should also be avoided. Some

patients find relief with broth-based soups, warm tea with mint, and ginger ale or other carbonated beverages.

Application to nursing. Nursing personnel manage many patients who are experiencing nausea and vomiting. Offering small meals at frequent intervals is a good place to start. Breathing exercises and repositioning may be helpful in some patients. Eliminate strong odors when possible. Good oral health is important, and patients can be given antiemetics (Zofran, Compazine, Phenergan) 30 to 60 minutes before meals are served.

⁕ **TEACHING TOOL**

Recommendations for Managing Nausea and Vomiting

- Chew foods slowly and thoroughly.
- Use ice chips.
- Sip on cool, clear, carbonated (allow to become "flat") beverages such as 7-Up and ginger ale.
- Avoid the caffeine of colas unless tolerated.
- Do not use acidic fruit juices such as orange, tomato, and grapefruit.
- Rest before and after meals. However, keep the head elevated to avoid reflux.

Peptic Ulcer Disease

Peptic ulcer disease (PUD) is the term used to describe a break or ulceration in the protective mucosal lining of the lower esophagus, stomach, or duodenum. Such ulcerations expose the submucosal areas to gastric secretions and autodigestion. Peptic ulcers can be acute or chronic and superficial (erosions) or deep. Deep ulcers may penetrate the muscularis mucosa and damage blood vessels, causing hemorrhage, or perforate the GI wall.

Infection with *Helicobacter pylori* and use of nonsteroidal anti-inflammatory drugs (NSAIDs) are the major causes of duodenal ulcers (Figure 13-5). *H. pylori* weakens the protective mucosal layer of the stomach and duodenum, allowing gastric acid to damage epithelial tissues, which leads to ulcerogenesis. Treatment goals focus largely on eradicating *H. pylori*, reducing stomach acidity, relieving symptoms, healing the ulcer, preventing reoccurrence, and avoiding complications. They are accomplished through *triple therapy,* a combination of antibiotics and acid-reducing medications (see Table 13-2) taken for at least 10 to 14 days. Triple therapy involves at least two antibiotics plus the acid reducers. The acid-reducing medications help relieve pain and also help the antibiotics work more effectively.

NSAIDs likely promote mucosal inflammation and ulcer formation through cellular damage, reducing gastric blood flow, reducing mucus and HCO_3 (bicarbonate) secretion, and decreasing the ability of cells to repair and replicate, leading to breakdown of mucosal defense mechanisms.

FIG 13-5 Chronic peptic ulcer. (From Damjanov I, Linder J, editors: *Anderson's pathology,* ed 10, vol 2, St. Louis, 1996, Mosby.)

Food and Nutrition Therapies

There is no evidence that a "bland diet" (or any specific diet) improves symptoms of ulcers or promotes their healing. Any dietary modifications must be individualized to include avoidance of foods that a patient can associate with symptoms. Some individuals avoid red and black pepper, chili pepper, coffee (caffeinated and decaffeinated), other caffeinated beverages, and alcohol.

Application to nursing. Foods and spices that are irritants, cause superficial mucosal damage, or worsen existing disease should be omitted. Patients need encouragement to take prescribed medications. Triple therapy often requires more than one round of treatment to eradicate *H. pylori* completely.

❋ **TEACHING TOOL**

Recommendations for Managing Ulcer Symptoms

- Regardless of the cause of an ulcer, smoking aggravates peptic ulcer disease. A smoking cessation program should be considered.
- Eating a good-quality diet is also important.

Dumping Syndrome

One of the functions of the stomach is to control the rate of gastric emptying of nutrients into the small intestine. The stomach empties according to signals from the stomach and duodenum. This process ensures efficient digestion, absorption, and metabolism. When part or all of the stomach (partial or total gastrectomy) is removed for treatment of stomach cancer or a severe ulcer or is bypassed to control obesity (Figure 13-6), dumping syndrome may develop.

Impairment of the normal reservoir function of the stomach causes a large volume of particles to be dumped rapidly into the small intestine. These hyperosmolar contents draw water into the lumen and stimulate bowel motility.

Some symptoms occur 10 to 20 minutes postprandially (early phase after a meal) and are characterized by feelings of epigastric fullness, abdominal cramps, nausea, or diarrhea. Vasomotor symptoms may also occur: tachycardia, postural hypotension, profuse sweating, weakness, flushing, and syncope. Patients may experience intestinal symptoms but not vasomotor symptoms, and vice versa. The late phase, which occurs less frequently than the early phase, develops about 1 to 3 hours postprandially; its symptoms are perspiration, hunger, nausea, anxiety, tremors, and weakness.

Food and Nutrition Therapies

Food and meals can be manipulated or restricted to help alleviate the symptoms of patients with dumping syndrome. Liquids should be consumed between rather than with meals to slow the movement of food from the stomach into the duodenum. Simple carbohydrates are limited because they may worsen the syndrome. Protein, fat, and complex carbohydrates are better tolerated. Over time, patients who have dumping syndrome often lose weight, so their nutritional status should be evaluated regularly by a registered dietitian; deficiencies of iron, vitamin B_{12}, protein, and vitamin D can occur (AND, 2013).

Application to nursing. Coping with dumping syndrome may seem overwhelming to newly diagnosed clients. Help them understand what is happening; discuss foods to avoid. Make sure patients consume adequate fluids between meals to prevent dehydration; I&O records will be important.

INTESTINAL DISORDERS

Intestinal Gas (Flatus)

Everyone's body produces and releases gas from the lower intestinal tract. Most gas leaves the GI tract without our awareness because it is odorless. Gas in the GI tract is caused by swallowing air, or by the fermentation of indigestible carbohydrates by bacteria in the large intestine. Everyone swallows a small amount of air when eating and drinking; however, the amount of air swallowed increases when people eat or drink too fast, smoke, chew gum, and drink carbonated beverages.

Indigestible carbohydrates are found in legumes, such as soybeans and black beans, and cruciferous vegetables, such as broccoli and cabbage. Another indigestible carbohydrate may be the lactose in milk. When the patient is missing the enzyme lactase, lactose begins to ferment, causing gas buildup, bloating, and diarrhea.

Food and Nutrition Therapies

Intestinal gas can probably be decreased through some simple changes of food-related behaviors. For many people, alcohol

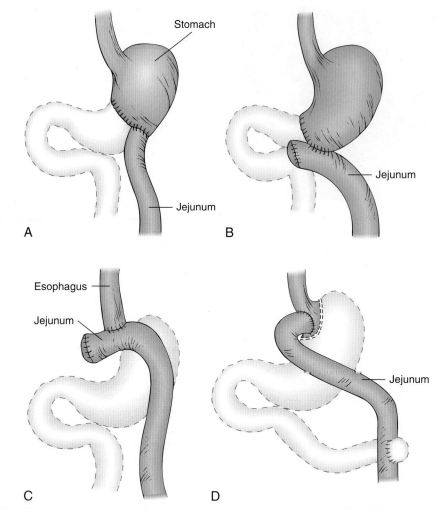

FIG 13-6 Typical gastric surgery resections. **A**, Partial gastrectomy, Billroth I (gastroduodenostomy). **B**, Partial gastrectomy, Billroth II (gastrojejunostomy). **C**, Total gastrectomy. **D**, Roux-en-Y bypass procedure. (**A-C** from Rolin Graphics.)

✳ TEACHING TOOL

Recommendations for Managing Dumping Syndrome

- Avoid drinking liquids with meals. Drink liquids 30 minutes before or 30 minutes after meals and limit servings to ½ to 1 cup.
- Carbonated beverages may cause excess gas formation and therefore are not recommended.
- Eat small, frequent meals to decrease intestinal distention caused by rapid emptying of large meals.
- Eat foods slowly, chew them well, and relax while eating.
- Avoid any foods that are not tolerated.
- Keep simple sugars (monosaccharides and disaccharides) to a minimum. Initially avoid sugar, honey, syrup, and other foods high in sugar; they may need long-term limitation.

- Food and liquids should be consumed at moderate temperatures (not too hot or too cold).
- Milk and milk products containing lactose may not be tolerated. Establish tolerance by gradually introducing them into the diet over time.
- Lie down for 15 to 30 minutes after meals to help decrease symptoms of dumping. If bothered by reflux, recline (at an angle) rather than lie flat.
- Pectin, a dietary fiber, may be helpful in delaying gastric emptying. Pectin can be purchased in powder form in grocery stores and supermarkets. Taking 1 teaspoon of pectin powder three times daily may be effective.

Data from Academy of Nutrition and Dietetics: *Nutrition care manual,* 2013. Accessed August 14, 2013, from www.nutritioncaremanual.org.

---

may be a problem; patients should omit or limit alcoholic beverages as needed.

Increase fluid intake and consume sufficient amounts of fiber to prevent constipation. To increase fiber intake, gradually add more fibrous foods such as legumes to allow the

system to adjust better and tolerate the increase. If there are effects after drinking milk, use small quantities over several weeks, working up to an 8-ounce glass. Note at what level gas may develop. If a problem occurs, consider eating other milk-related products such as yogurt, cheese, or lactose-reduced milk. Lactase enzyme is available in forms such as pills, tablets or drops.

Application to nursing. Encourage the patient to identify foods that are problematic. The cause of flatulence will be unique for each one. Over-the-counter products can be offered, including Gas-X, simethicone, and Mylanta®.

✳ TEACHING TOOL

Recommendations for Reducing Intestinal Gas

- Eat slower and chew foods more thoroughly.
- Avoid gum, carbonated beverages, and drinking out of a straw.
- Add new fiber-rich foods one at a time; evaluate for any discomfort before adding more new items.
- Drink plenty of liquids each day.
- Evaluate the effects of lactose from drinking milk.

Diarrhea

Diarrhea is the passing of loose, watery bowel movements that result when the contents of the GI tract move through too quickly to allow water to be reabsorbed in the colon. An occasional bout is not a problem. However, if diarrhea persists, fluid and electrolytes may be lost, leading to dehydration.

Acute diarrhea is typically of short duration and is usually the result of enteritis, effects of medications, changes in dietary habits or intake, or emotional stress. Diarrhea that lasts longer than 2 weeks is considered chronic; it is usually the result of malabsorption, which may necessitate permanent dietary changes. Chronic, persistent diarrhea may signify a more serious disease and should be evaluated by a physician.

Food and Nutrition Therapies

Nutrition therapy is based on the cause of diarrhea. In severe cases, the patient may be restricted to taking nothing by mouth to allow the GI tract to rest; however, it is usually unnecessary to withhold feedings.

Infants, young children, and older adults with diarrhea are at high risk for dehydration. Thus, fluids may be administered with enteral or parenteral fluids (carbohydrate and electrolytes). Enteral therapy may consist of oral rehydration solutions for 1 or 2 days before progressing to a low-fat, low-fiber, or low-lactose diet. Small, frequent meals are often better tolerated than three larger meals. The patient may return to the normal diet as soon as tolerated.

Application to nursing. Adequate hydration is essential in high-risk populations with diarrhea. Infants cannot easily communicate their thirst, and a greater proportion of their bodies consists of fluid; the excessive loss of fluid has serious consequences such as electrolyte imbalance and a distorted ability to maintain body temperature and functions. In older adults, the ability to detect thirst may be diminished. Disorientation, sometimes assigned to senility, may actually be a sign of dehydration. Because it is a symptom of illness,

diarrhea that lasts more than 2 days should be discussed with a primary care provider to uncover the cause.

✳ TEACHING TOOL

Recommendations for Managing Diarrhea

- Eat small meals frequently throughout the day.
- Chew with the mouth closed to avoid swallowing too much air.
- Drink liquids 30 minutes before or after meals.
- Limit use of apple juice, which may aggravate diarrhea (especially in children).
- Include foods that are low in fiber (bananas, rice, applesauce, dry toast, crackers).
- Progress to foods that are high in potassium when tolerated: oranges, grapefruit, bananas, apples, potatoes, dairy products, apricot nectar, baked squash, and sweet potatoes.
- Electrolyte solutions (Gatorade, Pedialyte, etc.) may be used to replenish lost sodium and potassium. Take only under medical advisement.
- If diarrhea is severe, the doctor may prescribe medication such as loperamide (Imodium). Avoid foods during that time that are:
  - Very hot—which might worsen diarrhea from increased natural movement of the intestines.
  - High in caffeine—such as coffee, colas, chocolate
  - High in fiber—whole-grain breads or cereals, raw fruits and vegetables, nuts, dried fruit, popcorn, salads, and bran.
  - Gas-forming—cabbage, onions, dried beans or lentils, carbonated beverages, broccoli, cauliflower, chewing gum.
- Get plenty of rest—lie down for 30-60 minutes after meals.
- Milk contains lactose, a natural sugar that may not be digested properly at this time. For some, this is a temporary situation.

Constipation

There is no clear definition of constipation. It is usually regard as difficulty and discomfort associated with defecation probably because of slow movement of feces through the colon. Individuals may interpret these terms differently and may vary in their natural urge to defecate. Not everyone needs to pass a bowel movement daily. Normal functioning ranges from three times a day to every 3 days. Generally, constipation is recognized as having fewer than three stools per week; in addition, people strain to pass hard, dry stools (National Institute of Diabetes and Digestive and Kidney Diseases [NIDDK], 2013).

Food and Nutrition Therapies

Water helps lubricate the intestines, making bowel movements easier to pass. To prevent dehydration and constipation, fluid intake should be approximately 8 to 10 glasses a day. Most of us need to consciously remember to drink water and other liquids to fulfill this need. The patient should use fiber-rich products such as psyllium (Metamucil), whole-grain breads and cereals, fruits, and vegetables. After intestinal fermentation, short-chain fatty acids and gas are produced that stimulate gastrointestinal sensation (Eswaran, et al, 2013).

Application to nursing. Chronic constipation is a distressing condition. Most patients in the hospital are at risk for constipation from decreased activity and the medications they are taking. Increasing physical activity and fluid are key factors.

Bulking agents, stool softeners, osmotic and stimulant laxatives, and probiotics may be used to prevent or alleviate constipation (Liu, 2011). Polyethylene glycol, sodium picosulfate, bisacodyl, prucalopride, lubiprostone, and linaclotide have been proven effective (Portalatin and Winstead, 2012); however, mineral oil should not be used because it depletes fat-soluble vitamins (A, D, E, and K) over time. Biofeedback therapy, a technique used to gain control over body functions, may be helpful (Collins and Norton, 2013). If these strategies do not relieve constipation, the physician should be consulted to rule out more serious disorders (see the *Personal Perspectives* box Constipation as a Warning?).

PERSONAL PERSPECTIVES

Constipation as a Warning?

A spouse or significant other is an observer of the health and illness of one's partner. As such, a spouse may note physical changes and remember medical history more clearly than the partner experiencing the symptoms. This is the perspective of a spouse about an early symptom of a neurologic disorder in her husband.

I remember the look of panic on his face. The simple act of "having a bowel movement" just wasn't happening for my husband. It had been several days. This was never a problem before, so the discomfort and panic increased. In 5 days we were to fly to the Netherlands to visit our son, whom we hadn't seen in almost a year.

After trying the usual over-the-counter laxatives with no reaction, he called his internist, who said to go to the emergency room. Emergency room! Now I have to admit I thought my husband was overreacting. Because he was so uncomfortable, I agreed we should go to the nearby hospital. After many hours of enemas, an overnight stay, and an emergency colonoscopy, my husband was released with follow-up instructions from a gastroenterologist. Diagnosis: unknown cause (an isolated incident). Nonetheless, he continues to need to use a prescriptive laxative.

We did visit our son in the Netherlands without any medical mishaps. However, about 2 years later, my husband was diagnosed with multiple system atrophy, a rare degenerative neurologic movement disorder. The original constipation problem was an early symptom of this serious disorder, which affects the sympathetic nervous system.

The moral of this story? A cluster of seemingly unrelated symptoms may be related and are important to communicate to health care providers. Keeping a record of symptoms, treatments, medications, and dates can be quite valuable.

Michele Grodner
Montclair, NJ

Copious amounts of fiber, particularly wheat bran, may result in the formation of bezoars in some people. Bezoars are physical obstacles created by tangles of fibrous material in the GI tract that may cause dangerous GI obstructions. They tend to occur more commonly in individuals who have diabetes and who suffer from gastroparesis.

TEACHING TOOL

Recommendations for Managing Constipation

- Listen to the body's signals and follow a schedule that allows time for a bowel movement to occur. Ignoring the natural urge to defecate causes feces to remain in the colon longer. This allows more water to be withdrawn, resulting in harder, drier feces.
- Exercise regularly. Lack of exercise can lead to a loss of tone in the muscles of the lower GI tract.
- Relax. Stress tightens muscles throughout the body and may inhibit proper bowel functioning.
- Consume regular meals. The body works best with an intake of nutrients and fiber throughout the day. Skipping meals should be avoided.

Celiac Disease and Gluten Sensitivity

Celiac disease is a chronic autoimmune disorder in which the mucosa of the small intestine, especially the duodenum and proximal jejunum, is damaged by dietary gluten. The gliadin fraction in wheat, secalin in rye, and hordein in barley are the specific prolamins (storage proteins), collectively known as *gluten,* that trigger the toxic reaction in genetically predisposed individuals (Escott-Stump, 2011). The resulting malabsorption of nutrients causes symptoms that can vary greatly depending on the duration and severity of the disease, the person's age, and the presence of extra-intestinal conditions. Although the classic symptoms are diarrhea, abdominal distention, fat malabsorption, and weight loss, many patients do not present with GI symptoms or are asymptomatic. Others may experience anemia, osteoporosis, infertility, or even lymphoma if their disease is untreated.

In the early stages of celiac disease, fat malabsorption (steatorrhea) is more typical than other forms of malabsorption. In severe cases, the digestion and absorption of proteins, fats, carbohydrates (especially lactose), calcium, vitamin D, vitamin K, iron, folate, and vitamin B_{12}, as well as other nutrients, become impaired. Severe nutritional deficiencies lead to osteopenia or osteoporosis, inadequate blood coagulation, easy bruising of skin due to lack of vitamin K, iron-deficiency anemia, and macrocytic anemia due to vitamin B_{12} and folate malabsorption (Escott-Stump, 2011).

Food and Nutrition Therapies

Once gluten is removed from the diet, symptoms gradually improve over the following weeks and months. Intestinal mucosa subsequently returns to a near normal condition. There is only one catch: Maintaining an asymptomatic state depends on lifelong avoidance of gluten. A diet that restricts these four grains can become monotonous. Table 13-3

TABLE 13-3 Sources of Gluten

Foods to include	Rice Corn Amaranth Quinoa Teff (or Tef) Millet Finger millet (ragi) Sorghum Indian rice grass (Montina) Arrowroot Buckwheat Flax Job's tears Sago Potato Soy Legumes Mesquite Tapioca Wild rice Cassava (Manloc) Yucca Nuts Seeds	Processed foods that may contain wheat, barley, or rye	Bouillon cubes Brown rice syrup Candy Cold cuts Communion wafers* French fries Gravy Hot dogs Imitation fish Licorice Matzoh Rice mixes Salami Sauces Sausage Seasoned snack foods (e.g., tortilla chips, potato chips) Seitan Self-basting turkey Soups Soy sauce Vegetables in sauce
Grains to avoid	Wheat, all varieties, including: • Einkorn • Emmer • Spelt • Kamut • Wheat bran • Wheat germ • Cracked wheat • Hydrolyzed wheat protein Barley Rye Cross-bread varieties such as triticale (cross between wheat and rye)		

*Communion wafers are generally made from wheat, although gluten-free wafers are manufactured by Ener-G Foods (www.ener-g.com). Low-gluten Communion wafers that conform to (Catholic) Canon law have been developed by the Benedictine Sisters of Perpetual Adoration (www.benedictinesisters.org).
Data from Academy of Nutrition and Dietetics: Celiac disease. In *Nutrition care manual,* Chicago, Author. Accessed August 14, 2013, from www.nutritioncaremanual.org.

summarizes sources of gluten. Note that "wheat starch" may be used (FDA, 2013).

Application to nursing. The restrictive diet required by celiac disease can be frustrating because of its limitations. Abstaining from wheat, oats, rye, and barley is difficult. Patients may need new coping skills. The diet will change many routines at home, school, and work for the patient's family as well.

Lactose Intolerance

The most common disaccharidase disorder is a deficiency of lactase, the intestinal brush-border enzyme that hydrolyzes lactose into glucose and galactose (see Chapter 4). This lactase deficiency leads to a condition called *lactose intolerance,*

⁂ TEACHING TOOL
Recommendations for Managing Celiac Disease

- Gluten-containing grains and products made from these grains are staples in the American diet. They are used as emulsifiers, thickeners, and other additives in commercially processed foods.
- Patients, with the help of registered dietitians and celiac disease support groups, must become ardent label readers to avoid unintentional ingestion of gluten.
- Availability of alternatives to wheat-based breads, crackers, and pasta is limited when one is eating away from home. Patients may need to pack lunches or snacks for a variety of events.

which is prevalent worldwide, in mostly non-European countries.

Lactose intolerance is investigated with a hydrogen breath test (HBT) or with genotyping in patients who have unexplained abdominal symptoms (Haberkorn, et al, 2011). Undigested lactose remaining in the intestine will, through osmotic effect, draw water into the digestive tract, resulting in abdominal cramping, flatulence, and diarrhea. The severity of these symptoms often depends on the amount of lactose ingested and the degree of intolerance an individual has. Lactase deficiency is sometimes secondary to acute or chronic diseases, such as celiac disease and Crohn's disease, or to small bowel or gastric surgery.

Food and Nutrition Therapies

Tolerance for lactose varies from population to population and from person to person. For individuals who have lactose intolerance or in whom it is suspected, health care professionals need to establish tolerance by gradually adding small amounts of lactose-containing foods to a lactose-free diet (Box 13-3). Most people can tolerate 6 to 9 g of lactose at a given time, which is the amount in 4 to 6 ounces of milk. These small amounts of lactose can generally be consumed on several occasions throughout the day. Individuals usually tolerate lactose if it is consumed along with other foods, rather than alone as a beverage or a snack. Yogurt may be better tolerated than milk, depending on brand and processing method. Cocoa and chocolate milk may also be better tolerated. *Lactobacillus acidophilus* milk is generally not tolerated.

Application to nursing. Restricting lactose-containing foods may pose a risk for calcium, riboflavin, and vitamin D deficiencies, depending on the degree of restriction. These nutrients can be provided at the Recommended Dietary Allowance (RDA) level with lactase-treated milk and milk products or with supplementation. Calcium is of particular importance to children and women of childbearing age. Vitamin D supplementation would be necessary for individuals whose serum levels of the vitamin are low.

✳ TEACHING TOOL

Recommendations for Lactose Intolerance

- Lactase enzyme is available as Lactaid or Dairy Ease and may be added to milk 24 hours in advance of ingestion. The tablet form is available and can be ingested just before eating a lactose-containing meal. Depending on the degree of intolerance, patients may use one-half to three tablets (Academy of Nutrition and Dietetics, 2013).
- Cheese and yogurt are dairy foods that are likely well tolerated; they can be used daily for calcium and riboflavin if milk is not included in the diet.

Irritable Bowel Syndrome

Irritable bowel syndrome (IBS) is a functional GI disorder involving disturbances between the brain and the gut. Patients

---

BOX 13-3 Lactose Content of Foods

Lactose content will vary, depending on portion size and product preparation. Most individuals can experiment with different lactose-containing foods to determine their level of tolerance. Although dairy products all contain lactose, processing reduces the lactose in some products.

High-Lactose Foods
Buttermilk
Cheesecake, cream pies
Cold cuts and hot dogs (some may contain varying amounts of lactose)
Cottage cheese (nonfat, low-fat, regular)
Cream
Cream cheese
Cream or milk soups
Creamy sauces (white sauce, Alfredo sauce, vegetables au gratin)
Evaporated milk
Half and half
Ice cream (regular and low-fat), ice milk, frozen yogurt
Milk (nonfat, skim, low-fat, whole)
Milk-related products
Powdered milk
Pudding, custard
Ricotta cheese
Salad dressings with milk
Sour cream
Yogurt

Low-Lactose Dairy Foods
Aged cheese (cheddar, Swiss)
Butter/margarine
Commercial bread and cake products (bread, muffins, pancakes, waffles, biscuits)
Drug preparations (tablets) (may contain lactose as filler, but usually tolerated)
Lactose-reduced milk (nonfat, skim, low-fat, whole)
Processed cheese (depending on milk solids added)
Processed foods containing dry milk solids or whey
Ready-to-eat cereals containing milk/lactose
Sherbet
Yogurt (may be tolerated)

---

with IBS can be divided into subgroups with alternating bowel habits (IBS-A), constipation-predominant IBS (IBS-C), and diarrhea-predominant IBS (IBS-D). Many patients with IBS attribute their symptoms to food allergies; others may have lactose maldigestion. Studies now suggest that some patients with IBS may have a nonceliac wheat or gluten sensitivity (Boettcher and Crowe, 2013). Thus, food allergies and intolerances seem to play a role.

Food and Nutrition Therapies

Depending on the individual's symptoms and food diary, lactose, gluten, or sugars may be eliminated from the diet. The low-FODMAP (fermentable oligosaccharides, disaccharides, monosaccharides, and polyols) diet is now accepted as a strategy. The low-FODMAP diet limits high sugar intake, which increases osmolarity. Foods containing fructose, sucrose, polyols (sorbitol and mannitol), and related carbohydrates would be restricted.

Application to nursing. Patients with IBS require medical attention when they have is fever, persistent diarrhea, anemia, rectal bleeding, and unintended weight loss.

✳ **TEACHING TOOL**

Irritable Bowel Syndrome

- A food diary is useful to note symptoms, specific foods, or dietary practices that cause problems.
- Dietitian-led education is necessary for use of the FODMAPS diet plan.
- Prebiotic or probiotic therapy may also be beneficial.

Inflammatory Bowel Disease

Inflammatory bowel disease (IBD) refers to two chronic inflammatory conditions of the intestines—ulcerative colitis (UC) and Crohn's disease (regional enteritis). UC is an inflammatory process confined to the mucosa of any or all of the large intestine. Crohn's disease is an inflammatory disorder that involves all layers of the intestinal wall and may affect the small intestine, large intestine, or both. It is associated with stricture formation, fistulous tracts, and abscesses.

Inflammatory bowel disorders are considered autoimmune conditions caused by a genetic predisposition followed by an environmental trigger. Both cause diarrhea, which may be profuse and bloody. Abdominal pain, intestinal bleeding, protein loss, and fever often result in nutritional depletion. Thus, decreased oral intake, malabsorption, increased nutrient loss, increased nutrient requirements, and drug-nutrient interactions must be addressed. Attention must be given to intestinal function, including any previous intestinal resections, site and extent of disease process (Figure 13-7), and anticipated medical and surgical treatment.

Food and Nutrition Therapies

The goals of nutrition therapy are to replace lost nutrients, correct deficits, and achieve energy, nitrogen, fluid, and electrolyte balance. During acute stages of IBD, nutrition therapy is individualized on the basis of food tolerance and affected portions of the GI tract. Diet and weight histories are essential to determine potential nutrient deficiencies. The

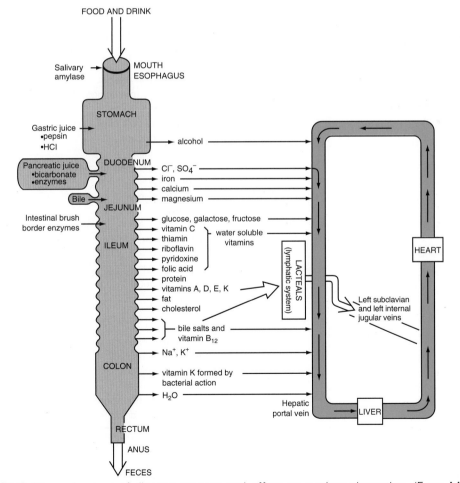

FIG 13-7 Site and extent of disease process and effect on nutrient absorption. (From Mahan LK, Escott-Stump S, Raymond JL: *Krause's food & nutrition therapy,* ed 13, Philadelphia, 2012, Elsevier.)

nutrients that most commonly may be poorly absorbed are minerals (iron, calcium, zinc, magnesium, selenium) and vitamins (folate, thiamine, riboflavin, pyridoxine, vitamin B_{12}, and vitamins A, D, and E). A high-calorie, high-protein diet divided into small, frequent meals is recommended (AND, 2013).

Application to nursing. Proper management requires nutritional maintenance and repletion along with therapies to facilitate healing of the inflamed bowel. Precise body weight measurements are necessary to detect the onset of malnutrition risk. Specific pharmacotherapy, surgery, and nutritional support are used. Although surgery is curative in ulcerative colitis, Crohn's disease tends to recur after surgical resection of affected sections; Box 13-4 and Table 13-4 summarize diets used for these disorders.

Ileostomies and Colostomies

Occasionally, when disease or obstruction cannot be resolved, all or a segment of the colon, including the rectum, is removed. An ileostomy consists of the removal of the entire colon and rectum. A surgical opening of the ileum onto the surface of the abdomen is created, through which fecal matter is emptied. A colostomy consists of the surgical creation of an artificial anus on the abdominal wall by incising the colon and bringing it out to the surface. It may be single-barreled (one opening) or double-barreled (distal and proximal loops open onto the abdomen).

Food and Nutrition Therapies

Appropriate nutrition therapy depends on which procedure, either an ileostomy or a colostomy, is performed. Goals are

---

BOX 13-4 Increasing Fiber Intake*

Excellent Sources of Fiber (10-16 g/cup)
All-Bran cereal
Bran Buds cereal
Grape Nuts cereal
Fiber One cereal
Baked beans
Black beans
Chickpeas (garbanzo)
Kidney beans, cooked
Split peas or lentils
Artichokes

Good Sources of Fiber (4-9 g per cup)
Apple with skin
Blueberries
Broccoli, cooked
Pear, with skin
Prunes
Raspberries
Green beans, frozen
Lima beans, cooked (1 cup)
Sweet potato with skin
Turnip greens, boiled (1 cup)
Barley, pearl, cooked (1 cup)
Peas, cooked
Black-eyed peas
Bran muffin
Bran Chex cereal
Corn Bran cereal
Graham crackers
Raisin Bran cereal
Oatmeal, cooked
Whole-wheat bread
Shredded wheat cereal

Sunflower seeds (1/4 cup)
Spaghetti, whole wheat

Fair Sources of Fiber (1-3 g/serving)
Banana
Pineapple, canned
Cheerios
Corn, whole kernel canned
Cauliflower
Carrots
Figs (2 medium dried)
Nuts–almonds, pistachios, pecans (1 oz)
Tomato, raw
Tomato paste (1/4 cup)
Brown rice (1 cup)
Potato with skin
Popcorn, air popped (3 cups)
Raisins (1 oz)
Strawberries, raw (1 cup)
Rye bread

Poor Sources
Celery
Cucumber
Lettuce (iceberg)
Mushrooms
Onions
Grapefruit
Fruit juices
Vegetable juices
Crisped rice cereal
Corn flakes cereal
Refined white flour products (white breads, rolls, bagels, most pastas, pizza crust, crackers)

NOTE: Increasing fiber without increasing fluid can lead to more constipation, abdominal pain, bloating, and gas. Fiber intake should be increased gradually, over a period of weeks while fluids are simultaneously increased.
*Current recommendations for Adequate Intake (AI) are for 25-38 g/day. This goal can be met by eating a well-balanced diet containing a variety of foods: 2-4 servings of fruit, 3-5 servings of vegetables, 6-11 servings of whole-grain breads or cereals, plenty of fluids.
Data from: Academy of Nutrition and Dietetics: *Nutrition care manual*, Chicago, Author Accessed August 14, 2013, from www.nutritioncaremanual.org; U.S.Department of Agriculture: *National nutrient database for standard reference, 2012.* Accessed August 14, 2013, from http://ndb.nal.usda.gov/.

TABLE 13-4	**Guidelines for Ostomy Patients**	
FOOD GROUP	RECOMMENDED FOODS	FOODS NOT RECOMMENDED
Dairy	Buttermilk Evaporated, skim, and low-fat milk Soy milk Yogurt with live active cultures Powdered milk Cheese	Yogurts with nuts or dried fruits Whole milk Half-and-half Cream Sour cream Regular (whole milk) ice cream
Grains Choose grains with <2 gm dietary fiber/serving	White flour Bread, bagels, rolls, crackers, pasta made from white or refined flour Cold or hot cereals made from white or refined flour	Whole-wheat or whole grain breads, rolls, crackers, or pasta Brown or wild rice Barley, oats, and other whole grains Cereals made from whole grains or bran Breads or cereals made with seeds or nuts Popcorn
Fruits and vegetables	Fruit juice without pulp, except prune juice Ripe bananas Canned soft fruits Most well-cooked vegetables without seeds or skins Potatoes without skin Lettuce Strained vegetable juice	All raw fruits and vegetables (except banana, melons, lettuce) Dried fruits, including prunes and raisins Fruit juice with pulp Canned fruit in heavy syrup Any fruits sweetened with sorbitol Prune juice Fried vegetables Beets Cruciferous vegetables (broccoli, Brussels sprouts, cabbage, cauliflower) Greens (collard, mustard, turnip) Corn Potato skins
Proteins	Tender, well-cooked meat, poultry, fish, eggs, or soy foods made without added fat Smooth nut butters	Fried meat, poultry, or fish Luncheon meats, such as bologna or salami Sausage or bacon Hot dogs Fatty meats Nuts Chunky nut butters
Beverages 8-10 cups of fluid is recommended each day; more may be needed to replace fluids lost to diarrhea	Decaffeinated coffee Caffeine-free teas Soft drinks without caffeine Rehydration beverages	Caffeinated beverages (coffee, tea, colas, energy drinks) Limit beverages containing high fructose corn syrup to 12 oz/day Avoid beverages sweetened with sorbitol Alcoholic beverages
Fats Other foods		Limit to <8 tsp/day Sugar alcohol such as xylitol and sorbitol Honey

Modified from Academy of Nutrition and Dietetics: Fiber-restricted nutrition therapy. In *Nutrition care manual*, Chicago, Author. Accessed August 14, 2013, from www.nutritioncaremanual.org

related to the liquidity of the effluent. In the case of an ileostomy, the effluent is more liquid because the ileocecal valve, which controls rate of movement from the small intestine to the large, is absent. Water, sodium, and other minerals that would otherwise be absorbed are lost, making fluid and electrolyte replacement an important goal. With a colostomy, the effluent liquid is proportional to the length of the remaining bowel (Figure 13-8).

Application to nursing. The more liquid the stool, the greater the loss of fluid and electrolytes. Any restrictions placed on the patient should be based solely on individual tolerance.

✳ TEACHING TOOL

Inflammatory Bowel Disease

- During acute episodes, bowel rest and a low-fiber diet (see Table 13-4) are frequently suggested to minimize symptoms.
- During periods of remission, avoid unwarranted restrictions. A high-fiber diet (see Box 13-4) can stimulate peristalsis and improve muscular tone of the walls of the GI tract, especially the colon.
- Prebiotic or probiotic therapy may be beneficial. The nurse should work with the medical and nutrition teams to evaluate products first.

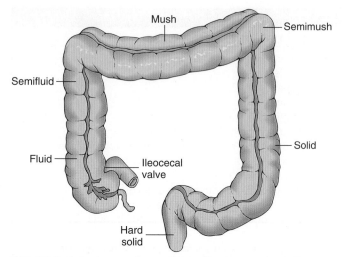

FIG 13-8 Colostomy site and its effect on output. Excess motility causes less absorption and diarrhea or loose feces. Poor motility causes more absorption, resulting in hard feces and constipation. (From Rolin Graphics. Modified from Guyton AC: *Textbook of medical physiology*, ed 11, Philadelphia, 2005, Saunders.)

✳ TEACHING TOOL

Recommendations for a Colostomy or Ileostomy

Meals can still be an enjoyable experience for patients with colostomies and ileostomies. Individual experimentation works best to determine the most appropriate dietary restrictions. The following are some strategies that may reduce negative symptoms:

Practices That May Cause Gas: Chewing gum, use of drinking straws, drinking carbonated beverages, smoking, chewing tobacco, eating quickly.

Eating Practices That May Reduce Discomfort: Take small bites of food and chew thoroughly. Eat smaller, frequent meals at regular times each day. Eat the largest meal in the middle of the day and a small evening meal.

Foods That May Help Control Odor or Gas: Buttermilk, parsley, yogurt, kefir, cranberry juice.

Foods That May Help Control Diarrhea: Applesauce, banana or banana flakes, pectin, pasta, potatoes, rice, cheese.

General Recommendations: Drink 8 to 10 cups of fluids each day, more during hot weather. Try new foods one at a time, and some more than one time.

Data from Academy of Nutrition and Dietetics: *Nutrition care manual*, 2013. Accessed August 14, 2013, from *www.nutritioncaremanual.org*

Short Bowel Syndrome

When large portions of the small intestine must be resected because of illness or injury, short bowel syndrome (SBS) may occur. The severity of SBS depends on the length and anatomy of the bowel resected and the health of the remaining tissue (Matarese, 2013). An inadequate absorptive surface results in malabsorption of vitamin B_{12} and other vitamins and less

than optimal nutritional status. Patients with SBS are prone to deficiencies in vitamins, minerals, and essential fatty acids; serum levels of these nutrients should be periodically monitored, and supplements provided as needed (Matarese, 2013).

Food and Nutrition Therapies

Nutritional management of the patient with SBS should take into consideration the individual's digestive and absorptive capabilities. Patients require parenteral nutrition (PN) or intravenous (IV) fluids in the immediate postresection period, but diet and enteral nutrition (EN) should be reintroduced as soon as possible (Matarese, 2013). Complex carbohydrates from whole grains, fruits, and vegetables should be used, but simple sugars should not.

MCT fats (oils) are specialized modular formulas made of medium-chain triglycerides that do not require pancreatic lipase or bile for digestion and absorption. They are absorbed directly into the portal vein (like amino acids and monosaccharides) rather than the lymphatic system like other lipids. Optimal fat intake varies with patient anatomy; patients with end-jejunostomies can tolerate a higher proportion of calories from dietary fat than patients with a remnant colon (Matarese, 2013).

Application to Nursing

Patients with SBS are at high risk of dehydration. Offer oral rehydration solutions to sip throughout the day. Because one of the primary goals is to reduce or eliminate dependence on parenteral or intravenous nutrition, optimized enteral nutrition and hydration will enhance successful weaning (Matarese, 2013).

✳ TEACHING TOOL

Recommendations for Managing Short-Bowel Syndrome

During the 2 years following resection, the remnant bowel undergoes an adaptation process that increases its absorptive capacity (Matarese, 2013). Frequent monitoring of nutritional status, especially fluid and electrolyte balance, is crucial. If a patient continues to fail on an oral diet, long-term parenteral nutrition at home may be indicated. Prebiotic or probiotic therapy may be beneficial, but more research is needed.

Diverticular Diseases

When the musculature of the bowel walls weakens, **diverticula** (pouchlike herniations protruding from the muscular layer of the colon) often develop, resulting in the condition **diverticulosis**. It is thought to develop as the result of long-term, low-fiber eating habits and increased intracolonic pressure such as that created with straining to have a bowel movement. Usually this condition remains undetected unless the diverticula become infected and inflamed from trapped fecal material and colon bacteria; the condition is then known as **diverticulitis**.

Food and Nutrition Therapies

When diverticula are inflamed, patients are given nothing by mouth, and then progress to liquids. After the inflammation abates, a high-fiber diet is recommended to reduce straining during defecation. High-fiber diets increase fiber-rich foods in the general diet by including fruits, vegetables, legumes, whole-grain breads, and cereals. Current fiber recommendations for Adequate Intake (AI) are 25 to 38 g/day.

Application to nursing. During periods of inflammation, the medical goal is to rest the bowel, allowing the infection to resolve. If constipation is a problem, stool softeners may be needed to avoid straining.

✳ TEACHING TOOL

Recommendations for Managing Diverticular Disorders

- There is no evidence-based research showing that nuts and seeds or popcorn worsen diverticular symptoms.
- Eating high-fiber foods is the only treatment for diverticulosis; see Box 13-4. Americans should consume at least five servings or cups of fruits/vegetables and six servings or ounces of whole-grain breads/cereals/legumes per day.
- Add more fiber gradually to allow the intestinal tract to adapt. This approach minimizes side effects such as abdominal distress, bloating, flatulence, cramps, and diarrhea, which are usually temporary.
- Care should also be taken to consume adequate amounts of fluid—at least 8 to 12 cups per day (Academy of Nutrition and Dietetics, 2013).

▌ S U M M A R Y

- Disorders of the GI tract include those that affect the esophagus, stomach, small intestine, and large intestine.
- Some disorders affect the muscular action of these sections of the GI tract, thereby affecting flow of sustenance through the GI tract; they include dysphagia and hiatal hernia.
- Peptic ulcer and diverticulitis can lead to site-specific tissue inflammation and pain.
- Several disorders may be caused by inability of the body to produce necessary digestive enzymes (e.g., lactase in lactose intolerance) or inability to metabolize nutrient substances (e.g., gliadin, resulting in severe reactions caused by celiac disease).

- Most disorders are also influenced by lifestyle behaviors that affect stress levels and alter dietary patterns.
- Prebiotics and probiotics show promise for the management of lower GI disorders, but the exact strains are not yet identified.
- Inflammatory bowel disorders are considered to be autoimmune conditions that have a genetic predisposition and an environmental trigger.
- All GI disorders require some level of nutrition therapy, which is individualized to meet the needs of each patient.

◎ THE NURSING APPROACH

Case Study: Dysphagia and Feeding Self-Care Deficit

Pierre, age 80, had a left-sided stroke 1 month ago and is in a rehabilitation center. He has been getting physical therapy for hemiparesis (one-sided weakness) in his right arm and leg. Initially after the stroke, he was evaluated by a speech therapist and received nourishment through a small-bore nasoduodenal feeding tube because of aphasia (language problems) and dysphagia (swallowing difficulties). Pierre has since been advanced to a soft diet (per doctor's orders), and he continues to work with a speech therapist in relation to expressive aphasia (knows what he wants to say but has trouble saying or writing what he means).

Assessment
Subjective (from Patient Statements)
The nurse is unable to understand Pierre's attempts to speak.

Objective (from Physical Examination)
- Coughs and chokes frequently when trying to eat or drink
- Clear lung sounds

- Pockets food in his cheeks
- Fed by nursing staff, does not assist with feeding, eats very slowly
- Can follow directions but has difficulty expressing himself

Diagnoses (Nursing)
1. Risk for aspiration related to impaired swallowing
2. Feeding self-care deficit related to weakness of right hand and arm, as evidenced by being fed by nurse; does not assist with feeding

Planning
Patient Outcomes
Short term (within 2 weeks):
- Pierre will be able to eat with minimal or no choking.
- Lung sounds will remain clear.
- He will not pocket food in his cheeks.
- He will be able to assist with his own feeding.

Continued

Long term (by discharge):
- He will not develop aspiration pneumonia.
- Pierre will be able to feed himself using adaptive equipment and assistance in setting up his food.

Nursing Interventions

1. Implement aspiration precautions.
2. Reinforce rehabilitation efforts by the health care team.

Implementation

1. Met with the health care team to design and implement an individualized rehabilitation care plan.
   The doctor prescribed the diet and therapies:
   - The dietitian planned nourishment consistent with physical limitations and nutrient needs.
   - The physical therapist strengthened the patient's weak arm to help with self-feeding.
   - The speech therapist taught the patient how to chew and swallow safely and to communicate needs.
   - The occupational therapist provided adaptive equipment for self-feeding and taught the patient how to become more independent.
   - The nurse helped facilitate schedules for the various therapies, helped feed the patient when team members from the other disciplines were not there, and reinforced teaching
   Team eforts enhance rehabilitation measures. Nurses are with the patient 24 hours per day and thus are in a position to coordinate necessary therapies and help implement the plan of care.
2. Tested Pierre's gag reflex and listened to lung sounds every morning before feeding him.
   Presence of the gag reflex reduces risk for aspiration. Assessment should be ongoing for any signs of aspiration pneumonia.
3. Positioned him in an upright position (high Fowler's) during meals and for 30 minutes after the meal.
   Gravity assists the passage of food and reduces the risk of choking and aspiration.
4. Reduced distractions such as television during mealtimes.
   Creating a focus for eating helps the patient concentrate on new swallowing and feeding techniques.
5. Assessed Pierre's food preferences by having him point to pictures of foods he likes that are part of the soft diet prescribed by the physician and at the recommendation of the dietitian.
   When the patient is able to make decisions about what to eat, he may feel some control of his situation. Foods that are easiest to chew and swallow include finely chopped meat and smooth textures. Nuts, tough skins, and dry, crispy, raw, or stringy foods are not allowed.
6. Added a commercial thickening agent to juices and water.
   Thin liquids provoke choking; thicker liquids are easier to swallow.
7. Used custard, gelatin, and liquid nutritional supplements between meals two or three times a day.
   Intake at mealtime is limited by patient tolerance and time. Between-meal snacks provide extra calories and fluids.
8. Instructed Pierre to follow specific steps when swallowing:
   A. Take a breath before swallowing
   B. Hold breath during swallowing
   C. Exhale forcefully after swallowing
   D. Swallow again
   This maneuver decreases the potential for aspiration by closing off the trachea.
9. Had suction equipment available during feedings.
   The nurse may need to remove fluids from the patient's mouth and throat by suction in order to prevent aspiration.
10. Provided mouth care before and after meals.
    A fresh mouth encourages appetite. Removal of pocketed food (food remaining in the weak side of the mouth) reduces danger of choking.
11. Encouraged Pierre to feed himself, using special plates and utensils.
    Adaptive equipment may facilitate success of the patient's attempts to feed himself.

Evaluation

Short term (at the end of 2 weeks):
- Pierre was beginning to feed himself.
- He was no longer pocketing food in his cheeks.
- He was still choking occasionally on his food and liquids, but his lungs remained clear.
  Goals partially met.

Discussion Questions

As Pierre started feeding himself, he sometimes left food on the same side of the plate as his weak arm. He also failed to see the nurse when she would come to assist feeding him if the nurse stood at his weak side. The nurse added the nursing diagnosis of "Unilateral neglect."

1. What causes this problem?
2. How could the nurse teach Pierre to compensate for this condition?
   NOTE: Periodic swallowing reevaluation is recommended. Swallowing dysfunction is different for every patient, and appropriate dietary modifications are determined by speech pathologists and registered dietitians.

Swallowing Exercise: Put Yourself in a Dysphagic Patient's Shoes

Most people take normal activities of daily living for granted. When something as simple as swallowing is impaired, eating and drinking become more difficult. To experience difficulty swallowing, tilt your head all the way backward so that you are looking up at the ceiling. Now try to swallow. Next, put your chin down toward your chest so that you are looking down. Again, try to swallow. Next, tilt your head all the way to the right side, and then swallow. Finally, look straight ahead with your head at a normal 90-degree angle and swallow. Can you tell the difference? Which was the easiest? As you can tell, it is much harder to swallow when your head is not aligned properly.

This is a simple exercise to demonstrate how difficult it can be for a patient with dysphagia to swallow. It also emphasizes the importance of ensuring that patients are sitting upright with their heads at a normal angle while eating and drinking. Not only does this positioning make swallowing easier, it also may allow for more independence and ease in self-feeding.

CRITICAL THINKING

Clinical Applications

Theresa, age 35, is admitted with microcytic anemia. Her medical history indicates that she underwent a total gastrectomy 2 years ago to treat bleeding ulcers. On admission she weighs 120 pounds, and she is 5 feet 9 inches tall. She has lost 30 pounds since the surgery. She has been taking ferrous sulfate and monthly injections of vitamin B_{12}. On admission her laboratory findings are as follows: hemoglobin 8 g/dL, hematocrit 26%, and serum albumin 2.7 g/dL. Her typical dietary intake is as follows:

Breakfast

1 egg scrambled in 1 teaspoon margarine

½ cup cream of wheat with 1 teaspoon margarine

1 slice white toast with 1 teaspoon margarine

1 cup black coffee

10 AM

6 saltine crackers

12-ounce can diet cola

Lunch

2 baked chicken wings

1 cup cooked carrots

1 medium boiled red potato

1 medium banana

12 ounces diet lemon-lime soda

3 PM

½ bagel with 1 tablespoon cream cheese

8 ounces chocolate milk

Dinner

1 broiled chicken breast

½ cup steamed broccoli

1 cup hot tea with artificial sweetener

9 PM

6 saltine crackers

1 tablespoon peanut butter

1 cup black coffee

1. What are common nutrition problems found in patients who have gastrectomies?
2. Which of these problems has Theresa experienced?
3. What factors explain the iron-deficiency anemia that develops after a gastrectomy? What is used to treat this anemia?
4. How do Theresa's laboratory values compare with normal values? What do they indicate?
5. Why is Theresa receiving monthly injections of vitamin B_{12}? Would you advise her to eat more foods high in B_{12}? Explain your rationale.
6. Review Theresa's usual dietary intake; what food groups and/or nutrients are lacking in her diet?
7. What suggestions would you offer Theresa concerning her dietary habits?
8. Should Theresa continue to consume six smaller meals and snacks? Why or why not?

WEBSITES OF INTEREST

Crohn's Disease/Ulcerative Colitis/Inflammatory Bowel Disease Pages

http://qurlyjoe.bu.edu/cduchome.html

Provides information on several digestive diseases; includes chat rooms, resources, retail items, and pharmaceutical links.

International Foundation for Functional Gastrointestinal Disorders (IFFGD)

www.iffgd.org

National Digestive Diseases Information Clearinghouse (NDDIC)

www.niddk.nih.gov/health/digest/nddic.htm

Sponsored by the National Institute of Digestive Diseases, this database contains health promotion and education materials not indexed elsewhere.

National Institute of Diabetes and Digestive and Kidney Diseases (NIDDK)

www.niddk.nih.gov

Contains information, resources, and related links on digestive diseases, diabetes, kidney and urologic diseases, and nutrition.

REFERENCES

Academy of Nutrition and Dietetics: *Nutrition care manual,* Chicago, 2013, Author. from: www.nutritioncaremanual.org. Accessed August 14, 2013.

Awosoqba T, et al: Prioritizing health disparities in medical education to improve care, *Ann N Y Acad Sci* 1287:17–30, 2013.

Boettcher E, Crowe SE: Dietary proteins and functional gastrointestinal disorders, *Am J Gastroenterol* 108:728–736, 2013.

Collins B, Norton C: Managing passive incontinence and incomplete evacuation, *Br J Nurs* 22:575–579, 2013.

Escott-Stump S: *Nutrition and diagnosis-related care,* ed 7, Baltimore, 2011, Lippincott-Williams & Wilkins.

Eswaran S, et al: Fiber and functional gastrointestinal disorders, *Am J Gastroenterol* 108:718–727, 2013.

FDA (Food and Drug Administration.): Food labeling: gluten-free labeling of foods. Final rule, *Fed Regist* 78:47154–47179, 2013.

Frazier TH, et al: Gut microbiota, intestinal permeability, obesity-induced inflammation, and liver injury, *JPEN J Parenter Enteral Nutr* 35:14S–20S, 2011.

Haberkorn BC, et al: Improving diagnosis of adult-type hypolactasia in patients with abdominal complaints, *Clin Chem Lab Med* 50:119–123, 2011.

Haughton B, Stang J: Population risk factors and trends in health care and public policy, *J Acad Nutr Diet* 112:35S–46S, 2012.

Kaspar K, Ekberg O: Identifying vulnerable patients: Role of the EAT-10 and the multidisciplinary team for early intervention and comprehensive dysphagia care, *Nestle Nutr Inst Workshop Ser* 72:19–31, 2012.

Liu LW: Chronic constipation: current treatment options, *Can J Gastroenterol* 25:22–28, 2011.

Matarese LE: Nutrition and fluid optimization for patients with short bowel syndrome, *JPEN J Parenter Enteral Nutr* 37:161–170, 2013.

Milazzo LS, et al: The swallowing process: Effects of aging and stroke, *Phys Med Rehabil State Art Rev* 3:489, 1989.

National Foundation of Swallowing Disorders: *Oral swallowing exercises,* n.d, from: www.swallowingdisorderfoundation.com/oral-swallowing-exercises/. Accessed August 14, 2013.

National Institute of Diabetes and Digestive and Kidney Diseases: *Constipation*, from: digestive.niddk.nih.gov/ddiseases/pubs/constipation/. Accessed September 19, 2013.

Nicholson JK, et al: Host-gut microbiota metabolic interactions, *Science* 336:1262, 2012.

Phan VH, et al: An update on ethnic differences in drug metabolism and toxicity from anti-cancer drugs, *Expert Opin Drug Metab Toxicol* 7:1395–1410, 2011.

Portalatin M, Winstead N: Medical management of constipation, *Clin Colon Rectal Surg* 25:12–19, 2012.

Stegemann S, et al: Swallowing dysfunction and dysphagia is an unrecognized challenge for oral drug therapy, *Int J Pharm* 430:197–206, 2012.

CHAPTER 14

Nutrition for Disorders of the Liver, Gallbladder, and Pancreas

Although the liver, gallbladder, and pancreas are not part of the digestive tract proper, little digestion, absorption, or metabolism would take place without them. You can live without a lung, but you cannot survive without a liver or a pancreas.

e http://evolve.elsevier.com/GRODNER/FOUNDATIONS

LEARNING OBJECTIVES

- Identify the importance of the liver, the gallbladder, and the pancreas for proper digestion.
- Describe disorders of the liver and the nutritional therapy to treat each disorder.
- Outline the specific nutrition therapy needs of each stage of liver transplantation.

- Discuss the nutrition approaches to reduce the symptoms of gallbladder disorders.
- Explain how pancreatitis alters digestion and absorption of dietary fats and protein.
- Review the potential need for enteral or parenteral nutrition support during treatment of pancreatitis.

NUTRITION IN LIVER HEALTH

Wellness requires well-functioning body organs. *Physical health* is crucially dependent on the liver, pancreas, and gallbladder; one malfunction can devastate nutritional status. Reasoning, an aspect of *intellectual health*, is required to make lifestyle decisions related to alcohol when a person is at risk for cirrhosis. A chronic life-threatening illness, such as pancreatitis, challenges *emotional health*. Restrictive dietary guidelines inhibit the ability to easily socialize with others, thereby diminishing *social health*. *Spiritual health* and religious beliefs will provide comfort when one is coping with serious physical disorders. The *environmental health* dimension encompasses striving for work and living surroundings that are free of toxic substances that could contaminate food, water, and air. Consumption of toxic substances can affect the health of the liver, which acts as a filter of toxins for the body.

LIVER DISORDERS

The liver, the largest organ in the body, lies beneath the diaphragm in the right upper quadrant of the abdomen and is responsible for the majority of biochemical functions that take place in the body. The liver manages bile production and its role in metabolism of carbohydrates, protein, lipids, and vitamins. Because this organ is such a workhorse, impaired liver function can result in major imbalances in metabolism and nutritional status. Progressive decline in nutritional status further impairs liver function. Figure 14-1 summarizes only a few of the liver's many roles in metabolism and nutritional status.

Hepatitis

Hepatitis is inflammation of the liver. Acute hepatitis can occur as the result of infectious mononucleosis, cirrhosis, toxic chemicals, or viral infection. Five types of hepatitis have been characterized. Their symptoms, signs, and presentation are similar, but their immunologic and epidemiologic characteristics are different (Table 14-1).

Hepatitis A virus (HAV) is typically transmitted through the fecal-oral route (contaminated food or water) but occasionally can be spread by transfusion of infected blood. It is frequently the result of poor hand washing or stool precautions and is widespread in overcrowded areas with poor sanitation (Box 14-1). Vaccination is recommended for persons at risk for HAV. Onset of HAV is rapid—4 to 6 weeks—and time to onset of symptoms may be dose related. Occurrence of disease manifestations and severity of symptoms directly correlate with the patient's age.

Treatment of acute HAV is generally supportive—usually consisting of bed rest—because no antiviral therapy is available. Hospitalization and intravenous (IV) fluids may be necessary for dehydration caused by nausea and vomiting. A balanced diet that excludes alcohol is recommended.

Hepatitis B virus (HBV) is an exceptionally resistant virus capable of surviving extreme temperatures and humidity. HBV is transmitted via blood, semen, vaginal mucus, saliva, and tears. Intravenous drug users, patients with hemophilia, those undergoing renal dialysis, and those who have undergone organ transplantation are at increased risk for HBV (Box 14-2). As a result, routine HBV vaccination is recommended for risk groups of all ages and for children up to age

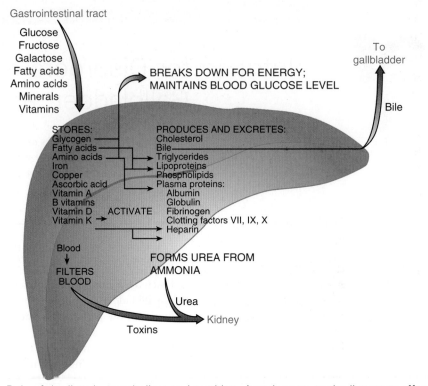

FIG 14-1 Role of the liver in metabolism and nutrition. Any damage to the liver may affect nutritional status. (From Rolin Graphics. Modified from Davis J, Sherer K: *Applied nutrition and diet therapy for nurses,* ed 2, Philadelphia, 1994, Saunders.)

TABLE 14-1 Comparison of Hepatitis Viruses

	HEPATITIS A (HAV)	HEPATITIS B (HBV)	HEPATITIS C (HCV)	HEPATITIS D (HDV)	HEPATITIS E (HEV)
Symptoms					
Jaundice	X	X	X	X	X
Low-grade fever	X	X	X	X	
Malaise	X	X	X	X	
Anorexia	X	X	X	X	
Dark urine	X	X	X	X	
Diarrhea	X	X	X	X	
Pale stools	X	X	X	X	
Hepatitis B surface antigen (HbsAg) in serum		X	X	X	
Can be asymptomatic			X	X	
Flu-like aches and pains					X
Transmission					
Fecal-oral	X				X
Foodborne	X				X
Sexual	X	X		X	
Parenteral		X		X	
Perinatal		Rare			
Contaminated food or water	X				X
Blood or serum			X		
Sharing contaminated needles, tattooing/piercing equipment			X		
Co-infected with HBV				X	
Prevention					
Hand washing	X	X	X	X	
Good personal hygiene	X	X	X	X	
Appropriate infection control measures	X	X	X	X	
Safe sex practices		X	X	X	
Not drinking contaminated water					X

BOX 14-1   Risk Factors for Hepatitis A Virus

- Travelers to areas where hepatitis A virus (HAV) is common
- Homosexual and male
- Sexual contact with infected people
- Use of injectable and noninjectable drugs
- Household contact with infected people
- Health care and public safety workers
- People, especially children, living in regions of the United States that have consistently increased rates of HAV

Data from Centers for Disease Control and Prevention: *Viral hepatitis,* Atlanta, 2013, Author. Accessed August 16, 2013, from www.cdc.gov/hepatitis/index.htm

---

BOX 14-2   Risk Factors for Hepatitis B Virus

- People with multiple sex partners or partners diagnosed with a sexually transmitted disease
- Homosexual men
- Sexual contact with infected people
- Use of injectable drugs
- Household contact with chronically infected people
- Infants born to infected mothers
- Infants and children of immigrants from areas with high rates of HBV infection
- Health care and public safety workers
- Patients receiving hemodialysis treatments

Data from Centers for Disease Control and Prevention: *Hepatitis B fact sheet,* Atlanta, 2013, Author. Accessed August 16, 2013, from www.cdc.gov/hepatitis/index.htm.

⊕ CULTURAL CONSIDERATIONS

Hepatitis B Virus Prevalence among Underserved Areas

Hepatitis B virus (HBV) occurs worldwide, especially where there are limited or primitive medical services. In Africa and Asia, widespread infection may occur in infancy and childhood. The overall carrier rates may be as high as 10% to 15%. HBV infection is prevalent in sub-Saharan Africa, where there are at least 65 million chronic carriers, 25% of whom are expected to die from liver disease (Burnett, et al, 2012). Many barriers prevent containment of the epidemic, including shortage of health care workers, poor medical infrastructures, and insufficient screening and poor access to care and treatment (Lemoine, et al, 2013). In developed countries, HBV is more common in high-risk groups. Contaminated and inadequately sterilized syringes and needles have led to outbreaks of hepatitis B among patients in clinics, physicians' offices, tattoo parlors, and acupuncturist offices. Occult HBV infection may occur in blood donors, especially immigrants. ***Application to nursing.*** Nurses working with clients who are at high risk for HBV can advocate for hepatitis B vaccinations for these individuals. Such clients include foreign-born individuals, individuals with alternative sexual orientation, people with histories of current or past drug abuse, and those exposed to or already diagnosed with human immunodeficiency virus.

Data from Burnett RJ, et al: An update after 16 years of hepatitis B vaccination in South Africa, *Vaccine* 3:45S-51S, 2012; Lemoine M, et al: Viral hepatitis in resource-limited countries and access to antiviral therapies: Current and future challenges, *Future Virol* 8:371-380, 2013; and World Health Organization: *Global Health Alert: Hepatitis B.* Accessed August 17, 2013, from http://www.who.int/csr/disease/hepatitis/whocdscsrlyo20022/en/index3.html.

---

18. The average incubation time of HBV is approximately 12 weeks. As with HAV, the majority of patients are asymptomatic. Those who acquire chronic HBV infection (determined by biopsy) can be healthy, asymptomatic carriers but remain infectious to others through parenteral or sexual transmission.

Chronic hepatitis B virus (HBV) is a major risk factor for hepatocellular carcinoma (Thein, et al, 2011). Chronic HBV is treated with interferon-α and lamivudine to reduce symptoms and prevent or delay progression of chronic hepatitis to cirrhosis or hepatocellular carcinoma (HCC). Hepatitis B immunoglobulin (HBIG) provides passive immunization. The hepatitis B vaccine is targeted to adolescents and adults in high-risk groups. Patients who need repeated transfusions, health care workers, patients and employees in hemodialysis centers, and nurses working in emergency departments or operating rooms should be vaccinated against HBV. Travelers to areas of the world where HBV is prevalent should be vaccinated; see the *Cultural Considerations* box Hepatitis B Virus Prevalence among Underserved Areas.

Hepatitis C virus (HCV) infection is increasing worldwide and is the major cause of hepatitis in the United States. It is transmitted through contaminated blood, saliva, or semen, although HCV is predominantly associated with blood exposure (e.g., transfusion, IV drug use, acupuncture, tattooing, and sharing razors). Onset is usually slow (i.e., approximately 8 weeks); HCV can develop into some form of chronic liver disease and is a risk factor for liver cancer.

Most cases of acute HCV are asymptomatic and infrequently detected. Chronic infection develops in 70% to 80% of infected people. Progression from HCV to cirrhosis may take 10 to 40 years. A more rapid disease progression is observed in older persons, those infected with human immunodeficiency virus (HIV) or HBV, and alcoholics. Chronic HCV is treated with a combination therapy of interferon-α and ribavirin. No special diet is recommended.

Hepatitis D virus (HDV) can occur only if an individual with HBV is subsequently exposed to HDV (co-infection or superinfection). The incubation period is 21 to 45 days but may be shorter in cases of superinfection. Clinical course varies, ranging from acute, self-limiting infection to acute fulminant liver failure. HDV is found throughout the world but is prevalent in the Mediterranean basin, Middle East, Amazon basin, and Asia. Of persons infected with HDV, 90% are likely to be asymptomatic. Parenteral transmission is understood to be the most common means of infection, making IV drug use a risk factor. Patients co-infected with HBV and HDV are less responsive to interferon therapy than patients infected with HBV alone. Diet does not need to be restricted.

Hepatitis E virus (HEV) is an enterically transmitted (oral-fecal route), self-limiting infection. The prevalence of HEV is generally attributed to travel in tropical climates, inadequate sanitation, and poor personal hygiene. The incubation period ranges from 15 to 60 days, and symptoms include myalgia, anorexia, nausea/vomiting, weight loss (typically 5 to 10 pounds), dehydration, jaundice, dark urine, and light-colored stools. Therapy should be predominantly preventive.

Travelers to endemic areas should avoid drinking water or other beverages that may be contaminated. Uncooked fruits and vegetables should not be eaten. No vaccines are available for HEV. Once infection occurs, therapy is limited to support.

Food and Nutrition Therapies

During periods of nausea and vomiting in patients with hepatitis, hydration via IV fluids may be necessary. Oral feedings should be initiated as soon as possible, with frequent feedings high in kcal and in high-quality protein, to promote adequate intake and minimize loss of muscle mass. Adequate protein, 1.0 to 1.2 g/kg body weight, is recommended for most persons. Dietary fats should not be limited unless they are not well tolerated (e.g., steatorrhea).

Fluid intake should be adequate to accommodate the high protein intake unless otherwise contraindicated. Supplementation with a multivitamin that includes vitamin B complex (especially thiamine and vitamin B_{12} because of decreased absorption and hepatic uptake), vitamin K (to normalize bleeding tendency), vitamin C, and zinc for poor appetite is recommended. Abstinence from alcohol is imperative.

Application to nursing. Patients should receive adequate hydration and electrolyte repletion. Hospitalization may be necessary for those unable to maintain an adequate oral intake. Bed rest and proper nutrition are the major constituents of therapy for all types of hepatitis. Treatment goals are as follows:

- Decrease viral replication or eradicate the infection
- Delay fibrosis and progression to cirrhosis
- Decrease incidence of liver cancer
- Ameliorate fatigue and joint pain
- Prevent hepatic decompensation and the need for liver transplantation.

✳ TEACHING TOOL

Suggestions for Coping with Hepatitis

- An adequate diet that excludes alcohol is recommended.
- For many individuals, loss of appetite, weight loss, and fatigue are common problems. Recommend rest periods before and after meals.
- Offer guidance and tips for increasing protein and calories without adding more total food volume. Sauces, gravies, desserts, milkshakes, and similar enhancements will help.

Fatty Liver and Nonalcoholic Steatohepatitis

Fatty liver (*hepatic steatosis*) is typically the result of an underlying problem. Bacterial overgrowth, immune dysfunction, alteration of the luminal factors, and altered intestinal permeability are all involved in the pathogenesis (Ilan, 2012). Fatty liver is an early form of alcoholic liver disease but can also be caused by obesity, complications of drug therapy (e.g., corticosteroids, tetracyclines), excessive parenteral nutrition, pregnancy, diabetes mellitus, inadequate intake of protein (in malnutrition) infection, or malignancy.

Fatty infiltration of the liver develops when hepatocytes are injured by toxic lipid molecules (lipotoxicity). This *nonalcoholic fatty liver disease (NAFLD)* is highly prevalent (15% to 45%) in modern societies, yet in only 10% to 25% of cases does hepatic fibrosis lead to cirrhosis, end-stage liver disease, or liver cancer develop (Farrell, et al, 2012).

Nonalcoholic steatohepatitis (*NASH*) is another name for the inflammatory fatty infiltration that occurs in the liver of people who drink little or no alcohol. NASH may manifest as fatigue, or it may progress to liver failure.

Food and Nutrition Therapies

A thorough diet history is essential, and a nutrition plan should be developed according to the etiology of the condition. If the problem is related to diabetes, glucose management would require carbohydrate counting or other measures. If the fatty liver occurs after initiation of parenteral nutrition, the amount and rate of administration should be altered.

Excess lipid accumulates and causes inflammation. Some studies suggest that high-fat and high-fructose intakes are problematic (Frazier, et al, 2011). Overnutrition, insulin resistance, hyperglycemia, and metabolic syndrome should be controlled (Farrell, et al, 2012). Patients may require control of dietary fat, carbohydrate, and alcohol or a combination of all three.

Weight loss may be needed. Meals should not be skipped in an effort to lose weight rapidly. Because this condition is common among the morbidly obese (body mass index [BMI] > 40), bariatric surgery may be required. If liver transplantation is needed, the effects of bariatric surgery, nutrition, pharmacotherapy, and immunosuppressive agents must be considered carefully (Charlton, 2013).

Application to nursing. A calorie-controlled diet limiting fats, fructose, and alcohol may be ordered. Adequate tracking of glucose and lipid levels will be needed. Whatever the cause, proper nutrition in the form of a well-balanced diet is important in reversing fatty infiltration.

Cirrhosis

Intestinal bacterial overgrowth and increased bacterial translocation of gut flora set patients up for bacterial infections, major complications, and chronic liver disorders like cirrhosis (Ilan, 2012). In cirrhosis, liver cells are replaced by fibrous connective tissue and fat infiltration (Figure 14-2). This damage can occur for a variety of reasons, including the following:

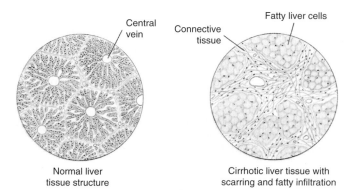

Central vein

Connective tissue

Fatty liver cells

Normal liver tissue structure

Cirrhotic liver tissue with scarring and fatty infiltration

FIG 14-2 Comparison of normal liver tissue structure with liver tissue changes from cirrhosis. (Medical and Scientific Illustration. From Williams SR: *Nutrition and diet therapy*, ed 8, St. Louis, 1997, Mosby.)

✳ TEACHING TOOL

Suggestions for Coping with Fatty Liver or Nonalcoholic Steatohepatitis (NASH)

- A balanced diet is important. It may require eliminating intake of alcohol and limiting total intake of fat or fructose.
- The assistance of a registered dietitian will be needed to guide this nutrition care plan successfully.
- Probiotics/prebiotics may be beneficial. They affect gut flora; certain forms may alleviate liver injury (Frazier, et al, 2011).

- Hepatitis (postnecrotic cirrhosis)
- Biliary cirrhosis disorders
- Chronic autoimmune disease
- Metabolic disorders (Wilson's disease or hemochromatosis)
- Chronic hepatotoxic drug use
- Alcoholic cirrhosis (see the *Health Debate* box Alcohol: Proscribe or Prescribe?)

Liver cell scarring can cause congestion of hepatic circulation (backing up of blood in the portal vein), which results in further decline of liver function, portal hypertension, and esophageal varices. Blood vessels tend to enlarge and bulge into the lumen of the esophagus, where they may rupture. Esophageal varices are usually the result of collateral circulation that develops around the esophagus when normal blood flow through the liver is blocked (Figure 14-3). The bleeding tends to recur and can eventually be fatal.

Another complication, ascites, is the accumulation of fluid in the peritoneal cavity. Fluid is trapped in the characteristic swollen or distended abdomen seen in patients with cirrhosis. As liver disease continues to progress, blood is shunted from portal circulation to systemic circulation. This causes blood to bypass the liver and could result in hepatic encephalopathy or hepatic coma. Hepatic encephalopathy is a "cerebral intoxication" caused by intestinal contents that

---

⚕ HEALTH DEBATE

Alcohol: Prescribe? Proscribe?

Alcohol is probably the most commonly used hepatotoxic drug. Next to caffeine, it is the most socially acceptable drug in the United States. Alcohol is legal, but its sales are regulated by state-controlled establishments. One drink equals 12 oz. beer, 5 oz. wine, or 1½ oz. hard liquor.

Alcohol use is linked with birth defects, domestic violence, and traffic accidents. Heavy alcohol intake (3+ drinks daily) causes damage to the liver, brain, and heart and increases the risk of cancer. Chronic, heavy drinking is associated with cancers of the mouth, throat, larynx, and liver. Moderate drinking has been linked with breast, prostate, and rectal cancers.

Could any possible good come from such a drug? Alcohol may actually decrease the risk of heart disease. Studies have found a lower coronary artery disease mortality risk among moderate drinkers (one or two drinks daily) than among nondrinkers. At first it looked as if red wine was the magic elixir, but white wine, beer, and hard liquor seem to be just as beneficial. So what's a person to do? If you're concerned about heart disease and drink small quantities of alcohol every day or every other day, you're probably okay.

Remember, alcohol is a drug. Like any drug, it is most effective when administered at the appropriate dosage. The dangers of excess outweigh any possible benefits. So ... don't begin if you do not currently drink, are pregnant or trying to conceive, are taking medication, are driving, or are unable to control your drinking.

Data from Brien SE, et al: Effect of alcohol consumption on biological markers associated with risk of coronary heart disease: Systematic review and meta-analysis of interventional studies, *BMJ* 342:636, 2011; Ronksley PE, et al: Association of alcohol consumption with selected cardiovascular disease outcomes: A systematic review and meta-analysis, *BMJ* 342:671, 2011.

---

have not been metabolized by the liver. In this condition, ammonia cannot be eliminated from the body. Patients experience changes in consciousness and behavior, loss of concentration and memory, confusion, apathy, personality changes, and other psychiatric symptoms. Neurologic changes include spasticity, muscle spasms, asterixis or flapping (involuntary jerky movements, especially of the hands), and rigidity of the limbs with flexion withdrawal of the lower limbs.

Neomycin is used to reduce the numbers of bacteria in the gastrointestinal (GI) tract, thus decreasing the amount of urea that can be converted to ammonia. Neomycin treatment allows more protein to be included in the diet for tissue regeneration, although protein intake might be mildly restricted. One disadvantage of neomycin is that it contributes to malabsorption of most nutrients and can cause nausea, vomiting, diarrhea, and nephrotoxicity.

Lactulose is a nonabsorbable disaccharide that is metabolized by intestinal bacteria, resulting in a lower-pH stool. The lowered pH traps ammonia in the colon; the ammonia is then excreted. This agent also has a laxative action, and diarrhea is common with its use.

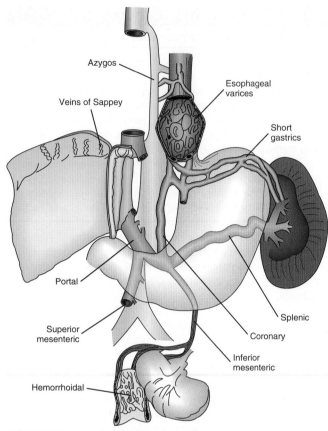

Azygos

Esophageal varices

Veins of Sappey

Short gastrics

Portal

Superior mesenteric

Splenic

Coronary

Inferior mesenteric

Hemorrhoidal

FIG 14-3 Varices related to portal hypertension. Portal vein, its major tributaries, and the most important shunts (collateral veins) between the portal and caval systems. (Redrawn from Kissane JM, editor: *Anderson's pathology,* ed 9, St. Louis, 1990, Mosby.)

Food and Nutrition Therapies

The most important aspect of nutrition therapy for cirrhosis to keep in mind is that each patient has individual nutritional needs that must be addressed. Protein and energy malnutrition is commonplace in patients with end-stage liver disease who have cirrhosis. A minimum of 0.8 g protein per kg body weight per day is essential. To promote positive nitrogen balance and avert breakdown of endogenous protein stores, 1.2 g protein/kg dry or appropriate body weight is recommended. Protein restriction should be avoided, because it could possibly worsen malnutrition.

If a patient appears to be protein sensitive (e.g., increased occurrence of encephalopathy), branched-chain amino acid–based formulas with restricted aromatic amino acids can be used to ensure a sustained level of protein intake. Plant proteins also produce less ammonia.

Patients with esophageal varices should eat soft, low-fiber foods. For ascites, a dietary sodium restriction (2000 mg) is used, usually with a fluid restriction. When diuretics are used, attention should be given to whether the drug depletes or spares potassium. If a potassium-depleting diuretic is used, potassium levels should be monitored carefully.

Application to nursing. Fluids are given in relation to input/output (I&O) records, daily weights, and electrolyte

values. Fluid restrictions are often necessary, beginning at 1500 mL/day. Limits may decrease to 1000 to 1200 mL/day, depending on the patient's response. The nurse may provide suggestions on how to cope with thirst in an effort to improve patient compliance with these kinds of fluid restrictions.

✳ TEACHING TOOL

Suggestions for Coping with Fluid Restriction

1. Salty and spicy foods make you thirsty; limit the amount of sodium and spicy foods in your diet.
2. Be aware of hidden fluids in foods: gelatin, watermelon, soup, gravy, and frozen treats like popsicles and ice cream.
3. Stay cool, especially in warmer weather. Try drinking cold liquids instead of hot beverages. Try snacking on approved vegetables and fruits that are ice cold.
4. Sip your beverages; use small cups or glasses for your beverages.
5. Drink to quench thirst only. Avoid drinking from habit or to be sociable.
6. Sliced lemon wedges can stimulate saliva and moisten a dry mouth.
7. Keep your mouth clean by brushing teeth frequently and rinsing mouth with water (do not swallow rinse water).
8. Battle dry mouth. Chew gum, suck sour hard candies, or use mints to stimulate saliva flow.
9. Freeze the allotted amount of fluid as ice. Sucking on ice is satisfying because it stays in the mouth longer. Add lemon to the ice cubes.
10. Limit fluids at mealtime; when appropriate, take medications with mealtime liquids or soft foods like applesauce.
11. Take medications with applesauce instead of liquid.
12. Take a small amount of fluid at one time.
13. If allowable, use high-fat foods such as gravies and margarine to moisten foods and make them easier to swallow.

Modified from Bio-Medical Applications of Carbondale, Dialysis Services Division, Carbondale, IL, 1995, Fresenius Medical Care; Davita: *Fluid control for kidney disease patients on dialysis.* Accessed August 17, 2013, from http://www.davita.com/kidney-disease/diet-and-nutrition/diet-basics/fluid-control-for-kidney-disease-patients-on-dialysis/e/5321.

Liver Transplantation

Liver transplantation is regarded as an appropriate treatment for end-stage liver disease. Nutritional goals for the patient awaiting organ transplantation depend on the individual's weight history and current status. Most patients in this condition show some indications of compromised nutritional status and therefore require special attention to nutritional needs.

It is difficult to assess nutritional status in patients with liver disorders because many parameters (e.g., body weight, nitrogen balance determination, total lymphocyte count, serum protein levels) are affected by edema, ascites, and hepatic necrosis. Therefore, it may be more appropriate to use subjective parameters, such as appetite, satiety level, taste changes, diet history, and GI symptoms. Weight change,

TABLE 14-2 Nutrition Care Guidelines after Liver Transplantation

NUTRIENTS/FLUIDS	SHORT-TERM	LONG-TERM
Energy	1.2-1.5 × BEE (use higher range if patient is severely underweight)	1.2-1.3 × BEE (basal energy expenditure) or as adequate to maintain weight
Protein	1.5-2 g/kg/day	0.8-1 g/kg
Carbohydrate		20-30 g dietary fiber/day
Fat		25%-35% kcal <10% kcal from saturated fats
Vitamins	History of alcoholism could suggest deficiencies in vitamins A, B_6, and B_{12}, niacin, thiamine, and folate	Recommended Dietary Allowance (RDA) amounts
	History of cholestatic liver disease could suggest preexisting deficiencies of fat-soluble vitamins and B_{12}	Consider supplementation/restriction based on pre-transplantation condition and diagnosis or post-transplantation complications
Minerals	Provide RDA in consideration of medical history	RDA
Electrolytes		Sodium <4 g/day Monitor potassium, phosphorus, magnesium Supplement/restrict as needed
Fluids	30-35 mL/kg, adjusting for increased losses or decreased needs	30-35 mL/kg; requirements higher in hot climates or with fever

COMMON LONG-TERM COMPLICATIONS	NUTRITION CARE
Excessive weight gain	Reduce kcal intake; aerobic exercise 3-5 times/week; reduce corticosteroid dose as able
Hyperlipidemia	Recommendations as above; change corticosteroid to tacrolimus; lipid-lowering medication used with caution
Diabetes mellitus	Diet and insulin or oral hypoglycemic agent to maintain glycemic control (fasting glucose <125 mg/dL, hemoglobin A_{1c} <7%); blood glucose self-monitoring; aerobic exercise 3-5 times/week; reduction of corticosteroid doses as possible
Osteoporosis	1000-1500 mg calcium/day; vitamin D supplements; weight-bearing exercise; discontinuation of smoking; moderate sodium and protein intake; hormone replacement therapy when appropriate

Data from Hasse JM: Adult liver transplantation. In Hasse JM, Blue LS, editors: *Comprehensive guide to transplant nutrition*, Chicago, 2002, American Dietetic Association.

however, is more often a reflection of fluid shifts rather than true weight loss. Physical examination findings such as temporal wasting of muscle and wasting of the upper extremities can be helpful to estimate the degree of malnutrition.

Food and Nutrition Therapies

Each phase of the transplantation procedure dictates specific nutritional requirements (Table 14-2). The primary objective in pre-transplantation nutrition therapy is to provide enough calories and protein to decrease protein catabolism and correct any nutritional deficiencies. The 4 to 8 weeks following surgery—the immediate post-transplantation period—require individualization of nutrition therapy according to the patient's needs. Ascites, edema, and excess fluid make using the patient's actual weight unreliable for determining energy and protein needs. Ideal (desirable) weight is a better reference point. Adequate calories and protein are necessary for the hypercatabolic (but not necessarily hypermetabolic) stresses that result from surgery and high doses of glucocorticoids.

Total parenteral nutrition (TPN) may be necessary if nutritional needs cannot be met enterally (feeding by mouth and/or with tube feeding). When oral intake is initiated, early satiety and altered tastes may prevent adequate intake. In such cases, between-meal feedings or supplements should be used to meet calorie and protein goals. Fluid losses from drains, nasogastric tubes, stool output, and urine should be considered in the determination of postoperative fluid needs.

Application to nursing. Over the long term after liver transplantation, a healthy, well-balanced diet is the nutrition goal. Because of common post-transplantation complications (e.g., excessive weight gain, hypertension, hyperlipidemia, diabetes), adjustments in intake of calories, fat, and concentrated carbohydrates may be necessary.

✳ TEACHING TOOL

Suggestions for Coping with Transplantation

- Patients will experience anxiety and depression after their transplantation.
- Support groups, social support, or therapy may be needed to make adjustments and improve quality of life.

GALLBLADDER DISORDERS

The gallbladder and the hepatic, cystic, and common bile ducts compose the biliary system (Figure 14-4). Bile is transported from the liver to the gallbladder via the common

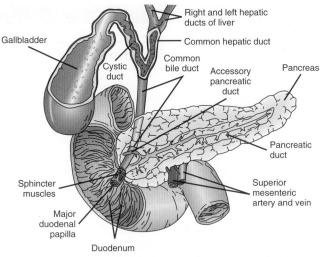

FIG 14-4 Gallbladder and bile ducts. Obstruction of either the hepatic or the common bile duct by stone or spasm prevents bile from being ejected into the duodenum. (From Rolin Graphics.)

FIG 14-5 Gallstones. (From Stevens A, Lowe J: *Pathology*, London, 1995, Mosby.)

hepatic duct system, where it is concentrated and stored until being released into the duodenum to expedite absorption of fats, fat-soluble vitamins, and certain minerals and to activate release of pancreatic enzymes. Gallstone disease (GSD) is common worldwide, but the prevalence in Western society is twice that in Asia (Chuang, et al, 2013). The *LITH* gene seems to play a role.

One of the main constituents of bile is cholesterol, which is also a major constituent of gallstones (*cholelithiasis*). Most gallstones (75%) are "silent" (asymptomatic), but individuals who experience symptoms are at higher risk for an inflamed gallbladder (*acute cholecystitis*) as well as biliary pancreatitis (Chuang, et al, 2013). If cholelithiasis is asymptomatic, no specific therapy is necessary. Symptoms usually manifest after consumption of a high-fat meal, with a mild, aching pain in the midepigastrium that may increase in intensity. Because the gallbladder lies directly beneath the right lobe of the liver, pain may radiate to the right upper quadrant and right subscapular region. Nausea, vomiting, tachycardia, and diaphoresis also may be present.

Gallstones are commonly found in women who are multiparous, are undergoing estrogen therapy, or use oral contraceptives; obese individuals; those with sedentary lifestyles; the aged; and those who have diabetes mellitus (Box 14-3). Gallstones form because of genetic tendencies, supersaturation of cholesterol in bile, and gallbladder hypomotility (after rapid weight loss). The amount of cholesterol in bile is determined in part by the amount of dietary fat consumed. Thus, long-term intake of high-fat foods increases risk for development of cholelithiasis (Figure 14-5).

People who lose a great deal of weight rapidly through very low-calorie diets (VLCDs) and some commercial weight-loss programs are at a high risk for development of gallstones. Following a diet too low in fat or going for long periods without eating (e.g., skipping breakfast) will decrease gallbladder contractions. If the gallbladder does not contract

---

BOX 14-3 **Risk Factors in Gallbladder Disease**

- Age 60
- Diabetes
- Diet that is high fat, high cholesterol, and/or low fiber
- Enzyme defects (mucin) and *LITH* gene
- American Indian or Mexican American ethnicity
- Family history of gallstones
- Female gender
- Hormonal imbalance (estrogen, progestin, insulin)
- Losing weight very quickly
- Medications (estrogen or oral contraceptives; clofibrate, cholestyramine, cholesterol-lowering)
- Obesity
- Pregnancy

Data from Mayo Clinic: *Disease and conditions: Gallstones*, 2013. Accessed August 18, 2013, from www.mayoclinic.com/health/gallstones/DS00165/DSECTION=risk-factors.

---

often enough to empty out the bile, gallstones may form. People considering losing a significant amount of weight should see a physician first to evaluate their medical history, individual circumstances, and the proposed method of weight loss.

Cholecystitis occurs when gallstones block the cystic duct or as the result of stasis, bacterial infection, or ischemia of the gallbladder. This inflammation is associated with pain, tenderness, and fever. Fat intolerance may manifest as regurgitation, flatulence, belching, epigastric heaviness, indigestion, heartburn, chronic upper abdominal pain, and nausea. Jaundice and steatorrhea may also be present. Recommended therapy for symptomatic cholelithiasis and cholecystitis is surgical removal of the gallbladder (cholecystectomy).

Food and Nutrition Therapies

Because cholelithiasis and cholecystitis usually produce rather painful symptoms, the main objective of nutritional care is to decrease the patient's discomfort. Most patients become acutely aware of foods that cause discomfort and thus avoid them. Low-fat diets are traditionally used to treat cholecystitis. During an acute attack, the hospitalized patient may receive IV fluids with nothing orally. Avoiding fatty foods is often advised, but no good evidence supports this recommendation.

Chronic cholecystitis with inflammation is usually treated with a fat-restricted diet. Individual food intolerances vary widely, but many patients omit foods that cause flatulence and bloating.

Application to nursing. Following cholecystectomy, bile enters the small intestine continually rather than in response to food in the GI tract. Immediately after an open laparotomy cholecystectomy, patients may receive either nothing orally or clear liquids until they can tolerate a regular diet. Some patients need to follow a low-fat diet for several weeks after surgery. The total amount of fat in the diet is more important than the type of fat consumed. The patient who undergoes laparoscopic cholecystectomy may consume a regular diet immediately after surgery.

✳ TEACHING TOOL

Suggestions for Coping with Gallbladder Disorders

- Without symptoms, a wait-and-see approach is recommended.
- For mild symptoms, follow a low-fat diet and lose weight slowly; the advice of a registered dietitian may be beneficial.
- For acute symptoms with pain and fever, most patients would be hospitalized for antibiotic therapy and pain management.
- If surgery is needed, laparoscopy is quite simple. See the *Personal Perspectives box* Cholecystectomy Before Laparoscopy.

PANCREATIC DISORDERS

Pancreatitis

The pancreas secretes hormones such as insulin and glucagon for glucose homeostasis. In addition to hormonal functions, the pancreas secretes enzymes necessary for protein, carbohydrate, and fat digestion. The pancreas also secretes sodium bicarbonate to neutralize acidic gastric contents as they enter the duodenum, providing the optimal pH for the activation of these enzymes.

Pancreatitis is an inflammatory process characterized by decreased production of digestive enzymes and bicarbonate with malabsorption of fats and proteins. This acute inflammation causes the local blood vessels to become exceptionally permeable, leaking fluid and plasma proteins into spaces between the cells. Edema and damage result. Pancreatic enzymes are ordinarily secreted into the intestinal lumen, where they are activated. However, if the pancreas is damaged,

---

👤 PERSONAL PERSPECTIVES

Cholecystectomy before Laparoscopy

I was just 25 years old, having taken the Graduate Record Examination (GRE) on a snowy Saturday in Pennsylvania. I lived on the top of a steep hill, so driving to and from the exam on slippery roads had made me even more anxious than the test itself. Finally, relief was in sight … but not for long! That night, after going to bed, I was awakened with severe colicky pain and nausea. I thought it was an ulcer, or even a heart attack from all of the recent stress. Fortunately, I was working as a clinical dietitian at the local hospital and was able to see my own doctor at work the following Monday. He immediately scheduled an X-ray for me, and surprisingly they found gallstones. The radiologist made a joke (he thought) by saying, "Ah too many French fries!" But I knew better. My diet was really healthy, except for skipping some meals and attempting to maintain a low body weight. I had been taking hormones to manage my irregular periods for several years, and I knew that most of the adults in my family had already had gallbladder surgery.

I had surgery the following summer, certain that it would be an easy recovery. I even asked the doctor whether I could leave the hospital the night before my surgery to go for my usual 2-mile run. So, overconfidence about the surgery reigned. But after the procedure, the pain was debilitating. The incision was about 10 inches long, and I had to wear a brace to be comfortable at home and eventually back at work. The healing process took longer than I had expected, and I can honestly say that I had abdominal pain in the scar area for a year after the surgery. Wearing any type of two-piece bathing suit became a thing of the past. Thus, when laparoscopy became available, I was an immediate advocate and continue to encourage that procedure for patients who must undergo gallbladder surgery.

Sylvia Escott-Stump

---

the enzymes are retained and activated within the pancreas, resulting in a form of autodigestion with severe pain.

When the enzymes amylase and lipase cannot be secreted into the intestine, they accumulate in the bloodstream. Thus, a highly elevated serum amylase value is an indication of pancreatitis. *Acute pancreatitis* is most commonly caused by excessive alcohol consumption or gallbladder disease. *Chronic pancreatitis* is usually associated with chronic alcohol consumption and is characterized by chronic pain and exocrine and endocrine insufficiency. Diabetes mellitus can occur as the result of chronic pancreatitis if beta cells are damaged, thus decreasing insulin production.

Food and Nutrition Therapies

The primary goal in pancreatitis is to provide for nutritional needs while minimizing pancreatic secretions. Traditionally, gut rest with IV fluids or parenteral nutrition has been standard practice. However, clinical evidence indicates that parenteral nutrition administered within 24 hours of admission worsens outcome by increasing the inflammatory response and impairing the immune response. Bowel rest leads to atrophy of intestinal mucosa and bacterial translocation. In contrast, early introduction of enteral nutrition promotes fewer infections, shorter hospital stays, and overall decreased medical costs.

Feeding into the lower small bowel, in the jejunum distal to the ligament of Treitz, allows areas associated with pancreatic stimulation to be bypassed. Low-fat, elemental formulas are recommended because they tend to reduce pancreatic stimulation. Patients receiving enteral feedings should be closely monitored for increases in pancreatic enzymes, abdominal pain, and discomfort. Enteral feedings should be terminated if any of these symptoms occurs.

Application to nursing. In addition to severe pain, patients with pancreatitis often experience nausea and vomiting.

The first 24 hours after admission for acute pancreatitis require rapid response. Evidence-based guidelines are used for appropriate fluid resuscitation and antibiotic therapy (Fisher and Gardner, 2012). Early enteral feeding is important. Placement of a percutaneous endoscopic gastro-jejunostomy feeding tube is commonly required for individuals who will need enteral feeding for longer than 30 days (Iqbal, et al, 2012). Parenteral support is recommended when there are contraindications to enteral feeding, such as small bowel obstruction (Iqbal, et al, 2012).

TEACHING TOOL
Suggestions for Coping with Pancreatitis

- Restricting fat to less than 50 g/day typically prevents symptoms of steatorrhea.
- A medium-chain triglyceride product such as MCT oil may be used to increase calories if needed.
- Consuming small meals in six feedings daily may facilitate adequate nutritional intake.
- In some cases, replacement pancreatic enzymes are taken orally with meals to control maldigestion and malabsorption.
- Complete abstinence from alcohol is essential.

SUMMARY

- The liver, gallbladder, and pancreas are important organs for proper digestion.
- Disorders of the liver include hepatitis, an inflammation of the liver, and cirrhosis, a chronic degenerative disease that causes fibrous connective tissue and fat infiltration of the liver.
- Nutrition therapy consists of bed rest and proper nutrition for hepatitis and individual nutrition plans for cirrhosis that ease liver function.
- Meeting nutrition therapy needs while still providing for adequate energy and RDA nutrient levels is challenging.
- Liver transplantations occur as treatment for end-stage liver disease, with specific nutrition therapies at each stage.
- Gallbladder disorders are characterized by the formation of gallstones within the gallbladder. Cholecystitis involves acute inflammation as well.
- Patients with gallbladder disease may require low-fat diets or calorie-controlled diets, but not all individuals gain relief from them.
- Pancreatitis affects production of digestive secretions, resulting in malabsorption of dietary fats and protein.
- In serious cases, pancreatitis requires enteral or parenteral nutrition support. If tube feeding is used, tube placement into the jejunum is usually tolerated.

THE NURSING APPROACH
Case Study: Cirrhosis of the Liver

Eric, aged 50 years, was diagnosed with cirrhosis subsequent to chronic hepatitis. As the liver damage progressed, he had frequent hospitalizations. At this admission, he is being treated with diuretics because of ascites (fluid in the peritoneal cavity) and peripheral edema. He is receiving lactulose to reduce levels of ammonia because of hepatic encephalopathy. The doctor has prescribed a 2000-kcal, 40-g protein, 1-g sodium diet with fluids restricted to 1200 mL per day.

Assessment
Subjective (from Patient Statements)
- "I don't have any appetite. You wouldn't either if you were feeling sick to your stomach and throwing up."
- "I'm thirsty."
- "Just leave me alone. Where am I anyway?"
- "Is it nighttime? I can't remember what I was doing."
- Usual weight 205 pounds when he doesn't have ascites.

Objective (from Physical Examination)
- Present weight 210 pounds
- Dark amber urine, jaundice of skin, and sclera
- Abdominal distention, ascites
- Peripheral edema in ankles and lower legs
- Muscle wasting of upper extremities and thighs
- Enlargement of the liver seen on radiograph
- Laboratory test results: Normal blood urea nitrogen, normal hematocrit, low albumin, and elevated liver enzymes
- Disoriented to date, time, and place

◎ THE NURSING APPROACH—cont'd

Diagnoses (Nursing)

1. Imbalanced nutrition: less than body requirements related to anorexia and nausea and vomiting, as evidenced by muscle wasting and loss of true body weight
2. Excess fluid volume related to intrahepatic pressure and decreased colloidal osmotic pressure, as evidenced by ascites and peripheral edema
3. Acute confusion related to toxicities in the brain, as evidenced by agitation; disorientation to date, time, and place; and short-term memory loss

Planning
Patient Outcomes

Short term (at the end of 1 week):
- Eating meals well
- Decrease of jaundice, nausea, and vomiting
- Loss of 1500 mL of body fluids, as evidenced by weight 207 pounds (loss of 3 pounds), output greater than intake on records, and decreases in abdominal girth and ankle edema
- Slight decrease of liver enzymes, and electrolytes within normal ranges
- No further muscle wasting of extremities
- Oriented to date, time, and place, and calmer

Nursing Interventions

1. Provide 2000-kcal diet with protein, sodium, and water restrictions as ordered.
2. Facilitate loss of excess fluid.
3. Orient Eric frequently.

Implementation

1. Asked the dietitian to assess Eric's nutritional status and food preferences in order to optimally implement the diet of 2000 kcal, 40 g protein and 1 g sodium, with 1200 mL fluid restriction.
   With patient assessment, the dietitian can individualize complex diets.
2. Helped deliver small frequent meals with high kcal, high carbohydrates, moderate fats, and restricted proteins (following the plan of the dietitian).
   Patients with nausea and distended abdomens usually tolerate small, frequent meals better than large meals. High kcal are needed for healing and prevention of catabolism of body proteins. Fat contains high kcal and fat-soluble vitamins but may not be metabolized well, causing steatorrhea (fat in the stools). Protein is needed for healing, but excess could increase ammonia production and make encephalopathy worse.
3. Removed noxious odors and unpleasant objects from the room before meals and gave antiemetic medication as ordered.
   Unpleasant smells and sights can trigger nausea, thus leading to anorexia. Antiemetics are given to prevent vomiting.
4. Restricted sodium to 1 g and planned with Eric how to restrict fluids to 1200 mL per day (300 mL with meals and 300 mL total between meals). Posted the plan on the bulletin board by Eric's bed and taught him, his family, and nursing staff the reasons for the fluid restriction.

Sodium is limited in order to decrease fluid retention. Fluid restriction is necessary to decrease portal hypertension, ascites, and peripheral edema. Involving the patient in planning encourages commitment and a sense of control. Dietary restrictions are easier to follow when purposes are understood. Written communication of the plan helps coordinate efforts.

5. Gave Eric ice, hard candy, and lemon wedges to reduce thirst.
   Thirst is minimized by spacing out fluid intake and providing treats that can dissolve slowly in the mouth.
6. Allowed no alcohol intake.
   Alcohol would further damage the liver and add to the patient's confusion.
7. Oriented Eric frequently to date, time, and place and gave him simple instructions and reminders. Wrote the date and name of the nurse on the white board by the patient's bed and clock.
   Confused patients become less agitated when told where they are, even if they forget quickly what the nurse just told them.
8. Asked dietary staff for herbs and spices that could be put on Eric's low-sodium food for flavoring.
   Low-sodium foods are bland without additional flavoring.
9. Provided supplemental vitamins and liquids (such as Ensure and Ensure Plus).
   Nutrient-dense supplements increase nourishment and kcal. Drinking liquid nourishment requires less energy than chewing foods.
10. Gave diuretic medicines as ordered.
    Diuretics cause increased urine output, thus reducing body fluids, ascites, and peripheral edema.
11. Gave lactulose as ordered.
    Ammonia is produced when intestinal bacteria metabolize protein. Ammonia going to the brain (because the liver cannot detoxify it) contributes to hepatic encephalopathy. Lactulose is a synthetic nonabsorbable disaccharide that is given to reduce ammonia in the intestines. Lactulose is metabolized in the intestines, releasing organic acids and lowering the pH; this enables trapping of ammonia in the stool, where it can be excreted. Lactulose also causes diarrhea, limiting time for intestinal bacteria to produce ammonia.
12. Carefully measured and recorded intake and output each shift; measured and recorded patient weights and abdominal girth daily.
    Ongoing assessment of fluid balance helps evaluate effectiveness of treatment.
13. Monitored lab reports for changes.
    Diarrhea from lactulose may lead to loss of fluids and electrolytes. Some diuretics cause loss of potassium.

Evaluation

At the end of 1 week:
- Eating meals well
- No change in muscle wasting of extremities
- Jaundice, nausea, and vomiting decreased
- Liver enzymes slightly decreased and electrolytes within normal ranges

Continued

◎ THE NURSING APPROACH—cont'd

- Quickly forgot about his water restriction even with frequent reminders
- Exceeded water intake (about 1400 mL rather than 1200 mL per day)
- Body fluids decreased by 1000 mL, as evidenced by weight of 208 pounds (loss of 2 pounds), output greater than intake on records, and decreased abdominal girth and ankle edema
- Oriented to place but not date and time
Goals partially met.

Discussion Questions

During a follow-up appointment with the physician, the nurse asked Eric how he was doing with his diet. His response was "Not very well. I really don't know what foods I am supposed to eat."
1. What other questions should the nurse ask? What nursing diagnosis will the nurse probably identify?
2. Should the nurse suggest to the doctor that he refer Eric to a dietitian? Why?

❓ CRITICAL THINKING*

Clinical Applications

Chronic alcohol abuse is usually the cause of chronic liver disease (cirrhosis and hepatic encephalopathy) and chronic pancreatitis. One way to evaluate the risk of alcohol-related liver disease is to assess the pattern, quantity, and duration of alcohol intake; usual dietary intake; and socioeconomic factors affecting eating habits. Data can be collected from the patient or a reliable friend or family member and evaluated to determine amount (grams) and the kcal value of alcohol consumed. When consumed in large quantities, alcohol can provide the majority of the day's kcal intake. Professionals working with individuals who consume excessive amounts of alcohol advise that self-reported intakes may constitute about half of what is actually consumed. Therefore, double-checking any information obtained from a patient about alcohol intake with a reliable family member or friend is recommended.

Alcohol provides 7 kcal/g.[†] The average percent alcohol content (based on weight per volume) of various forms of alcoholic beverages is as follows:

Beer = 4% to 6%

Wine = 9% to 12%

Distilled alcohol (whiskey, rum, gin, or brandy) = 35% to 50%

The concentration of alcohol in distilled beverages (hard liquor) is usually referred to as *proof*. One proof equals 0.5% alcohol, which means that 80-proof tequila contains 40% alcohol. Hard liquor is routinely measured in a jigger or shot, which holds 1½ ounces or 45 mL.
1. How many grams of alcohol and kcal would two shots of 80-proof tequila provide?
2. What is the best way to obtain information from an individual about his/her alcohol consumption?
3. You obtain the following information from the alcohol intake questionnaire and diet history: Alcohol is consumed 7 days/week at home, work, and bars. A typical day's intake consists of a Bloody Mary (1 cup tomato juice,

two shots 80-proof vodka) first thing in the morning, followed by 5 cups of black coffee (some at home, some at work). Three more shots of 80-proof vodka are consumed at work. Lunch is usually a fast-food double cheeseburger, small fries, and a cup of black coffee. After work, four 12-ounce bottles of beer (4% alcohol) and pretzels (about 30) are consumed at the local bar with friends. Dinner at home consists of a lunchmeat sandwich (usually two slices white bread, 2 ounces bologna, 1 teaspoon mustard), 10 potato chips, and two more 12-ounce beers. Total intake for the day is approximately 3200 kcal.
   a. How many grams of alcohol are consumed? _____ grams alcohol
   b. How many kcal are provided by the alcohol? _____ kcal from alcohol
   c. What percent of the kcal are provided by alcohol? _____ % energy from alcohol

Alcohol Intake Assessment Tool

1. How many days a week do you drink alcoholic beverages?
   Circle number of days: 0 1 2 3 4 5 6 7
2. Where do you drink? Circle all that apply:
   a. At home
   b. At a friend's
   c. At a bar
   d. At work
   e. In the car
   f. Other (specify)
3. Which alcoholic beverages do you consume? Circle all that apply:
   a. Beer
   b. Wine
   c. Sherry or port
   d. Gin
   e. Whiskey
   f. Vodka
   g. Rum
   h. Other (specify)
4. How do you determine how much you drink? Circle all that apply:
   a. Count the number of beer cans
   b. Count the number of wine glasses
   c. Count the number of shots poured

---

*Modified from Roe DA, Lasswell AB: Nutritional assessment and tools. In Lasswell AB, et al, editors: *Nutrition for family and primary care practitioners*, Philadelphia, 1986, F. Stickley.

[†]Any beverages used as mixers should be included in the estimated kcal intake.

d. Count the number of bottles of wine

e. Count the number of bottles of liquor used a day or week

f. I don't know exactly how much I drink

g. Other method of deciding alcohol intake (specify)

5. On any drinking day, how many drinks do you have? Circle letter(s) indicating drinks consumed and number within each category consumed to indicate number of drinks per day:

a. Beer	1	2	3	4	5	>5
b. White, red, or rosé wine	1	2	3	4	5	>5
c. Sherry or port	1	2	3	4	5	>5
d. Gin	1	2	3	4	5	>5
e. Whiskey	1	2	3	4	5	>5
f. Vodka	1	2	3	4	5	>5
g. Rum	1	2	3	4	5	>5
h. Other (specify)	1	2	3	4	5	>5

6. For how long have you been drinking this quantity?

7. Do you drink this amount on a regular basis?

WEBSITES OF INTEREST

Alcoholics Anonymous

www.alcoholics-anonymous.org

Dedicated to the self-help approach for overcoming alcoholism, including links for teenagers, newcomers, health professionals, and the AA Grapevine.

American Liver Foundation

www.liverfoundation.org

Devoted to research, education, and support groups related to hepatitis and all liver diseases.

Centers for Disease Control (CDC)

http://www.cdc.gov/hepatitis/

Useful for obtaining tips and statistics for the five types of hepatitis.

National Institute on Alcohol Abuse and Alcoholism

www.niaaa.nih.gov

Provides leadership for the national effort to reduce alcohol-related problems through research, collaborative endeavors of agencies and organizations, and educational resources.

REFERENCES

Charlton M: Evolving aspects of liver transplantation for nonalcoholic steatohepatitis, *Curr Opin Organ Transplant* 18:251–258, 2013.

Chuang SC, et al: Genetics of gallstone disease, *Adv Clin Chem* 60:143–185, 2013.

Farrell GC, et al: NASH is an inflammatory disorder: Pathogenic, prognostic and therapeutic implications, *Gut Liver* 6:149–171, 2012.

Fisher JM, Gardner TB: The "golden hours" of management in acute pancreatitis, *Am J Gastroenterol* 107:1146–1150, 2012.

Frazier TH, et al: Gut microbiota, intestinal permeability, obesity-induced inflammation, and liver injury, *JPEN J Parenter Enteral Nutr* 35:14S–20S, 2011.

Ilan Y: Leaky gut and the liver: A role for bacterial translocation in nonalcoholic steatohepatitis, *World J Gastroenterol* 18:2609–2618, 2012.

Iqbal S, et al: Endoscopist's approach to nutrition in the patient with pancreatitis, *World J Gastrointest Endosc* 4:526–531, 2012.

Thein HH, et al: Trends in incidence of hepatocellular carcinoma after diagnosis of hepatitis B or C infection: A population-based cohort study, 1992–2007, *J Viral Hepat* 18:232–241, 2011.

Nutrition for Diabetes Mellitus

Once thought of as a disease of the West, the prevalence of diabetes mellitus is increasing at alarming rates in many other areas of the world. The heterogeneity of the disease has been demonstrated both through anthropometric and genetic studies. Despite this heterogeneity, some treatments, particularly lifestyle interventions, have been found to have a positive impact on the disease.

David W. Lam and Derek Leroith (2012)

(e) http://evolve.elsevier.com/GRODNER/FOUNDATIONS

LEARNING OBJECTIVES

- Define diabetes mellitus (DM).
- Compare and contrast type 1 DM (T1DM) with type 2 DM (T2DM).
- Explain the main goal of diabetes treatment and how it can be achieved.
- Discuss the composition and process of the diabetes management team.
- Describe current nutrition therapy guidelines.
- Identify groups for whom special care and individualized goals are needed.

WELLNESS AND DIABETES

Serious *physical health* complications may be avoided if hyperglycemia is controlled through dietary and lifestyle modifications. The ability of the individual to understand the condition; to be compliant on a regular basis regarding insulin injections, if required; and to follow dietary and exercise recommendations depends on *intellectual health*. Not only must the individual deal with a chronic lifelong condition, but changes in dietary habits may necessitate the loss of favorite foods, which affects *emotional health*. Support, especially from family members and friends, is a crucial part of *social health*. Finally, people who eat certain foods according to their religious or spiritual beliefs may need special adaptations for *spiritual health* while living with diabetes. The *environmental health* dimension can support diabetes management based on the availability and means to access diabetes management health care.

DEFINITION

Diabetes mellitus represents a group of conditions characterized by either a relative or complete lack of insulin secretion by the beta cells of the pancreas or by defects of cell insulin receptors, which result in disturbances of carbohydrate, protein, and lipid metabolism. Although many cases of diabetes are undiagnosed, the medical community is aware that the condition is prevalent and growing in all age groups (Figure 15-1).

Diabetes is usually diagnosed and characterized by elevated fasting blood glucose values (>126 mg/dL if found on at least two occasions) or hyperglycemia. The main goal of treatment is achievement of insulin/glucose homeostasis (Figure 15-2). In addition to everyday maintenance necessary to control blood glucose levels, diabetes mellitus is associated with disability and premature death because of the disease's effect on structural and functional alterations in many body systems, especially large and small blood vessels. Ranked as one of the most costly health problems in America, diabetes mellitus is often a "silent killer."

Complications

Everyone with diabetes mellitus is vulnerable to long-term complications (Table 15-1) and premature death. Many of these complications may be preempted with control of hyperglycemia (Table 15-2). Macrovascular effects of diabetes increase the risk of coronary artery disease, peripheral vascular disease, and stroke. Unfortunately, cardiovascular disease is often established by the time diabetes is diagnosed; metabolic disturbances seem to make a permanent impression on blood vessels, called "metabolic memory" that is not easily reversed (Porter and Riches, 2013). In fact, two out of three people with diabetes die from cardiovascular diseases (American Diabetes Association [ADA], n.d.).

Microvascular effects include nephropathy (kidney disorder) and retinopathy (eye disorder from blood vessel changes). As a result of nephropathy, chronic kidney disease (CKD) and renal failure requiring dialysis develop in approximately half of all individuals with type 1 diabetes mellitus. Retinopathy is the leading cause of blindness in North America. In addition, neuropathy complications affect peripheral circulation, causing decreased sensations in extremities that may result in

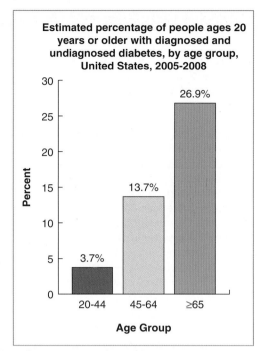

FIG 15-1 Estimated number of new cases of diagnosed diabetes in people aged 20 years or older, by age group, in the United States in 2010. (From National Diabetes Information Clearinghouse: *National diabetes statistics, 2011* (NIH Publ 11-3892), 2011. Accessed August 18, 2013, from diabetes.niddk.nih.gov/dm/pubs/statistics/.)

injury without the patient's knowledge. Healing is impaired because of the effects of diabetes on the circulatory system; gangrene may develop, and amputation may be necessary (Figure 15-3).

Autonomic effects may include orthostatic hypotension, persistent tachycardia, gastroparesis, neurogenic bladder (urinary bladder dysfunction from neurologic damage), impotence, and impairment of visceral pain sensation that can obscure symptoms of angina pectoris or myocardial infarction. Development of these long-term complications is believed to be correlated to the level and frequency of hyperglycemia experiences throughout the life span of a person with diabetes.

CLASSIFICATION

Glucose intolerance is classified primarily as type 1 diabetes mellitus (T1DM)* and type 2 diabetes mellitus (T2DM). Other types are latent autoimmune diabetes of adults (LADA), gestational diabetes mellitus (GDM), impaired glucose tolerance (IGT), and other forms. These classifications are based on etiology, treatment needs, and symptoms (Table 15-3). More than 90% of people with diabetes have T2DM. Figure 15-4 shows a checklist for diabetes risk.

---

*The terms *insulin-dependent diabetes mellitus, non-insulin-dependent diabetes mellitus, IDDM,* and *NIDDM,* should no longer be used because they are confusing and classify patients based on treatment rather than etiology.

FIG 15-2 Glucose-insulin homeostasis. (From endocrineweb.com: Normal regulation of blood glucose, n.d. Accessed June 14, 2014 from www.endocrineweb.com/conditions/diabetes/normal-regulation-blood-glucose.)

FIG 15-3 Neuropathy ulceration. (From Lewis SM, Heitkemper MM, Dirksen SL: *Medical-surgical nursing: Assessment and management of clinical problems,* ed 6, St. Louis, 2004, Mosby.)

TABLE 15-1 Clinical Complications of Diabetes Mellitus

COMPLICATION	MANIFESTATION	INCIDENCE
Dental disease	Periodontitis	Those with diabetes mellitus (DM) are often at twice the risk of those without diabetes. Almost 30% of people with diabetes have severe periodontal disease with loss of attachment of gums to the teeth measuring 5 mm or more.
Pregnancy	Congenital malformations	Poorly controlled diabetes before conception and during the first trimester of pregnancy can cause major birth defects in 5%-10% of pregnancies and spontaneous abortions in 15%-20% of pregnancies. Poorly controlled diabetes during second and third trimesters of pregnancy can result in excessively large newborns.
Microvascular*	Retinopathy	Leading cause of blindness in adults between 20 and 74 years of age
	Nephropathy	Kidney disease will develop in more than 30% of people with type 1 diabetes mellitus (T1DM), compared with perhaps 10% of those with T2DM. Risk of end-stage renal disease in people with T1DM is 15 times that in those with T2DM.
Macrovascular†	Coronary artery disease	Patients with DM are two to four times more likely to have heart disease; heart disease deaths are also two to four times higher than in adults without DM.
	Peripheral vascular disease	
	Cerebrovascular disease	Patients with DM are two to four times more likely to suffer stroke than people without DM
Neuropathy	Peripheral	Approximately 60%-70% of people with diabetes have mild to severe forms of nerve damage. Neuropathy is a major contributing factor in foot and leg amputations among people with the disease. Risk of leg amputation is 15-40 times greater for a person with DM.
	Autonomic (postural hypotension, persistent tachycardia, neurogenic bladder, incontinence, gastroparesis, impotence)	Impotence occurs in approximately 13% of men who have T1DM and 8% of men with T2DM. Some reports indicate that men older than 50 years have impotence rates as high as 50%-60%.
Skin conditions	Atherosclerosis	As blood vessels narrow, the skin changes. It becomes hairless, thin, cool, and shiny. Toes become cold. Toenails thicken and discolor.
	Fungal infections (*Candida albicans*)	Common fungal infections are "jock itch," "athlete's foot," ringworm, and vaginal infections, all of which can cause itching.
	Bullosis diabeticorum (diabetic blisters)	Rare condition that can occur on backs of hands, fingers, toes, feet, and sometimes legs or forearms. They look like burn blisters, are painless, and have no redness. Often occur in people with neuropathy; the only treatment is to bring blood glucose levels under control.
	Diabetic dermopathy	Light brown scaly skin patches often mistaken for age spots; occurs most often on the fronts of both legs. Patches do not hurt, open up, or itch.
	Necrobiosis lipoidica diabeticorum (NLD)	Rare condition. Similar to diabetic dermopathy; however, spots are fewer but larger and deeper. Often start as dull, red raised area. Sometimes itchy and painful; spots may crack open.
	Eruptive xanthomatosis	Firm, yellow, pealike enlargements in the skin. Occurs most often on backs of hands, feet, arms, legs, and buttocks. Usually occurs in young men with T1DM who have high serum levels of cholesterol and lipids. Usually disappear when glucose levels are controlled.
	Digital sclerosis	Tight, thick, waxy skin on backs of hands. Finger joints become stiff. Occurs in about 30% of those with T1DM. The only treatment is to control blood glucose levels.
	Disseminated granuloma annulare	Sharply defined ring- or arc-shaped raised areas on skin that can be red, red-brown, or skin colored. Occurs most often on distal parts of the body.
	Acanthosis nigricans	Tan or brown raised areas on sides of the neck, axilla, and groin. May sometimes occur on hands, elbows, and knees. Usually manifests in the obese.

*Compounds effects of macrovascular problems.
†Exacerbated by concurrent hypertension, hypercholesterolemia, smoking, and aging.
Data from Centers for Disease Control and Prevention: *Diabetes report card 2012*, 2012. Accessed August 18, 2013, from http://www.cdc.gov/diabetes/pubs/reportcard.htm; National Diabetes Information Clearinghouse: *National diabetes statistics, 2011* (NIH Publ 11-3892), 2011. Accessed August 18, 2013, from http://diabetes.niddk.nih.gov/dm/pubs/statistics/index.htm.

TABLE 15-2 Criteria for Diagnosing Diabetes and Prediabetes*

Boold Test Levels for Diagnosis of Diabetes and Prediabetes

	A1C (Percent)	Fasting Plasma Glucose (mg/dL)	Oral Glucose Tolerance Test (mg/dL)
Diabetes	6.5 or above	126 or above	200 or above
Prediabetes	5.7 to 6.4	100 to 125	140 to 199
Normal	About 5	99 or below	139 or below

Definitions mg = milligram, dL = deciliter
For all three tests, within the prediabetes range, the higher the test result, the greater the risk of diabetes.

*In the past, the hemoglobin A_{1c} test was used to monitor blood glucose levels but not for diagnosis. The A_{1c} test has now been standardized, and in 2009, an international expert committee recommended that it be used for diagnosis of type 2 diabetes and prediabetes.
From National Diabetes Information Clearinghouse: *Diagnosis of diabetes and prediabetes* (NIH Publ 12-4642), 2012, National Institute of Diabetes and Digestive and Kidney Diseases. Accessed August 19, 2013, from diabetes.niddk.nih.gov/dm/pubs/diagnosis/. Adapted from American Diabetes Association: Standards of medical care in diabetes—2012, *Diabetes Care* 35(Suppl 1):S12, 2012.

TABLE 15-3 Metabolic Goals in Diabetes Management

	GOAL
Glycemic control	
Hemoglobin A_{1c}	<7.0%
Preprandial capillary plasma glucose (mg/dL)	90-130
Peak postprandial capillary plasma glucose (mg/dL)*	<180
Cardiovascular	
Blood pressure (mm Hg)	<139/80
Triglycerides (mg/dL)	<150
Low-density lipoprotein cholesterol (mg/dL)	<100
High-density lipoprotein cholesterol (mg/dL)	
Males	>40
Females	>50

*Measurement should be made 1 to 2 hours after the beginning of the meal. Reinforce lifestyle interventions at every visit and check A_{1c} every 3 months until A_{1c} is <7% and then at least every 6 months. The interventions should be changed if A_{1c} is ≥7%.
Data from American Diabetes Association: Standards of medical care in diabetes: 2010, *Diabetes Care* 33:11-61S, 2010.

TYPE 1 DIABETES MELLITUS

Onset of T1DM is usually sudden. Cells use glucose for energy, and without endogenous insulin, they literally begin to starve. The body responds by sending signals to eat because cells are hungry, but because the end product of digestion (glucose) cannot enter cells, glucose builds up in the bloodstream. It is common for the person to experience weight loss while consuming large quantities of food (polyphagia). Because glucose cannot enter cells and it builds up in the bloodstream, blood becomes hypertonic, and the body tries to get rid of the excess glucose by increasing urine output (polyuria). In reaction to increased excretion of urine, the body again responds by increasing thirst (polydipsia) to replace lost fluids.

T1DM is an autoimmune disease resulting in beta-cell destruction. Autoantibodies to beta-cell proteins form as a byproducts of the autoimmune destruction of the beta cells, rather than having an active role in its pathogenesis (Hampe, 2012). Genetic predisposition and environmental factors are involved. One or more autoantibodies are present in the majority of individuals diagnosed with T1DM (Hampe, 2012).

The rate of beta-cell destruction is variable, being rapid in infants and children and slow in adults. In fact, the first manifestation of T1DM may be diabetic ketoacidosis (DKA). Adults may retain enough residual beta-cell function to prevent ketoacidosis for many years, but when they eventually become dependent on insulin, they also are at risk for DKA. Although the majority of individuals diagnosed with T1DM are usually 20 years of age or younger, a growing number of cases are documented in older individuals. If a person chooses wisely, he or she can live healthfully with T1DM. See the *Personal Perspectives* box Type 1 Diabetes Mellitus: A Tale of Longevity.

PERSONAL PERSPECTIVE

Type 1 Diabetes Mellitus: A Tale of Longevity

Childhood diabetes is now aggressively approached with an array of gadgets to assist in controlling the disorder. But imagine trying to maintain blood glucose levels when the pancreas is producing little if any insulin and the means to self-inject insulin is not yet available or still is being refined as treatment. When Robert Cleveland was diagnosed as a young boy and his brother, Gerald, at age 16, his mother could depend on only diet and exercise to treat her sons. Now at 86 years old, Robert has lived with the disease for almost 81 years, and Gerald—at 90—is the oldest known individual with type 1 diabetes mellitus. Robert and Gerald's successful longevity probably has to do with their methodical practice of lifestyle habits. For all these years, they've restricted their intake of simple starches and sweets, exercised, maintained healthy body weights, and continually tracked and recorded their glucose levels, food intake, and insulin dosages, testing their blood glucose many times a day. Such determination plus a positive attitude is reflected by Gerald's comment, "My main reason to stay alive is to prove to young people there's a way to live with diabetes, to live well."

Data from Pérez-Peña R: Diabetic brothers beat odds with grit and luck, *New York Times*, February 5, 2006, section A1, pp 1, 30.

ARE YOU AT RISK FOR
TYPE 2 DIABETES?

American Diabetes Association

Diabetes Risk Test

1 **How old are you?**
Less than 40 years (0 points)
40—49 years (1 point)
50—59 years (2 points)
60 years or older (3 points)

Write your score in the box.

2 **Are you a man or a woman?**
Man (1 point)   Woman (0 points)

3 **If you are a woman, have you ever been diagnosed with gestational diabetes?**
Yes (1 point)   No (0 points)

4 **Do you have a mother, father, sister, or brother with diabetes?**
Yes (1 point)   No (0 points)

5 **Have you ever been diagnosed with high blood pressure?**
Yes (1 point)   No (0 points)

6 **Are you physically active?**
Yes (0 points)   No (1 point)

7 **What is your weight status?**
(see chart at right)

Height	Weight (lbs.)		
4' 10"	119-142	143-190	191+
4' 11"	124-147	148-197	198+
5' 0"	128-152	153-203	204+
5' 1"	132-157	158-210	211+
5' 2"	136-163	164-217	218+
5' 3"	141-168	169-224	225+
5' 4"	145-173	174-231	232+
5' 5"	150-179	180-239	240+
5' 6"	155-185	186-246	247+
5' 7"	159-190	191-254	255+
5' 8"	164-196	197-261	262+
5' 9"	169-202	203-269	270+
5' 10"	174-208	209-277	278+
5' 11"	179-214	215-285	286+
6' 0"	184-220	221-293	294+
6' 1"	189-226	227-301	302+
6' 2"	194-232	233-310	311+
6' 3"	200-239	240-318	319+
6' 4"	205-245	246-327	328+
(1 Point)	(2 Points)	(3 Points)

You weigh less than the amount in the left column (0 points)

Add up your score.

Adapted from Bang et al., Ann Intern Med 151:775-783, 2009.
Original algorithm was validated without gestational diabetes as part of the model.

If you scored 5 or higher:
You are at increased risk for having type 2 diabetes. However, only your doctor can tell for sure if you do have type 2 diabetes or prediabetes (a condition that precedes type 2 diabetes in which blood glucose levels are higher than normal). Talk to your doctor to see if additional testing is needed.

Type 2 diabetes is more common in African Americans, Hispanics/Latinos, American Indians, and Asian Americans and Pacific Islanders.

For more information, visit us at www.diabetes.org or call 1-800-DIABETES

Visit us on Facebook
Facebook.com/AmericanDiabetesAssociation

Lower Your Risk

The good news is that you can manage your risk for type 2 diabetes. Small steps make a big difference and can help you live a longer, healthier life.

If you are at high risk, your first step is to see your doctor to see if additional testing is needed.

Visit diabetes.org or call 1-800-DIABETES for information, tips on getting started, and ideas for simple, small steps you can take to help lower your risk.

STOP DIABETES.

FIG 15-4 Risk test for diabetes mellitus. (From Diabetesforecast.org: *Are you at risk for type 2 diabetes?* Accessed June 14, 2014, from http://www.diabetes.org/assets/pdfs/at-risk/risk-test -paper-version.pdf.)

Treatment

Insulin

Everyone with T1DM requires exogenous insulin to maintain normal blood glucose levels and to survive. Some individuals with T2DM may require insulin to optimize blood glucose control. Regardless of the type of diabetes, the goal of insulin therapy, in conjunction with nutrition therapy and physical activity, is to mimic physiologic insulin delivery. Optimal insulin management can be realized only by evaluating blood glucose monitoring records, adjusting food and exercise activities, and proposing insulin adjustments.

Bioengineered human insulin is the only insulin available for use in the United States. Types of insulin are classified into three groups according to duration of their action: rapid or short acting, intermediate acting, and long acting. Figure 15-5 shows a list of insulins used in the United States.

Patterns of insulin administration vary with type of diabetes and desired glycemic control. As you can see in Figure 15-6, a single dose of insulin is rarely capable of providing optimal glycemic control in T1DM. The three basic types of insulin administration regimens are described here.

Conventional or standard insulin therapy is composed of a constant dose of intermediate-acting insulin combined with short- or rapid-acting insulin, or a mixed dose of insulin. Insulins may be mixed by the patient or purchased premixed (for example, 30 units of 70/30 insulin). Administration of insulin (Figure 15-7) and food intake must be synchronized to avoid hypoglycemia (ADA, 2013).

Flexible or intensive insulin therapy is composed of multiple daily injections (MDIs) of short- or rapid-acting insulin before meals, as well as intermediate-acting insulin once or twice daily. This approach allows insulin to be adjusted to correspond with food intake, imitating endogenous insulin

Insulins Used in the United States

Generic Name (U-100, except where noted)	Brand Name	Form	Manufacturer	Cloudy or Clear
Rapid-acting				
insulin glulisine	Apidra*	analog	Sanofi-Aventis	clear
insulin lispro	Humalog*	analog	Eli Lilly	clear
insulin aspart	NovoLog*	analog	Novo Nordisk	clear
Regular				
regular	Humulin R†, ReliOn (Wal-Mart)	human	Eli Lilly	clear
regular	Novolin R	human	Novo Nordisk	clear
Intermediate-acting				
NPH	Humulin N*, ReliOn (Wal-Mart)	human	Eli Lilly	cloudy
NPH	Novolin N	human	Novo Nordisk	cloudy
Long-acting				
insulin detemir	Levemir*	analog	Novo Nordisk	clear
insulin glargine	Lantus*	analog	Sanofi-Aventis	clear
Mixtures				
70% NPH/30% regular	Humulin 70/30*, ReliOn (Wal-Mart)	human	Eli Lilly	cloudy
70% NPH/30% regular	Novolin 70/30‡	human	Novo Nordisk	cloudy
50% lispro protamine/50% insulin lispro	Humalog Mix 50/50*	analog	Eli Lilly	cloudy
75% lispro protamine (NPL)/25% lispro	Humalog Mix 75/25*	analog	Eli Lilly	cloudy
70% aspart protamine/30% aspart	NovoLog Mix 70/30*‡	analog	Novo Nordisk	cloudy
Less commonly used insulins				
regular	Humulin R U-500†§	human	Eli Lilly	clear
50% NPH/50% regular	Humulin 50/50	human	Eli Lilly	cloudy

* Available in prefilled, disposable pens or cartridges for reusable pens.
† Note difference between Humulin R and Humulin R U-500.
‡ Note difference between Novolin 70/30 (70% NPH/30% regular) and NovoLog Mix 70/30 (70% aspart protamine/30% aspart).
§ U-500 and U-100 are different concentrations of insulin. U-500 is typically used in very insulin-resistant people.

FIG 15-5 Types of insulin used in the United States. (From Diabetesforecast.org: *Insulins used in the United States,* revised 2011. Accessed August 18, 2013, from www.forecast.diabetes.org/files/images/Insulin_Chart_Rev_8-2-11.pdf?loc=dorg-insulin-basics.)

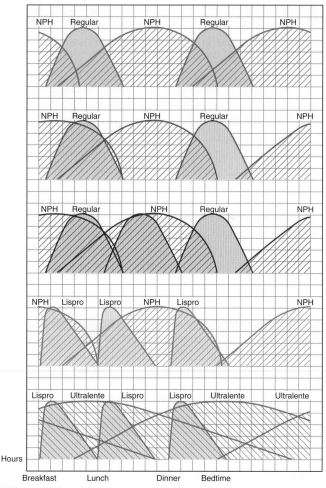

FIG 15-6 Typical patterns of insulin use. (Designed by Lisa Siegel. From Copstead-Kirkhorn L-E, Banasik J: *Pathophysiology,* ed 3, Philadelphia, 2005, Saunders.)

FIG 15-7 Self-injection sites for insulin. (Redrawn from BD, Diabetes Learning Center: *Injection sites,* n.d. Accessed January 1, 2014 from http://www.bd.com/us/diabetes/page.aspx?cat=7001&id=7261.)

secretion in a person without diabetes. Insulin doses can also be adjusted to treat hyperglycemia, inconsistent carbohydrate intake, or modification in usual physical activity. Insulin regimen must be integrated with the patient's lifestyle. Individuals who use intensive therapy should know the basic insulin doses for both insulins they use. This knowledge allows them to fine-tune short- and rapid-acting insulin doses when they deviate from usual meal plans and/or exercise programs. This intensive therapy may not be appropriate for everyone.

Continuous subcutaneous insulin infusion is a form of intensive therapy. Rapid- or short-acting insulin is pumped continuously in micro-amounts through a subcutaneous catheter and is monitored 24 hours a day (Figure 15-8). Boluses of rapid- or short-acting insulins are given before meals.

Exercise

Exercise, like insulin, lowers blood glucose levels, assists in maintaining normal lipid levels, and increases circulation. For most individuals, consistent and individualized exercise helps reduce the therapeutic dose of insulin. People with

T1DM who do not have complications and are in good blood glucose control can perform all levels of exercise, including leisure activities, recreational sports, and competitive sports. To do so safely, the patient must possess the ability to collect self-monitored blood glucose data (during exercise) and then use these data to adjust the therapeutic regimen (insulin and medical nutrition therapy).

General guidelines for regulating the glycemic response to exercise are summarized as follows:

Metabolic control before exercise: Avoid exercise if fasting glucose levels are greater than or equal to 250 mg/dL and ketosis is present or if glucose levels are greater than 300 mg/dL, regardless of whether ketosis is present. Ingest added carbohydrate if glucose levels are less than 100 mg/dL. Patients with T1DM should not perform exercise at the time insulin is at its peak. Ideally, they should exercise when blood glucose levels are between 100 and 200 mg/dL or about 30 to 60 minutes after meals. They should also avoid exercising when blood glucose is greater than 250 mg/dL or when ketones are present in the urine.

Blood glucose monitoring before and after exercise: Identify when changes in insulin or food intake are necessary. Learn the blood glucose response to different exercise conditions.

Food intake: Consume added carbohydrate as needed to avoid hypoglycemia. Carbohydrate-based foods should be readily available during and after exercise (Box 15-1).

FIG 15-8 Insulin injection using an insulin pump. (From Peckenpaugh NJ: *Nutrition essentials and diet therapy*, ed 9, Philadelphia, 2003, Saunders.)

BOX 15-1 Foods Containing 15 Grams of Carbohydrate per Serving

Grains, Breads, Cereals, Starches
1 slice bread
¾ cup dry cereal
½ cup cooked cereal
⅓ cup cooked rice or pasta

Milk and Yogurt
1 cup milk
⅓ cup (6 ounces) unsweetened or sugar-free yogurt

Fruits
1 small fresh fruit
½ cup canned fruit (canned in juice)
1 cup melon or berries
¼ cup dried fruit
½ cup unsweetened fruit juice

Vegetables
½ cup cooked potatoes, peas, or corn
3 cups raw vegetables
1½ cups cooked vegetables
Small portions (½ cup) of nonstarchy vegetables are free

Sweets and Snack Foods
½ cup or ¾ ounce snack food (pretzels, chips)
4 to 6 snack crackers
1 ounce sweet snack (2 small cookies)
½ cup regular ice cream
1 tablespoon sugar

Derived from American Diabetes Association: *Understanding carbohydrates,* 2013. Accessed August 19, 2013, from www.diabetes.org/food-and-fitness/food/planning-meals/carb-counting/.

Glucose control can be compromised if proper adjustments are not made in food intake or insulin administration.

Hypoglycemia can occur during exercise that lasts longer than 1 hour and for up to 24 hours after unusually strenuous, prolonged, and/or sporadic exercise. Blood glucose levels should be monitored, and carbohydrates should be increased and/or insulin adjustments should be made.

TYPE 2 DIABETES MELLITUS

Type 2 DM is an insidious disease. People with it have gradual onset of polyuria and polydipsia, are easily fatigued, and have frequent infections (especially of the urinary tract).

Some of the first symptoms that cause individuals to seek medical attention are actually complications (heart attack, stroke, and neuropathic problems) associated with diabetes. It is not uncommon for a person to have T2DM years before diagnosis.

The primary metabolic problem in T2DM is insulin resistance (failure of cells to respond to insulin produced by the body) or defects in insulin secretion. Family history and obesity are the two strongest risk factors for T2DM. The genetic tendency for diabetes leads to beta-cell exhaustion and hyperglycemia in some, but not all, obese people. Thus, nutrition is an important environmental factor that modulates expression of genes involved in metabolic pathways associated with obesity and T2DM (Phillips, 2013).

Upper body obesity is an even greater risk factor for diabetes than extent of obesity or BMI. *Upper body obesity,* defined as a waist-to-hip ratio greater than 0.8 for women and 0.95 to 1 for men, is a risk factor not only for diabetes but also for heart disease and hypertension (see also the *Cultural Considerations* box Prevalence of Type 2 Diabetes Mellitus).

Treatment: Oral Glucose-Lowering Medications

Oral glucose-lowering medications are used to treat T2DM when diet and physical activity alone cannot control hyperglycemia. Medications used to manage T2DM utilize different pharmacologic approaches: stimulating insulin production, reducing hepatic gluconeogenesis, slowing polysaccharide

🌐 CULTURAL CONSIDERATIONS

Prevalence of Type 2 Diabetes Mellitus

T2DM poses a major health threat worldwide. Mean fasting plasma glucose levels and diabetes prevalence are high in North America, Oceania, Asia, Latin America, the Caribbean, north Africa, and the Middle East (Danaei et al, 2011). Nearly 26 million Americans have diabetes, and 79 million have prediabetes (CDC, 2013). T2DM develops in East Asian patients at a lower mean body mass index (BMI); visceral body fat levels are higher in such patients than in those of European descent (Ma and Chan, 2013).

Several other population groups remain at high risk for diabetes. Among ethnic groups significantly at risk for T2DM are African Americans, Hispanic/Latino Americans, Native Americans, and Pacific Islanders. For adults in 2010, diabetes rates were 16.1% for American Indians/Alaska Natives, 12.6% for blacks, 11.8% for Hispanics, 8.4% for Asian-Americans, and 7.1% for non-Hispanic whites (CDC, 2013). Factors influencing preventive and diabetes management care among minority groups in the United States include limited access to health care, cultural attitudes and behaviors related to medicine, and self-care.

Application to nursing. For minority and cultural groups, language barriers, health care access, level of acculturation, practices of diabetes self-care, and possible genetic variations may contribute to higher risk of long-term diabetes complications. East Asian patients with T2DM have a higher risk for development of cancer, renal disorders, and stroke (Ma and Chan, 2013). Thus, nurses will want to tailor educational sessions for such patients in culturally appropriate ways (Carter et al, 2013). Evidence suggests that patients with diabetes who participate in a group education program have lower hemoglobin $_{1c}A_{1c}$ levels, better lipid profiles, higher quality of life scores, and improved diabetes knowledge and problem-solving ability (Erlich et al, 2013).

Data from Carter BM, et al: Culturally tailored education for African Americans with type 2 diabetes, *Medsurg Nurs* 22(2):105-109, 2013; and Erlich DR, et al: Diabetes update: population management, *FP Essent* 408:25-33, 2013.
See also Centers for Disease Control and Prevention: *Frequently asked questions: Groups especially affected by diabetes,* Atlanta, Author. Accessed August 18, 2013, from www.cdc.gov/diabetes/consumer/groups.htm.

digestion, and increasing insulin sensitivity in muscle, liver, and fat to achieve euglycemia (Unger, et al, 2013). Metformin continues to be first-line therapy. The variety of new drugs for treatment of diabetes has greatly expanded during the past several years (Table 15-4).

MANAGEMENT OF DIABETES

Blood Glucose Monitoring

Controlled blood glucose levels are the cornerstone of diabetes management. Improved control is correlated with sustained reduced rates of retinopathy, nephropathy, and neuropathy. Follow-up studies of the Diabetes Control and Complications Trial–the Epidemiology of Diabetes Intervention and Complications Study (DCCT-EDIC), and the United Kingdom Prospective Diabetes Study (UKPDS) emphasize the role of glycemic control early in the course of the disorder. Even transient exposure to hyperglycemia results in long-lasting epigenetic modifications (the legacy effect) with changes in chromatin structure and altered gene expression (Pirola, et al, 2010).

The goals of glycemic control are similar for various age groups, but the elderly require fewer diabetic medications for the same level of glycemic control (Thompson, et al, 2013). Glycemic control can be monitored by measurement of glycosylated hemoglobin, or hemoglobin A_{1c} (A_{1c}), along with self-monitoring of blood glucose (SMBG).

A_{1c} is formed through an irreversible process. As red blood cells (RBCs) circulate in the bloodstream, hemoglobin combines with glucose, forming glycosylated hemoglobin. The amount of glycosylated hemoglobin formed depends on the amount of glucose in the bloodstream circulation during the RBCs' 120-day life span. The more glucose an RBC was exposed to, the higher the value. This value is not affected by short-term factors such as food intake, exercise, or stress, so the blood sample can be drawn at any time. A_{1c} samples are easier to obtain than the fasting blood glucose samples. Table 15-5 shows the correlation between mean plasma glucose levels and A_{1c} levels.

Self-monitoring and charting are useful in evaluating glycemic control, physical activity, and effectiveness of the meal plan in meeting the goals of medical nutrition therapy. SMBG can be performed in the individual's home with blood glucose meters, which can be purchased at pharmacies. A droplet of blood is obtained through a finger stick on a regular basis to monitor glucose levels before and after meals and at bedtime.

SMBG is recommended three or more times daily for nearly all individuals with T1DM and for pregnant women taking insulin. Individuals with T2DM who take insulin usually need to perform SMBG more often than those not taking it. Records should be kept of SMBG levels for review by the health care team to determine food, insulin, and exercise needs. This approach allows for individualized treatment, especially with meal plans. Blood glucose levels are often regulated as follows:

- Before meals: 70-130 mg/dL
- Two hours after meals: less than 180 mg/dL (expect a 30- to 50-point rise from premeal glucose)
- Bedtime: 90-150 mg/dL

Hypoglycemia

Hypoglycemia (below-normal blood glucose levels) usually results from taking too much insulin, skipping meals, or engaging in too much exercise without a concomitant increase in food intake. Onset is sudden, and the complication can be fatal if left untreated. Usually, hypoglycemia occurs at a time when plasma insulin (or oral hypoglycemic agents) levels peak or during the night while the patient sleeps (fasting). Box 15-2 lists the symptoms of hypoglycemia.

TABLE 15-4 Oral Hypoglycemic Agents

DRUG CLASS	DRUG NAME(S)	ACTION	TARGET ORGAN(S)	SIDE EFFECTS	HOW TAKEN
Alpha-glucosidase inhibitors(AGIs)	*Acarbose:* Precose *Miglitol:* Glyset	Delay absorption of glucose from gastrointestinal tract	Small intestine	Excess flatulence, diarrhea (particularly after high-carbohydrate meal); abdominal pain, may interfere with iron absorption	Must be taken with meals 3 times/day
Biguanides	*Metformin:* Glucophage	Decrease hepatic glucose production and intestinal glucose absorption; improve insulin sensitivity	Liver, small intestine, and peripheral tissues	Weight gain less likely, weight loss possible; anorexia, nausea, diarrhea, metallic taste; biguanides may reduce absorption of vitamin B_{12} and folic acid and are rarely suitable for adults >80 yr of age	Taken with first main meal
Meglitinides (nonsulfonylurea insulin releasers)	*Nateglinide:* Starlix *Repaglinide:* Prandin	Stimulate secretion of insulin	Pancreatic beta cells	Hypoglycemia and weight gain; *repaglinide* has a lightly increased risk for cardiac events	Taken with meals
Sulfonylureas	First-generation: *Acetohexamide:* Dymelor *Tolazamide:* Tolinase *Tolbutamide:* Orinase *Chlorpropamide:* Diabinese Second-generation: *Glimepiride:* Amaryl *Glyburide:* DiaBeta, Micronase, Glynase PresTabs	Stimulate secretion of insulin	Pancreatic beta cells	Hypoglycemia and weight gain; *tolbutamide* may be associated with cardiovascular complications; *chlorpropamide* can cause hyponatremia and should not be used by women who are pregnant or nursing, or by individuals allergic to sulfa drugs; sulfonylurea interacts with many other drugs (prescription, over-the-counter, and alternative); *Diabinese:* avoid alcohol	Taken before or with meals
Thiazolidinediones (TZDs)	*Pioglitazone:* Actos *Rosiglitazone:* Avandia	Improves insulin sensitivity	Activate genes involved with fat synthesis and carbohydrate metabolism	Possible liver damage, weight gain, mild anemia	Once or twice daily

Data from Nelms MN, et al: *Nutrition therapy and pathophysiology*, ed 2, Belmont, CA, 2010, Cengage/Thomson.

BOX 15-2 Symptoms of Hypoglycemia

- Cool, clammy, pale skin
- Confusion
- Erratic behavior
- Hunger
- Trembling, shaking

Symptoms usually occur when blood glucose drops below 50 mg/dL or there is a relatively significant drop in the level. For example, if a patient is in a consistent state of hyperglycemia (e.g., 180 to 200 mg/dL) and the blood glucose level is brought down to 90 mg/dL, the patient may experience hypoglycemia even though the blood glucose level is in the normal range. The key is that for this patient, the usual blood glucose is too low.

Diabetic Ketoacidosis

When glucose cannot be used by cells, or when endogenous sources of energy are unavailable, the body breaks down fats and proteins for energy, possibly leading to ketosis. Ketosis is an abnormal accumulation of ketones caused by metabolism of fatty acids for energy with little carbohydrate metabolism occurring.

Diabetic ketoacidosis (DKA) is a life-threatening condition caused by insulin deficiency. Common conditions that

TABLE 15-5 Correlation Between Mean Plasma Glucose Levels and Hemoglobin A₁c Levels

MEAN PLASMA GLUCOSE (mg/dL)	A₁c (%)
60	4
90	5
120	6
150	7
180	8
210	9
240	10
270	11
300	12
330	13

Data from Rickheim P, et al: *Insulin basics,* Minneapolis, 2001, International Diabetes Center.

BOX 15-3 Symptoms and Clinical Signs of Diabetic Ketoacidosis

- Dehydration and metabolic acidosis
- Dry, flushed skin and mucous membranes
- Fruity (acetone) breath
- Generalized weakness
- Nausea
- Polydipsia
- Polyphagia
- Polyuria
- Vomiting
- Weakness, fatigue
- Weight loss

BOX 15-4 Symptoms and Clinical Signs of Hyperglycemic Hyperosmolar Nonketotic Syndrome

- Polyuria
- Polyphagia
- Weight loss
- Nausea
- Dry, flushed skin and mucous membranes
- Dehydration secondary to osmotic diuresis
- Polydipsia
- Possible seizures and tremors
- Generalized weakness
- Vomiting
- Fatigue

precipitate DKA are insufficient or interrupted insulin therapy, too much food, infection, and other stresses (e.g., trauma, surgery, emotional stress, myocardial infarction). The resulting hyperglycemia causes osmotic diuresis, dehydration, and lactic acidosis. Lowered pH, resulting from the acidosis, stimulates the respiratory center and produces deep, rapid respirations known as Kussmaul's respirations.

Large amounts of ketone bodies in the body produce a fruity, acetone odor to the breath (a person suffering from DKA could be mistaken for someone who is inebriated). Box 15-3 lists symptoms and clinical signs of DKA. If this condition is not recognized and treated promptly, the acidosis and dehydration may lead to loss of consciousness and possibly coma and death.

Hyperglycemic Hyperosmolar Nonketotic Syndrome

Hyperglycemic hyperosmolar nonketotic syndrome (HHNS), like DKA, is a life-threatening emergency caused by a relative or actual insulin deficiency resulting in severe hyperglycemia. Most often HHNS is triggered by trauma or infection that increases the body's demand for insulin. Although enough insulin may be present in the plasma to prevent formation of ketones and acidosis, there may not be enough to prevent hyperglycemia. If hyperglycemia is left untreated, serum becomes hyperosmolar. Osmotic diuresis causes significant loss of electrolytes via urine. The mortality rate for HHNS is 10% to 25%. Symptoms and clinical signs of the disorder are listed in Box 15-4.

Food and Nutrition Therapies

There is no ideal "diabetic" or "ADA diet." In the past it typically meant a physician-determined calorie level with specific percentages of carbohydrate, protein, and fat based on the exchange lists. The American Diabetes Association no longer endorses any particular meal plan or specific percentages of nutrients. Diet orders such as "no concentrated sweets," "no sugar added," "low sugar," and "liberal diabetic" are not considered suitable because they do not reflect diabetes nutrition recommendations and pointlessly restrict sucrose. Such meal plans propagate the false notion that merely restricting sucrose-sweetened foods will improve blood glucose control.

Nutrition therapy is an essential element of glycemic control and *diabetes self-management education (DSME)*. Individualized nutrition therapy is required to achieve treatment goals. The basis for nutrition therapy and DSME involves a comprehensive nutrition assessment, a self-care treatment plan, and the client's health status, learning ability, readiness to change, and current lifestyle. The key is to tailor the meal planning approach to each individual's needs. Individuals using intensive insulin therapy have flexibility in when and what they eat, whereas people using conventional insulin therapy must be consistent with timing of meals and amounts of food consumed.

Recommendations for total fat, saturated fat, cholesterol, fiber, vitamins, and mineral intakes are the same for individuals with diabetes as those for the general population. Carbohydrate recommendations are based on the individual's eating habits, blood glucose, and lipid goals. Blood glucose control is not impaired by the use of sucrose in the meal plan, but sucrose-containing foods should only be eaten as an occasional substitute for other carbohydrate foods and should not be eaten in addition to a meal plan. Protein intake can range

TABLE 15-6 Historical Perspective of Nutrition Recommendations for Diabetes Mellitus

YEAR	CARBOHYDRATE	FAT	PROTEIN
Pre-1921	Starvation diets		
1921	20% of total energy	70% of total energy	10% of total energy
1950	40% of total energy	40% of total energy	20% of total energy
1971	45% of total energy	35% of total energy	20% of total energy
1986	≤60% of total energy	<30% of total energy	12%-20% of total energy
1994	Based on nutrition assessment and treatment goal	Based on nutrition assessment and treatment goals; <10% of energy from saturated fats	10%-20% of total energy
2002	Patients should receive individualized nutrition therapy as needed to achieve treatment goals, preferably provided by a registered dietitian familiar with components of diabetes nutrition therapy (NT).		
	Whole grains, fruits, vegetables, and low-fat milk should be included in a healthy diet.	<10% of energy from saturated fat	Ingested protein is just as potent a stimulant of insulin secretion as carbohydrate
	Total amount of carbohydrate in meals or snacks is more important than source or type of carbohydrate.	~10% of energy from polyunsaturated fat	Protein requirements may be >0.8 g/kg/day for individuals with less-than-optional glycemic control
	Sucrose and sucrose-containing foods should be eaten in the context of a healthy diet (they do not need to be restricted, but should be occasionally consumed instead of other carbohydrate sources or covered with insulin or other glucose-lowering medication).	Intake of *trans* fat should be minimized <300 mg cholesterol/day Fat intake should be individualized and designed to fit ethnic and cultural backgrounds	Usual protein intake (15%-20% of total energy) need not be modified if renal function is normal
	Individuals receiving intensive insulin therapy should adjust their pre-meal insulin dosages on basis of carbohydrate content of meals.		
	Individuals receiving fixed daily insulin dosages should be consistent in day-to-day carbohydrate intake.		
2010	Of U.S. residents 65 years and older,10.9 million, or 26.9%, had diabetes in 2010. 57 million Americans (categorized as "prediabetic") are at risk for development of diabetes in the next 10 years if they don't make appropriate lifestyle changes.		

Adapted from Defeat Diabetes Foundation: *Diabetes ABCs*, n.d. Accessed August 19, 2013, from www.defeatdiabetes.org/about_diabetes/text.asp?id=Diabetes_Timeline.

from 15% to 20% of daily kcal from animal and vegetable protein sources. *If* diabetes is well controlled, blood glucose levels are not affected by moderate alcohol use. Alcohol kcal ought to be regarded as additional kcal, and no food should be omitted. Alcohol should be consumed with food to reduce the risk of hypoglycemia.

The latest recommendations are shown in Table 15-6. Carbohydrate counting is a very effective method for most individuals to maintain glycemic control (Figure 15-9). Goals of nutrition therapy that apply to all individuals with diabetes are as follows:

1. Attain and maintain optimal metabolic outcomes, including:
   a. Glucose level in normal range, or as close to normal range as is safely possible to prevent or reduce risk of complications
   b. Lipid or lipoprotein profile that reduces risk for macrovascular disease
   c. Blood pressure levels that reduce risk for vascular disease (Box 15-5)
2. Modify nutrient intake and lifestyle as appropriate for prevention and treatment of obesity, dyslipidemia, cardiovascular disease, hypertension, and nephropathy.
3. Enhance health using healthy food choices and physical activity.
4. Address individual nutritional needs with regard to personal and cultural preferences and lifestyles while respecting the individual's wishes and willingness to change.

A registered dietitian who is knowledgeable and skilled in implementing nutrition therapy into diabetes management is the medical team member responsible for providing *medical nutrition therapy (MNT)*, especially if the patient's health care team is coding and billing for services with Medicare or Medicaid.

It is essential that other health care team members be knowledgeable about the implications of dietary choices in diabetes, and supportive of the patient with diabetes who needs to make these important lifestyle changes.

Nutrition therapy is an integral component of diabetes management and DSME. It involves conducting a nutrition

**Diabetes Care
and Education**
a diecetic practice group of the
Academy of Nutrition
and Dietetics

Ready, Set, Start Counting!

Carbohydrate Counting — a Tool to Help Manage Your Blood Glucose

When you have diabetes, keeping your blood glucose in a healthy range will help you feel your best today and in the future. Carbohydrate counting — or "carb counting" — is a flexible meal-planning tool (not a diet) that helps you understand how your food choices affect your blood glucose level.

Carbohydrate and blood glucose

Any carbohydrate food you eat (e.g., milk, fruit, bread and pasta) is digested into glucose, which causes your blood glucose level to increase. That said, it's still important to eat carbohydrates throughout the day because they provide energy and essential nutrients for your body. To better manage your blood glucose, energy levels and weight, pay attention to how much carbohydrate you eat.

Maintaining the right balance between carbohydrate and insulin (whether you make it or take it) regulates your blood glucose level. Determining when and how much you eat — and whether or not you have snacks — should be based on your lifestyle, medications and meal-planning goals. A registered dietitian (RD) may consider the following factors in helping you determine the healthiest plan for you:

- **Consistency:** If you use diabetes medications or insulin, it is important to eat the same amount of food and carbohydrate at the same time each day. Doing this can keep your blood glucose from getting too high or too low.

- **Maximums:** Setting a meal-time maximum for carbohydrates along with focusing on a healthy lifestyle, and/or taking diabetes medications, is another way you can help keep your blood sugar from getting too high.

- **Matching:** If your insulin plan includes varying your dose based on what you are eating, it is important to know how much carbohydrate you are eating.

Foods that contain carbohydrate:
- Grains (e.g., breads, crackers, rice, hot and cold cereals, tortillas and noodles)
- Starchy vegetables (e.g., potatoes, peas, corn, winter squash, lentils and beans)
- Fruit and juices
- Milk and yogurt
- Sweets and desserts

Non-starchy vegetables (e.g., carrots, broccoli and tomatoes) contain only a small amount of carbohydrates and will not affect blood glucose when eaten in small portions.

FIG 15-9 Carbohydrate counting.

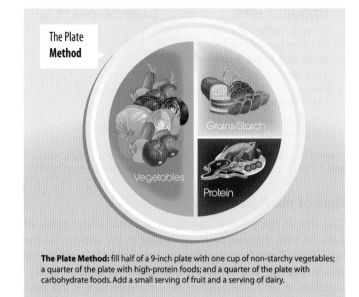

The Plate Method: fill half of a 9-inch plate with one cup of non-starchy vegetables; a quarter of the plate with high-protein foods; and a quarter of the plate with carbohydrate foods. Add a small serving of fruit and a serving of dairy.

FIG 15-10 The Plate Method for planning menus in diabetes management. (From A to Z Health: *Living with diabetes: The plate method,* n.d. Accessed August 20, 2013, from diabetes.atozhealth.com/healthy-eating/meal-planning/the plate method.)

assessment to evaluate a patient's food intake, metabolic status, lifestyle, and willingness to make changes; goal setting; nutrition education; individualized counseling; monitoring and evaluation. To enhance compliance, the medical nutrition therapy plan should be individualized and should take into consideration the patient's lifestyle, cultural background, and financial situation. Patients with diabetes require assessment by a registered dietitian to determine an appropriate nutrition prescription and plan for DSME.

Nutrition therapy should consider a person's usual eating habits and other lifestyle factors. Maintaining consistency within an eating pattern, rather than following an arbitrary eating style, will result in lower glycosylated hemoglobin levels. Other related nutrient issues include use of nutritive and nonnutritive sweeteners. Although fructose creates a smaller rise in plasma glucose than sucrose and other carbohydrates, large amounts of fructose provide no advantage as a sweetener. Other nutritive sweeteners, such as corn sweeteners, fruit juice or juice concentrate, honey, molasses, dextrose, and maltose, affect glycemic response and caloric content much like sucrose does. The sugar alcohols (sorbitol, mannitol, and xylitol) result in lower glycemic responses than other simple and complex carbohydrates, but ingesting large amounts of them may have a laxative effect.

Nonnutritive sweeteners approved for use by the U.S. Food and Drug Administration (FDA), such as saccharin, aspartame, and acesulfame K, are considered safe for consumption by individuals with diabetes. Each product has undergone rigorous testing and scrutiny before approval. All have been shown to be safe when consumed by the public, including people with diabetes and pregnant women. For more information, visit the resource websites at fnic.nal.usda.gov/food-composition/nutritive-and-nonnutritive-sweetener-resources.

Nutrition and diet are considered by both patients and health professionals to be the most difficult problems in the management of diabetes. The plate method and glycemic index are two methods for planning. Glycemic index (GI) is rather complicated, and each person responds uniquely to a "low-GI" or "high-GI" food. So an individual person with diabetes may want to keep track of how different foods affect his or her blood glucose levels. The plate method asks you to draw an imaginary line on your plate and then try to fill it with half nonstarchy vegetables; the remaining sections can be protein foods and starches. Add a glass of low-fat milk and a small portion of fruit (Figure 15-10).

Although no longer used on a regular basis, food exchange lists provide a good estimation of nutrient and calorie content for planning meals. Such lists show foods with their serving sizes, which are usually measured after cooking, and the amount of calories they provide from the macronutrients (carbohydrate, protein, and fat). It is useful to measure the size of each serving to learn to "eyeball" correct serving sizes. The following chart shows the amount of nutrients in one serving from each exchange group or list:

GROUPS/LISTS	CARBOHYDRATE (g)	PROTEIN (g)	FAT (g)	CALORIES
Carbohydrate Group				
Starch	15	3	0-1	80
Fruit	15	—	—	60
Milk				
Fat-free, low-fat	12	8	0-3	90
Reduced-fat	12	8	5	120
Whole	12	8	8	150

GROUPS/LISTS	CARBOHYDRATE (g)	PROTEIN (g)	FAT (g)	CALORIES
Other carbohydrates	15	Varies	Varies	Varies
Nonstarchy vegetables	5	2	—	25
Meat and Meat Substitutes Group				
Very lean	—	7	0-1	35
Lean	—	7	3	55
Medium-fat	—	7	5	75
High-fat	—	7	8	100
Fat Group	—	—	5	45

From American Diabetes Association: www.diabetes.org/food-and-fitness/food/planning-meals/diabetes-meal-plans-and-a-healthy-diet.html; Mayo Clinic: www.mayoclinic.com/health/diabetes-diet/DA00077.

Role of the Nurse

The role of the nurse in caring for the nutritional needs of patients with diabetes varies according to the setting and the age of the client. However, the general approach is to become aware of and to help assess the patient's knowledge of, understanding of, and adherence to the prescribed diet. When possible, observing meals and food choices as well as monitoring glucose levels can give the nurse important clues to the level of compliance.

When adherence is faulty, the nurse needs to offer information and support. Knowledge deficits can be remedied by the nurse or the dietitian; lack of motivation is harder to handle. For example, adolescents with diabetes may not believe that long-term complications are related to diet and may be more motivated to eat like their peers, or older adults with diabetes may be set in lifelong eating habits and may not want to change them as long as they take medication for hyperglycemia.

When a trusting relationship exists between the nurse and patient, discussions about motivations and concerns can take place. The nurse may then influence the patient to be more concerned about his or her long-term welfare. See the *Teaching Tool* box Helping Clients Follow Instructions. Additional forms of support may be provided by community agencies and associations; see Box 15-6 and the Websites of Interest section at the end of this chapter.

BOX 15-6 Making Lifestyle Changes: Tips for Enhancing Conviction and Confidence

Enhancing Conviction

If conviction is very low, emphasize patient autonomy. "Perhaps now is not the right time to talk about this ... I don't want to push you into a decision, it's clearly up to you. I suggest you take time to think about it...."

If conviction is very low, ask permission to provide new information. Avoid giving the same old lecture—vary the message.

Expand on limited conviction. "You said it was somewhat important that you change this behavior. Why did you score a 4 and not a 1? What would have to happen to move you up to a 6 or 7?"

Identify ambivalence. Avoid hard confrontation, which causes the patient to defend the attacked position. Identifying ambivalence helps the patient believe you understand his or her perspective: "So, you have considered this before, but you do not like people telling you what to do."

Identify barriers to considering change. Brainstorm replacements: "Watching television seems to help you relax. What else have you noticed helps you relax? How might you combine your goals of relaxing and improving physical fitness?"

Brainstorm around obstacles. "What will make it hard to increase your activity level?"

Address stated worries directly. "Because you are uncomfortable exercising in public, let's think of some other ways to increase your physical activity."

Discuss pros and cons. Have the patient list the benefits and costs of no change versus change. Start with benefits of no change—there are obviously benefits to the patient or he or she would not be continuing that behavior. Summarize and let the patient draw conclusions.

Help the patient take a hypothetical look "over the fence." "So you're not too sure about changing your diet. Let's imagine for a moment that you did make this change. How would that make you feel?"

Enhancing Confidence

Review previous change successes, praising positive steps and exploring obstacles. "Have you tried this before? How long did you continue that effort? What helped you succeed for that long? What do you think will work for you now? What obstacles were there? What might help with those obstacles now? Tell me about some of the things you have successfully changed in the past."

Expand on limited confidence. "You said you had some confidence that you could change this. Why did you score a 4 and not a 1? What would have to happen to move you up to a 6 or 7?"

Brainstorm solutions, coaching patient to select small, easy steps based on patient's previous experiences and preferences.

Facilitate the shift from success or failure to a stage model. "Most people have partial success several times before they succeed for good. Previous attempts to change increase the odds of success. People go through a period of not wanting to think about it, thinking about it, considering options, deciding to change, struggling to change, struggling with temptations or slips, and finally feeling like it's behind them. Sometimes people cycle through all or parts of that process several times before changing for good."

Address relapse prevention. Discuss "slips" rather than failures; brainstorm ways to break any pattern of slips that leads to a sense of failure; anticipate triggers and plan solutions.

From Koenigsberg MR, et al: Facilitating treatment adherence with lifestyle changes in diabetes, *Am Fam Physician.* 69(2):309-316, 2004. Accessed August 20, 2013, from http://www.aafp.org/afp/2004/0115/p309.html?printable=afp.

Helping Clients Follow Instructions

Diabetes is on the rise. English is a second language for many patients, and education may be limited for others (e.g., reading at a fourth- or fifth-grade level). Nearly 50% of Americans have low literacy skills, which affect their ability to understand their disease and treatment instructions. Because diabetes requires long-term behavioral changes and monitoring, adherence is important. The following care plan provides guidance for the team. Patients who are empowered with knowledge about their disease and treatment can take an active role in their diabetes care and are more likely to achieve blood glucose

Continued

and hemoglobin A_{1c} goals (White, 2012). Health professionals can improve understanding and compliance by (1) using patient education materials that are simple and concise, (2) using culturally appropriate graphics showing step-by-step instructions, and (3) involving family members. Educational strategies such as interactive teaching, problem solving, and individualized education have a positive impact (White, 2012). A care plan that meets the patient's social, psychologic, and physical needs is then developed as a result of collaboration among the nurse, physician or primary health care provider, dietitian, and patient.

From http://www.nutrition411.com/clinical-nutrition/care-algorithms/item/643-interdisciplinary-nutrition-care-plan-diabetes-mellitus.

SPECIAL CONSIDERATIONS

Illness

During periods of illness, blood glucose values may become elevated, and diabetes control may worsen. These changes are caused by an increase in hepatic production of glucose that has been stimulated by infection, illness, injury, or stress (specifically by the release of epinephrine, norepinephrine, glucagon, and cortisol). Under such conditions, this hyperglycemia increases insulin requirements. Although illness increases the need for insulin, decreased appetite and food intake are common. Liquids and soft foods are often better tolerated, provide some energy, and prevent dehydration. See the *Teaching Tool* box Sick Day Guidelines.

✳ **TEACHING TOOL**

Sick Day Guidelines

The following guidelines have been used by patients with diabetes who have brief illness, only during that emergency,—for a maximum of 3 days:

1. Monitor blood glucose at least four times a day (before each meal and at bedtime). If you are too ill, have someone else check it for you. Write your levels down in case you need to discuss them with your doctor.
2. Test urine for ketones (if blood glucose is 250 mg/dL or higher). Write down these levels as well.
3. Stick to your normal meal plan if possible.
4. Drink lots of sugar-free liquid (water, broth, tea) to prevent dehydration.
5. Call your physician if any of the following occurs:
   - Vomiting or diarrhea for more than 2 hours
   - Fever of 100.0°F or higher
   - Blood glucose levels 250 mg/dL or higher after two checks, or if levels do not go down after extra insulin
   - Spilling of moderate or large amounts of ketones in your urine
6. Medications to control blood glucose should not be omitted. Dosages may need to be adjusted when food intake is reduced. If you take insulin, you must continue to take your usual dose to prevent ketoacidosis. Your need for insulin continues or may increase during illness. If you take oral hypoglycemic agents (tablets), continue to take your usual dose unless you are vomiting.
7. If you cannot tolerate regular foods, replace carbohydrates in the meal plan with liquid, semiliquid, or soft foods. A general rule is to consume approximately 15 g carbohydrates every 1 to 2 hours; the following list has good suggestions.

Foods Containing 15 g Carbohydrates
½ cup orange or grapefruit juice
⅓ cup grape or apple juice
½ cup ice cream
½ cup cooked cereal
¼ cup sherbet
⅓ cup regularly sweetened gelatin
1 cup broth-based soups (reconstituted with water)
1 cup cream soup
¾ cup regular soft drink (ginger ale, cola)
¼ cup milkshake
1½ cups milk
½ cup eggnog (commercial)
⅓ cup tapioca pudding
½ cup custard
1 cup plain yogurt
1 slice toast
6 saltine crackers

Adapted from Joslin Diabetes Center: *Stay healthy with diabetes: Sick days*, n.d. Accessed August 20, 2013, from http://www.joslin.org/info/Sick_Days.html.

Gastroparesis

Approximately 20% to 30% of individuals with diabetes experience gastroparesis. Delayed gastric emptying can manifest as heartburn, nausea, abdominal pain, vomiting, early satiety, and weight loss. Gastroparesis occurs as a result of vagal autonomic neuropathy and occurs more often in T1DM. Dietary treatment of gastroparesis involves careful monitoring of intake. Carbohydrates should be replaced with foods of soft or liquid consistency. Six small meals may be better tolerated than three large meals. If constipation or diarrhea occurs, fiber intake is altered according to patient needs. A low-fat diet may be useful to prevent delay in gastric emptying. If metoclopramide (Reglan) is used to increase gastric contractions and relax the pyloric sphincter, the patient may experience the side effects dry mouth and nausea. If the patient complains of dry mouth, fluids can be increased and food moistened with broth. Insulin should be matched with meals to regulate delayed absorption and glucose changes. Bezoar formation is common if oranges, coconuts, green beans, apples, figs, potato skins, Brussels sprouts, and sauerkraut are eaten. If problems are severe, a temporary jejunostomy tube feeding may be indicated.

Eating Disorders

Eating disorders in T1DM are somewhat common. Once insulin therapy is initiated, weight gain occurs. What is dangerous is insulin restriction to keep weight under control. Warning signs of a potential eating disorder include changes in usual eating pattern, unexplained elevations in A_{1c}, excessive exercising, amenorrhea, and frequent episodes of DKA, which may be fatal. Body image problems have been nicknamed "diabulimia" in the media, but there is nothing amusing about these disorders. Referral to a mental health professional is needed.

Metabolic Syndrome

Disproportionate fat deposition in the abdomen leads to excessive secretion of cytokines and chronic low-grade inflammation (Dulloo and Montani, 2012). Adipose tissue contributes to type 2 diabetes, cardiovascular diseases, and the metabolic syndrome. See Box 15-7 for further information.

BOX 15-7 Metabolic Syndrome

Metabolic syndrome (MetS) is a cluster of metabolic abnormalities characterized by central obesity, dyslipidemias, hypertension, high fasting glucose value, chronic low-grade inflammation, and oxidative stress; about 34 % of American adults have this condition (Andersen and Fernandez, 2013).

Criteria for MetS consist of the presence of any three of the following:

- Enlarged waist circumference (according to population and country-specific definitions)
- High-density lipoprotein cholesterol <40 mg/dL in men and <50 mg/dL in women.
- Blood pressure 130/85 mm Hg or greater
- Fasting glucose value 100 mg/dL or greater

Treatment is vital because diabetes, coronary artery disease, and stroke quickly develop in individuals with MetS.

Treatment is multifaceted, consisting of diet, exercise, and pharmacologic treatment, including with statins, fibrates, angiotensin-converting enzyme (ACE) inhibitors, and thiazolidinediones. Because a significant risk factor is central obesity, successful strategies include energy restriction and weight loss; manipulation of dietary carbohydrates and fat; enrichment in beneficial fatty acids, functional foods, and bioactive nutrients; and adherence to the Mediterranean diet and diet/exercise regimens.

Data from Andersen CJ, Fernandez ML: Dietary strategies to reduce metabolic syndrome, *Rev Endocr Metab Disord* 14:241-254, 2013; Kassi E, et al. Metabolic syndrome: definitions and controversies. BMC Med. 9:48, 2011.

DIABETES MANAGEMENT THROUGH THE LIFE SPAN

Nutrition therapy is crucial for optimal blood glucose control and will be affected by various life stages: growth and development in children, growth spurts in teens, pregnancy, even the chronic conditions of aging.

Pregnancy

Women with preexisting diabetes who become pregnant are vulnerable to fetal complications, and maternal health can be compromised when complications of diabetes occur. Occasionally the stress of pregnancy may induce *gestational diabetes (GDM),* a form of glucose intolerance with onset during pregnancy. Whether the mother has preexisting diabetes or GDM, risk of fetal abnormalities and mortality is increased in the presence of hyperglycemia, so every effort should be made to control blood glucose levels. Ideally women with diabetes should achieve excellent glycemic control 3 months before conception.

Changes that take place during pregnancy greatly affect diabetes control and insulin use. Some hormones and enzymes produced by the placenta are antagonistic to insulin, thus reducing its effectiveness. Maternal insulin does not cross the placenta, but glucose does. The fetal pancreas increases insulin production if blood glucose levels get too high. The increased production of insulin causes macrosomia, the typical "large for gestational age (LGA)" infant (Pham, et al, 2013). LGA newborns may experience respiratory difficulties, hypocalcemia, hypoglycemia, hypokalemia, or jaundice.

Individualization of nutrition therapy is contingent on maternal weight and height. Adequate calories and nutrients must meet the needs of the pregnancy and should be consistent with established maternal blood glucose goals. SMBG presents important information about the impact of food on blood glucose levels. At the start, minimal SMBG four times a day should be planned (fasting and 1 or 2 hours after each meal), but it is not uncommon for pregnant women with diabetes to test blood glucose levels eight times per day. Blood glucose goals during pregnancy are as follows:

- Fasting: ≤95 mg/dL
- 1 hour postprandial: ≤140 mg/dL
- 2 hours postprandial: ≤120 mg/dL

Guidelines for all pregnant women can be used because there are no unique weight gain recommendations for women with diabetes. Desired weight gain goals are based on prepregnancy BMI and should be steady and progressive (Table 15-7). Thin women should gain more weight than overweight/obese women. Given that women with GDM are often overweight or obese, an average weight gain of 15 pounds (6.8 kg) can be recommended.

No calorie adjustments are needed for the first trimester. During the second and third trimesters, an increased energy intake of approximately 100 to 300 kcal/day is recommended. High-quality protein should be increased by 10 g/day and can be supplied easily with one or two extra glasses of low-fat or

TABLE 15-7 Desired Weight Gain Goals for Pregnant Women*			
BMI RANGE	**PRE-PREGNANCY BMI**	**RECOMMENDED WEIGHT GAIN**	**KCAL REQUIREMENTS**
Obese	30 and greater	11-20 lbs total	12-18 kcal/kg prepregnancy weight
Overweight	25-29.9	15-20 lbs total	24 kcal/kg prepregnancy weight
Normal weight	18.5-24.9	First trimester: ≈3 to 5 lbs/month	30 kcal/kg prepregnancy weight
		25-35 lbs total	
Underweight	Less than 18.5	28-40 lbs total	36-40 kcal/kg prepregnancy weight

Adapted from Institute of Medicine: *Weight gain during pregnancy: Reexamining the guidelines,* 2009. Accessed August 19, 2013, from www.iom.edu/Reports/2009/weight-Gain-during-pregnancy-Reexamining-the-Guidelines.aspx
*The effects of gestational weight gain on pregnancy outcome depend on the woman's pre-pregnancy body mass index (BMI). Women in whom gestational diabetes mellitus (GDM) develops tend to have higher gestational weight gain. Gestational weight gain is a significant risk factor for GDM in the overweight or obese patient but not in patients who are underweight or have a normal BMI before pregnancy (Gibson, et al, 2012).

skim milk, or 1 to 2 ounces of meat or meat substitute. As with any pregnancy, 400 μg/day of folic acid is recommended for prevention of neural tube defects and other congenital abnormalities. Alcohol should not be consumed in any amount.

Energy restriction in the diabetic patient who is pregnant must be cautious. A minimum of 1700 to 1800 kcal/day of carefully selected foods has been shown to prevent ketosis. Intakes below this level are not advised. Each patient with GDM should be evaluated individually by a registered dietician; her care plans should be adjusted, and she should be provided patient education as needed to achieve weight goals.

Overt Diabetes in Pregnancy

A successful pregnancy for a woman who has diabetes requires planning and commitment. Because most fetal malformations occur during the first trimester of pregnancy, achieving and maintaining excellent glycemic control before conception and during early pregnancy are essential. The optimal period of care for a woman with diabetes is *before* conception.

Ideally, preconception counseling should begin during puberty and continue through the childbearing years. Glycosylated hemoglobin levels should be normal or as close to normal as possible before conception is attempted. Insulin requirements rise during the second and third trimesters because of higher blood glucose levels caused by increased production of pregnancy-associated hormones that are insulin antagonists. Successful preconception care programs have used the following preprandial and postprandial goals:

Before meals: Capillary whole-blood glucose 70 to 100 mg/dL or capillary plasma glucose 80 to 110 mg/dL

2 Hours postprandial: Capillary whole-blood glucose less than 140 mg/dL or capillary plasma glucose less than 155 g/dL

Pregnancy will require greater attention to nutrition on a day-to-day basis. Guidance during early pregnancy should address food cravings and nausea. The meal plan should be individualized, evolving throughout the pregnancy to meet changing nutritional needs and insulin requirements. Three meals and three snacks are usually recommended. Use of frequent home blood glucose monitoring is necessary to help the patient maintain normal fasting and postprandial glucose levels and avoid frequent or severe hypoglycemic reactions.

Gestational Diabetes

GDM develops in about 5% to 6% of all pregnancies (Vandorsten, et al, 2013). It occurs more frequently among American Indian, African American, and Hispanic/Latina American women. Women in whom GDM develops are often obese, but weight reduction should not be attempted at this time. Nutrition recommendations for GDM are summarized in Table 15-8.

Good glucose control is usually accomplished by individualization of intake and graphing of weight gain. Often, insulin may be prescribed in addition to medical nutrition therapy to reduce the risks of fetal macrosomia, neonatal hyperglycemia, and perinatal mortality. The FDA has not approved any oral hypoglycemic agents for use during pregnancy. Glucose levels usually revert to normal following delivery, but there is an increased risk for later development of T2DM.

Type 2 Diabetes in the Young

Incidence and prevalence of T2DM in children, especially ethnic minority populations, have increased 30-fold over the past 20 years, causing the term *epidemic* to be used to describe the phenomenon. The burden of diabetes and its accompanying complications will affect many more individuals, putting an enormous drain on the country's health care resources. More Americans will be taking potent medications, which have side effects, for most of their lives. What has accompanied this epidemic of T2DM in children across the United States? The answer apparently lies within another epidemic: childhood obesity.

Obesity is the most prominent clinical risk factor for T2DM in children and adolescents. About one third of children with T2DM have BMIs greater than 40, indicating morbid obesity, and 17% have BMIs greater than 45 (normal BMI range for the pediatric population is 35 to 39). Children and adolescents diagnosed with T2DM are generally between 10 and 19 years old, are obese, have a strong family history for T2DM, and have insulin resistance (Centers for Disease Control and Prevention [CDC], 2011).

TABLE 15-8 Nutrition Recommendations for Gestational Diabetes Mellitus

NUTRIENT	RECOMMENDATIONS
Energy*	Sufficient to promote adequate, but not excessive, weight gain and to avoid ketonuria
Carbohydrate	Base effect of intake on glycemic control; intake should be distributed throughout the day
Protein	0.8 g/kg (Recommended Dietary Allowance) desirable body weight per day + 25 g/day or 1.1 g/kg desirable body weight
Fat	Limit saturated fat
Sodium	Not routinely restricted
Fiber	Adequate intake along with fluid for prevention of constipation
Nonnutritive sweeteners	Use in moderation
Vitamins and minerals	Preconception folate intake; assess for individual needs; multivitamin throughout pregnancy; iron at 12 weeks; calcium in last trimester and during lactation
Caffeine	Limit to <300 mg/day
Alcohol	Avoid

*Recommendations to patients are based on prepregnancy BMI. For BMI levels <18.5, 18.5-24.9, 25-29.9, and >30 kg/m^2, weight gain ranges are suggested at 28-40, 25-35, 15-25, and 11-20 pounds, respectively, and the recommended rates of weight gain are 1-1.3, 0.8-1, 0.5-0.7, and 0.4-0.6 pounds/week (Bloomgarden, 2010).
Data from Reader D: Diabetes in pregnancy and lactation. In Ross TA, Boucher JL, O'Connell BS, editors: *American Dietetic Association guide to diabetes: Medical nutrition therapy and education,* Chicago, 2005, American Dietetic Association.

Besides morbid obesity, clinical signs that may indicate risk for T2DM include the following:

- Acanthosis nigricans (hyperpigmentation and thickening of the skin into velvety irregular folds in the neck and flexural areas), which reflects chronic hyperinsulinemia
- Polycystic ovary syndrome (PCOS), which is associated with insulin resistance and obesity (Box 15-8)
- Hypertension, which may occur in 20% to 30% of patients with T2DM

American Indian children are at highest risk (CDC, 2011). Girls appear to be more susceptible than boys to T2DM, regardless of race. In addition, adolescents with T2DM generally have obese parents who themselves tend to have insulin resistance or overt T2DM. Although there are currently insufficient data to make definite T2DM screening recommendations for children or adolescents, a panel of experts on children with diabetes developed the recommendations outlined in Box 15-9.

As with T2DM in adults, the ideal treatment goal is normalization of blood glucose values and A$_{1c}$. Successful control of associated comorbidities, such as hypertension and hyperlipidemia, is also important. The ultimate goal is to decrease

BOX 15-8 Polycystic Ovary Syndrome

Polycystic ovary syndrome (PCOS) is the most common hormonal reproductive problem a woman of reproductive age can have. It can affect her menstrual cycle, fertility, hormones, insulin production, heart, blood vessels, and appearance. Clinical features include the following:

- Acanthosis nigricans
- Adult acne
- Dyslipidemia, hypercholesterolemia
- High level of male hormones (hyperandrogenism)
- Hirsutism
- Hyperinsulinemia, peripheral insulin resistance, or diabetes
- Infertility or recurrent pregnancy loss
- Luteinizing hormone hypersecretion
- Menstrual dysfunction or anovulation
- Possible development of small cysts in ovaries
- Sleep apnea
- Weight gain or obesity with upper body fat distribution

Approximately 5% to 10% of women in the United States have PCOS. Obesity is present in half, and approximately 10% of this group will have T2DM by age 40 years. Women with PCOS may be at increased risk for endometrial hyperplasia or cancer. They are also at increased risk for diabetes and heart disease. There is no single test to diagnose PCOS, and there is no cure. Treatment is based on an individual's symptoms.

Data from Womenshealth.gov: *Polycystic ovary syndrome (PCOS) fact sheet,* 2012. Accessed August 19, 2013, from http://womenshealth.gov/publications/our-publications/fact-sheet/polycystic-ovary-syndrome.hml.

BOX 15-9 Testing for Type 2 Diabetes Mellitus in Children

Criteria
Overweight (body mass index [BMI] > 85th percentile for age and gender, or weight for height > 85th percentile, or weight > 120% of ideal for height)
 PLUS Any two of the following risk factors:
- Family history of the disease in first- or second-degree relative
- Race/ethnicity (Native American, African American, Latino, Asian American, Pacific Islander)
- Signs of insulin resistance or conditions associated with insulin resistance (acanthosis nigricans, hypertension, dyslipidemia, or PCOS)

Age of Initiation
10 years or at onset of puberty, if puberty occurs at a younger age

Frequency
Every 2 years

Test Preferred
Fasting plasma glucose measurement

Modified from American Diabetes Association: Standards of medical care in diabetes: 2010, *Diabetes Care* 33:11S-61S, 2010.

risk of the acute and chronic complications associated with diabetes.

Generally, children and adolescents with type 2 diabetes have poor glycemic control, with A_{1c} values around 10% to 12% (CDC, 2011). Initial treatment depends on clinical symptoms. The range of disease at diagnosis varies from asymptomatic hyperglycemia to DKA and hyperosmolar HHNS. Both DKA and HHNS are associated with high morbidity and mortality in children. Nutrition therapy and exercise are obvious first-line treatments, but most children diagnosed with T2DM require drug therapy. Although insulin is the only FDA-approved drug for treatment of diabetes in children, oral agents are most often used for children with T2DM.

The American Academy of Pediatrics (AAP) recommends integrating lifestyle modifications (diet and exercise) with medication (Copeland, et al, 2013). All children with T2DM should receive comprehensive self-management education, including SMBG, referral to a registered dietitian with knowledge and experience in nutritional management of children with diabetes, behavior modification strategies for lifestyle changes, increased daily physical activity, and decreased sedentary activity (e.g., TV viewing and computer use). Referral to experts trained in the care of children and adolescents with T2DM is appropriate when treatment goals are not met or when therapy with insulin is initiated (Copeland, et al, 2013).

Type 2 Diabetes in the Elderly

Older adults with diabetes are at risk for development of macrovascular and microvascular complications, with higher overall risk for cardiovascular disease. Key factors to consider are as follows (Up-to-Date, n.d.).

- Common problems in the elderly are polypharmacy, functional disabilities, cognitive impairment, depression, urinary incontinence, falls, and chronic pain.
- The appropriate target for A_{1c} in fit elderly patients who have a life expectancy of more than 10 years should be <7%.
- The goal for A_{1c} should be somewhat higher (≤8%) in frail older adults with multiple medical and functional comorbidities and in those whose life expectancy is less than 10 years.
- Individualized goals should include efforts to preserve quality of life and to avoid hypoglycemia and the complications of impaired cognition and function.
- Individualized counseling should be offered regarding lifestyle modification, including a medical nutrition evaluation and nutrition prescription (tailored on the basis of medical, lifestyle, and personal factors).
- In the absence of specific contraindications, metformin is the initial therapy. In patients with contraindications and/or intolerance to metformin, a short-acting sulfonylurea such as glipizide is an alternative option.

SUMMARY

- Diabetes mellitus is a group of conditions characterized by either a relative or complete lack of insulin secretion by the beta cells of the pancreas or defects of cell insulin receptors, which results in disturbances of carbohydrate, protein, and lipid metabolism and hyperglycemia.
- Long-term complications often lead to disability and premature death.
- Complications may be related to the level and frequency of hyperglycemia experiences throughout the life span in addition to genetic and environmental factors.
- The two primary categories of glucose intolerance are T1DM and T2DM.
- T1DM symptoms appear suddenly and include polyphagia, polyuria, polydipsia, and weight loss.
- Everyone with T1DM requires exogenous insulin to maintain normal blood glucose levels.
- The primary metabolic problem in T2DM is insulin resistance.
- Family history and obesity are the two strongest risk factors for T2DM.
- The gradually occurring symptoms of T2DM are polyuria, polydipsia, fatigue, and frequent infections.
- Some individuals with T2DM may require insulin to optimize blood glucose control.
- Additional types of diabetes are GDM, impaired glucose tolerance, and other less common forms.

- Related conditions that may occur are hypoglycemia, DKA, HHNS, and eating disorders.
- Control of blood glucose levels is the cornerstone of diabetes management.
- The main goal of diabetes treatment is maintenance of plasma insulin/glucose homeostasis. Treatment may include the use of insulin or other medicines, nutrition therapy, and exercise.
- Blood glucose can be monitored several ways: (1) fasting blood glucose determination by reputable laboratories, (2) glycosylated hemoglobin determination by reputable laboratories, and (3) self-monitoring with standardized devices.
- Nutrition therapy is an essential component of successful diabetes management, and the complexity involved requires a team approach.
- The diabetes management team should include a registered nurse, a physician or primary health care provider, a registered dietitian, and the person with diabetes. As needed, family members should be included for education and counseling.
- For successful nutrition therapy, the diabetes management team conducts a thorough assessment, encourages the patient's role in goal setting, implements nutrition intervention, monitors results, and regularly evaluates the nutrition care plan.

- The current guidelines include (1) planning for near normal blood glucose levels and optimal lipid levels; (2) individualizing diet plans; (3) having the patient reach a reasonable weight; and (4) if desired, enabling the patient to consume some sugar and foods that contain sugar if they are occasionally used instead of other carbohydrate foods.
- Nutrition recommendations for total fat, saturated fat, cholesterol, fiber, vitamins, and minerals are the same for individuals with diabetes as for the general population.

- Recommendations are modified for protein, carbohydrates, sucrose, and alcohol because of the nature of diabetes in relation to carbohydrate metabolism or the effects of diabetic complications.
- Special care is needed for diabetes in children, teens, and the elderly and during pregnancy. Individualized goals should include efforts to preserve quality of life, manage hyperglycemia, avoid hypoglycemia, and prevent complications.

◎ THE NURSING APPROACH

Case Studies: Type 1 and Type 2 Diabetes Mellitus

Case Study 1: Type 1 Diabetes Mellitus

Jason, age 15, has come to diabetes camp this summer for the first time. Diagnosed with type 1 diabetes mellitus (T1DM) 2 years ago, he is the only one in his family who has diabetes. He lives with his parents, a younger brother, and a younger sister. The camp nurse assessed Jason's situation and created a successful plan of care.

Assessment

Subjective (Information Told Directly to the Camp Nurse)
- "My blood sugar has been bouncing all over the place."
- "The nurse practitioner suggested that I come to diabetes camp. I want to control my blood sugar so I can feel better."
- "I have been thinking about getting an insulin pump. I hate checking my blood sugar and giving myself shots. I take four shots a day now. I'd like a pump that will measure my blood sugar and give me insulin automatically."
- "I want to be the same as my friends. They can eat whatever they want whenever they want. I don't want to be different."

Objective (Information from His Camp Admission Record)
- Jason injects Lantus insulin (long acting) at bedtime and Humalog insulin (rapid acting) immediately before meals.
- He has not seen a dietitian since he was first diagnosed and does not follow any special meal plan.
- Last hemoglobin A_{1c} value was 8% (normal 4.4% to 6.7%)

Diagnoses (Nursing)
1. Health-seeking behaviors as evidenced by participation in diabetes camp and "I want to control my blood sugar so I can feel better"
2. Deficient knowledge: insulin pumps related to misinformation as evidenced by "I'd like a pump that will measure my blood sugar and give insulin automatically" and "I hate checking my blood sugar and giving myself shots" four times a day

Planning

Patient Outcomes

Short term (by the end of day 2 at camp):
- Jason will follow camp rules and participate fully in all activities and education sessions.
- He will have few or no episodes of hypoglycemia.

- He will observe how some campers use insulin pumps and will express interest in learning more.

Long term (by the end of camp in 5 days):
- He will make friends and express the desire to return to camp next summer.
- He will set a goal to continue at home to follow his meal plan and to check his blood glucose and give himself insulin before each meal and at bedtime.
- He will have few or no episodes of hypoglycemia.
- He will recognize that an insulin pump does not measure blood glucose and is not automatic.

Nursing Interventions
1. Set rules for camp and participate with campers in activities.
2. Give a presentation during an education session.
3. Be a role model by following a meal plan.
4. Be on call for emergencies.

Implementation
1. Established the following rules for diabetic campers. Each camper will:
   - Demonstrate to a counselor the correct technique for injecting insulin and using the camper's personal blood glucose meter.
   - Check and record blood glucose before each meal and at bedtime.
   - Follow the meal plan established by the camp dietitian.
   - Follow the prescription for insulin determined by the camp doctor and meet with the camp doctor and nurse daily to discuss possible insulin adjustments.
   - Report any blood glucose level below 60 mg/dL to a counselor or the camp nurse and consume crackers and juice as needed.
   - Participate in all planned group activities and education sessions.
   - Seek treatment for illness and injuries at the camp medical cabin.
   Rules are set to create order, safety, and a learning environment.
2. Accompanied campers to activities: swimming, boating, hiking, dancing, singing, and skits.
   Activities provide fun and opportunities for campers to make friends. Campers learn how to recognize and treat

Continued

◎ THE NURSING APPROACH—cont'd

hypoglycemia that may occur following exercise. The nurse is present to treat emergencies and mingle socially with the campers.

3. Taught classes regarding sick-day management and recognition and treatment of hypoglycemia.

   Camp provides practical diabetes education and prepares campers to recognize and report problems of hyperglycemia and hypoglycemia.

4. Wore a fanny pack containing blood glucose testing equipment, glucose tablets, glucagon, and glucose for intravenous administration.

   Quick action is needed to treat hypoglycemia, as follows:

   • If a camper's blood glucose results are below 60 mg/dL and the camper is alert, he or she can eat glucose tablets or food containing 15 g of carbohydrate. After waiting 15 minutes, the camper should recheck the blood glucose level. If it is still low, the camper should again eat 15 g of food.

   • When a camper is not responsive enough to take glucose, glucagon can be given subcutaneously.

   • If necessary, a needle can be inserted into a vein for immediate injection of concentrated glucose.

5. Was on call for emergencies each night.

   Many episodes of hypoglycemia occur during the night. Sometimes a camper may fall from his or her bed with severe hypoglycemia, and this occurrence awakens counselors or other campers so they can seek help.

6. Served as a role model, following a meal plan established by the camp dietitian. Selected foods according to serving sizes and number of carbohydrates in an individualized meal plan. Measured foods, using measuring cups and spoons.

   Campers need good role models. They learn serving sizes by measuring foods.

Evaluation (by the Camp Nurse)

Short term (at the end of 2 days):

• Jason had made friends and was having fun at activities.

• He checked his blood glucose level four times a day, followed his meal plan, and gave himself insulin before each meal and at bedtime, based on his doctor's prescription.

• He had no episodes of hypoglycemia.

• Jason expressed interest in learning more about insulin pumps.

Goals met.

Long term (at the end of camp on day 5):

• Jason stated he wanted to keep in touch with friends from camp and return to camp next summer.

• He said he wanted to continue measuring his blood glucose four times a day, follow his meal plan, and give insulin four times a day at home.

• He learned a lot about insulin pumps from friends at camp. He recognized that a pump does not measure blood glucose and is not automatic. He said he wants to learn more about carbohydrate counting and insulin pumps.

• He had one episode of hypoglycemia late at night after hiking and swimming, and he treated it successfully with juice, crackers, and cheese.

Goals met.

Discussion Questions

Risk for hypoglycemia is another nursing diagnosis that could be added to Jason's care plan. Jason witnessed the nurse giving one of the campers a glucagon injection when the camper's blood glucose level was low and he was not alert enough to eat anything.

1. How does a glucagon injection raise blood glucose? After a client becomes more alert, what food should be given? Why?

2. How could Jason begin to learn about carbohydrate servings by reading exchange lists for diabetes?

Case Study 2: Type 2 Diabetes Mellitus

Juanita, age 47, is from Mexico and has been newly diagnosed with type 2 diabetes mellitus (T2DM). She speaks only a few words in English. Juanita's daughter, Maria, has accompanied her to the health clinic because she is bilingual and can act as an interpreter. Maria works as an accountant and is computer literate. Juanita was given a nutrition instruction sheet by the doctor; however, she could not read the English words, so she came to the clinic to learn what she should eat. Because the dietitian would not be available to meet with Juanita until 2 weeks later, the nurse gave initial instructions to Juanita and Maria.

Assessment

Subjective (Directly from Juanita or Interpreted by Her Daughter)

• "My daughter told me what the instruction sheet said, but it doesn't have any of the foods I usually eat. Do I have to change everything I eat?"

• "The doctor said I shouldn't eat sugar anymore."

• "If I eat right, I don't need to take any diabetes medicine."

• "I usually cook tacos or enchiladas or burritos for my family. Can't I just eat what they eat?"

• "I don't go walking very often. I usually stay home."

Objective (from Physical Exam and Juanita's Medical Record)

• Height 5 feet, weight 135 pounds

• Blood glucose 160 mg/dL today 1 hour after eating lunch

• The doctor diagnosed diabetes after treating Juanita for a vaginal yeast infection and obtaining lab work needed for a diagnosis of diabetes.

• No diabetes medicine was prescribed.

Diagnoses (Nursing)

1. Deficient knowledge: dietary management of diabetes related to new diagnosis as evidenced by desire to know what to eat, "Do I have to change everything I eat?" and "The doctor said I shouldn't eat sugar anymore."

2. Imbalanced nutrition: more than body requirements related to excess food and inadequate exercise as evidenced by 135% ideal body weight

Planning

Patient Outcomes

Short term (by the end of this visit):

• Juanita will understand that the main dietary focuses are healthy food choices and weight loss.

THE NURSING APPROACH—cont'd

- She will agree to read the Spanish resources about diabetes.
- She and her daughter will make an appointment to meet with the dietitian as soon as possible.

Nursing Interventions

1. Stress the importance of healthy food choices and weight loss.
2. Provide resources about diabetes in Spanish.

Implementation

1. Told Juanita that she could still eat foods she prepares for her family, although it would be healthy for all to limit fat and sugar and salt.

   Meal plans are designed for individuals on the basis of usual eating patterns and preferences. Healthy food choices are applicable to the entire family.

2. Explained that Juanita should focus on small serving sizes in order to lose weight, which would improve diabetes control and general health.

   When an overweight or obese person with T2DM loses weight, glucose resistance is reduced, and cardiovascular health is improved.

3. Gave Juanita a Spanish pamphlet on meal planning from the American Diabetes Association.

   This guide is a good introduction to healthy eating for people with diabetes, preparing the patient to meet with a dietitian. Brochures are generally helpful when written in the patient's language.

4. Informed Maria that the American Diabetes Association has Spanish educational materials at www.diabetes.org.

   Authoritative resources are available for Hispanic/Latino patients who are newly diagnosed with diabetes. Many resources at American Diabetes Association are free, and cooking books for Latinos may be purchased.

5. Wrote down government websites for Spanish pamphlets about diabetes:
   - National Diabetes Education Program at www.ndep.nih.gov.
   - National Institute of Diabetes & Digestive & Kidney Diseases at www.diabetes.niddk.nih.gov.

   Many free Spanish resources are available from the government to help patients understand diabetes and what to eat.

6. Encouraged Juanita and her daughter to make an appointment to meet with the dietitian as soon as possible.

   The dietitian can design an individualized meal plan for the patient.

7. Suggested that Juanita make an appointment with the doctor for follow-up diabetes management and to ask about safe exercise, such as walking.

   Regular visits to the doctor are important to good diabetes management. The level of exercise should be determined by the doctor who knows about the patient's medical condition.

Evaluation

Short term (at the end of the visit):

- Juanita and her daughter identified healthy food choices and weight loss as the main focuses for eating.
- They agreed to read the Spanish version of the meal planning guide.
- Maria indicated that she would visit the websites suggested.
- They made appointments with the dietitian and the doctor. Goals met.

Discussion Questions

1. What are the basic differences between a healthy food pyramid and a diabetes food pyramid?
2. How could you help Maria explain the importance of appropriate serving sizes?

CRITICAL THINKING

Clinical Applications

Alan, age 75, is a white man admitted to the hospital following a cerebrovascular accident. He has a history of T2DM, hypertension, moderate obesity, and possible alcohol abuse. Medications on admission are furosemide (Lasix), hydrochlorothiazide, propranolol (Inderal), and chlorpropamide (Diabinese) 500 mg bid. Alan comes to the clinic regularly, and at his last visit, he complained of blurred vision, polydipsia, polyuria, and a weight loss of 8 pounds in the past 2 weeks. He was admitted to the hospital with a diagnosis of urinary tract infection and hyperglycemic hyperosmolar nonketotic (HHNS) syndrome. Physical examination revealed the following:

- Height: 5 feet 11 inches
- Weight: 215 pounds
- Blood pressure: 160/82 mm Hg
- Cholesterol: 380 mg/dL
- Triglycerides: 300 mg/dL
- Blood sugar: 750 mg/dL
- Family history: Sister has had T2DM for 10 years

1. Explain how Alan's blood glucose level could become so high without producing ketones.
2. If this patient's HHNS is not treated, how would you expect his disease to progress?
3. What are Alan's blood glucose and lipid goals?
4. What is the purpose of the prescribed medications? Are there any possible drug-nutrient interactions?
5. How frequently should blood glucose levels be monitored?
6. What are possible complications?

WEBSITES OF INTEREST

American Association of Diabetes Educators (AADE)

aadenet.org

The accreditation association for diabetes educators, AADE educates and supports diabetes educators as they lead clients to self-management of diabetes and related chronic conditions.

American Diabetes Association (ADA)

www.diabetes.org

Educates and sponsors community services and research to prevent, cure, and manage diabetes.

National Diabetes Information Clearinghouse (NDIC)

www. diabetes.niddk.nih.gov/

Functions as a diabetes information dissemination service of the National Institute of Diabetes and Digestive and Kidney Diseases (NIDDK), National Institutes of Health (NIH).

REFERENCES

American Diabetes Association: *Living with diabetes*, n.d. From: www.diabetes.org/living-with-diabetes/. Accessed August 18, 2013.

Bloomgarden JT: Gestational diabetes mellitus and obesity, *Diabetes Care* 33:e60–e65, 2010.

Centers for Disease Control and Prevention, CDC Newsroom: Press release: Number of Americans with diabetes rises to nearly 26 million, January 26, 2011. From: www.cdc.gov/media/releases/2011/p0126_diabetes.html. Accessed August 18, 2013.

Copeland KC, et al: Management of newly diagnosed type 2 diabetes mellitus (T2DM) in children and adolescents, *Pediatrics* 131:364–382, 2013.

Danaei G, et al: National, regional, and global trends in fasting plasma glucose and diabetes prevalence since 1980: Systematic analysis of health examination surveys and epidemiological studies with 370 country-years and 2·7 million participants, *Lancet* 378:31–40, 2011.

Dulloo AG, Montani JP: Body composition, inflammation and thermogenesis in pathways to obesity and the metabolic syndrome: An overview, *Obes Rev* 13:1S–5S, 2012.

Gibson KS, et al: Maternal weight gain in women who develop gestational diabetes mellitus, *Obstet Gynecol* 119:560–565, 2012.

Hampe CS: Protective role of anti-idiotypic antibodies in autoimmunity—lessons for type 1 diabetes, *Autoimmunity* 45:320–331, 2012.

Lam DW, Derek Leroith D: The worldwide diabetes epidemic, *Curr Opin Endocrinol Diabet Obes* 19:93–96, 2012.

Ma RC, Chan JC: Type 2 diabetes in East Asians: similarities and differences with populations in Europe and the United States, *Ann N Y Acad Sci* 1281:64–91, 2013.

Pham MT, et al: Risk of childhood obesity in the toddler offspring of mothers with gestational diabetes, *Obstet Gynecol* 121:976–982, 2013.

Phillips CM: Nutrigenetics and metabolic disease: current status and implications for personalized nutrition, *Nutrients* 5:32–57, 2013.

Pirola L, et al: Epigenetic phenomena linked to diabetic complications, *Nat Rev Endocrinol* 6:665–675, 2010.

Porter KE, Riches K: The vascular smooth muscle cell: A therapeutic target in type 2 diabetes? *Clin Sci (Lond)* 125:167–182, 2013.

Thompson A, et al: Evaluation of type 2 diabetes mellitus medication management and control in older adults, *Consult Pharm* 28:296–306, 2013.

Unger J, et al: Putting medications where they belong: Practical advice for managing type 2 diabetes in clinical practice, *J Am Acad Nurse Pract* 25:65–76, 2013.

Up-To-Date: Treatment of type 2 diabetes mellitus in the older patient, n.d. From: www.uptodate.com/contents/treatment-of-type-2-diabetes-mellitus-in-the-elderly-patient#H34. Accessed August 20, 2013.

Vandorsten JP, et al: NIH consensus development conference: Diagnosing gestational diabetes mellitus, *NIH Consensus State Sci Statements* 29(1):1–31, 2013.

White RD: Patient empowerment and optimal glycemic control, *Curr Med Res Opin* 28:979–989, 2012.

CHAPTER 16

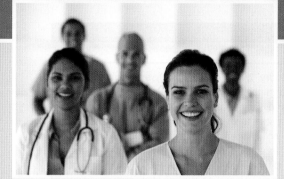

Nutrition in Metabolic Stress: Burns, Trauma, and Surgery

The patient with burns, trauma, sepsis, or major surgery has increased energy and nutrient needs. The stress response to injury and any preexistent malnutrition alter the healing rate and may lead to severe morbidity. A decrease in lean body mass is of particular concern as this component is responsible for all protein synthesis necessary for healing. Nutrition assessment and support need to be well orchestrated and precise.

RH Demling

(e) http://evolve.elsevier.com/GRODNER/FOUNDATIONS

LEARNING OBJECTIVES

- Outline the responses of the body to starvation.
- Explain metabolic changes in uncomplicated stress and in hypermetabolic state of stress.
- Discuss the relationships among function of the immune system, nutritional status, and metabolic stress.
- List nutrients that are required for immune system functions.

- Describe systemic inflammatory response syndrome (SIRS) and identify conditions under which SIRS may occur.
- Define multiple organ dysfunction syndrome (MODS), including the rationale for close monitoring of nutrition support.

METABOLIC RESPONSE TO STRESS

It is important for nurses to understand metabolic changes that occur as a reaction to stress, both in uncomplicated stress that is present when patients are at nutritional risk and in severe stress brought about by trauma or disease.

IMMUNE SYSTEM AND INFLAMMATION

When metabolic stress develops, hormonal and metabolic changes subdue the immune system's ability to protect the body. This activity is further depressed if impaired nutritional status accompanies the metabolic stress. A deadly cycle often develops: impaired immunity leads to increased risk of disease, disease impairs nutritional status, and compromised nutritional status further impairs immunity. Recovery requires that this cycle be broken.

Role of Nutrition

For optimal immunity, adequate nutrients must be available. A well-nourished body will not be ravaged by infections the way a poorly nourished body will be. Changes in socioeconomic status, cultural traditions, population growth, and agriculture have affected diets worldwide and will continue to impact the provision of health care in a multicultural society (Kau, et al, 2011); see the *Cultural Considerations* box The Process of Balance for a multicultural perspective on balanced eating for good health.

Diet and nutritional status influence our gut microbial communities as well as our innate and adaptive immune systems (Kau, et al, 2011) (Figure 16-1). Various dietary components modulate key inflammatory pathways: Sympathetic activity, oxidative stress, and proinflammatory cytokine production all affect the immune response (Kiecolt-Glaser, 2010).

Compromised nutritional status makes it difficult for the body to mount both a stress response and an immune response when confronted with a metabolic stressor such as a virus, surgery, or trauma.

Malnutrition affects each part of the immune system. Integrity of the skin and mucous membranes are compromised, and wound healing is slowed. In the gastrointestinal (GI) tract, microvilli become flat, reducing nutrient absorption. Damage to the GI tract increases the risk that infection-causing bacteria will spread outside the intestinal system (*bacterial translocation*). T-lymphocyte (T-cell) distribution is depressed. More time is needed for phagocytosis kill time and lymphocyte activation. Finally, antibodies are fewer in number and less effective.

A number of nutrients are known to affect immune system functioning. For example, omega-3 fatty acids, vitamins A

🌐 CULTURAL CONSIDERATIONS

The Process of Balance

What is a balanced way of eating for good health? To most Americans, the response is to eat foods from each of the food groups, with particular emphasis on fruits and vegetables. Among other cultures, foods consumed to achieve balance and good health do not follow the American food categories. The Chinese system of *yin-yang* sorts foods into *yin* (bean curd or tofu, bean sprouts, bland and boiled foods, broccoli, carrots, duck, milk, potatoes, spinach, and water) and *yang* (bamboo, beef, broiled meat, chicken, eggs, fried foods, garlic, ginger-root, green peppers, and tomatoes). Foods should be selected from each group to achieve balance. Which foods belong in each group may vary by region, but some foods, such as rice and noodles, are considered neutral. The overall goal is to maintain the harmony of the body with adjustments for climate variations and physiologic factors.

Balance is also the focus of the hot-cold classification of foods practiced in the Middle East, Latin American, India, and the Philippines. This concept is derived from Greek humoral medicine, which is based on the four natural world characteristics of air-cold, fire-hot, water-moist, and earth-dry as related to the body humors of hot and moist (blood), cold and moist (phlegm), hot and dry (yellow/green bile), and cold and dry (black bile). Although this concept is related to the development of disease and their remedies, it also applies to foods. The hot and cold aspects of specific foods are emphasized. This concept does not relate to the actual temperatures of the foods but to their innate characteristics. To achieve balance, eating cold foods offsets hot foods. The list of foods in each category varies among subgroups within each culture. Often, younger generations follow this concept but without knowing that it is based on the hot-cold theory of balance.

Application to nursing. Each of the cultures subscribing to the *yin-yang* concept and the hot-cold theory has a sizable population in the United States. In the treatment of members of these cultures, these concepts of food selection may affect client food choices and recovery. Although healthy foods are often selected, subtle behavioral responses may occur. For example, within the hot-cold theory, pregnancy and vitamins are considered "hot." Consequently, vitamins are not taken during pregnancy because to do so would not restore balance. If a client seems unwilling to follow dietary and supplement recommendations, ways to remedy the situation can be discussed.

Data from Kittler PG, Sucher KP, Nelms M: *Food and culture,* ed 6, Belmont, CA, 2011, Wardsworth.

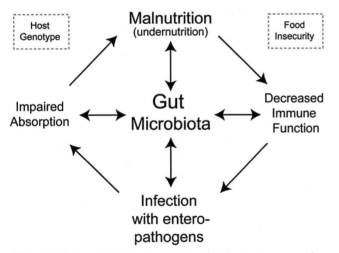

FIG 16-1 Gut microbiota serve as a barrier to enteropathogenic infections; the barrier may be disrupted by malnutrition. (From Kau AL, et al: Human nutrition, the gut microbiome and the immune system, *Nature* 474:327-336, 2011.)

and C, and zinc each play a significant part in immunity. It is difficult to determine which exact nutrient deficiency results in symptoms when a patient is malnourished because of overlapping nutrient deficiencies, illness, weakness, anorexia, and infection. Table 16-1 outlines how specific nutrient deficiencies affect the immune system.

THE STRESS RESPONSE

The body's response to metabolic stress depends on the magnitude and duration of the stress. Stress sets up a chain reaction involving hormones and the central nervous system that affects the entire body. Hormones altered by stress include:

- Aldosterone—corticosteroid that causes renal sodium retention
- Antidiuretic hormone (ADH)—stimulates renal tubular water absorption to conserve water and salt to support circulating blood volume.
- Adrenocorticotropic hormone (ACTH)—acts on adrenal cortex to release cortisol (mobilizes amino acids from skeletal muscles)
- Catecholamines—epinephrine and norepinephrine from renal medulla stimulate hepatic glycogenolysis, fat mobilization, gluconeogenesis

Whether stress is uncomplicated (altered food intake or activity level) or complicated by trauma or disease, metabolic changes take place throughout the body. The metabolic response to stress differs from the metabolic response to starvation.

Effects of Stress on Nutrient Metabolism

The body's constant response to minor changes brought about by needs or environment was first called the "fight or flight" response, or *general adaptation syndrome (GAS).* The body constantly adapts to minor environmental changes to maintain homeostasis. The stress response involves an integrated series of actions that involve the hypothalamus and hypophysis, sympathetic nervous system, adrenal medulla, and adrenal cortex. Significant effects of this response to stress are outlined in Table 16-2. These responses to stress produce multiple changes in metabolic processes throughout the body (Figure 16-2).

TABLE 16-1 Role of Nutrients and Nutritional Status on Immune System Components

IMMUNE SYSTEM COMPONENT	EFFECTS OF MALNUTRITION	VITAL NUTRIENTS
Mucus	Decreased antibody secretions	Vitamin B_{12}, biotin, vitamins B_6, and C
Gastrointestinal tract	Flat microvilli, increased risk of bacterial spread to outside gastrointestinal tract	Arginine, omega-3 fatty acids
Skin	Integrity compromised, density reduced, wound healing slowed	Protein, vitamins A and C, niacin, zinc, copper, linoleic acid, vitamin B_{12}
T lymphocytes	Depressed T-cell distribution	Protein, arginine, omega-3 fatty acids, vitamins A, B_{12}, and B_6, folic acid, thiamine, riboflavin, niacin, pantothenic acid, zinc, iron
Macrophages and granulocytes	Longer time for phagocytosis kill time and lymphocyte activation	Protein, vitamins A, C, B_{12}, and B_6, folic acid, thiamine, riboflavin, niacin, zinc, iron
Antibodies	Reduced antibody response	Protein, vitamins A, C, B_{12}, and B_6, folic acid, thiamine, biotin, riboflavin, niacin

TABLE 16-2 Effects of the Stress Response*

TARGET ORGAN	HORMONAL RESPONSE	PHYSIOLOGIC RESPONSE	SIGNS/SYMPTOMS
Sympathetic nervous system and adrenal medulla	Norepinephrine	Vasoconstriction	Pallor, decreased glomerular filtration rate, nausea, elevated blood pressure
Adrenal medulla	Epinephrine	Vasoconstriction	See above
		Increased heart rate	Elevated blood pressure
		Vasodilation	Increased skeletal muscle function
		Central nervous system (CNS) stimulation	More alert, increased muscle tone
		Bronchodilation	Increased O_2
		Glycogenolysis, lipolysis, gluconeogenesis	Increased blood glucose
Adrenal pituitary and cortex	Cortisol/glucocorticoids	CNS stimulation	Increased blood glucose,
		Protein catabolism, gluconeogenesis	increased serum amino acids, delayed wound healing
		Stabilize cardiovascular system	Enhance catecholamine action
		Gastric secretion	Ulcers
		Inflammatory response decreased	Decreased white blood cells (WBCs)
		Allergic response decreased	
		Immune response decreased	
	Aldosterone/ mineralocorticoid	Increased blood pressure	Retained sodium and water, increased blood volume
Posterior pituitary	Antidiuretic hormone (vasopressin) and aldosterone	Water reabsorbed, increased blood volume, increased blood pressure	

*Possible complications include hypertension, tension headaches, insomnia, diabetes mellitus, infection, heart failure, peptic ulcer, and fatigue.
Data from Gould BE: *Pathophysiology for the health-related professions,* ed 3, Philadelphia, 2006, Saunders.

Effects of Starvation

If someone must involuntarily go without food, his or her state can be described as *starvation.* If we withhold food from ourselves for a period of time, that act can be described as *fasting.* Whatever the cause of inadequate food intake and nourishment, results are the same. After a brief period of going without food or an interval of nutrient intake below metabolic needs, the body extracts stored carbohydrate and fat, as well as protein from muscles and organs, to meet energy demands.

Liver glycogen is used to maintain normal blood glucose levels to provide energy for cells. Although readily available, this source of energy is limited, and glycogen stores are usually depleted in 24 hours. Unlike glycogen stores, lipid (triglyceride) stores may be substantial, and the body also begins to mobilize this energy source. As the amount of liver glycogen decreases, mobilization of free fatty acids from adipose tissue increases to provide energy needed by the nervous system. After approximately 24 hours without energy intake (especially carbohydrates), the prime source of glucose is from gluconeogenesis.

FIG 16-2 The body changes that occur with the initial response to stress.

TABLE 16-3 **Metabolic Responses to Severe Stress**	
INITIAL INJURY (EBB) PHASE	**RECOVERY (FLOW) PHASE**
↓ Oxygen consumption	↑ Oxygen consumption
↓ Cardiac output	↑ Cardiac output
↓ Plasma volume	↑ Plasma volume
Hypothermia	Hyperthermia
	↑ Nitrogen excretion
↓ Insulin levels	Normal or elevated insulin levels
Hyperglycemia	Hyperglycemia
Hypovolemia	Normal volume
Hypotension	Usual blood pressure
↑ Lactate	Normal lactate
↑ Free fatty acids	↑ Free fatty acids
↑ Catecholamines, glucagon, cortisol	↑ Catecholamines, glucagon, cortisol
Insulin resistance	↑ Insulin resistance

↑, Increased; ↓, decreased.

Some body cells, brain cells in particular, use mainly glucose for energy. During early starvation (about 2 to 3 days), the brain uses glucose produced from muscle protein. As muscle protein is broken down for energy, the levels of branched-chain amino acids (BCAAs), consisting of leucine, isoleucine, and valine, increase in circulation, although BCAAs are primarily metabolized directly inside muscle.

The body does not store any amino acids as it does glucose and triglycerides. The only internal sources of amino acids are lean body mass (muscle tissue), vital organs including heart muscle, and other protein-based constituents such as enzymes, hormones, immune system components, and blood proteins. By the second or third day of starvation, approximately 75 g of muscle protein is catabolized each day, a level inadequate to supply full energy needs of the brain. At this point, other sources of energy become more available. Fatty acids are hydrolyzed from the glycerol molecule, and both free fatty acids and glycerol are released into the bloodstream. Free fatty acids are used, and glycerol can be used by the liver to generate glucose (gluconeogenesis).

If starvation is prolonged, the body preserves proteins by mobilizing more and more fat for energy. Production of ketone bodies from fatty acids is accelerated, and the body's demand for glucose decreases. Although some glucose is still vital for brain cells and red blood cells, these and other body tissues obtain the major proportion of their energy from ketone bodies. Muscle protein is still being catabolized but at a much lower rate, which prolongs survival.

An additional defense mechanism of the body to conserve energy is to slow its metabolic rate, thereby decreasing energy needs. As a result of declining metabolic rate, body temperature drops, activity level decreases, and sleep periods increase—all to allow the body to preserve energy. If starvation continues, intercostal muscles necessary for respiration are lost, possibly leading to pneumonia and respiratory failure. Starvation will continue until adipose stores are exhausted. Figure 16-3 shows the phases.

Severe Stress

Whether stress is accidental (broken bones, trauma, or burns) or necessary (surgery), the body reacts to it as well. During starvation, the body's metabolic rate slows, becoming hypometabolic. During severe stress, the body's metabolic rate rises profoundly, thus becoming hypermetabolic. This response to stress involves most metabolic pathways, with accelerated metabolism of LBM, negative nitrogen balance, and muscle wasting. Once the systemic response is activated, the physiologic and metabolic changes that follow may lead to septic shock.

The body's response to stress can be summarized as two phases: immediate post-injury and then recovery. During the *immediate post-injury (ebb) phase*, decreased oxygen consumption, tissue hypoxia, decreased cardiac output, hypothermia (lowered body temperature), and lethargy occur (Table 16-3). Insulin levels drop because the glucagon level is elevated. The major medical concern during this time is to maintain cardiovascular effectiveness and tissue perfusion.

As the body responds to injury, recovery begins about 36 to 48 hours after injury. The *recovery (flow) phase* follows fluid resuscitation and is characterized by increased oxygen consumption, hyperthermia (increased body temperature), increased cardiac output, and nitrogen excretion, as well as expedited catabolism of carbohydrate, protein, and triglycerides to meet the higher metabolic demands. Marked rises in glucose production, free fatty acids, and circulating hormones (insulin/glucagon/cortisol) occur. Recovery will last for days, weeks, or months, until the injury is healed.

Multiple stresses result in increased catabolism and even greater loss of body proteins. If the patient is in poor nutritional status before the stress of surgery, he or she is at greater risk for development of pneumonia or a wound infection accompanied by fever as a result of decreased protein synthesis. As in starvation, energy requirements will be met from endogenous sources (within the body) if exogenous sources

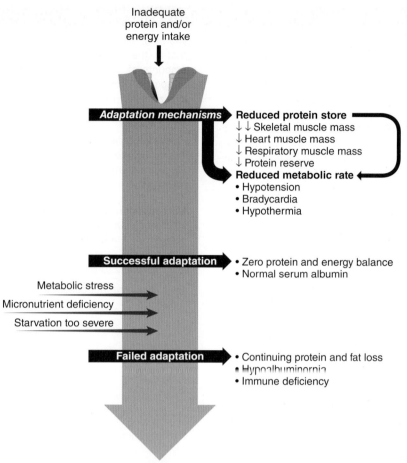

Inadequate protein and/or energy intake

Adaptation mechanisms → **Reduced protein store**
↓↓ Skeletal muscle mass
↓ Heart muscle mass
↓ Respiratory muscle mass
↓ Protein reserve
Reduced metabolic rate ←
• Hypotension
• Bradycardia
• Hypothermia

Successful adaptation → • Zero protein and energy balance
• Normal serum albumin

Metabolic stress
Micronutrient deficiency
Starvation too severe

Failed adaptation → • Continuing protein and fat loss
• Hypoalbuminemia
• Immune deficiency

Death

FIG 16-3 Metabolic changes in starvation. (From Hoffer LJ: Clinical nutrition: Protein-energy malnutrition in the inpatient, *CMAJ* 165:1345-1349, 2001. Accessed August 23, 2013, from www.cmaj.ca/content/165/10/1345.figures-only.)

(food, outside the body) are not available or adequate. Intercostal muscles may be depleted, leading to pneumonia, or inadequate amino acid levels will impair antibody production and the immune response to infection. Either complication has a negative impact on metabolic demands.

Food and Nutrition Therapies

Nutrients affected by hypermetabolic stress include protein, vitamins, and minerals; there are also related nutritional concerns about total energy and fluid intake. During moderate metabolic stress, protein requirements have been reported to increase from 0.8 g/kg body weight (normal recommendation for an average healthy adult) to 1 to 1.5 g/kg body weight. In severe stress (e.g., thermal injuries exceeding 20% total body surface area or deep stage IV pressure ulcers), protein requirements may rise to 1.5 to 2 g/kg body weight. These levels allow for protein synthesis if sufficient energy is also provided from carbohydrate and fat.

Requirements of vitamins and minerals all increase during stress. Tissue repair especially depends on adequate intakes of vitamin C, zinc, calcium, magnesium, manganese, and copper. At the least, Dietary Reference Intake (DRI) levels of nutrients should be consumed, preferably from foods or tube

feeding rather than from vitamin or mineral supplements. Achieving requirements through food supports provision of sufficient energy to meet increased demands during critical illness.

Several formulas have been used to determine the resting metabolic rate (RMR) and energy needs of patients experiencing hypermetabolic stress. However, handheld (Medgem) calorimeters are more accurate than predictive equations based on gender, age, and ethnicity and are a viable alternative (Hipskind, et al, 2011). Registered dietitians, in collaboration with the medical team, use these tools or formulas to determine energy requirements.

Fluid requirements during hypermetabolic stress are based on age, reflecting age-related modifications of body composition. For adults younger than 55 years, fluid needs are calculated at 35 to 40 mL/kg body weight. Adults between ages 55 and 65 years require a lower amount, 30 mL/kg body weight.

Box 16-1 provides some general guidelines used in determining nutrition and fluid needs in metabolic stress. The objectives for optimal metabolic and nutritional support in injury, trauma, burns, and sepsis are to:

• Detect and correct preexisting malnutrition
• Prevent progressive protein-calorie malnutrition

BOX 16-1   Nutrition Therapy for Metabolically Stressed Patients

Energy requirements are highly individual and may vary widely from person to person. Total kcal requirements depend on the basal energy expenditure (BEE) plus the presence of trauma, surgery, infection, sepsis, and other factors. The most accurate method to determine energy needs is indirect calorimetry. When indirect calorimetry cannot be performed, use of predictive formulas is necessary. The formulas with the best prediction accuracy for critically ill patients are the Ireton-Jones energy equations. Other formulas do not have adequate prediction accuracy because they were developed for the healthy population.

Ireton-Jones Energy Equations (IJEEs)

$$\text{Spontaneously breathing (s)} = 629 - 11(A) + 25(W) - 609(O)$$

$$\text{Ventilator dependent IJEE (v)} = 1925 - 10(A) + 5(W) \\ + 281(S) + 292(T) + 851(B)$$

Age (A) in years; body weight (W) in kilograms (kg); sex (S, male = 1, female = 0); diagnosis of trauma (T, present = 1, absent = 0); diagnosis of burn (B, present = 1, absent = 0); obesity >30% above initial body weight from body mass index >27 (present = 1, absent = 0).

Protein Requirements

Additional protein is required to synthesize the proteins necessary for defense and recovery, to spare lean body mass, and to reduce the amount of endogenous protein catabolism for gluconeogenesis.

Vitamin/Mineral Needs

Needs for most vitamins and minerals increase in metabolic stress; however, no specific guidelines exist for provision of vitamins, minerals, and trace elements. It is commonly believed that if the increased kcal requirements are met, adequate amounts of most vitamins and minerals are usually provided. In spite of this belief, vitamin C, vitamin A or beta carotene, and zinc may need special attention.

Fluid Needs

Fluid status can affect interpretation of biochemical measurements as well as anthropometry and physical examination. Fluid requirements can be estimated using several different methods.

Micronutrient Supplementation

Vitamin C: 500 to 1000 mg/day in divided doses
Vitamin A: 1 multivitamin tablet containing vitamin A, one to four times daily
Zinc sulfate: 220 mg, one to three times daily

Fluid requirements based on:		Water (mL)
Weight		100 mL/kg for first 10 kg
		50 mL/kg for next 10 kg
		20 mL/kg for each kg above 20 kg
Age and weight	16-30 yr (active)	40 mL/kg/day
	20-55 yr	35 mL/kg/day
	55-75 yr	30 mL/kg/day
	>75 yr	25 mL/kg/day
Energy needs	1 mL/kcal	
Fluid balance	Urine output + 500 mL/day	

Data from Academy of Nutrition and Dietetics, Evidence Analysis Library: *Critical Illness Evidence-Based Nutrition Practice Guideline.* Accessed August 22, 2013, from www.andevidencelibrary.com.

- Optimize patient's metabolic state by managing fluid and electrolytes.
- Initiate specialized nutrition support (SNS) when it is anticipated that the critically ill patient will be unable to meet nutrient needs orally for a period of 5 to 10 days. Enteral nutrition is the preferred route of feeding over parenteral nutrition whenever possible.
- Indirect calorimetry is the standard for determination of RMR in critically ill patients because RMR based on measurement is more accurate than estimation using predictive equations (Academy of Nutrition and Dietetics, Evidence Analysis Library [EAL], 2013).
- Because overfeeding is more problematic than underfeeding, some clinicians use an adjusted calculation of 20-21 kcal/kg actual BW in obese patients.
- Clinical judgment must play a major role in the decision to begin or continue nutrition support.

Effects of Stress on Nutrient Metabolism
Protein Metabolism

Even if adequate carbohydrate and fat are available, protein (skeletal muscle) is mobilized for energy (amino acids are

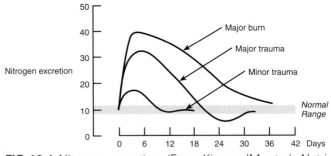

FIG 16-4 Nitrogen excretion. (From Kinney JM, et al: *Nutrition and metabolism in patient care,* Philadelphia, 1988, Saunders.)

converted to glucose in the liver). There is decreased uptake of amino acids by muscle tissue, and increased urinary excretion of nitrogen (Figure 16-4).

In highly stressed patients, 1.5 to 2.0 g/kg/day is given to start. Close monitoring is needed to end negative nitrogen balance and its detrimental effects. To date, no studies have demonstrated a significant difference in infection, length of

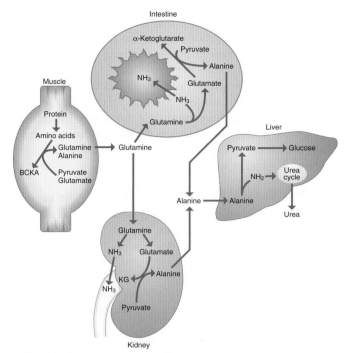

FIG 16-5 Glutamine metabolism. Glutamine is generated by skeletal muscle from glutamate by transamination. Glutamine is taken up by the intestine and kidney, where deamination and ammonia elimination occur. The glutamate formed is transaminated with pyruvate to form alanine, which goes to the liver for gluconeogenesis, and alpha-ketoglutarate (KG), which can be used for energy production by the muscle or kidney. *NH₂,* amine; *NH₃,* ammonia. (From Simmons RL, Steed DL: *Basic science review for surgeons,* Philadelphia, 1992, Saunders.)

stay, or mortality rates on the basis of the level of protein intake or method of protein delivery (EAL, 2013).

Some nonessential amino acids become "conditionally essential" during episodes of metabolic stress. During stress, glutamine is mobilized in large quantities from skeletal muscle and lung to be used directly as a fuel source by intestinal cells (Figure 16-5). Glutamine also plays a significant role in maintaining intestinal immune function and enhancing wound repair by supporting lymphocyte and macrophage proliferation, hepatic gluconeogenesis, and fibroblast function.

Carbohydrate Metabolism

Hepatic glucose production is increased and disseminated to peripheral tissues, although proteins and fats are being used for energy. Insulin levels and glucose use will increase, but hyperglycemia occurs that is not necessarily resolved by the use of exogenous insulin. It appears, to some extent, to be driven by an elevated glucagon-to-insulin ratio.

In general, carbohydrate should provide 60% to 70% of total calories. If carbohydrate is given parenterally, note that the maximum rate of glucose oxidation is 5 to 7 mg/kg/min or 7 g/kg/day. Overfeeding should not occur. Blood glucose levels should be monitored and nutrition regimen and insulin adjusted to keep the serum glucose level below 150 mg/dL.

Fat Metabolism

To support hypermetabolism and increased gluconeogenesis, fat is mobilized from adipose stores (lipolysis) to provide energy. Lipolysis is the result of elevations of catecholamines along with a concurrent decrease in insulin production. If hypermetabolic patients are not fed during this period, fat stores and proteins are rapidly depleted. This malnutrition increases susceptibility to infection and may contribute to multiple organ dysfunction syndrome (MODS), sepsis, and death.

Fat should be sufficient to prevent essential fatty acid (EFA) deficiency and to provide extra energy. In general, fat should provide 15% to 40% of total calories. However, in stressed patients, high-fat feedings (long-chain fatty acids) may cause immunosuppression. Newer formulas focus more on omega-3 fatty acids.

Hydration/Fluid Status

Increased fluid losses can result from fever, increases in perspiration or urine output, diarrhea, draining wounds, or diuretic therapy. An average calculation is 1 to 1.5 mL/kcal expended, or 30 to 40 mL/kg of body weight. Requirements may be decreased in the presence of heart, renal, or liver failure. Input and output (I&O) records are essential at this time.

Vitamins and Minerals

Just as energy needs increase in hypermetabolic conditions, provision of most vitamins and minerals must also be increased. If calorie needs are met, the patient will most likely receive adequate amounts of most vitamins and minerals. Special attention, however, should be given to vitamin C (ascorbic acid), vitamin A or beta-carotene, and zinc. Vitamin C is crucial for the collagen formation necessary for optimal wound healing. Supplements of 500 to 1000 mg/day are recommended. Vitamin A and beta-carotene (the vitamin A precursor) play an important role in the healing process and as antioxidants.

Zinc increases the tensile strength (force required to separate the edges) of a healing wound. Supplements of 220 mg/day zinc sulfate (orally) are commonly used when the patient is stabilized. Additional zinc may be necessary with large intestinal losses, as in ileostomy drainage. It should not be used for longer than 2 weeks at a time, however; excessive zinc will suppress immunity. Immune-enhancing formulas may reduce infectious complications in critically ill patients but do not alter mortality overall (EAL, 2013).

SURGERY AND TRAUMA

In a perfect world, all patients undergoing surgery would be at optimal nutritional status to help them tolerate the physiologic stress of the surgery and temporary starvation that follows. But all too often, surgical patients may be malnourished secondary to the medical condition causing the need for surgery. Additionally, they may experience anorexia, nausea, or vomiting, which decreases their ability to eat. Fever may increase their metabolic rate. Or nutritional needs may not be met because of malabsorption.

For surgery to be successful, patients who are malnourished or in danger of malnutrition must be identified early so corrective action may be arranged. Undernutrition can lead to decreased protein synthesis, weakness, organ failure (MODS), or even death.

Once admitted for surgery, patients are typically held at NPO (nothing by mouth) status for 8 hours before the operation. Oral intake is generally resumed when bowel sounds return, usually 24 to 48 hours after surgery. The postoperative diet is "diet as tolerated" for most patients. Some people prefer a liquid diet, but it is no longer mandatory or recommended. There is no physiologic reason to withhold solid foods once small amounts of liquids are tolerated.

Special Considerations
Bariatric Surgery

Because obesity has become such a worldwide epidemic, bariatric surgery has become quite common. Fortunately, type 2 diabetes mellitus (T2DM) improves after gastric bypass surgery via several mechanisms: change of meal pattern, rapid nutrient transit, enhanced hormonal (incretin) release, improved insulin secretion, changes in bile acids and microbiota, and insulin sensitivity that improves over time as a function of weight loss (Laferrere, 2012).

Bariatric surgery is generally scheduled for patients with a body mass index (BMI) >40 or for those individuals with a BMI >35 if they have comorbidities. Optimal outcomes for patients are achieved with Center of Excellence–designated surgeons and facilities (Glatt and Sorenson, 2011). A multidisciplinary approach is also essential, and the team should include the dietitian, exercise physiologist, psychologist, and bariatric nurse coordinator (Glatt and Sorenson, 2011). Discharge teaching and relevant instruction sheets are important (Table 16-4).

The Roux-en-Y gastric bypass (RYGB) has been used to resolve T2DM in morbidly obese patients. In obese patients with uncontrolled T2DM, 12 months of medical therapy plus bariatric surgery achieves better glycemic control than medical therapy alone (Schauer, et al, 2012).

Unfortunately, gastroenterologists are seeing more patients with malabsorption or dumping syndrome after RYGB (Hammer, 2012). Deficiency of oral dietary intake, lack of gastric secretions, and exclusion of proximal duodenum and jejunum may contribute to these problems.

TABLE 16-4 Dietary Sequence After Bariatric Surgery

DIET ORDER	TIMING
Clear liquids (no more than 1/2 cup total)	1-2 days after surgery
Full liquids (gradually increase to no more than 3/4 cup total)	Days 3-21
Puréed (gradually increase to no more than 1 cup total)	3-6 weeks after surgery
Regular (small meals and snacks with no more than 1 cup total; 2 oz total meat)	6 weeks on

Gastrointestinal Surgery

Poor preoperative nutritional status has been linked consistently with an increase in postoperative complications and poorer surgical outcome (Burden, et al, 2012). When possible, preoperative nutrition support should be administered to malnourished patients for 7 to 14 days if the operation can be safely postponed. Some protocols may also be started 24 hours prior to surgery, with carbohydrate loading and early oral or enteral feeding given to patients the first day after surgery (Burden, et al, 2012).

High-Risk Surgical Procedures and Trauma

Hip replacement, open heart surgery, and prostatectomy are considered high-risk procedures. Patients at high risk for malnutrition who undergo these procedures have significantly longer lengths of hospital stay and mortality rates than well-nourished patients. Preoperative nutrition and postoperative nutrition must be carefully planned and managed. See Figure 16-6 for an interdisciplinary care plan for hip fracture.

In traumatic brain injury (TBI), patients are severely hypermetabolic and catabolic. The more severe the head injury, the greater the release of catecholamines (norepinephrine and epinephrine) and cortisol, and the greater the hypermetabolic response. A swallowing evaluation is needed prior to any oral feeding to determine safety and risk of aspiration. Patients with multiple traumas in addition to spinal cord injury (SCI), may have higher nutritional needs. Over months, the recovering patient with TBI or SCI will need a lower calorie intake to prevent excessive weight gain.

SYSTEMIC INFLAMMATORY RESPONSE SYNDROME

Systemic inflammatory response syndrome (SIRS) describes the inflammatory response that occurs in infection, pancreatitis, ischemia, burns, multiple trauma, shock, and organ injury. For diagnosis, the site of infection must be established, and at least two of the following are present: body temperature >38° C or <36° C, heart rate >90 beats/minute, respiratory rate >20 breaths/min (tachypnea), $Paco_2$ <32 mm Hg (hyperventilation), white blood cell (WBC) count >12,000/mm^3 or <4000/mm^3. SIRS may be caused by bacterial translocation. Patients with SIRS are hypermetabolic, and their nutrient needs increase significantly. At the same time, higher volume may not be tolerated.

MULTIPLE ORGAN DYSFUNCTION SYNDROME

Multiple organ dysfunction syndrome (MODS) involves the progressive failure of two or more organ systems (e.g., the renal, hepatic, cardiac, or respiratory systems) at the same time. It may occur after SIRS. MODS usually results from an uncontrolled inflammatory response that progresses to organ failure. MODS commonly begins with lung failure, which is followed by failure of the liver, intestine, and kidney.

Interdisciplinary Nutrition Care Plan

Hip Fracture

Client Name: _____ #: _____ Initiated by: _____ Date: _____

Screen
Nutrition Screen diagnosis: Hip Fracture
Signed: _____ Date: _____

Assess *(Check any/all)*
❏ Impaired mobility
❏ Poor strength
❏ Infection (eg, pneumonia, UTI, URI)
❏ Pressure ulcers/wounds
Weight/BMI
  ❏ Weight loss >3 lb/wk or >5%/mo or
    >10%/6 mo
  ❏ BMI <20 (High Risk)
  ❏ BMI >27
❏ Dehydration
Poor Oral Intake Symptoms
  ❏ Nausea   ❏ No appetite
  ❏ Vomiting   ❏ Diarrhea
  ❏ Complex   ❏ Depression/anxiety
    diet order
Signed: _____ Date: _____

1 or more

High Risk Interventions *(Check any/all)*
❏ Food Record provided and explained
❏ Fluid intake stressed
Obtain Dr. orders as needed:
  ❏ RD referral for home visits
  ❏ Social Services referral for home visits
  ❏ PT referral for home visits
  ❏ Monitor weight q: _____
  ❏ Monitor I & O q: _____
  ❏ BID/TID supplements
❏ Other: _____
  (See notes for documentation.)

Signed: _____ Date: _____

Next visit

Assess Response *(Check any/all)*
❏ Decreased mobility
❏ Decreased strength
❏ Weight change not appropriate per goal
❏ Continued dehydration
❏ Onset of new infection
❏ Other: _____
  (See notes for documentation.)
Signed: _____ Date: _____

1 or more

Outcomes Not Achieved
Reassess/evaluate need for EN/PN (refer to Tube
Feeding Nutrition Care Plan). Document on
Nutrition Variance Tracking form.

Goals (check any/all):
❏ Maintain or improve mobility in _____ (goal time).
❏ Maintain or improve nutritional status in _____ (goal time).
❏ Increase strength in_____ (goal time).
Weight ❏ maintained, or ❏ loss/❏ gain of _____ lb in _____ (goal time).

None

Moderate Risk Interventions
(Check any/all)
❏ Food Record provided and explained
❏ Fluid intake encouraged
Obtain Dr. orders as needed:
  ❏ RD chart consult
  ❏ Social Services chart consult
  ❏ PT chart consult
  ❏ Monitor weight q: _____
  ❏ BID/TID supplements
❏ Other: _____
  (See notes for documentation.)

Signed: _____ Date: _____

Next visit

Assess Response *(Check any/all)*
❏ Decreased mobility
❏ Decreased strength
❏ Weight change not appropriate per goal
❏ Onset of new infection
❏ Dehydration
❏ Other: _____
  (See notes for documentation.)
Signed: _____ Date: _____

None

Outcomes Achieved
❏ Mobility maintained or improved
❏ Strength maintained or improved
❏ Weight maintained or improved
❏ Hydration status maintained or improved
❏ Other: _____
  (See notes for documentation.)
❏ Repeat Nutrition Risk Screen in _____ days
Signed: _____ Date: _____

Outcomes Achieved
❏ Mobility maintained or improved
❏ Strength maintained or improved
❏ Weight maintained or improved
❏ Hydration status maintained or improved
❏ Other: _____
  (See notes for documentation.)
❏ Repeat Nutrition Risk Screen in _____ days
Signed: _____ Date: _____

Review Date 12/12 • G-1435

FIG 16-6 Interdisciplinary nutrition care plan—hip fracture. (From http://www.nutrition411.com/clinical-nutrition/care-algorithms/item/647-interdisciplinary-nutrition-care-plan-hip-fracture.)

TABLE 16-5 Nutritional Concerns in Multiple Organ Dysfunction Syndrome

SYSTEM	EFFECTS
Pulmonary	Acute respiratory distress syndrome (ARDS): patients requiring ventilator support may need higher lipid content in their diets (even with cardiac failure)
Gastrointestinal	Abdominal distention and ascites Intolerance to internal feedings Paralytic ileus Diarrhea Ischemic colitis Mucosal ulceration Bacterial overgrowth in stool
Liver	Increased serum ammonia level Hepatic encephalopathy
Hypermetabolism	Decreased lean body mass Muscle wasting Severe weight loss Negative nitrogen balance Hyperglycemia
Central nervous system	Lethargy Altered level of consciousness
Immune	Fever: increased energy needs Infection: increased energy needs Decreased lymphocyte count Anergy
Gallbladder	Abdominal distention Unexplained fever: increased kcal needs Decreased bowel sounds

Data from Escott-Stump S: *Nutrition and diagnosis-related care,* ed 7, Baltimore, 2011, Lippincott Williams & Wilkins.

Myocardial failure generally manifests later, but central nervous system changes can occur at any time.

The pathogenesis of MODS is complex but usually results in the initiation of the stress response and release of catecholamines, producing a hypermetabolic state in the patient. Higher levels of calories and protein are necessary to meet increased metabolic demands. Early enteral feedings (see Chapter 12) appear to maintain gut mucosal mass and barrier function and to promote normal enterocytic growth in the gut. These achievements are not possible with parenteral feedings (Table 16-5).

BURNS (THERMAL INJURY)

Burns are customarily defined as electrical, thermal, chemical, or radioactive. They produce tissue destruction that results in circulatory and metabolic alterations requiring the compensatory response to injury. Thermal burns are usually characterized as contact (hot solid object), flame (direct contact with flames), or scald (heated liquid) injuries. Nonthermal causes include chemical, electrical, and radioactive sources. These events have significant effects on nutritional status.

Burns are generally classified by physical appearance and symptoms associated with the affected skin and are often described in terms of percent of body surface burned (Figure 16-7). First-degree burns (or partial-thickness injury) involve only the epidermis, resulting in simple reddening of the area with no injury to underlying dermal or subcutaneous tissue. Sunburns are an example of first-degree burns caused by ultraviolet radiation damage to skin; these burns heal within 3 to 5 days without scarring.

Second-degree burns (superficial partial-thickness injury and deep partial-thickness injury) involve two categories of burn depth. Superficial partial-thickness burns are characterized by redness and blistering that affects the epidermis and some dermis. Deep partial-thickness burns are characterized by destruction of epidermis and dermis (resulting in a waxy, white, mottled appearance), leaving only skin appendages such as hair follicles and sweat glands. Second-degree burns take weeks to months to heal.

Third-degree burns (full-thickness injury) are characterized by destruction of the entire epidermis, dermis, and, frequently, the underlying subcutaneous tissue. Occasionally, muscle or bone tissue may be destroyed. Third-degree burns cannot heal and will require skin grafts.

In addition to pain management, wound care, and infection control, nutrition support is one of the most significant considerations in care of burned patients. The first 24 to 48 hours of treatment for such patients are dedicated to replacement of fluid and electrolytes. Fluid needs are based on the patient's age and weight, and the extent of the burn. Total body surface area (TBSA), used to estimate the extent of the burn, can be estimated using the "rule of nines" (Figure 16-8).

Thermal injury wounds heal only if the patient is in an anabolic state. Therefore, feeding should be initiated as soon as the patient has been hydrated. The American Burn Association practice guidelines state that enteral feedings should be initiated between 4 and 24 hours after injury to prevent ileus, stress ulceration, and the effects of hypermetabolism (Mosier, et al, 2011). Placement of the feeding tube in the small bowel should be considered when patient is in supine position or under heavy sedation. Nutritional goals for patients with burns are outlined in Table 16-6. Early enteral nutrition may allow the following objectives to be achieved:

- Nutrient needs satisfied
- Improved feeding tolerance
- Decreased incidence of bacterial translocation
- Decreased number of infectious episodes
- Decreased antibiotic therapy
- Improved nitrogen balance
- Reduced urinary catecholamines
- Diminished serum glucagon
- Suppressed hypermetabolic response
- Enhanced visceral protein status.

Energy needs vary according to the size of the burn. Several methods may be used to estimate energy and protein needs in burned patients when indirect calorimetry is not available.

TISSUE LAYER	SKIN THICKNESS (inches)	DEPTH OF BURN
Epidermis	0.010	1
Dermis	0.020	2
Subcutaneous tissue	0.035	3
Muscle	0.060	4

FIG 16-7 Interpretation of burn classification based on damage to the integument. (From Mahan LK, Escott-Stump S: *Krause's food & nutrition therapy*, ed 12, Philadelphia, 2008, Saunders.)

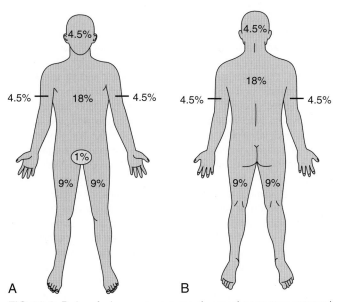

FIG 16-8 Rule of nines—a commonly used assessment tool with estimates of the percentages (in multiples of nine) of the total body surface area burned. **A,** Adults (anterior view). **B,** Adults (posterior view). (From Thompson JM, et al: *Mosby's clinical nursing*, ed 5, St. Louis, 2002, Mosby.)

One of the simplest and easiest to use is the Curreri formula (adults), as follows:
- (25 kcal × kg of body weight) + (40 kcal × %TBSA)
- 16 to 18 kcal × kg body weight if patient >125% regular body weight
- Burns >50%: use a maximum value of 50% TBSA.

TABLE 16-6 Nutritional Goals for Burned Patients

GOAL	ACTION(S)
Minimize metabolic response	Control environmental temperature Monitor fluid and electrolyte balance Control pain and anxiety Cover wounds early
Meet nutritional needs	Provide adequate kcal to prevent weight loss >10% of usual body weight Provide adequate protein for positive nitrogen balance and maintenance or repletion of visceral protein stores
Prevent Curling's ulcer	Provide antacids or continuous enteral feedings

Modified from Winkler MF, Malone AM: Medical nutrition therapy for metabolic stress: Sepsis, trauma, burns and surgery. In Mahan LK, Escott-Stump S, Raymond JL, editors: *Krause's food & nutrition therapy*, ed 13, Philadelphia, 2012, Elsevier.

Estimates using the Curreri formula may exceed actual energy needs, but it is not uncommon for a patient to need 4000 to 5000 calories per day.

Protein is lost through urine and wounds, increased gluconeogenesis, and healing in burned patients. It is therefore important that calories from protein are not calculated into total energy needs. Carbohydrates and fats provide protein sparing as nonprotein energy sources. Whether a patient receives adequate amounts of energy or protein is evaluated by wound healing rate, graft "take," and basic nutritional assessment parameters. The risk of sepsis is reduced in burned patients who are supported by earliest possible enteral nutrition (Lu, et al, 2011).

In conjunction with increased energy demands, vitamin and mineral needs are increased in burn patients, but exact requirements are not known (Academy of Nutrition and Dietetics, Nutrition Care Manual, 2013.). Most patients receive vitamins in excess of the recommended intake because of their high calorie intakes, but special consideration should be given to vitamin C (collagen synthesis, immune function) and vitamin A (immune function and epithelialization). Supplements are commonly recommended.

Regardless of nutritional interventions, the outcome after burn injury is a multidimensional concept affected by three psychometrically sound health domains—function, skin involvement, and affect and relations—that can be evaluated over time (Willebrand and Kidal, 2011). See the *Personal Perspectives* box Love, Greg & Lauren for one couple's struggle with the aftermath of severe burns.

PERSONAL PERSPECTIVES

Love, Greg & Lauren

On September 11, 2001, at 8:48 AM, Lauren Manning, a senior vice president, partner, and director of global data sales for Cantor Fitzgerald, was entering the lobby of One World Trade Center in New York City. As the first of two planes dove into the World Trade Center buildings, an explosive fireball ran through the lobby. Lauren was burned on more than 82.5% of her body. The following is an excerpt from her husband's day-by-day e-mail account in the months following the tragedy of Lauren's struggle to heal and survive for her son, Tyler, and her husband. Consider the effect of serious injuries on patients, their families, and the medical personnel who assist in the healing process.

Date: Saturday, September 29, 2001, 12:40 AM
Subject: Lauren Update for September 28 (Friday)

Today was a stable day. Lauren still has the septic infection, which they are fighting with antibiotics, but her lungs are functioning well, as is her stomach, two very important factors. The oxygen and the protein intake she is receiving through a feeding tube are needed to build new tissue and for her skin to heal.

I have a better understanding now of something the doctor told me about doing Lauren's grafts. He said he would "mesh 3-1" when doing autografts. Basically, a special machine is used to create a mesh pattern in the donor skin—her own skin—that permits it to cover an area three times as large as the site from which it was taken. The homograft, or skin-bank skin, is then placed over this mesh, creating a layer that enables the autograft beneath to heal better. The goal is for the mesh to take and for healing to occur in the open spots. More than one graft is often necessary.

The grafts already done look good, which means the majority have probably taken. Unfortunately, the infection does have an adverse effect on the healing process, both of the grafts and of the donor sites. That is why Lauren's time in the burn ICU is such a balancing act. Negative factors have to be controlled so that positive factors can win out. The good aspect for Lauren is that she was strong and healthy going in, so she has managed to keep herself mostly stable, a word that has become very important for the families of all the burn patients.

Her nurse explained to me tonight how Lauren's various systems were adjusting on their own to maintain stability. For example, her heart was pumping faster to maintain her blood pressure despite a slight dilation of blood vessels due to infection. A glass-half-full type of sign.

I put two pictures—of Lauren and of Lauren, Tyler, and my dad—up on her wall. The pictures are an important way for the nursing staff to make a connection to her. They are all looking forward to meeting her when she is more awake, later in her treatment course.

That alone should tell you how difficult the work is that these nurses do. The patients arrive gravely injured, frequently unable to communicate, and highly critical. The medical and nursing staffs often fight for weeks to keep the patient improving; this is well before they have a chance to encounter the patient's personality. The staff first gets to know the patient through the family visitors, and the photographs help the staff connect with the life they are trying to help the patient return to.

The WTC disaster families have been there for 17 days now, and we know each other well. This bonding between families is due to the utter stress of the situation. We have all spent days, now weeks, and hopefully months, worrying minute to minute about a loved one's condition. It is the same as if a surgical procedure were to last for weeks on end. We learn to read the facial expressions and voices of doctors and nurses.

So we, the waiting, speak to each other, and to the staff psychologists and chaplain and the Red Cross volunteers who wander through, and we are visited by Good Samaritans of all types, who provide food. ... And in the end, we alone understand what we are going through: we are the loved ones of critically injured patients from a massive tragedy in which most victims either died or walked out under their own power.

We, the waiting, are therefore at somewhat of a disconnect from the world at large, which is pursuing closure (not my favorite word), whether coping with loss of a family member; coming to terms with having one's life saved by something so trivial as arriving late for work; or honoring the heroism of lost firefighters and police.

Most of the world is already viewing the attacks from a distance, but we are pretty much still there at Time Zero, with the outcome unknown. However, we are all making it through, with the help of the huge support networks that have sprung up all around us. Including y'all. ... It really does help us, me and Lauren, to know how many people care.

Love, Greg & Lauren

Update: Lauren Manning left home for work on September 11, 2001, and returned home on March 16, 2002. She continues to regain the life she had, including running, biking, getting back to work, and just being there with and for her son as he grows up.

From Manning G: *Love, Greg & Lauren,* New York, 2002, Bantam Books.

Nursing Approach

In fluid-resuscitated, critically ill patients, enteral nutrition (EN) started within 24 to 48 hours following injury or admission to the intensive care unit (ICU) reduces the incidence of infectious complications (EAL, 2013). Nurses can alert the registered dietitian to ensure adequate energy provision when the patient's status changes, as with new fever or skin breakdown. It is also important to closely monitor blood glucose levels. Hyperglycemia is associated with infection, morbidity, even mortality. The goal is to keep blood glucose between 140 and 180 mg/dL (American Society for Parenteral and Enteral Nutrition [ASPEN], 2013). Insulin drip and sliding scale should be used, with conversion to subcutaneous insulin as possible.

Evaluating patient position should be part of the monitoring plan for tube-fed patients. To decrease the incidence of aspiration pneumonia and reflux of gastric contents into the esophagus and pharnyx, a 45-degree head of bed elevation should be used in critically ill patients, if not contraindicated.

Weight may be difficult to obtain and inaccurate owing to fluid shifts and dressings. Scales must be recalibrated on a schedule to ensure accuracy. Regular documentation of weights and I&O records becomes essential because many complications arise during the recovery process. For example, refeeding syndrome involves physiologic and metabolic complications associated with reintroducing nutrition (refeeding) too rapidly to a malnourished person. These complications include glucose and electrolyte shifts that lead to cardiac insufficiency, heart failure, respiratory distress, convulsions, coma, or even death (Box 16-2).

Evaluating *gastric residual volume* (GRV) in critically ill patients is an optional part of a monitoring plan to assess tolerance of EN. Blue dye should never be used to detect

---

BOX 16-2   Refeeding Syndrome

Overfeeding a patient with protein-energy malnutrition can result in many complications or death if not initiated correctly. Introduction of excess carbohydrate can overload various enzymatic and physiologic functions that were adapted during malnutrition. As feeding is initiated, rapid changes occur in thyroid and endocrine function, increasing oxygen consumption, cardiac output, insulin secretion, and energy expenditure. Electrolyte shifts are the most dangerous changes and are described here.

Phosphorus

During starvation, total phosphorus is greatly reduced. With feeding, increased cellular influx of phosphorus occurs, leading to severe extracellular **hypophosphatemia**. This will occur in enteral and parenteral feeding but can be prevented by a slower rate of nutrient infusion. Cardiac decompensation occurs when sodium shifts also play a role. In addition, hypophosphatemia can lead to tissue hypoxia and, subsequently, altered tissue function.

Potassium

Potassium is greatly reduced from tissue. During feeding, extracellular fluid levels fall (hypokalemia), possibly leading to life-threatening arrhythmias.

Magnesium

Magnesium is greatly reduced in tissue. Under the anabolic condition of feeding, extracellular fluid levels drop (hypomagnesemia), leading to cardiac depression, arrhythmias, neuromuscular weakness, irritability, and hyporeflexia.

Glucose Metabolism

When high-glucose feedings are given, the starved patient loses the stimulus for gluconeogenesis (an important adaptive mechanism during nutritional depletion). Suppression of gluconeogenic glucose production leads to a corresponding decrease in amino acid use and negative nitrogen balance.

Hyperglycemia can precipitate osmotic diuresis, dehydration, hypotension, hyperosmolar nonketotic coma, ketoacidosis, and metabolic acidosis (see Chapter 15).

Fluid Intolerance

Refeeding with carbohydrate results in sodium and water excretion. With concurrent sodium ingestion, such excretion can lead to a rapid expansion of extracellular fluid volume, fluid retention, and subsequent weight gain. This enhanced fluid retention may in turn be exacerbated by the loss of tissue mass resulting from starvation.

Preventing Refeeding Syndrome

Nutrients should be reintroduced to the malnourished patient while medical and metabolic status is closely monitored. Careful estimation of energy requirements should be made through a complete nutritional assessment. The notion of "starting low and going slow" daily is not relevant; avoiding a high proportion of carbohydrate appears to be more important than the absolute number of calories (Kohn, et al, 2011). Care should also be taken to minimize fluid retention (weight gain >1 kg/wk can be assumed to be fluid retention and should be avoided) and to provide adequate repletion of phosphorus, potassium, and magnesium on a daily basis. Weight and fluid balance should be monitored daily to assess the rate of weight regain.

Refeeding syndromes are associated more with parenteral nutrition than enteral feeding via the gastrointestinal tract (see Chapter 12). Formulas (whether enteral or parenteral) must contain adequate amounts of vitamins and minerals. Greater than routine amounts are not necessary, but the absence of these nutrients may be lethal. After 1 week, intake of kcal, fluid, and sodium can be liberalized without fear of consequences because the various metabolic equilibrations should have taken place. Thus, common sense and discretion are of key importance in the feeding of semistarved and chronically ill patients.

Data from Boateng AA, et al: Refeeding syndrome: Treatment considerations based on collective analysis of literature case reports, *Nutrition* 26:156-167, 2010; Kohn MR, et al: Refeeding in anorexia nervosa: Increased safety and efficiency through understanding the pathophysiology of protein calorie malnutrition, *Curr Opin Pediatr* 23:390-394, 2011.

aspiration. EN should be withheld when a GRV greater than or equal to 250 mL is documented on two or more consecutive occasions. Note that holding EN when GRV is less than 250 mL is associated with delivery of less EN.

Responses to a feeding protocol include evaluations of intake and output (both stooling and fluid balance), tolerance of feeding regimen (abdominal examination, gastric residuals), amount of nutrition prescription actually delivered (note of any interruption due to surgery, dressing changes, intolerance, or therapy). The nurse should work with the dietitian when nutrition support is withheld for prolonged periods; a more suitable product or volume must be identified.

SUMMARY

- The stress response of the body also affects nutritional status.
- Whether the stress response is caused by physiologic or psychologic determinants, the entire body is affected.
- Starvation leads to decreased energy expenditure, use of alternative fuels, decreased protein wasting, and use of stored glycogen in 24 hours.
- In late starvation, fatty acids, ketones, and glycerol provide energy for all tissues except brain, nervous system, and RBCs.
- Metabolic changes occur in uncomplicated stress, which is present when patients are at nutritional risk, or in severe stress caused by trauma or disease.
- In a hypermetabolic state, stress causes accelerated energy expenditure, glucose production, and glucose cycling in liver and muscle. Hyperglycemia can occur from either insulin resistance or excess glucose production via gluconeogenesis. Muscle breakdown is also accelerated.
- Many hormone levels are altered by stress.

- The functioning of the immune system is affected by the hormonal and metabolic changes that occur. The immune system cannot protect the body when impaired nutritional status accompanies metabolic stress.
- A number of nutrients are known to affect immune system functioning: omega-3 fatty acids, vitamins A and C, and zinc.
- Systemic inflammatory response syndrome (SIRS) describes the inflammatory response that occurs in infection, pancreatitis, ischemia, burns, multiple trauma, shock, and organ injury. Patients with SIRS are hypermetabolic.
- Multiple organ dysfunction syndrome (MODS) results from direct injury, trauma, or disease or as a response to inflammation; the response is usually in an organ distant from the original site of infection or injury.
- It is essential to closely monitor patients receiving nutrition support. Input and output, stooling patterns, signs of intolerance, and long periods of holding should be discussed with the dietitian to determine whether a new plan is needed.

◎ THE NURSING APPROACH

Case Study: Nutritional Needs during Physical Stress

Daniel, age 65, had pneumonia 2 days after his left hip replacement. He is receiving physical therapy, intravenous (IV) antibiotics, supplemental oxygen, and a high-kcal, high-protein diet. The hospital dietitian met with Daniel to individualize his diet on the basis of his Orthodox Jewish religion.

Assessment
Subjective (from Patient Statements)
- "The muscles in my chest ache from coughing, and my hip hurts."
- Pain rating: 3 of 10
- "I don't feel like eating, but if I have to eat, I want to observe dietary laws for an Orthodox Jew."
- "I feel tired and sometimes short of breath."

Objective (from Physical Examination)
- Eats small amounts of food, then pushes the food tray away
- Drinks about 1200 mL of fluid per day (mostly water)
- Tympanic temperature 101.2° F
- Crackles in lungs bilaterally
- O₂ saturation 90% with oxygen at 6 liters via cannula
- White blood count 12,000/mm³
- Productive cough, with thick yellow sputum
- Surgical wound on left hip intact without redness or drainage

Diagnosis (Nursing)
Imbalanced nutrition: less than body requirements related to inadequate food intake (secondary to shortness of breath and discomfort) and increased metabolic stresses (surgery, infection, and fever), as evidenced by "I don't feel like eating," eats small amounts then pushes meal tray away, drinks about 1200 mL of fluid per day

Planning
Patient Outcomes
Short term (by discharge to a rehabilitation center in 5 days):
- Eating moderate amounts of food, especially protein-rich and nutrient-dense foods
- Drinking at least 2000 mL per day
- No weight loss
- No shortness of breath, O₂ saturation 95% without supplemental oxygen
- Afebrile (no fever)
- White blood cell (WBC) count below 10,000/mm³
- Decrease or absence of crackles in lungs
- No signs of infection of surgical wound on left hip

Nursing Interventions
1. Provide high-kcal, high-protein diet.
2. Maintain dietary intake according to Orthodox Jewish kosher dietary laws.

⊚ THE NURSING APPROACH—cont'd

Implementation

1. Asked Daniel's family to bring in kosher ground meat and special serving dishes.
   Ground meat provides high protein and requires little energy for chewing. If the hospital does not have a kosher kitchen, kosher meals may be ordered from special suppliers. Family members may be able to obtain kosher food and reassure the patient that it is truly kosher. Meat (no pork or shellfish) must be properly slaughtered, blessed by a rabbi, and cooked in a kosher kitchen. Dishes reserved for meat must be separated from dishes for milk, and meat cannot be served in the same meal as milk.

2. Asked Daniel and his family to inform nursing or dietary staff about special dietary needs, particularly for upcoming holidays and the Sabbath.
   Culturally sensitive staff will ask individuals and families how they can meet special dietary needs.

3. Provided rest periods and oral care before meals, and gave pain medicine as needed.
   Rest helps increase patient energy, and a fresh mouth promotes appetite. Patients eat more food when comfortable.

4. Pointed out the high-protein and nutrient-dense foods on meal trays and encouraged Daniel to eat them first.
   When patients can eat only small amounts of food, nourishment is better if they choose nutrient-dense foods.

5. Conferred with the dietitian and physician concerning high-kcal, high-protein snacks between meals.
   Increased kcal are needed to compensate for metabolic stresses, and additional protein is needed for healing and building up immunity. Frequent small meals are easier to consume than large meals when the patient is short of breath. Some doctors prefer to limit milk products for patients with respiratory problems because of potential phlegm. Milk-based supplements must be served several hours before or after meats, according to Jewish dietary laws.

6. Provided a vitamin/mineral supplement, as prescribed by the physician.
   Bone healing requires adequate calcium and vitamin D. Vitamins A and C help promote wound healing. B vitamins are needed in stressful conditions.

7. Offered water frequently between meals and encouraged drinking 2000 mL of fluid per day.
   Fluid intake is needed to replace fluids lost during fever. Additional fluids help thin sputum, making it easier for the patient to cough up the sputum. Liquids during meals should be minimized if patient feels full after eating little food.

8. Recorded intake and output and weighed the patient daily.
   Records can help show balance or imbalance of fluid intake (by mouth and by intravenous fluid) and fluid output (urine). Adequate nutrition is needed to prevent weight loss.

9. Encouraged Daniel to get a pneumonia shot this year and a flu shot every year.
   Serious respiratory infections may be prevented by immunizations. Generally, only one pneumonia shot is given, preferably when an adult becomes 65 years old. Influenza shots must be received by the patient annually, usually in the fall. Health promotion is an important nursing responsibility.

Evaluation

Short term (at discharge to the rehabilitation center on the fifth day):

- Daniel was eating moderate amounts of food.
- He was drinking 2000 mL of fluids per day.
- No weight loss.
- No shortness of breath, O_2 saturation 95% without supplemental oxygen.
- Tympanic temperature 99° F.
- WBC 9500/mm³.
- Decreased crackles in lungs.
- No signs of infection of surgical wound on left hip.
Goals met.

Discussion Questions

1. How would Daniel's diet plan be different if he did not request a kosher diet?
2. Compare and contrast a diet for a patient with pneumonia versus a patient with severe burns.

❔ CRITICAL THINKING

Clinical Applications

Kristin, age 19, is a member of her college's cheerleading team and was involved in a serious motor vehicle accident when the team was returning from a game. She was admitted through the emergency department of your hospital suffering from multiple fractures and contusions. Kristin is 5 feet 5 inches tall and weighed 120 pounds before the accident. Because she is young, looked healthy, and is somewhat muscular from being a cheerleader, the physician did not request a consult for the dietitian to evaluate Kristin's nutritional status. After she had been in intensive care 2 weeks, pneumonia developed. The nurse learned that before the automobile accident, Kristin had been using a commercial weight loss product and was consuming approximately 400 kcal/day for 3 months before the accident in an attempt to "make weight" so that she could remain on the cheerleading team.

1. How did the very low-calorie diet (VLCD) affect Kristin's nutritional status?
2. Why did pneumonia develop?
3. Describe the variety of stresses Kristin experienced.
4. Could the pneumonia have been prevented? How?

▪ WEBSITES OF INTEREST

American Society for Enteral and Parenteral Nutrition

http://www.nutritioncare.org/
A key resource for tips on enteral and parenteral nutrition for the critically ill patient.

Burnsurgery.org

www.burnsurgery.org

Offers up-to-date educational tools on burn care and treatment for health professionals.

KidSource OnLine!

www.kidsource.com/kidsource/content2/ecoli/anna.1.html

Presents support and resources on parenting resources including a parent's personal account of her daughter's experience with MODS caused by an *Escherichia coli* infection.

REFERENCES

Academy of Nutrition and Dietetics: *Nutrition care manual: Burns: calculations for nutrition assessment.* From: www.nutritioncaremanual.org. Accessed August 22, 2013.

Academy of Nutrition and Dietetics, Evidence Analysis Library: *Critical illness evidence-based nutrition practice guideline.* from: www.andevidencelibrary.com. Accessed August 22, 2013.

American Society for Parenteral and Enteral Nutrition: *Nutrition support of adult patients with hyperglycemia,* from: www.nutritioncare.org/Professional_Resources/Guidelines_and_Standards/Guidelines/. Accessed August 23, 2013.

Burden S, et al: Pre-operative nutrition support in patients undergoing gastrointestinal surgery, *Cochrane Database Syst Rev* (11):CD008879, 2012.

Glatt D, Sorenson T: Metabolic and bariatric surgery for obesity: A review, *S D Med* Spec No:57–62, 2011.

Hammer HF: Medical complications of bariatric surgery: Focus on malabsorption and dumping syndrome, *Dig Dis* 30:182–186, 2012.

Hipskind P, et al: Do handheld calorimeters have a role in assessment of nutrition needs in hospitalized patients? A systematic review of literature, *Nutr Clin Pract* 26:426–433, 2011.

Kau AL, et al: Human nutrition, the gut microbiome and the immune system, *Nature* 474:327–336, 2011.

Kiecolt-Glaser JK: Stress, food, and inflammation: Psychoneuroimmunology and nutrition at the cutting edge, *Psychosom Med* 72:365–369, 2010.

Laferrere B: Gut feelings about diabetes, *Endocrinol Nutr* 59:254–260, 2012.

Lu G, et al: Influence of early post-burn enteral nutrition on clinical outcomes of patients with extensive burns, *J Clin Biochem Nutr* 48:222–225, 2011.

Mosier MJ, et al: Early enteral nutrition in burns: Compliance with guidelines and associated outcomes in a multicenter study, *J Burn Care Res* 32:104–109, 2011.

Schauer PR, et al: Bariatric surgery versus intensive medical therapy in obese patients with diabetes, *N Engl J Med* 366:1567–1576, 2012.

Willebrand M, Kidal M: Burn specific health up to 24 months after the burn: A prospective validation of the simplified model of the burn specific health scale—brief, *J Trauma* 71:78–84, 2011.

CHAPTER 17

Nutrition for Cardiopulmonary Diseases

Chronic diseases (heart disease, stroke, diabetes) are leading causes of morbidity and mortality in the United States. Half of adults have at least one cardiovascular risk factor, yet not even 1% of the population attains ideal cardiovascular health (Kones, 2011). Engaging in healthy behaviors and accessing preventive health care services can reduce morbidity, medical costs, and mortality.

http://evolve.elsevier.com/GRODNER/FOUNDATIONS

LEARNING OBJECTIVES

- List the diseases and conditions that constitute cardiovascular disease (CVD).
- Identify the CVD risk factors that are controllable, noncontrollable, and predisposing.
- Discuss the goals of nutrition therapy for CVD.
- Describe the two types of hypertension (HTN) and the treatment regimens.

- Explain the focus of nutrition therapy to reduce risk of myocardial infarctions (MI) and heart failure (HF).
- Identify the two categories of pulmonary disorders and the importance of nutritional status.
- Describe the goal of nutrition therapy for chronic obstructive pulmonary disease (COPD).

HEART AND LUNG HEALTH

The *physical health* dimension is affected as CVD affects the heart, an essential organ; this disease impairs functioning of many other body systems. Determining one's own risk factors and devising a program to reduce the effects will depend on *intellectual health. Emotional health* is stressed when client denial occurs; many individuals view heart problems as something that happens only to other people! Because of increased education through the work of health associations and health departments, many restaurants and resorts serve "heart healthy" entrées; with careful selections, *social health* can continue as usual. *Spiritual health* is manifested through an optimistic attitude that taking care of our bodies is a sacred task. *Environmental health* impacts health status by increasing risk of chronic bronchitis, asthma, and emphysema if air is polluted or if lifestyle behaviors such as smoking damages the body.

CARDIOVASCULAR DISEASES

Coronary Artery Disease

Cardiovascular disease encompasses a group of diseases and conditions that affect the heart and blood vessels: coronary artery disease (CAD) (also called *coronary heart* disease [CHD]), hypertension, peripheral artery disease (PAD), heart failure, and congenital heart diseases. CVD continues to be the leading cause of death for American men and women in all ethnic and racial groups. Although death rates from CVD have declined, the burden of the disease remains high; Box 17-1 lists the top ten facts that everyone should know.

Most people who have heart attacks die before they ever reach a hospital for treatment, a situation that emphasizes the need for prevention of heart disease. In 2013, the American Heart Association and American College of Cardiology published new cholesterol guidelines (NHLBI, 2014.)

Health professionals cannot assume that patients newly diagnosed with CAD, regardless of education or socioeconomic level, are knowledgeable about the disorder and relevant treatments. Primary prevention is a public health effort. Secondary prevention behaviors reduce the effects of a disease or illness. For CVD, reducing risk factors can minimize negative health effects. The purpose of tertiary prevention is to minimize further complications or to assist in the restoration of health. For CVD, these efforts may involve significant lifestyle changes combined with medication and other medical care. Learning more about the disorder is often helpful for patients and their families (see the *Personal Perspectives* box Go Red for Women and Figure 17-1).

BOX 17-1 Top Ten Things to Know About Heart Disease and Stroke Statistics

1. From 1999 to 2009, the cardiovascular disease (CVD) death rate declined by 33%. However, CVD still takes the lives of more than 2150 Americans each day, an average of 1 death every 40 seconds.

2. During that same time, the relative rate of stroke death fell by 37%, and the actual number of stroke deaths declined by 23%. Still, stroke is a leading cause of disability in the United States.

3. Smoking—18% of students grades 9-12 report being current smokers. Among adults, 21% of men and 17% of women are smokers.

4. Physical activity—Only 21% of adults meet the federal guidelines for physical activity. Among ninth through twelfth graders, only 28% meet the recommendations.

5. Healthy diet—Less than 1% of U.S. adult intakes meet the definition for "ideal healthy diet"; essentially no children's intakes meet the goal. Of the 5 components of a healthy diet, reducing sodium and increasing whole grains are the biggest challenges.

6. Body mass index—The estimated prevalence of overweight and obesity in U.S. adults is 155 million, which represents 68% of this group. Among children, 32% are overweight and obese (24 million children), and 17% are obese (13 million children).

7. Cholesterol—An estimated 32 million adults have total serum cholesterol levels ≥240 mg/dL, with a prevalence of 14%.

8. Hypertension—An estimated 78 million U.S. adults are hypertensive. About 82% are aware of their condition, and 75% are using antihypertensive medication, but only in 53% of those is the condition controlled.

9. Diabetes—An estimated 20 million adults have physician-diagnosed diabetes. An additional 8 million adults have undiagnosed diabetes, and about 87 million adults have prediabetes.

10. Over the past decade, there have been improvements in both children and adults in prevalence of ideal levels of smoking, blood pressure, and cholesterol and declines in ideal rates of body mass index and fasting glucose.

Modified from Go AS, et al: Heart disease and stroke statistics—2013 update: a report from the American Heart Association. *Circulation* 127:e6-e245, 2013. Accessed from circ.ahajournals.org/lookup/doi/10.1161/CIR.0b013e31828124ad. © 2012, American Heart Association.

FIG 17-1 Debbie Phelps kissing Olympian son Michael Phelps at the Red Dress Event, New York City, 2012. (Photo courtesy of S. Escott-Stump.)

Atherosclerosis

Atherosclerosis is the chronic inflammatory process in which damage to the arterial wall can lead to coronary artery disease, stroke, and peripheral artery disease (Figure 17-2). Atherosclerosis begins early in life and advances seamlessly throughout life (Kones, 2011).

The most common and serious manifestation is development of lesions in coronary arteries that can cause angina pectoris if blood flow is partially occluded by a thrombus. If blood flow to the heart is completely occluded, then a myocardial infarction occurs. If thrombosis occurs in a cerebral artery, a cerebrovascular accident (CVA) or stroke occurs. Peripheral artery disease (PAD) occurs when atherosclerosis in the abdominal aorta, iliac arteries, and femoral arteries produces temporary insufficient blood flow in the arteries on exertion (intermittent claudication) or ischemic necrosis of the extremities, which may lead to gangrene.

👤 PERSONAL PERSPECTIVES

Go Red for Women

Go Red for Women is a national campaign of the American Heart Association. The movement encourages women to engage in heart-healthy activities to reduce their personal risk of heart disease, the number one killer of women. The message of the movement, Love Your Heart, spreads awareness that prevention is possible—one heart at a time through the empowerment of women. Go Red for Women local events take place in most communities. The National Wear Red Day, the major event of the campaign, asks everyone to wear something red in February to highlight ways to reduce risks by simple acts such as the following:

• Seeing a health care provider
• Consuming a healthier diet
• Being more physically active
• Educating others about heart disease

When you wear red blouses, dresses, ties, lipstick, shoes, or jackets, think "I Love My Heart!" For more information, check out the American Heart Association: Go red for women webpage at www.goredforwomen.org.

The Coca Cola Company and the National Heart Lung and Blood Institute (NHLBI) have partnered on behalf of women and heart disease. Every year in February, they sponsor a Heart Truth Red Dress Event at the beginning of Fashion Week in New York City. Movie stars and media personalities are invited to participate in a runway event, all wearing designer red dresses. I had the privilege of representing the Academy of Nutrition and Dietetics at this event in 2012. Figure 17-1 shows a kiss between Debbie Phelps and her son, Michael, whose presence sent a great message to all women to take care of their hearts for family and loved ones. For the Heart Truth Red Dress event information, go to http://www.nhlbi.nih.gov/educational/hearttruth/.

Sylvia Escott-Stump
Winterville, NC

FIG 17-2 Risk factors for coronary artery disease. (Modified from http://emedicine.medscape.com/article/164163-overview)

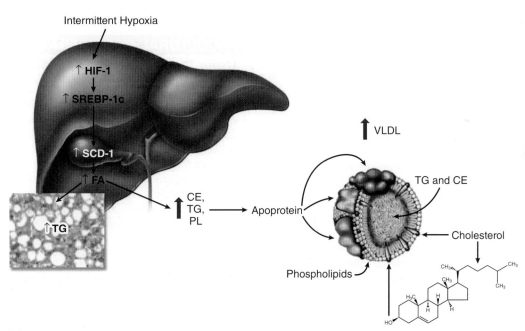

FIG 17-3 Effects of hypoxia on serum lipids. *CE,* Cholesterol ester; *FA,* fatty acid; *HIF-1,* hypoxia-inducible factor-1; *PL,* phospholipid; *SCD-1,* stearoyl CoA desaturase 1; *SREBP-1c,* sterol regulatory element binding protein-1c; *TG,* triglyceride; *VLDL,* very low-density lipoprotein. (From Drager, et al: Obstructive sleep apnea and dyslipidemia: Implications for atherosclerosis. *Curr Opin Endocrinol Diabetes Obes* 17:161-165, 2010.)

Dyslipidemia

The most common approach in assessing CAD risk is to measure the proportions of different types of plasma lipoproteins. Altered serum lipids lead to a condition called dyslipidemia. Later studies suggest that intermittent hypoxemia from sleep apnea may also trigger dyslipidemia (Figure 17-3).

Cholesterol is an essential component of cell membranes and a precursor of bile acids, steroid hormones, and vitamin D. Cholesterol is a not actually a lipid, but it travels in the bloodstream in *lipoprotein* spheres, which contain lipids and proteins. Plasma lipoproteins are usually measured from a fasting individual; they may include very low-density

TABLE 17-1 Classification of Serum Lipid Values*

CATEGORY	TRIGLYCERIDE LEVELS	LDL CHOLESTEROL LEVELS	TOTAL CHOLESTEROL
Optimal		<100 mg/dL	<200 mg/dL
Normal	<150 mg/dL	100-129 mg/dL	
Borderline high	150 to 199 mg/dL	130-159 mg/dL	
High	200 to 499 mg/dL	160-189 mg/dL	
Very high	>500 mg/dL	>190 mg/dL	

*Goal: Reduce elevated lipid values: keep total cholesterol value below 200 mg/dL, triglyceride values below 200 mg/dL, high-density lipoprotein (HDL) cholesterol values between 40 and 60 mg/dL, and low-density lipoprotein (LDL) cholesterol values between 100 and 129 mg/dL.
Adapted from National Cholesterol Education Program (NCEP): *Third report of the NCEP expert panel on detection, evaluation, and treatment of high blood cholesterol in adults (Adult Treatment Panel III),* Washington, DC, 2001, National Institutes of Health, National Heart, Lung, and Blood Institute.

lipoproteins (VLDLs), low-density lipoproteins (LDLs), and high-density lipoproteins (HDLs). LDLs contain approximately 60% to 70% of total serum cholesterol (TC), and high serum levels are related to increased risk of CAD. HDLs usually contain 20% to 30% of the total cholesterol, and serum levels are inversely correlated with risk for CAD. VLDLs are largely composed of triglyceride. Elevated triglyceride values, small LDL cholesterol particles, and low HDL cholesterol values are often seen in people with premature CHD.

Triglyceride is the most common type of fat found in the bloodstream. The body gets triglyceride directly from foods and produces more in the liver. Serum triglyceride levels range from about 50 to 250 mg/dL (Table 17-1). Factors that may cause elevations of triglycerides are as follows:

- Long-term, excessive alcohol intake
- Overweight and obesity
- Physical inactivity
- Cigarette smoking
- Very high carbohydrate intake (>60% of total energy)
- Other diseases (type 2 diabetes mellitus, chronic renal failure, nephrotic syndrome)
- Certain drugs (corticosteroids, protease inhibitors for human immunodeficiency virus/acquired immunodeficiency syndrome [HIV/AIDS], β-adrenergic blocking agents, estrogens)
- Genetic factors

Plasma levels of total cholesterol and HDL have a strong heritability factor of 40% to 60%. Indeed, genetic transcription factors are the master regulators of cholesterol, triglyceride, and fatty acid synthesis (Liu, et al, 2013).

Genetic mutations, such as *apolipoprotein E (ApoE)* polymorphisms, contribute to CAD. Blood lipid response to diet or the inflammatory process of obesity will vary according to a person's *APOE* genotype. In addition, elevated plasma levels of *lipoprotein(a)* and *coronary artery calcification (CAC)* promote atherosclerosis (Jiang, et al, 2013). Lipoprotein(a) seems to be more of a factor in Asian populations than in Caucasians (Sharma, et al, 2011).

HDL cholesterol counteracts the detrimental, proinflammatory effects of LDL cholesterol. Low HDL is defined as a level of less than 40 mg/dL in men and 50 mg/dL in women. Increasing the activity of cholesteryl ester transfer protein (CETP) may be as one way to increase HDL (Shinkai, 2012;) (Figure 17-4). Furthermore, oxidative stress contributes to

CVD and atherosclerosis. Pharmacological doses of niacin can lower total cholesterol (TC), triglycerides, and VLDL and LDL levels and increase HDL levels (Hamoud, et al, 2013). However, long-term trials have not proven safety and efficacy.

We know right now that obesity (especially abdominal obesity), insulin resistance, and physical inactivity are detrimental to cardiac health. The heart is a muscle and requires exercise. Thus, lifestyle modifications such as weight control and increased physical activity are primary treatments (see the *Cultural Considerations* box Using T'ai Chi to Reduce Cardiovascular Risk Factors).

🌐 CULTURAL CONSIDERATIONS

Using T'ai Chi to Reduce Cardiovascular Risk Factors

A common risk factor for cardiovascular disease (CVD) is physical inactivity. Interventions that are age and culturally appropriate to increase physical activity can reduce associated risks and enhance quality of life. In China, T'ai chi is a form of exercise favored by older adults. T'ai chi is a mind-body practice that began as a martial art. One moves slowly while focusing on breathing deeply and clearing the mind of distracting thoughts. In Western societies, T'ai chi is part of health practices associated with traditional, complementary and alternative medicine (TCAM). T'ai chi exercise is a good option for heart patients with very limited exercise tolerance and can be an adjunct to rehabilitation programs for patients with CHD or heart failure (Ng, et al, 2012). Community-based T'ai chi exercise programs may reduce disability from chronic disorders such as CVD and may improve physical ability in older adults.
Application to nursing. Community-based interventions on CVD risk factors such as diet, smoking, and exercise need to be provided in a culturally appropriate format. Although T'ai chi has Chinese origins, it is appropriate as a form of exercise for older adults of any ethnic and cultural background. Yoga therapy as another effective complementary treatment in the management of high blood pressure because it modulates the heart rate and reduces blood glucose level, cholesterol level, and body weight (Okonta, 2012).

Data from Ng SM, et al: Tai chi exercise for patients with heart disease: A systematic review of controlled clinical trials, *Altern Ther Health Med* 18:16-22, 2012; Okonta NR: Does yoga therapy reduce blood pressure in patients with hypertension? An integrative review, *Holist Nurs Pract* 26:137-141, 2012.

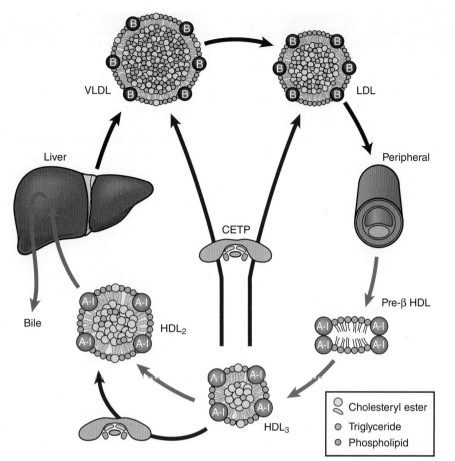

FIG 17-4 Cholesterol transport includes CETP (cholesteryl ester transfer protein), HDL (high-density lipoprotein), LDL (low-density lipoprotein), and VLDL (very low-density lipoprotein). HDL_2 and HDL_3 are HDL subfractions. (From Shinkai H: Cholesteryl ester transfer-protein modulator and inhibitors and their potential for the treatment of cardiovascular diseases, *Vasc Health Risk Manag* 8:323-331, 2012.)

Other Risk Factors

Several nonlipid risk factors are associated with increased CHD risk and are targets for preventive efforts. Fixed risk factors (increasing age, male gender, genes, and family history of premature CHD) cannot be modified, and their existence implies need for intensive lowering of LDL. Modifiable nonlipid risk factors include hypertension, cigarette smoking, diabetes, obesity, physical inactivity, and atherogenic diet. Table 17-2 summarizes CHD risk factors.

Food and Nutrition Therapies

Patients with or at risk for CHD should be referred to registered dietitians for nutrition therapy. Thought should be given to adequate nutrition therapy before the addition of LDL-lowering medications. Overall, the composition of the *Therapeutic Lifestyle Changes (TLC)* diet is consistent with recommendations of the *Dietary Guidelines for Americans*. See Table 17-3 and Box 17-2.

LDL should be measured at 6-week intervals to evaluate response to the TLC diet described here. If the goal has not been achieved, nutrition guidance can be re-explained

and reinforced; further therapeutic dietary options can be added. Response to nutrition therapy should be assessed in another 6 weeks. Achievement of the LDL target indicates that current intensity of nutrition intervention should continue indefinitely.

The TLC protocol focuses on
- Altered intake of types of fats
- Plant stanols and sterols, increased soluble fiber
- Weight reduction
- Increased regular physical activity

Saturated Fat

Reducing saturated fat intake is the foundation of the TLC diet.

Monounsaturated Fat

Substitution of monounsaturated fat for saturated fats at an intake level of up to 20% of total energy intake is recommended. Monounsaturated fats lower LDL levels without decreasing HDL. Almonds, walnuts, pistachios, extra-virgin olive oil, and canola oil are especially beneficial.

TABLE 17-2 Major Risk Factors in Cardiovascular Disease

Known	Age (men >45 yr, women after menopause)
	Diabetes and prediabetes
	Ethnicity (African Americans, Mexican Americans, American Indians, native Hawaiians, some Asian Americans)
	Family history
	Dyslipidemia (high low-density lipoprotein and low high-density lipoprotein cholesterol levels)
	High blood pressure
	High stress levels
	Obesity
	Physical inactivity
	Sex (all men, but women mostly after menopause)
	Smoking
	Unhealthy diet
Further research needed	Elevated homocysteine levels
	Elevated C-reactive protein
	High fibrinogen levels
	Lipoprotein(a)
	Sleep apnea

Data from American Heart Association: *Coronary artery disease—coronary heart disease,* n.d. Accessed August 26, 2013, from www.heart.org/HEARTORG/Conditions/More/MyHeartandStrokeNews/Coronary-Artery-Disease—The-ABCs-of-CAD_UCM_436416_Article.jsp; Mayo Clinic: *Diseases and conditions: Coronary artery disease,* n.d. Accessed August 26, 2013, from www.mayoclinic.com/health/coronary-artery-disease/DS00064/DSECTION=risk-factors; and National Heart, lung and Blood Institute: *What are coronary heart disease risk factors?* 2011. Accessed August 26, 2013, from www.nhlbi.nih.gov/health/health-topics/topics/hd/.

Polyunsaturated Fats

When used instead of saturated fats, polyunsaturated fats, in particular linoleic acid, reduce LDL levels but also reduce HDL. Liquid vegetables oils, semiliquid margarines, and other margarines low in *trans* fatty acids are best sources of polyunsaturated fats.

Carbohydrate

When saturated fats are replaced with complex carbohydrates, LDL decreases.

Protein

Although dietary protein, as a rule, has a negligible effect on serum LDL level, substituting plant-based proteins for animal proteins appears to be beneficial. Plant-based protein foods (e.g., legumes, dry beans, nuts, whole grains, and vegetables) lack saturated fat content. Good choices of animal proteins include fat-free or low-fat dairy products, egg whites, fish, skinless poultry, and lean cuts of beef and pork.

Soluble Fiber, Sterols, and Stanols

When 5 to 10 g of soluble fiber from oats, barley, psyllium, pectin-rich fruit, and beans is added to the daily diet, there is

TABLE 17-3 Components of Therapeutic Lifestyle Changes (TLC) Program

COMPONENT	RECOMMENDATION
LDL Cholesterol–Raising Nutrients	
Saturated fats	<7% of total energy intake
Dietary cholesterol	<200 mg/day
Therapeutic Options for Lowering LDL Cholesterol	
Plant stanols/sterols	2 g/day
Soluble fiber	10 to 25 g/day
Total dietary fiber	20 to 30 g/day
Total energy (kcal)	Adjust total energy intake to maintain desirable body weight and prevent weight gain
Physical activity	Include enough moderate exercise to expend at least 200 kcal/day
Polyunsaturated fat	Up to 10% total energy intake
Monounsaturated fat	Up to 20% total energy intake
Total fat	25% to 35% total energy intake
Carbohydrate (whole grains, fruits, vegetables)	50% to 60% total energy intake

LDL, Low-density lipoprotein.
Adapted from National Cholesterol Education Program (NCEP): *Third report of the NCEP expert panel on detection, evaluation, and treatment of high blood cholesterol in adults (Adult Treatment Panel III),* Washington, DC, 2001, National Institutes of Health, National Heart, Lung, and Blood Institute.

a roughly 5% reduction in LDL. Daily intakes of 2 to 3 g of plant stanols or sterol esters (isolated from soybean and tall pine tree oils) present an additional therapeutic option. Products on the market that contain stanols include some brands of orange juice, cereals, and spreads such as Take Control and Benecol.

Mediterranean Diet

Many dietary factors have an additive effect. Components such as plant stanols and sterols, soy protein, β-glucans from oats or mushrooms, canola oil, almonds, and tree nuts can reduce the need for pharmaceutical interventions (Lin, et al, 2013; Harland, 2012). Among persons at high cardiovascular risk, a Mediterranean diet supplemented with extra-virgin olive oil or nuts can really reduce the number of major cardiovascular events (Estruch, et al, 2013). The Mediterranean diet has the following components:

- Fresh fruits and vegetables, whole grains, nuts, garlic, fish, and wine in moderation
- Meat and animal products in very small amounts
- Dairy products used sparingly; if cheese is consumed, Feta cheese is the choice
- Up to 4%0 of calories coming from fat, especially olive oil

Drug Therapy

If treatment with dietary change is unsuccessful after 3 months, drug treatment may be required. Use of medications does not negate the need for dietary changes that also lower

---

BOX 17-2 Therapeutic Lifestyle Changes (TLC) Program: Healthy Lifestyle Recommendations For a Healthy Heart

Food Items to Choose More Often

Breads and cereals: ≥6 servings per day, adjusted to kcal needs; breads, cereals, especially whole grains; pasta; rice; potatoes; dry beans and peas; low-fat crackers and cookies

Vegetables: 3 to 5 servings per day fresh, frozen, or canned without added fat, sauce, or salt

Fruits: 2 to 4 servings per day fresh, frozen, canned, dried

Dairy products: 2 to 3 servings per day fat-free, ½%, or 1% milk, buttermilk, yogurt, cottage cheese, fat-free and low-fat cheese

Eggs: 2 egg yolks per week; egg whites or egg substitute

Meat, poultry, fish: <5 ounces per day; lean cuts(loin, leg, round), extra-lean hamburger; cold cuts made with lean meat or soy protein; skinless poultry; fish

Fats and oils: Amount adjusted to kcal level: unsaturated oils; soft or liquid margarines and vegetable oil spreads; salad dressings, seeds, and nuts

Stanol/sterols and soluble fiber: Stanol/sterol-containing margarines; soluble-fiber food sources: barley, oats, psyllium, apples, bananas, berries, citrus fruits, nectarines, peaches, pears, plums, prunes, broccoli, Brussels sprouts, carrots, dry beans, soy products (tofu, miso)

Food Items to Choose Less Often

Breads and cereals: Many baked products, including doughnuts, biscuits, butter rolls, muffins, croissants, sweet rolls, Danish, cakes, pies, coffee cakes, cookies; many grain-based snacks, including chips, cheese puffs, snack mix, regular crackers, buttered popcorn

Vegetables: Vegetables fried or prepared with butter, cheese, or cream sauce

Fruits: Fruits fried or served with butter or cream

Dairy products: Whole or 2% milk, whole-milk yogurt, ice cream, cream, cheese

Eggs: >3egg yolks/week, whole eggs

Meat, poultry, fish: Higher-fat meat cuts: ribs, T-bone steak, regular hamburger, bacon, sausage; cold cuts: salami, bologna, hot dogs; organ meats: liver, brains, sweetbreads; poultry with skin; fried meat; fried poultry; fried fish

Fats and oils: Butter, shortening, stick margarine, chocolate, coconut

Recommendations for Weight Reduction
Weigh Regularly
Record weight, body mass index (BMI), and waist circumference

Lose Weight Gradually
Goal: lose 10% of body weight in 6 months; lose ½ to 1 pound per week

Develop Healthy Eating Patterns
Choose healthy foods (see "Food Items to Choose More Often"):
- Reduce intake of less healthy foods (see "Food Items to Choose Less Often")
- Limit number of eating occasions
- Avoid second helpings
- Identify and reduce hidden fat by reading food labels to choose products lower in saturated fat and kcal, and ask about ingredients in ready-to-eat foods prepared away from home
- Identify and reduce sources of excess carbohydrates such as fat-free and regular crackers, cookies and other desserts, snacks, and sugar-containing beverages

Recommendations for Increased Physical Activity
Make Physical Activity Part of Daily Routine
- Reduce sedentary time
- Walk, wheel, or bike-ride more; drive less. Take the stairs instead of an elevator. Get off the bus a few stops early and walk the remaining distance. Mow the lawn with a push mower. Rake leaves. Garden. Push a stroller. Clean the house. Do exercises or pedal a stationary bike while watching television. Play actively with children. Take a brisk 10-minute walk or wheel before work, during your work break, and after dinner.

Make Physical Activity Part of Exercise or Recreational Activities
- Walk, wheel, or jog. Bicycle or use an arm-pedal bicycle. Swim or do water aerobics. Play basketball. Join a sports team. Play wheelchair sports. Golf (pull cart or carry clubs). Canoe. Cross-country ski. Dance. Take part in an exercise program at work, home, school, or a gym.

Modified from the National Cholesterol Education Program (NCEP): *Third report of the NCEP expert panel on detection, evaluation, and treatment of high blood cholesterol in adults (Adult Treatment Panel III),* Washington, DC, 2001, National Institutes of Health, National Heart, Lung, and Blood Institute.

CHD risks. Major drugs used to treat dyslipidemia include statins, niacin, bile-acid resins, fibric acid derivatives, and cholesterol absorption inhibitors (Table 17-4).

MYOCARDIAL INFARCTION

Heart attacks (myocardial infarctions) are the single largest killer of adult men and women in the United States. An American suffers a heart attack every 20 seconds, and someone dies from one every minute. Disability or death can result after a myocardial infarction (MI), depending on how much heart muscle is damaged.

Food and Nutrition Therapies

The purpose of nutrition therapy for patients suffering from an MI is to reduce the workload of the heart. This is also a good time to initiate education about modification of diet-related cardiovascular risk factors. The patient may start with liquids and progress, as tolerated, to foods of regular consistency. Smaller, frequent meals are usually better tolerated

TABLE 17-4 Major Drugs Used to Treat Dyslipidemia

DRUG CLASS	AVAILABLE DRUGS	LIPID/LIPOPROTEIN EFFECTS	POTENTIAL NUTRITIONAL SIDE EFFECTS AND CAUTIONS
Statins (HMG CoA reductase inhibitors)	Lovastatin (Altocor, Mevacor), pravastatin (Pravachol), simvastatin (Zocor), fluvastatin (Lescol), atorvastatin (Lipitor)	↓ LDL cholesterol and triglycerides; moderately HDL cholesterol	Avoid St. John's wort; avoid grapefruit juice with Lipitor, Zocor, Mevacor Nausea, dyspepsia, abdominal pain, constipation, diarrhea, flatulence Avoid substantial alcohol
Bile acid sequestrants	Cholestyramine (Questran), colestipol (Colestid), colesevelam (WelChol)	↓ LDL cholesterol	Tongue irritation, belching, constipation, dyspepsia, nausea/vomiting, flatulence, diarrhea Fat-soluble in water-miscible form Folacin supplement recommended with long-term use
Nicotinic acid (niacin)	A variety of prescription or over-the-counter preparations available in three forms: immediate-release, timed-release, extended-release nicotinic acid (Niaspan)	↑ HDL cholesterol and ↓ LDL cholesterol and triglycerides	Flushing of face and neck, nausea, vomiting, diarrhea, gout, high blood glucose, peptic ulcers
Fibrates (fibric acid derivatives)	Fenofibrate (Lofibra, Tricor), gemfibrozil (Lopid)	↓ Triglycerides and modestly HDL cholesterol	Take with meals; nausea/vomiting, constipation, flatulence, avoid alcohol
Cholesterol absorption inhibitors	Ezetimibe (Zetia)	↓ LDL cholesterol and slightly ↓ both triglycerides and HDL cholesterol	Diarrhea, stomach pain, fatigue
Combination cholesterol absorption inhibitor and statin	Ezetimibe/simvastatin (Vytorin)	↓ LDL cholesterol and triglycerides and moderately ↑ HDL cholesterol	Same as statins and cholesterol absorption inhibitors

HDL, High-density lipoprotein; *HMG CoA,* 3-hydroxy-3-methylglutaryl coenzyme A; *LDLC,* low-density lipoprotein; ↑, increase; ↓, decrease.
Data from Citkowitz E: *Hypercholesterolemia, familial,* n.d. Accessed August 26, 2013, from www.emedicine.com/med/topic1072.htm#section~AuthorsandEditors; Pronsky ZM: *Food-medication interactions,* ed 17, Birchrunville, PA, 2008, 2012, Food-Medication Interactions.)

than large meals. Large meals can raise myocardial oxygen demand by increasing splanchnic (visceral) blood flow. Caffeine-containing beverages are sometimes restricted to avoid myocardial stimulation. However after recovery, coffee and other antioxidant-rich foods (fruits, vegetables, whole grains) help prevent future heart attacks (Rautiainen, et al, 2012). Consuming omega-3 fatty acids appears to reduce the risk of blood clots that may cause an MI. Sources of omega-3 fatty acids include fish such as tuna, salmon, halibut, sardines, and lake trout.

Overall, sodium, saturated fats, fluid, and calories are controlled according to the patient's needs. Active intervention with either a low-fat or a Mediterranean-style diet benefits overall and cardiovascular event–free survival after MI (Tuttle, et al, 2008).

HYPERTENSION

Nearly one in three U.S. adults, or 68 million persons, has hypertension; in half of those, the condition is not under control (Centers for Disease Control and Prevention [CDC], 2012). Not only is it a cardiovascular disorder itself, but HTN is also a risk factor for CAD. Hypertension (HTN)

contributes to about 50% of cardiovascular events worldwide and 37% of cardiovascular-related deaths in Western populations (Ried, et al, 2012). According to the American Heart Association (n.d.), the incidence of HTN is higher in the following groups:

- Until age 45, a higher percentage of men than women
- From ages 45 to 54, the percentage of women with HTN increases
- For those older than 54, a higher percentage of women than men
- African Americans, Puerto Ricans, Cuban Americans, and Mexican Americans

In about 95% of cases of HTN, cause is not known, so the condition is called essential or primary hypertension. For some individuals, an overactive hormonal renin-angiotensin-aldosterone system plays a part in altered vascular tone, salt and water homeostasis, and cardiac functioning.

A diseased heart has numerous adverse effects on kidney function, and vice versa (Figure 17-5). We know that prematurity, low birth weight, infections, and poor nutrition can lead to inadequate kidney development (Carmody and Charlton, 2013). Thus, prenatal nutrition and maternal health are of great significance for health later in a person's life.

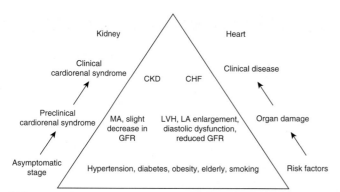

FIG 17-5 Common pathophysiologies affect cardiac and renal function, structure, and overt disease. *CHF,* Congestive heart failure; *CKD,* chronic kidney disease *GFR,* glomerular filtration rate; *LA,* left atrial; *LVH,* left ventricular hypertrophy; *MA,* microalbuminuria. (From Tsioufis C, et al: Preclinical cardiorenal interrelationships in essential hypertension, *Cardiorenal Med* 3(1):38-47, 2013.)

TABLE 17-5 Classification of Blood Pressure for Adults

CATEGORY	CYCTOLIO (mm Hg)		DIAOTOLIC (mm Hg)
Normal	<120	And	<80
Prehypertensive	120 to 139	Or	80 to 89
Stage 1 hypertension	140 to 159	Or	90 to 99
Stage 2 hypertension	≥160	Or	≥110

Data from *The seventh report of the joint national committee on prevention, detection, evaluation, and treatment of high blood pressure* (NIH Pub No 04-5230), Washington, DC, 2004, National Institutes of Health, National Heart, Lung, and Blood Institute.

Secondary hypertension is the term used when a specific cause of elevated blood pressure can be identified, such as Cushing's syndrome and primary aldosteronism. Although sometimes called a "silent killer," HTN is easily detected and usually controllable. Classifications of blood pressure are shown in Table 17-5. Prescribed treatment regimens for HTN are individualized and vary because the disease differs in degree of severity.

Food and Nutrition Therapies

Weight loss is the most effective means of lowering blood pressure. Other lifestyle modifications are decreasing alcohol consumption, increasing physical activity if one is sedentary, terminating cigarette smoking, decreasing sodium intake, and increasing intake of potassium, magnesium, and calcium. Box 17-3 summarizes lifestyle modifications that help reduce high blood pressure and overall cardiovascular risk.

Weight reduction facilitates lower blood pressure even when it is only a loss of 10 to 15 pounds. Weight reduction and sodium restriction also augment the effects of antihypertensive medications. Diet for weight loss and control should include an energy restriction and an aerobic exercise prescription, such as for walking or swimming.

BOX 17-3 Lifestyle for Hypertension Prevention and Management

- Lose weight if overweight. Maintain normal body weight (body mass index 18.5-24.9).
- Limit alcohol intake to no more than 1 ounce (30 mL) ethanol (e.g., 24 oz [720 mL] beer, 10 oz [300 mL] wine, or 2 oz [60 mL] 100-proof whiskey) per day or 0.5 oz (15 mL) ethanol per day for women and lighter-weight people.
- Engage in aerobic physical activity (at least 30 minutes most days of the week).
- Reduce sodium intake to no more than 100 mmol per day (2.4 g sodium or 6 g sodium chloride).
- Adopt DASH eating plan. Consume dietary pattern of fruits, vegetables, and low-fat dairy products and reduce intake of saturated fat and total fat.
- Stop smoking for overall cardiovascular health.

Data from *The seventh report of the joint national committee on prevention, detection, evaluation, and treatment of high blood pressure* (NIH Pub No. 04-5230), Washington, DC, 2004, National Institutes of Health, National Heart, Lung, and Blood Institute.

Reducing sodium intake to 2300 mg/day potentially could prevent 11 million cases of hypertension and save billions of dollars in health care expenditures; reducing sodium intake further would yield additional benefits (CDC, 2012). Sodium reduction results in a 3.5% decrease in hypertension, a significant increase in plasma renin, plasma aldosterone, plasma adrenaline, and plasma noradrenaline levels (Graudal, et al, 2011).

The average sodium intake among persons in the United States aged 2 years or older is 3266 mg/day, excluding table salt (CDC, 2012). Most comes from sodium added during processing and manufacturing of foods. The other main source of dietary sodium is the discretionary use of table salt (sodium chloride). A small portion of dietary sodium also comes from natural sodium content of foods.

Public policies and culturally appropriate dietary patterns that support the "total diet approach" should be used to empower individuals to make positive lifestyle changes (Freeland-Graves, et al, 2013). The U.S. National High Blood Pressure Education Program recommends trying lifestyle modifications for 3 to 6 months in patient with mild to moderate HTN. A diet rich in fruits, vegetables, and low-fat dairy products along with reduced saturated and total fats has been found to significantly lower blood pressure.

The DASH (Dietary Approaches to Stop Hypertension) diet is recommended for prevention and management of HTN (National Institutes of Health, National Heart, Lung, and Blood Institute, 2006). If the diet works, it will show effectiveness in lowering blood pressure within 2 weeks. Among children and teens, intake of 2 or more cups per day of dairy products lowers high blood pressure; this intake would support the dietary guideline recommendations (Yuan, et al, 2013).

TABLE 17-6 DASH Diet Pattern*

FOOD GROUP	DAILY SERVING(S) (EXCEPT WHERE NOTED)	SERVING SIZES	EXAMPLES AND NOTES	SIGNIFICANCE TO THE DASH DIET PATTERN
Grains and grain products	7-8	1 slice bread 1 ounce dry cereal[†] ½ cup cooked rice, pasta, or cereal	Whole-wheat bread, English muffin, pita bread, bagel; cereals; grits; oatmeal	Major source of energy and fiber
Vegetables	4-5	1 cup raw, leafy vegetables ½ cup cooked vegetables 6 ounces vegetable juice	Tomatoes, potatoes, carrots, peas, squash, broccoli, turnip greens, collards, kale, spinach, artichokes, beans, sweet potatoes	Rich sources of potassium, magnesium, and fiber
Fruits	4-5	6 ounces fruit juice 1 medium fruit ¼ cup dried fruit ½ cup fresh, frozen, or canned fruit	Apricots, bananas, dates, grapes, oranges, orange juice, tangerines, strawberries, mangoes, melons, peaches, pineapple, prunes, raisins	Important sources of potassium, magnesium, and fiber
Low-fat or free dairy foods	2-3	8 ounces milk 1 cup yogurt 1½ ounces cheese	Fat-free or 1% milk, fat-free or low-fat buttermilk; nonfat or low-fat yogurt; part-skim mozzarella cheese, nonfat cheese	Major sources of calcium and protein
Meats, poultry, and fish	≥2	3 ounces cooked meats, poultry, or fish	Select only lean meats; trim away visible fats; broil, roast, or boil, instead of frying; remove skin from chicken	Rich sources of protein and magnesium
Nuts, seeds, and legumes	4-5 per week	1½ ounces or ½ cup nuts ½ ounce or 2 tablespoons seeds ½ cup cooked legumes	Almonds, filberts, mixed nuts, peanuts, walnuts, sunflower seeds, kidney beans, lentils	Rich sources of energy, magnesium, potassium, protein, and fiber
Fats and oils[‡]	2-3	1 teaspoon soft margarine 1 tablespoon low-fat mayonnaise or salad dressing 2 tablespoons light salad dressing 1 teaspoon vegetable oil	Soft margarine, low-fat mayonnaise, light salad dressing, vegetable oil (e.g., olive, corn, canola, or safflower)	DASH has 27% of kcal as fat, including that in or added to foods
Sweets	5 per week	1 tablespoon sugar 1 tablespoon jelly or jam ½ ounce jelly beans 8 ounces lemonade	Maple syrup, sugar, jelly, jam, fruit-flavored gelatin, jelly beans, fruit punch, sorbet, ices, hard candy	Sweets should be low in fat

*The DASH diet is based on 2000 kcal/day. This table indicates the number of recommended daily servings from each food group with examples of food choices. The number of servings may increase or decrease, depending on individual calorie needs.
[†]Equals ½ to 1¼ cups depending on cereal type. Check the product's nutrition label.
[‡]Fat content changes serving counts for fats and oils. For example, 1 tablespoon of regular salad dressing equals 1 serving; 1 tablespoon of low-fat dressing equals ½ serving; 1 tablespoon of fat-free dressing equals 0 servings.
From U.S. Department of Health and Human Services, Public Health Service, National Institutes of Health, National Heart, Lung, and Blood Institute: *Your guide to lowering your blood pressure with DASH* (NIH Publication No. 06-4082), Bethesda, MD, 2006, Author. Accessed August 26, 2013, from www.nhlbi.nih.gov.

The DASH eating plan described in Table 17-6 is based on 2000 kcal/day. The number of daily servings from each group can be modified according to individual energy needs (see the *Teaching Tool* box Strategies for Adopting DASH). See Figure 17-6, which shows a family enjoying a DASH-designed meal together.

An even larger drop in blood pressure is seen when the DASH eating plan is combined with sodium restriction (Table 17-7). The largest reduction in blood pressure is seen in those using the DASH eating plan with the sodium intake level of 1500 mg/day (Box 17-4). For many, a sodium intake of 1500 mg/day would be a moderately severe restriction.

Current dietary guidelines recommend reducing consumption of sodium to less than 2300 mg/day. African Americans, persons 51 years or older, and anyone with hypertension, diabetes, or chronic kidney disease (about half of the

✳ TEACHING TOOL

Strategies for Adopting DASH

Dietary changes are best achieved through small changes in food selections. Use this list of tips as a way to initiate discussion and encourage dietary compliance.

Change gradually:

- If you now eat one or two vegetables a day, add a serving at lunch and another at dinner.
- If you don't eat fruit now or have only juice at breakfast, add a serving to your meals or have it as a snack.
- Gradually increase your use of fat-free and low-fat dairy products to three servings a day. For example, drink milk with lunch or dinner instead of soda, sugar-sweetened tea, or alcohol. Choose low-fat (1%) or fat-free (skim) dairy products to reduce your intake of saturated fat, total fat, cholesterol, and kcal.
- Read food labels on margarines and salad dressings and choose those lowest in saturated fat. Some margarines are now *trans* fat–free.

Treat meat as one part of the whole meal, instead of the focus:

- Limit meat to 6 ounces a day (two servings)—all that's needed. A serving of 3 to 4 ounces is about the size of a dook of oardo.
- If you currently eat large portions of meat, cut portion sizes back gradually—by a half or a third at each meal.

- Include two or more vegetarian-style (meatless) meals each week.
- Increase servings of vegetables, rice, pasta, and dry beans in meals. Try casseroles, pasta, and stir-fry dishes, which have less meat and more vegetables, grains, and dry beans.

Use fruit or other foods low in saturated fat, cholesterol, and kcal as desserts and snacks:

- Fruits and other low-fat foods offer great taste and variety. Use fruits canned in their own juice. Fresh fruits require little or no preparation. Dried fruits are a good choice to carry with you.
- Try these snacks ideas: unsalted pretzels or nuts mixed with raisins; graham crackers; low-fat, fat-free, or frozen yogurt; popcorn with no salt or butter added; and raw vegetables.

Try the following other tips:

- Choose whole-grain breads, cereals, and pasta to get added nutrients, such as minerals and fiber.
- If you have trouble digesting dairy products, try taking lactase enzyme pills or drops (available at drugstores and groceries) before eating dairy foods, or buy lactose-free milk or milk with lactase enzyme added to it.
- Use fresh, frozen, or sodium-free canned vegetables.

From U.S. Department of Health and Human Services, Public Health Service, National Institutes of Health, National Heart, Lung, and Blood Institute: *Your guide to lowering your blood pressure with DASH* (NIH Publication No 06-4082), Bethesda, MD, 2006, Author. Accessed August 25, 2013, from www.nhlbi.nih.gov.

FIG 17-6 Family members of all ages can enjoy a heart-healthy diet.

U.S. population and the majority of adults) should reduce sodium intake to 1500 mg/day (CDC, 2012). Maintaining sodium consumption at this level is a challenge, given the amount of sodium added to foods during processing and manufacturing. Salt adds its own salty flavor to foods, alters other tastes and flavors, and conceals bitterness without necessarily causing the foods to taste salty. As a result, when salt is reduced or removed from a food, the saltiness and other flavors of that food are changed.

Although there is currently no acceptable substitute for salt that provides similar taste satisfaction, a salt substitute may be prescribed for some patients. The *Teaching Tool* box Seven Sneaky Sodium Stowaways gives tips on helping patients recognize foods potentially high in sodium.

✳ TEACHING TOOL

Seven Sneaky Sodium Stowaways

Provide patients with an easy way to remember categories of foods that may be high in sodium. Label reading is often an absolute necessity. Consider that sodium hides in seven categories of foods in the form of salt or as part of an added ingredient. Following are the seven sneaky categories of sodium stowaways:

*S*nacks (corn chips, potato chips, pretzels, peanuts, certain crackers)

*S*easonings and nonnutritive sweeteners (monosodium glutamate, sodium saccharin)

*S*oups (especially canned and dried mixes)

*S*auces (dried mixes and bottled, including ketchup)

*S*moked meats and fish (smoked ham and lox)

*S*auerkraut and other pickled foods (pickles, relishes, and pickled herring)

*S*odium-processed luncheon meats (bologna, salami, ham, corned beef)

TABLE 17-7 Where's the Sodium?*

FOOD GROUPS	SODIUM (mg)
Grains and Grain Products	
Cooked cereal, rice, pasta, unsalted, ½ cup	0-5
Ready-to-eat cereal, 1 cup	100-360
Bread, 1 slice	110-175
Vegetables	
Fresh or frozen, cooked without salt, ½ cup	1-70
Canned or frozen with sauce, ½ cup	140-460
Tomato juice, canned, ¾ cup	820
Fruit	
Fresh, frozen, canned, ½ cup	0-5
Low-Fat or Fat-Free Dairy Foods	
Milk, 1 cup	120
Yogurt, 8 ounces	160
Natural cheeses, 1½ ounces	110-450
Processed cheeses, 1½ ounces	600
Nuts, Seeds, and Dry Beans	
Peanuts, salted, ⅓ cup	120
Peanuts, unsalted, ⅓ cup	0-5
Beans, cooked from dried or frozen, without salt, ½ cup	0-5
Beans, canned, ½ cup	400
Meats, Fish, and Poultry	
Fresh meat, fish, poultry, 3 ounces	30-90
Tuna canned, water pack, no salt added, 3 ounces	35-45
Tuna canned, water pack, 3 ounces	250-350
Ham, lean, roasted, 3 ounces	1,020

*Only a small amount of sodium occurs naturally in foods. Most sodium is added during processing. The table gives examples of varying amounts of sodium that occur in foods before and after processing.
From U.S. Department of Health and Human Services, Public Health Service, National Institutes of Health, National Heart, Lung, and Blood Institute: *Your guide to lowering your blood pressure with DASH* (NIH Publication No. 06-4082), Bethesda, MD, 2006, Author. Accessed August 26, 2013, from www.nhlbi.nih.gov.

HEART FAILURE

Heart failure is a form of cardiac decompensation. Left ventricle failure produces pulmonary congestion, whereas right ventricular failure results in systemic congestion that causes poor perfusion to all organ systems.

Food and Nutrition Therapies

If heart failure is caused by a valve problem, most dietary measures will not be effective. If excessive sodium intake has been part of the etiology, then nutrition therapy focuses on restricting dietary sodium. Patients with mild to moderate heart failure (HF) are often prescribed a sodium restriction of 3000 mg/day. People whose disease is unresponsive to this level or who have severe HF are more likely to benefit from sodium restriction to 2000 mg/day. Fluid restriction of 1 to 2 L is sometimes indicated when hyponatremia is present. Fluid requirements depend on medical status and use of diuretics.

Cardiac Cachexia

Energy requirements are 20% to 30% above basal needs in people with HF because of increased cardiac and pulmonary energy demands and increased metabolic rate. Protein and energy intake should be sufficient to maintain body weight. Meeting these increased nutrient and energy requirements is problematic. In HF, early satiety, gastrointestinal congestion, shortness of breath, anorexia, and nausea are common concerns, often leading to cardiac cachexia. If the patient has cardiac cachexia, additional calories and protein are needed to prevent further catabolism.

Caution must be used so as not to overfeed the patient. Calorie-dense (1.5 kcal/mL) nutritional supplements may be helpful to increase energy and protein intake. Enteral or parenteral nutrition may be necessary for patients who cannot meet their nutritional needs through oral intake. If enteral nutrition support is required, continuous rather than bolus feedings are favored because they reduce myocardial oxygen consumption. Concentrated enteral formulas are available if fluid restriction is necessary.

ROLE OF NURSING

Although dietitians are responsible for developing the medical nutrition plan and for diet education and counseling, nurses reinforce that teaching and answer any additional questions of patients and their families. Nurses play a major role in teaching people how to reduce cardiovascular risk factors, including reinforcement of dietary modifications. The emphasis has shifted away from standardized information sheets toward an individualized, tailored approach. Thus, familiarity with key dietary principles will make the discussions easier.

Family Education

Modifications in lifestyle are easier to follow when the entire family is supportive and compliant. Dietary education should include individuals who buy and prepare meals or snacks for the patient. By including all family members in the educative process, not only is the health of the individual with CAD enhanced but primary risk factors for younger family members may be decreased. Lists of health associations, community hospitals, and other organizations offering cooking courses and of bookstores or public libraries with available heart-healthy cookbooks are excellent adjuncts for nutrition counseling. Lifelong health promotion habits that develop early can benefit everyone.

Demystifying Labels

Label reading is an important skill for all of us but is especially so for someone with diet-related illnesses, including

BOX 17-4 DASHing with Less Salt: A Sample Menu

This sample menu provides five fruit servings, five vegetable servings, and four dairy servings.

2300-mg SODIUM MENU	SODIUM (mg)	SUBSTITUTIONS TO REDUCE SODIUM TO 1500 mg	SODIUM (mg)
Breakfast			
¾ cup bran flakes	220	¾ cup shredded wheat cereal	1
1 slice whole-wheat bread	149	½ cup fruit yogurt, fat free, no sugar added	86
1 cup low-fat milk	107		
1 teaspoon soft (tub) margarine	26	1 teaspoon soft (tub) margarine, unsalted	0
Lunch			
¾ cup chicken salad	179	Omit salt from recipe	120
2 slices whole-wheat bread	299		
1 tablespoon Dijon mustard	373	1 tablespoon regular mustard	175
½ cup fruit cocktail, juice pack	5		
Salad:			
½ cup fresh cucumber slices	1		
½ cup tomato wedges	5		
1 tablespoon sunflower seeds	0		
1 teaspoon Italian dressing, reduced calorie	43		
Dinner			
3 ounces spicy baked fish	50	Omit salt from recipe	
1 cup green beans, cooked from frozen, without salt	12		
1 small baked potato	14		
2 tablespoons fat-free sour cream	21		
1 tablespoon chopped scallions	1		
2 tablespoons grated cheddar cheese, natural, reduced fat	67	2 tablespoons cheddar cheese, natural, reduced fat, low sodium	1
1 small whole-wheat roll	148	1 teaspoon soft margarine, unsalted	0
1 teaspoon soft margarine	26		
1 medium peach	0		
1 cup low-fat milk	107		
Snack			
1 cup orange juice	5		
⅓ cup almonds, unsalted	0		
¼ cup raisins	4		
1 cup fruit yogurt, fat free with no sugar added	173		

Spicy Seasoning Mix

Mix together the following ingredients and store in airtight container for other recipes: 1½ teaspoons white pepper, ½ teaspoon cayenne pepper, ½ teaspoon black pepper, 1 teaspoon onion powder, 1¼ teaspoons garlic powder, 1 tablespoon dried basil, 1½ teaspoons dried thyme.

From U.S. Department of Health and Human Services, Public Health Service, National Institutes of Health, National Heart, Lung, and Blood Institute: *Your guide to lowering your blood pressure with DASH* (NIH Publication No. 06-4082), Bethesda, MD, 2006, Author. Accessed August 25, 2013, from www.nhlbi.nih.gov.

HTN and CVD. Educating patients about use of food label information helps demystify the process of limiting dietary fat and sodium. Food labels may display two types of messages about packaged food: nutrient content claims and health claims. Federal regulations formulated by the U.S. Food and Drug Administration (FDA) control how certain terms can be used in labeling. Table 17-8 defines terms related to sodium, dietary cholesterol, and fat—nutrients of concern for patients with CVD.

PULMONARY DISEASES

Disorders of the pulmonary system are classified into two categories. The first consists of disorders that result in chronic long-term changes in pulmonary function, such as chronic obstructive pulmonary disease (COPD), a collective phrase for chronic bronchitis, asthma, and emphysema. COPD is the second leading cause of disability in the United States. The goal of nutrition therapy for this category is to maintain respiratory muscle strength and function and to prevent or correct malnutrition.

The second category contains disorders that cause acute changes in pulmonary function, such as respiratory distress syndrome (RDS) and acute respiratory failure (ARF). These disorders can develop in patients who are critically ill, in shock, or severely injured, or who have sepsis. For ARF and RDS, the goal of nutrition therapy is to inhibit tissue destruction by providing extra nutrients for hypermetabolic

TABLE 17-8 Nutrient Content Claims

TERM	FAT	SATURATED FAT	CHOLESTEROL	SODIUM	KCAL
Free ("zero," "no," "without," "trivial source of," or "dietarily insignificant source of")	<0.5 g per reference amount*	<0.5 g saturated fat and <0.5 g *trans* fatty acids per reference amount	<2 mg per reference amount and per labeled serving	<5 mg per reference amount and per labeled amount	<5 kcal per serving
Low ("little," "few" for kcal, "contains a small amount of," "low source of")	≤3 g per serving	≤1 g per serving	≤20 mg per serving	≤140 mg per serving	≤40 kcal per serving
Light or lite	A product has one third fewer kcal than a comparable product or 50% of the fat found in a comparable product, or the sodium content of a low-kcal, low-fat food has been reduced by 50% ("light" may still be used to describe properties of food such as texture and color).				
Reduced/Less	A nutritionally altered product that contains 25% less of a nutrient or kcal than the regular product (this claim cannot be made on a product if the regular food already meets the requirement for "low").				
Free	A product contains virtually none of one or more of these: fat, saturated fat, cholesterol, sodium, sugars, and kcal.				
Lean†	<10 g fat, *plus*	4 g saturated fat	*And* <95 mg of cholesterol per serving and per 100 g		
Extra lean†	<5 g fat, *plus*	<2 g saturated fat	*And* <95 mg of cholesterol per serving and per 100 g		

*"Reference amount" is amount customarily consumed at one seating.
†Used to describe the fat content of meat, poultry, seafood, and game meats
Data from U.S. Food and Drug Administration: *Food labeling guide: guidance for industry,* Washington, DC, updated 2008, Author. Accessed August 26, 2013, from www.fda.gov/Food/GuidanceComplianceRegulatoryInformation/GuidanceDocuments/FoodLabelingNutrition/FoodLabelingGuide/default.htm.

conditions without contributing to the decline in pulmonary function.

Chronic Obstructive Pulmonary Disease

Energy required for breathing is something most of us often take for granted. High energy demands, however, occur in patients with COPD while they are just breathing. These patients therefore have an increased likelihood of malnutrition. It is common to see significant weight loss from both fat stores and muscle mass. Muscle wasting is most evident in the diaphragm and respiratory muscles. Thus, the presence of malnutrition contributes to the patient's decline.

Food and Nutrition Therapies

Malnutrition of individuals with COPD is multifactorial. Contributing factors include altered taste because of chronic mouth breathing and excessive sputum production, fatigue, anxiety, depression, increased energy requirements, frequent infections, and the side effects of multiple medications. Preventing malnutrition will not only help preserve muscle strength needed for pulmonary function but also maintain the integrity of the immune system. The first step in this prevention is to provide adequate nutrition. Anorexia, early satiety, nausea, and vomiting are all common in these patients. Box 17-5 discusses maximizing food intake in COPD.

Energy expenditure is usually elevated, but it will vary according to a person's level of physical activity. Moreover, energy balance and nitrogen balance go hand in hand;

visceral and somatic proteins can only be conserved if optimal energy balance is maintained. Indirect calorimetry is the most accurate method of determining energy expenditure for hospitalized patients with COPD. Adequate but not excessive protein stimulates the ventilatory drive. Patients may require 1.2 to 1.9 g protein per kg of body weight for maintenance and 1.6 to 2.5 g/kg for repletion.

Providing nutrients in proper combination is also important to reduce production of carbon dioxide and maintain pulmonary function. This issue is particularly crucial for the ventilator-dependent patient. When each type of macronutrient is metabolized, carbon dioxide and water are produced.

Respiratory Quotient

The respiratory quotient (RQ) is the ratio of carbon dioxide produced to the amount of oxygen consumed. Carbohydrate metabolism produces the greatest amount of carbon dioxide and therefore has the highest RQ. Physiologic range for RQ is 0.67 to 1.3. Fat metabolism produces the least amount of carbon dioxide and has the lowest RQ (0.7). An RQ greater than 1 may indicate that carbohydrate is the primary energy source, and it is evidence of accumulating carbon dioxide, making respiration that much more difficult for a patient with COPD. Nonprotein kcal should be divided evenly between fat and carbohydrate. The important issue is to provide adequate nutrition without overfeeding the patient. Overfeeding also produces an excessive amount of carbon dioxide and would be reflected in a RQ greater than 1.

BOX 17-5 Maximizing Food Intake in Chronic Obstructive Pulmonary Disease (COPD)

Although well-balanced, nutritionally sound meals are provided, it is sometimes difficult for patients with COPD to consume adequate amounts of nutrients, particularly in the home setting. Here are ideas to make mealtimes easier and more nutritious by increasing energy and protein without increasing the amount of food eaten.

Feeding the Patient with COPD

- Suggest that patients consume small, frequent meals.
- Encourage patients to eat the most when well rested, such as the first meal of the day.
- Encourage the use of high-calorie, high-protein supplements.
- Teach patients to swallow as little air as possible when eating.
- Encourage the use of easily prepared or convenience foods to decrease any fatigue.

In clinical and home health care settings:

- Eat high-calorie foods first.
- Try more frequent meals and snacks.
- Add margarine, butter, mayonnaise, sauces, gravies, and peanut butter to foods.

- Limit liquids at mealtimes.
- Try cold foods, which can give a more reduced sense of fullness than hot foods.
- Rest before meals.

In home health care settings:

- Keep favorite foods and snacks on hand.
- Keep ready-prepared meals available for periods of increased shortness of breath.
- Eat larger meals when you are not as tired.
- Avoid foods that you know cause gas.
- Add skim milk powder (2 tablespoons) to regular milk (8 oz) to add protein and kcal.
- Use milk or half-and-half instead of water when making soups, cereals, instant puddings, cocoa, or canned soups.
- Add grated cheese to sauces, vegetables, soups, and casseroles.
- Choose dessert recipes that contain egg, such as sponge cake, angel food cake, egg custard, bread pudding, and rice pudding.

Cystic Fibrosis

Cystic fibrosis (CF) is an autosomal recessive inherited disease of the mucus-producing exocrine glands. CF is characterized by high levels of sodium and chloride in saliva, tears and sweat, and highly viscous secretions in the pancreas, bronchi, bile ducts, and small intestine that may be obstructive. CF occurs in about 1 of every 3300 live births of white infants and 1 in every 15,300 nonwhite births. Physical signs such as growth retardation, failure to gain weight, abdominal protuberance, lack of subcutaneous fat, and poor muscle tone are common findings. Frequent pulmonary infections, pancreatic insufficiency, and gastrointestinal (GI) malabsorption put individuals with CF at great nutritional risk.

The average survival for a patient with CF in the United States is 37 years. Death most often results from malnutrition, bronchopneumonia, lung collapse, and cor pulmonale. The *Personal Perspectives* box Ways of Coping summarizes one young man's experience dealing with CF.

Food and Nutrition Therapies

Nutrition is of prime importance in the treatment of CF. Nutritional requirements vary depending on the age of the patient and severity of disease. Poor nutritional status because of undernutrition contributes to poor growth, pulmonary complications, and susceptibility to infection. The primary goal of nutritional therapy for patients with CF is to exceed the Dietary Reference Intakes (DRI) for kcal and all other nutrients by 1.2 to 2 times. Dietitians estimate individual energy requirements on the basis of basal metabolic rate, activity level, lung function, and fat absorption.

Improvements in pancreatic enzyme replacement therapy now allow higher amounts of dietary fat intake in patients with CF, which were previously prohibited. Because fat provides such a concentrated source of energy, it does not need

to be restricted as long as pancreatic enzyme replacement therapy is individualized according to the patient's intake. Although the sodium requirement may be considerably higher for patients with CF, routine sodium supplementation appears unnecessary because the average American diet contains an overabundance. Multivitamin supplements should be prescribed for all patients with CF. Additional fat-soluble vitamins may be prescribed as well, in a water-miscible form if fat malabsorption is severe.

Infants. Pancreatic enzyme replacement therapy should be used along with all types of milk products, including breast milk, in infants with CV. Supplemental fat or carbohydrate may be necessary for some infants to increase calorie density above 20 kcal/ounce. Introduction of solid food is no different from that in infants without CF.

Childhood to adulthood. Nutritional adequacy of the diet, compliance with pancreatic enzymes, and growth patterns should be closely monitored because as the child with CF becomes older and more independent, compliance may become questionable. Reevaluation of the patient's diet is important to ascertain whether recommendations are adequate to support growth and maintain nutritional status. As changes occur in the disease process and growth continues, nutritional needs also change. Weight gain, linear growth, and level of pancreatic enzyme replacement therapy should also be closely monitored and assessed during this time. The young adult with CF will continue to require pancreatic enzymes and extra calories and micronutrients.

Regular evaluation by a registered dietitian should be scheduled. Poor clinical outcomes are often associated with undernutrition; complicated clinical situations that directly affect nutrition include lung transplantation, cystic fibrosis–related diabetes, and bone health (Kalnins and Wilschanski, 2012).

Acute Respiratory Failure and Respiratory Distress Syndrome

Most patients in acute respiratory failure require mechanical ventilation, so in such cases, nutrition support may be provided via enteral or parenteral nutrition. Almost half of all patients with acute respiratory failure suffer from malnutrition, which impairs recovery and prolongs weaning from mechanical ventilation. A diet that minimizes carbon dioxide production while maintaining good nutrition is recommended.

Food and Nutrition Therapies
Malnutrition and the method of feeding will influence the outcome in respiratory disease or respiratory failure. Nutrition therapy is important to maintain or replenish nutritional status and can positively or negatively influence weaning from mechanical ventilation. Because a significant number of patients with pulmonary disease or respiratory failure have

clinically relevant malnutrition, nurses and other health care professionals caring for them should always be alert to alterations in nutritional status.

Nutrition support should be initiated as soon as possible to help wean the patient from the ventilator. Nutritional recommendations are similar to those for patients with COPD: high kcal, high protein, moderate to high (50% nonprotein kcal) fat, with moderate (50% nonprotein kcal) carbohydrate.

Enteral nutrition. Commercial formulas that provide 40% to 50% of total kcal from fat are available. Higher-caloric density formulas may be necessary when fluid is restricted in these patients. Low-osmolality feedings are started slowly to avoid gastric retention and diarrhea. Continuous administration is recommended unless otherwise contraindicated. Because patients with ARF or RDS are at risk for aspiration, special precautions, such as elevating the head of the bed or using a tube placed into the duodenum or jejunum, are necessary.

Parenteral nutrition. Parenteral nutrition may be needed in the treatment of acute respiratory failure. High glucose concentrations can lead to excess carbon dioxide production, making weaning from the ventilator more difficult; therefore, they should be avoided. The optimal parenteral solution should provide adequate protein to maintain nitrogen balance and 1 to 2 g of lipid per kilogram of body weight. Remaining caloric needs can then be met by carbohydrates. It is additionally recommended to infuse nutrition support for these clients over the whole 24 hours period, not just intermittently.

Nutrition status monitoring in the critically ill is best managed by qualified team members. Daily calorie counts, daily weights, and biochemical parameters are necessary to assess response to nutrition support. A comparison of nutritional intake with indirect calorimetry provides useful guidance to monitor the adequacy of nutrition support. Collaboration with clinical dietitians is best to monitor transition from parenteral to enteral feedings to conventional feeding.

Asthma

Oxidative stress plays a role in asthma; antioxidant dietary approaches might be valuable (Grieger, et al, 2013). Intake of fruits, vegetables, and whole grains other than wheat and rice provide dietary fibers, iron, magnesium, and phosphorus from natural sources and should be used often (Ruel, et al, 2013). In addition, vitamin D, fish oil, and vitamin C are protective nutrients. A healthy diet during pregnancy, childhood, and aging may reduce asthma exacerbations in this vulnerable population. Table 17-9 provides insight into a naturally antioxidant-rich diet. Figure 17-7 shows colorful antioxidant foods.

Tuberculosis

With the increasing prevalence of HIV/AIDS throughout the world, tuberculosis has returned as a significant health threat.

Nutrition support should be initiated as soon as possible in the patient with tuberculosis to prevent or correct weight loss and signs of malnutrition. Medications are many in this population, and strict adherence to scheduled administration will help achieve resolution of the disease. However, compliance is often a challenge.

Tuberculosis (TB) has been declared a global health emergency by the World Health Organization (Musa, et al, 2009). Nearly one third of the world's population is infected, and with international travel and immigration, more individuals will be exposed. Evidence supports the role of type 2 diabetes as an individual-level risk factor for TB (Goldhaber-Fiebert, et al, 2011). Interestingly, vitamin D may play a part in both conditions; low serum levels should be corrected in patients with T2DM to protect against TB infection.

TABLE 17-9 Antioxidant-Rich Foods	
FOOD	**ANTIOXIDANT NUTRIENTS**
Acorn squash, pumpkin, winter squash	Beta carotene
Apples	Catechins
Apricots, cantaloupe, peaches	Beta carotene
Beans	Catechins, vitamin E
Beets	Anthocyanins
Bell peppers	Beta carotene, vitamin C
Berries	Anthocyanins, catechins, ellagic acid (in raspberries and strawberries), resveratrol (in blueberries), vitamin C
Broccoli, greens, spinach	Beta carotene, lutein, vitamin C
Brown rice	Selenium
Carrots	Beta carotene
Chicken	Selenium
Citrus fruits	Vitamin C
Corn	Lutein
Egg	Lutein (in yolks); selenium, vitamin A
Eggplant	Anthocyanins
Garlic and onions	Selenium
Grapefruit, pink	Lycopene, vitamin C
Grapes, red wine	Anthocyanins (in red and purple grapes), resveratrol
Mango and papaya	Beta carotene, vitamin C
Milk	Vitamin A
Nuts, nut butters, oils, seeds	Vitamin E
Oatmeal	Selenium
Peanuts	Resveratrol
Prunes	Anthocyanins
Salmon, tuna, seafood	Selenium
Sweet potatoes	Beta carotene, vitamin C
Tea, black or green	Catechins
Tomatoes (canned)	Lycopene, vitamin C
Watermelon	Lycopene, vitamin C
Wheat germ, whole grains	Selenium, vitamin E

FIG 17-7 Colorful antioxidant foods for healthy lungs.

SUMMARY

- Cardiovascular disease consists of a group of diseases and conditions that affect the heart and blood vessels; they include CAD, HTN, PAD, CHF, and CHD.
- CVD risk factors are categorized into three groups: controllable, noncontrollable, and predisposing.
- Controllable or lifestyle factors include tobacco use, diet, and physical inactivity. Noncontrollable factors are gender, age, and family history.
- Predisposing conditions may be diabetes mellitus, hypertension, obesity, and dyslipidemia.
- Atherosclerosis is the chronic inflammatory development of lesions in coronary arteries that can lead to arteriosclerosis, angina pectoris, or myocardial infarction.
- If thrombosis occurs in a cerebral artery, a cerebrovascular accident or hemorrhagic stroke occurs.
- CAD risk is assessed through measurement of the total blood cholesterol and the proportions of the different types of lipoproteins that carry cholesterol in the blood.
- Plasma lipoproteins are synthesized in the liver; contain varying amounts of triglycerides, cholesterol, phospholipids, and proteins; and are classified according to composition and density.
- Kinds of plasma lipoproteins: chylomicrons, high-density lipoproteins (HDLs), low-density lipoproteins (LDLs), and very low-density lipoproteins (VLDLs).
- Lowering total cholesterol and LDL cholesterol can be achieved by dietary intervention, including weight loss and exercise.
- Goals of nutrition therapy are to reduce total fat, saturated fat, *trans* fatty acids, and cholesterol intake in an attempt to reduce plasma total cholesterol, LDL cholesterol, and triglyceride levels.
- HTN for which the cause is not known is called *primary* or *essential HTN*.
- In *secondary HTN*, the cause of elevated blood pressure can be identified.
- Prescribed treatment regimens for HTN are individualized and vary because the disease differs in its degree of severity.
- First line of treatment is usually nonpharmacologic, or focused on lifestyle modifications.

- Weight reduction and sodium restriction augment antihypertensive medications.
- MIs are the single largest killer of adults in the United States. The purpose of nutrition therapy in patients who have experienced them is to reduce the workload of the heart.
- CAD, lung disease, complications of hypothyroidism, or damage to the myocardial or cardiac muscle can cause cardiac failure.
- HF is characterized by decreased blood flow to the kidneys and retention of sodium and fluid. Patients with HF often experience edema of the feet and ankles and shortness of breath.
- To lessen the workload of the heart, also desirable in HF, nutrition therapy focuses on restricting dietary sodium.
- Pulmonary disease is characterized by wasting and malnutrition, largely due to the effect of the disorder or the secondary consequences of treatment on the GI tract.
- Two categories of pulmonary disorders cause either chronic changes in pulmonary function, such as COPD and cystic fibrosis, or acute changes in pulmonary function, such as RDS and ARF.
- The goal of nutrition therapy for COPD is to maintain respiratory muscle strength and function while preventing or treating existing malnutrition.
- As pulmonary disorders progress, nutritional status tends to decline and malnutrition exacerbates, reducing respiratory muscle function and ventilatory drive.
- ARF and RDS may develop in patients who are critically ill, in shock, or severely injured, or have sepsis.
- For ARF and RDS, the function of nutrition therapy is to inhibit tissue destruction by providing the extra nutrients required for hypermetabolic conditions.
- Malnutrition and the method of refeeding influence the outcome in pulmonary disease or respiratory failure.
- Cystic fibrosis, tuberculosis, asthma, and related pulmonary disorders warrant regularly scheduled contact with a registered dietitian, especially patients at high risk for malnutrition and those with multiple disorders.

THE NURSING APPROACH

Case Study: Hypertension and Heart Failure

The home health nurse visited Reba, a 70-year-old African American woman who had been diagnosed with heart failure and hypertension. Lab tests revealed elevated triglycerides, cholesterol, and LDL cholesterol. The nurse had first become acquainted with Reba when Reba was discharged from the hospital after an acute episode of pulmonary edema. The physician advised Reba to begin a walking program, starting slowly.

The physician prescribed a 2-gram-sodium, low-fat, low-calorie diet. Several medications had been prescribed, including digoxin, a diuretic, and a vasodilator. In a previous visit, the nurse instructed Reba to monitor her pulse and blood pressure daily, and to weigh herself daily. The purpose of this follow-up visit was to determine the patient's compliance with the treatment plan and to assess her current health status.

THE NURSING APPROACH—cont'd

Assessment

Subjective (from Patient Statements)

- "Sometimes I forget whether I have taken my medicines."
- "I've kept a record of my pulse, blood pressure, and weight almost every day."
- "Today I weighed 2 pounds more than I did when I was in the hospital."
- "I feel really tired. I get short of breath when I climb stairs (dyspnea). I haven't been going for walks."
- "I have trouble breathing when I lie down at night" (orthopnea).
- "I usually warm up a can of soup or a frozen dinner because I am too tired to cook. I like it when my granddaughter brings me cake and doughnuts."

Objective (from Physical Examination)

- Height 5 feet 8 inches, weight 182 pounds with truncal obesity
- Blood pressure 162/85 mm Hg, temperature 98°F, pulse 92 irregular; respirations 18, unlabored
- Lung sounds clear
- Pitting edema in ankles
- Jugular venous distention

Diagnoses (Nursing)

1. Excess fluid volume related to decreased cardiac output and excess sodium intake as evidenced by blood pressure 162/85, pitting edema of ankles, jugular venous distention, weight 2 pounds higher than during hospitalization
2. Decreased cardiac output related to hypertension, weakened cardiac muscles, and obesity as evidenced by pulse 92 irregular, fatigue, shortness of breath with activity, and orthopnea

Planning

Patient Outcomes

Short term (at the end of this visit):

- Reba will agree to meet with a dietitian to learn about an individualized nutrition plan and healthy food choices.
- She will commit to read labels and choose foods lower in sodium and fat.
- She will plan to obtain a small medicine organizer.

Long term (at follow-up visit in 1 month):

- Weight 178 pounds; blood pressure 140/85
- Edema absent or nonpitting, lungs clear
- Reports less fatigue; walking short distances regularly
- Electrolyte values within normal range and lipid levels reduced

Nursing Interventions

1. Check Reba's home records of blood pressure, pulse, and weight.
2. Teach her about general dietary measures to reduce her edema.
3. Set up an appointment with a dietitian for an individualized plan.
4. Review her medications and teach her when to notify the doctor.

Implementation

1. Measured vital signs, reviewed the log that Reba had recorded, and praised Reba for her conscientious efforts.
   Vital signs help determine the effectiveness of treatments for heart failure and hypertension. Praise often motivates a patient to continue positive behaviors.
   a. Asked Reba to demonstrate how she takes her pulse and blood pressure, using her home blood pressure monitoring equipment.
   b. Compared Reba's results with the nurse's.
   In order to look for valid trends in results, accuracy of measurement technique is needed.
2. Reviewed Reba's record of daily weights and explained how weight increases with excessive sodium intake.
   a. Taught Reba that sodium causes the body to retain fluid, contributing to weight gain, edema, and dyspnea (difficulty breathing).
   b. Showed Reba how to read labels and choose soups and frozen dinners that are lower in sodium.
   c. Gave her a list of foods that are high in sodium and thus should be limited or avoided.
   d. Told her about herbs that can be used in place of salt to flavor food.
   Patients are more likely to comply with nutrition therapy if they understand the reasons for restrictions and are given practical suggestions as to how to adhere to guidelines.
3. Taught Reba guidelines for making healthy food choices based on fat and calories.
   a. Recommended eating fish and chicken instead of red meat as well as increasing whole grains, fruits and vegetables, and skim milk (with lactase if needed).
   Omega-3 fatty acids from fish may reduce clot formation, reducing the risk of coronary occlusion. Red meat is a source of cholesterol. Soluble fiber can help reduce LDL cholesterol levels. Lactase additives can be added to milk if necessary because many African Americans have lactose intolerance.
   b. Explained that low-fat, low-cholesterol foods help minimize fatty deposits in the blood vessels and heart.
   A decrease in saturated fats, cholesterol, and trans fats minimizes formation of atherosclerosis.
   c. Recommended nutritious low-calorie foods to help Reba lose weight and thus decrease the workload of the heart.
   Obesity increases peripheral resistance and cardiac workload. Reducing high-fat desserts can help with weight loss and reduction of lipid levels.
11. Referred Reba to the American Heart Association for additional information and simple recipes.
12. Recommended small, frequent meals rather than large meals, with rest periods before meal preparation and eating.
   Small meals require less energy for eating and digesting food. Rest periods can reduce oxygen consumption, relieve shortness of breath and fatigue, and help increase appetite.
5. Asked Reba to show the nurse her medications, and recommended placing medications in a small weekly organizer.

Continued

◎ THE NURSING APPROACH—cont'd

Small medicine holders may designate the days of the week, alerting the patient to whether medicine has been taken on a particular day.

 a. Asked Reba to tell the nurse the purpose of each medicine and when each should be taken.

  Verifying a patient's understanding of prescribed medications is important for safety and effectiveness

 b. Informed Reba about special precautions needed when taking her medications.

  Digoxin increases stroke volume by strengthening cardiac muscles, but if doses are excessive, nausea and vomiting may occur, and the pulse rate may drop too low. The patient should withhold the medicine if the pulse is below 60. Diuretics promote loss of sodium and fluid but may also waste potassium. Frequent lab tests are necessary to determine digoxin and potassium levels. Vasodilators decrease peripheral resistance, but they can produce orthostatic hypotension. Patients should be advised to rise slowly from bed to avoid becoming dizzy.

6. Drew blood for the lab to check digoxin and electrolyte levels. Told Reba that she may need to eat more foods high in potassium because of the diuretic she was taking.

  Some diuretics waste potassium, but other medicines may conserve potassium. Electrolytes need to be checked regularly because there is danger of death if the potassium levels are too high or too low. Low potassium contributes to digoxin toxicity, so a potassium supplement may be prescribed. Foods high in potassium include fruits (especially bananas and citrus), vegetables (especially green leafy), dairy products, meats, and legumes.

7. Instructed Reba regarding when to call the doctor—for example, when she gains 3 pounds or more in 2 days, when she has difficulty breathing, and when edema gets worse. Also, she should call if her blood pressure is 180/90 or higher and/or her pulse is below 60.

A gain of 1 kg of weight (2.2 pounds) could indicate retention of 1 L of fluid. Hypertension may lead to a stroke, so medications may need to be adjusted.

8. Set up an appointment with a dietitian for an individualized nutrition plan.

 Because the diet combines several components, it could be confusing to the patient. The DASH (Dietary Approaches to Stop Hypertension) diet focuses on low sodium. The TLC (Therapeutic Lifestyle Changes) diet and low-calorie diets focus on low fat.

9. Encouraged her to begin a walking program for 10 minutes each day, as approved by the doctor.

 Regular exercise strengthens cardiac muscle and increases peripheral vascular blood flow. It also helps with weight reduction.

Evaluation

Short term (at the end of the visit):

- Reba agreed to meet with a dietitian.
- She said she would read labels and choose foods lower in sodium and fat.
- She planned to ask her granddaughter to buy a small medicine organizer at the drugstore for her.
- Reba made an appointment with the nurse for a visit in 1 month.

Goals met.

Discussion Questions

1. Compare and contrast the basic principles of the TLC diet and the DASH diet.
2. *Trans* fats increase LDL levels and decrease HDL cholesterol levels, so they should be restricted. Which foods are likely to contain *trans* fats and thus should be avoided?

？CRITICAL THINKING

Clinical Applications

Kevin, age 69, is admitted to the coronary care unit of your hospital. He is 6 feet tall, has a medium frame, and weighs 210 pounds. He has gained 30 pounds since he retired 4 years ago, which he attributes to boredom and lack of exercise. Three months before admission, Kevin began to experience chest pain that radiated up his neck and down to his stomach. He has a history of hypertension and elevated serum cholesterol levels. After admission to the hospital, Kevin is diagnosed with having had an acute myocardial infarction.

Test results for serum lipids are as follows:

Cholesterol: 300 mg/dL

LDL-c cholesterol: 200 mg/dL

HDL-c cholesterol: 30 mg/dL

Triglycerides: 600 mg/dL

Medications prescribed after admission: atenolol (Tenormin), diltiazem (Cardizem), nitroglycerin

Diet order: TLC diet

1. What are the risk factors for cardiovascular disease?

2. What are Kevin's risk factors?
3. Define the term *myocardial infarction* and describe what happens when a myocardial infarction occurs.
4. What specific guidelines are included in the National Cholesterol Education Program's (NCEP) TLC diet recommendations?

While caring for Kevin you learn that he snacks on high-fat cheeses, ice cream, potato chips, corn chips, peanuts, and crackers. He also drinks whole milk and eats a lot of butter on his bread at every meal. What characteristics of Kevin's intake contradict the NCEP's TLC diet recommendations? What are some alternative foods that are appealing to Kevin that he could eat for snacks?

▮ WEBSITES OF INTEREST

American Heart Association (AHA)

www.americanheart.org

Contains resources, interactive educational materials, and everyday strategies and support for prevention and treatment of heart disease and stroke.

National Cholesterol Education Program (NCEP)

www.nhlbi.nih.gov/chd

Makes available the wide ranges of educational and research programs of NCEP.

World Hypertension League (WHL)

www.worldhypertensionleague.org

Advocates for the detection, prevention, and treatment of HTN in populations globally through association with the World Health Organization.

REFERENCES

American Heart Association: Heart and stroke facts, n.d. from: www.americanheart.org/presenter.jhtml?identifier=3000333. Accessed August 25, 2013.

Carmody JB, Charlton JR: Short-term gestation, long-term risk: Prematurity and chronic kidney disease, *Pediatrics* 131:1168–1179, 2013.

Centers for Disease Control and Prevention: CDC grand rounds: Dietary sodium reduction—time for choice, *MMWR Morb Mortal Wkly Rep* 61:89–91, 2012.

Drager LF, et al: Obstructive sleep apnea and dyslipidemia: Implications for atherosclerosis, *Curr Opin Endocrinol Diabetes Obes* 17:161–165, 2010.

Estruch R, et al: Primary prevention of cardiovascular disease with a Mediterranean diet, *N Engl J Med* 368:1279–1290, 2013.

Freeland-Graves JH, et al: Position of the Academy Of Nutrition and Dietetics: Total diet approach to healthy eating, *J Acad Nutr Diet* 113:307–317, 2013.

Goldhaber-Fiebert JD, et al: Diabetes mellitus and tuberculosis in countries with high tuberculosis burdens: Individual risks and social determinants, *Int J Epidemiol* 40:417–428, 2011.

Graudal NA, et al: Effects of low sodium diet versus high sodium diet on blood pressure, renin, aldosterone, catecholamines, cholesterol, and triglyceride, *Cochrane Database Syst Rev* (11):CD004022, 2011.

Grieger JA, et al: Improving asthma during pregnancy with dietary antioxidants: The current evidence, *Nutrients* 5:3212–3234, 2013.

Hamoud S, et al: Niacin administration significantly reduces oxidative stress in patients with hypercholesterolemia and low levels of high-density lipoprotein cholesterol, *Am J Med Sci* 345:195–199, 2013.

Harland JI: Food combinations for cholesterol lowering, *Nutr Res Rev* 25:249–266, 2012.

Jiang Y, et al: Serum lipoprotein(a) positively correlates with coronary artery calcification in low-risk Chinese Han patients: A study from a single center, *PLoS ONE* 8:e71673, 2013.

Kalnins D, Wilschanski M: Maintenance of nutritional status in patients with cystic fibrosis: New and emerging therapies, *Drug Des Devel Ther* 6:151–161, 2012.

Kones R: Primary prevention of coronary heart disease: Integration of new data, evolving views, revised goals, and role of rosuvastatin in management: A comprehensive survey, *Drug Des Devel Ther* 5:325–380, 2011.

Lin L, et al: Evidence of health benefits of canola oil, *Nutr Rev* 71:370–385, 2013.

Liu Y, et al: Nuclear transport modulation reduces hypercholesterolemia, atherosclerosis, and fatty liver, *J Am Heart Assoc* 2:e000093, 2013.

Musa TL, et al: The tuberculosis structural genomics consortium: A structural genomics approach to drug discovery, *Adv Protein Chem Struct Biol* 77:41, 2009.

National Institutes of Health, National Heart, Lung, and Blood Institute: DASH eating plan: Lower your blood pressure *(NIH Publ 06-4082)*, 2006. From: www.nhlbi.nih.gov/health/public/heart/hbp/dash/new_dash.pdf. Accessed August 28, 2013.

NHLBI: Management of Blood Cholesterol in Adults: Systematic Evidence Review from the Cholesterol Expert Panel. Accessed July 20, 104 at http://www.nhlbi.nih.gov/guidelines/cholesterol/ser/.

Rautiainen S, et al: Total antioxidant capacity from diet and risk of myocardial infarction: A prospective cohort of women, *Am J Med* 125:974–980, 2012.

Ried K, et al: Effect of cocoa on blood pressure, *Cochrane Database Syst Rev* (8):CD008893, 2012.

Ruel G, et al: Association between nutrition and the evolution of multimorbidity: The importance of fruits and vegetables and whole grain products, *Clin Nutr* 33(3):513–520, 2013.

Sharma A, et al: Abnormal lipoprotein(a) levels predict coronary artery calcification in Southeast Asians but not in Caucasians: Use of noninvasive imaging for evaluation of an emerging risk factor, *J Cardiovasc Transl Res* 4:470–476, 2011.

Shinkai H: Cholesteryl ester transfer-protein modulator and inhibitors and their potential for the treatment of cardiovascular diseases, *Vasc Health Risk Manag* 8:323–331, 2012.

Tsioufis C, et al: Preclinical cardiorenal interrelationships in essential hypertension, *Cardiorenal Med* 3(1):38–47, 2013.

Tuttle KR, et al: Comparison of low-fat versus Mediterranean-style dietary intervention after first myocardial infarction (from The Heart Institute of Spokane Diet Intervention and Evaluation Trial), *Am J Cardiol* 101:1523–1530, 2008.

Yuan WL, et al: Influence of dairy product consumption on children's blood pressure: results from the QUALITY cohort, *J Acad Nutr Diet* 113:936–941, 2013.

18 | CHAPTER

Nutrition for Diseases of the Kidneys

The chief life-preserving function of the kidneys is to maintain chemical homeostasis in the body.

e http://evolve.elsevier.com/GRODNER/FOUNDATIONS

LEARNING OBJECTIVES

- State the primary function of the kidneys.
- Discuss the cause and potential results of nephrotic syndrome.
- Identify determinates of nutrition needs in acute renal failure (ARF).
- Describe chronic kidney disease (CKD) and the focus of management during CKD and end-stage renal failure.

- Summarize the factors and objectives to be considered in the implementation of the National Renal Diet.
- Explain the composition of renal calculi and ways to reduce risk of stone formation.

THE KIDNEY IN HEALTH

Although often taken for granted, kidneys filter approximately 1 L of blood per minute to remove excess fluid and more than 200 waste products from the body. They also perform vital metabolic and hormonal functions. Because kidneys play so many roles in wellness, kidney disease has serious consequences. The nutritional needs of patients with kidney disease are complex, ever-changing, and demanding. These factors present a challenge to doctors, nurses, dietitians, and other health care team members.

Functions of the kidneys affect total physical well-being. Nutrition therapy is essential for enhancing the *physical health* dimension. *Intellectual health* requires clients to understand their own anatomy and physiology, to fully comprehend their kidney disorder, and to follow a complicated diet. The chronic nature and potentially life-threatening aspects of kidney disorders may be *emotionally* draining. *Social health* is also strained. Significant others are worn down by the responsibility of caring for loved ones with renal disorders. Dialysis disrupts normal routines and social relationships. *Healthy spirituality* may lower blood pressure and actually enhance the physical response to treatment. *Environmental health* may be affected by the presence of excessive amounts of sodium and other minerals in the water supply.

KIDNEY FUNCTION

The chief life-preserving function of the kidneys is to maintain chemical homeostasis in the body. They process components within the blood to maintain fluid, electrolyte, and acid-base balance by eliminating wastes in the urine. Each kidney has approximately 1 million "microscopic" workhorses called *nephrons* (Figure 18-1).

Each nephron filters and resorbs essential blood constituents, secretes ions as needed to maintain acid-base balance, and excretes fluid and other substances as urine. Other important functions of kidneys are manufacturing hormones to regulate blood pressure (renin), stimulating production of red blood cells (erythropoietin), and regulating calcium and phosphorus metabolism in the final step of vitamin D synthesis. Kidneys also detoxify some drugs and poisons (Box 18-1).

Various inflammatory, obstructive, and degenerative diseases affect kidneys in different ways. These disorders interfere with nephron regulation of the products of metabolism. Ultimately, kidney failure could lead to homeostatic failure and, if not relieved, death. There are 4.4 million noninstitutionalized U.S. adults with diagnosed kidney disease, and kidney diseases rank eighth as a cause of death in Americans (Centers for Disease Control and Prevention [CDC], 2012).

NEPHROTIC SYNDROME

Nephrotic syndrome describes a complex of symptoms that can occur as a result of damage to the capillary walls of the glomerulus. Glomerular damage results in increased urinary excretion of protein (proteinuria), which leads to decreased serum levels of albumin (hypoalbuminemia), hyperlipidemia, and edema. Nephrotic syndrome is often the result of a secondary disease process: primary glomerular

FIG 18-1 The nephron. Blood flows into the glomerulus, and some of its fluid is absorbed into the tubule. Waste products are filtered and passed through the tubule into the bladder. The fluid and dissolved substances needed by the body are resorbed in vessels alongside the tubule. (From Ignatavicius DD, Workman L: *Medical-surgical nursing: Patient-centered collaborative care,* ed 7, St. Louis, 2013, Elsevier Saunders.)

BOX 18-1 Kidney Functions

- Maintain fluid, electrolyte, and acid-base balance
- Eliminate waste products
- Regulate blood pressure
- Stimulate red blood cell production
- Regulate calcium and phosphorus metabolism
- Eliminate many drugs
- Release important hormones: renin, erythropoietin, calcitriol

Adapted from National Kidney Center: *Chronic kidney disease: Facts,* n.d. Accessed September 23, 2013, from www.nationalkidneycenter.org/chronic-kidney-disease/facts/

---

disease (glomerulonephritis), nephropathy secondary to amyloidosis (accumulation of waxy starchlike glycoprotein), diabetes mellitus, systemic lupus erythematosus (SLE) (a chronic inflammatory disease affecting many body systems), or infectious disease. The syndrome may be treated with corticosteroid or immunosuppressive medications, but in some patients, it is resistant to treatment and may progress to renal failure.

Food and Nutrition Therapies

Primary goals are to control hypertension, minimize edema, decrease urinary albumin losses, prevent protein malnutrition and muscle catabolism, supply adequate energy, and

---

BOX 18-2 Foods High in Sodium

Condiments
Pickles, olives (black and green), salted nuts, meat tenderizers, commercial salad dressings, monosodium glutamate (MSG, Accent), steak sauce, ketchup, soy sauce, Worcestershire sauce, horseradish sauce, chili sauce, commercial mustard, salt, seasoned salts (onion, garlic, celery), butter salt

Breads/Starches
Salted crackers, potato chips, corn chips, popcorn, pretzels, dehydrated potatoes

Meats/Meat Substitutes
Cured, smoked, and processed meats (ham, bacon, corned beef, chipped beef, hot dogs, luncheon meats, bologna, salt pork, canned salmon, and tuna); all cheeses except low-sodium and cottage cheese; convenience foods (microwave and TV dinners); peanut butter

Beverages
Commercial buttermilk, instant hot cocoa mixes

Soups
Canned soups, dehydrated soups, bouillon

Vegetables
Sauerkraut, hominy, pork and beans, canned tomato and vegetable juices

For more detail, see University of California San Francisco Medical Center: *Guidelines for a low sodium diet,* n.d. Accessed September 23, 2013, from www.ucsfhealth.org/education/guidelines_for_a_low_sodium_diet/.

---

slow the progression of renal disease. Patients need to consume adequate amounts of protein (0.7 to 1 g/kg/day) and energy (35 kcal/kg/day) to prevent malnutrition from catabolism of lean body tissue. Complex carbohydrates should provide the majority of a patient's kcal because protein may have to be limited. In addition, reducing dietary sodium intake may be necessary to control hypertension and edema (see Chapter 17).

Role of Nursing

It is essential for nursing personnel to monitor and document patient weights and intake and output (I&O); I&O should be recorded at least during every shift. Indeed, the nurse and dietitian often develop the care plan together. They partner in educating patients about dietary advice, including foods high in sodium (Box 18-2).

A high dietary sodium intake is detrimental to the nephron, often contributing to high blood pressure and a more rapid decline in renal status (Ruta, et al, 2010). Commercial preparation of processed foods often adds substantial amounts of sodium. Hidden sources of salt may also be found in the water supply, medications, even oral hygiene products. Because toothpaste and mouthwash often contain a significant amount of sodium, patients should be instructed not to

BOX 18-3	Hidden Sources of Sodium

- Baking powder
- Drinking and cooking water
- Medications:
  - Antacids
  - Antibiotics
  - Cough medicines
  - Laxatives
  - Pain relievers
  - Sedatives
- Mouthwash
- Toothpaste

BOX 18-4	Foods High in Potassium

- Apricots, melons
- Banana; 1 medium: 422 mg
- Broccoli; 1 cup, cooked: 457 mg
- Cantaloupe; cubed, 1 cup: 431 mg
- Carrots, raw
- Chicken breast; 3 ounces, cooked: 218 mg
- Dried fruits
- Halibut; 3 ounces, cooked: 490 mg
- Lentils; half cup, cooked: 366 mg
- Milk; 1% low fat, 8 ounces: 366 mg
- Orange juice (100%); 8 ounces: 496 mg
- Pistachios; shelled, 1 ounce, dry roasted: 295 mg
- Pork tenderloin; 3 ounces, cooked: 382 mg
- Potato; medium, baked with skin: 610 mg
- Raisins; quarter cup: 250 mg
- Salmon; farmed Atlantic, 3 ounces, cooked: 326 mg
- Sweet potato; medium, baked with skin: 694 mg
- Tomatoes, tomato juice, tomato sauce
- Tuna; light, canned, drained, 3 ounces: 201 mg
- White beans; canned, drained, half cup: 595 mg
- Winter squash; cubed, 1 cup, cooked: 896 mg
- Yogurt; fat-free, 1 cup: 579 mg

From WebMD. *Food & recipes. Are you getting enough potassium?* n.d. Accessed September 23, 2013, from www.webmd.com/food-recipes/features/potassium-sources-and-benefits?page=2

swallow them (Box 18-3). For more specific sodium content of foods, consult the Food Composition Table on the Evolve website.

ACUTE RENAL FAILURE

Acute renal failure (ARF) is characterized by an abrupt loss of renal function that may or may not be accompanied by oliguria or anuria. The most common cause of ARF is either acute tubular necrosis (ATN), which is injury after a decreased blood supply, or a nephrotoxic cause, such as certain medications. Although a few patients do not experience any reduction in urine output, many experience the following three stages:

Oliguric phase (24 to 48 hours after initial injury, lasting approximately 1 to 3 weeks): Manifested by retention of excessive amounts of nitrogenous compounds in the blood, acidosis, high serum potassium and phosphorus levels, hypertension, anorexia, edema, and risk of water intoxication (indicated by low sodium levels).

Diuretic phase (lasts 2 to 3 weeks): Urinary output is gradually increased.

Recovery phase (lasts 3 to 12 months): Kidney function gradually improves, but there may be some residual permanent damage.

Most patients with ARF require at least a short period of dialysis. Dialysis allows diffusion of waste particles to move from an area of high to one of lower concentration, osmosis of fluid across the membrane, and movement of fluid (urine) across the membrane as a result of an artificially created pressure differential.

Food and Nutrition Therapies

The underlying cause of the ARF will be one determinant of nutrient requirements. Patients may be hypermetabolic if renal failure is caused by trauma, burns, septicemia, or infection. These conditions and renal failure have a negative affect on the patient's appetite, thus increasing the risk for rapid nutritional decline. Nonprotein calories should be provided in sufficient amounts for weight maintenance and to meet the demands of the stress of ARF, usually 30 to 40 kcal/kg. Fats, oils, simple carbohydrates, and low-protein starches are given.

If dialysis is not necessary for treatment, 0.6 g to 0.8 g of protein per kg body weight is often provided.

When dialysis is used as part of the medical treatment, protein intake can be liberalized to 1.0 to 1.4 g/kg. In either situation, use of high-quality proteins (high biologic value, usually animal sources) will be recommended. Diets containing less than 60 g of protein per day may be deficient in niacin, riboflavin, thiamine, calcium, iron, vitamin B_{12}, and zinc, and these nutrients may need to be supplemented during convalescence.

During the oliguric phase, sodium may be restricted to 1000 to 2000 mg and potassium to 1000 mg per day. Both sodium and potassium, the principal electrolytes, may be lost during the diuretic phase or during dialysis. Therefore, losses should be replaced as needed, depending on urinary volume, serum levels, and frequency of dialysis. Box 18-4 lists foods high in potassium.

Another nutrient of great importance is phosphorus. Over time, diets that are not controlled for phosphorus, potassium, and protein-energy malnutrition are associated with a greater risk for bone and heart diseases. High phosphorus intakes in excess of basic nutrient needs of a healthy population may significantly disrupt the hormonal regulation of phosphate, calcium, and vitamin D, leading to impaired kidney function (Calvo an Uribarri, 2013).

Role of Nursing

Fluids are usually restricted to the amount of the patient's output (urine, vomitus, and diarrhea) plus 500 mL during

TABLE 18-1   **Treatments and Major Concerns for Pre–End-Stage Renal Disease (ESRD), Hemodialysis, and Peritoneal Dialysis**

	PRE-ESRD	HEMODIALYSIS	PERITONEAL DIALYSIS
Treatment modalities	Diet + medication	Diet + medication + hemodialysis Dialysis using vascular access for waste product and fluid removal	Diet + medication + peritoneal dialysis Dialysis using peritoneal membrane for waste product and fluid removal
Duration concerns	Indefinite Hypertension, glycemic control in patients with diabetes mellitus	3-4 hours 3 days/week Bone disease, hypertension	3-5 exchanges 7 days/week Bone disease, weight gain, hyperlipidemia, glycemic control in patients with diabetes mellitus
	Glomerular hyperfiltration, rise in blood urea nitrogen, bone disease	Amino acid loss, interdialytic electrolyte and fluid changes	Protein loss into dialysate, glucose absorption from dialysate
	Anemia, cardiovascular disease	Anemia, cardiovascular disease	Anemia, cardiovascular disease

Data from Academy of Nutrition and Dietetics: *Chronic kidney disease nutrition management module 1—Chronic kidney disease basics: Epidemiology, identification and monitoring and medical nutrition therapy,* Chicago, 2013, Author.

the oliguric phase. During the diuretic phase, large amounts of fluid may be needed to replace losses. Close monitoring of intake and output is essential. Nurses should be watchful for constipation as a result of restricted intake of fluids and fresh fruits (most are high in potassium), bed rest, and medication side effects.

Nurses help coordinate patient and family education with the renal dietitian. Complex nutrition education often involves reduced protein, sodium, potassium, phosphorus, and fluid intake. The Food Composition Table on the Evolve website lists the specific protein, sodium, potassium and phosphorus content of foods. The nurse should encourage patients to reduce consumption of highly processed foods, especially restaurant meals, fast foods, and convenience foods (Calvo and Uribarri, 2013).

CHRONIC KIDNEY DISEASE

Chronic kidney disease (CKD) involves progressive, irreversible loss of kidney function over days, months, or years. Many causes are possible, but some of the most common are glomerulonephritis, nephrosclerosis (necrosis of the renal arterioles from hypertension), obstructive diseases (kidney stones, tumors, congenital birth defects of kidneys and urinary tract), diabetes mellitus, SLE, and illicit use of analgesics or street drugs. Regardless of the cause, results will include retention of nitrogenous waste products and fluid and electrolyte imbalances that affect all body systems.

Before dialysis is required, management focuses on slowing the progression and minimizing complications. Once CKD reaches end-stage renal disease (ESRD), management centers on reducing uremia (excessive amounts of urea and other nitrogenous waste products in the blood) by various renal replacement treatments: hemodialysis, peritoneal dialysis (PD), or renal transplantation.

Food and Nutrition Therapies

Medical nutrition therapy (MNT) is a legal term regulated by the federal government that allows Medicare recipients to have "pre–end-stage renal disease" nutrition counseling from a qualified renal dietitian. The goal is to slow or prevent the progression to the need for dialysis. Ideally, all individuals at risk for renal failure should be given personalized nutrition counseling and advice. Planning requires the renal dietitian to evaluate the results of laboratory assessments (blood urea nitrogen [BUN], creatinine, sodium, potassium, phosphorus, glucose). The next step is to determine current versus ideal fluid, energy, protein, lipid, phosphorus, potassium, sodium, vitamin, and mineral intakes from meals or nutrition support.

Nutritional management depends on method of treatment in addition to medical and nutritional status of the patient (National Kidney Foundation, 2013.). Table 18-1 provides a comparison of the treatment methods and primary concerns associated with each. The National Kidney Foundation (NKF) provides updated guidelines as new evidence suggests (see http://www.kidney.org/professionals/kdoqi/guidelines_commentaries.cfm). For example, the Kidney Disease Outcomes Quality Initiative (KDOQI) updated its guidance for managing CKD and diabetes in 2012 (NKF, 2012).

The exact point at which nutrition therapy should begin is variable, but dietary modifications (Table 18-2) should start as early as possible to minimize uremic toxicity, delay progression of renal disease, and prevent wasting and malnutrition. This can be accomplished by limiting foods in which metabolic byproducts add to buildup of such toxic substances and by providing adequate kcal to prevent body tissue catabolism.

It is important to design food combinations that include necessary nutrients and foods that the patient accepts and enjoys. This task is complicated, but there are renal dietitian specialists who are credentialed (Board Certified Specialist in Renal Nutrition [CSR]) and enjoy the challenge. High–biologic value proteins (eggs, meats, poultry, game, fish, soy, and dairy products) are the preferred protein sources for patients with renal disease. Some protein foods in vegan diets are of low biologic value. Ovo-vegetarian and ovo-lacto vegetarian diets include high–biologic value protein sources, but they also tend to be high in phosphorus. Thus, careful planning is required. Box 18-5 provides a sample menu based on tips from the National Renal Diet.

TABLE 18-2 Nutrition Guidelines for Chronic Renal Failure (CRF) Without Dialysis, CRF With Hemodialysis or Peritoneal Dialysis

NUTRIENT	CRF WITHOUT DIALYSIS	HEMODIALYSIS	PERITONEAL DIALYSIS	COMMENTS
Energy	30-35 kcal/kg ideal body weight (IBW)	35 kcal/kg IBW if <age 60; 30-35 kcal/kg IBW if >age 60	30-35 kcal/kg IBW	
Protein	0.6-1.0 g/kg IBW	1.2 g/kg IBW	1.2-1.3 g/kg IBW	At least 50% from high–biologic value animal plant sources
Sodium	Individualized, 2-3 g/day	2-3 g/day	2-4 g/day	
Potassium	Individualized to cover losses with diuretics	2-3 g/day	3-4 g/day	
Phosphorus	8-12 mg/kg IBW or 0.8-1.2 g/day	0.8-1.2 g/day or <17 mg/kg IBW	0.8-1.2 g/day	May require phosphate binder
Fluid	As desired	750-1000 mL + urine output/day	Unrestricted if weight and blood pressure controlled and residual renal function is 2-3 L/day	
Vitamin/mineral supplementation	As appropriate	As appropriate	As appropriate	Supplements designed specially for patients undergoing dialysis are available; supplements of vitamin C should not exceed 100 mg/day to prevent hyperoxalemia; vitamin A supplementation is not recommended; in patients receiving recombinant human erythropoietin (rHuEPO), iron supplementation is almost always required; zinc supplementation may be helpful for patients with impaired taste

Data from National Kidney Foundation, Kidney Dialysis Outcomes Quality Initiative: *KDOQI clinical practice guidelines for nutrition in chronic renal failure,* 2000. Accessed August 29, 2013, from www.kidney.org/professionals/kdoqi/guidelines_updates/doqi_nut.html.

In view of the fact that malnutrition is so clearly associated with mortality in renal failure, continuing to assess nutritional status and dietary compliance is important. One point of emphasis is that the renal guidelines and food lists are only a starting point for individualized meal plans and education. Patient compliance is enhanced by designing meal plans to meet the specific needs of each patient.

An interesting fact about sodium must be considered. The neutralization of dietary acid with sodium bicarbonate (along with increased potassium intake from fruits and vegetables) will decrease kidney injury and slow the decline of the glomerular filtration rate (GFR) in patients with CKD (Goraya, et al, 2012). Thus, it is important to teach about the proper intake of both sodium and potassium needed for acid-base balance.

Role of Nursing

Patients often find the renal diet difficult to follow for a long period. Motivation, support, and encouragement are crucial. Nurses play an important role in helping patients maintain good nutritional status, weight, morale, and appetite by reinforcing the nutrition education. Through formal and informal teaching, nurses can help patients appreciate the need for the stringent diet.

There is a direct relationship between adherence to the diet and symptoms that reduce quality of life. Because patients may find that foods "don't taste like they used to," nurses should encourage the use of spices such as garlic, onions, and oregano to enhance the flavor of allowed foods. They should also discuss any patient concerns with the renal dietitian so they can be resolved.

HEMODIALYSIS

During hemodialysis, blood is shunted from the patient's body by way of a special vascular access or shunt (usually in the nondominant forearm), thinned with heparin, cleansed of excess fluid and waste products through a semipermeable membrane, and then returned to the patient's circulation (Figure 18-2). The dialysate (dialysis solution) is an electrolyte solution similar in composition to normal plasma. Each constituent may be varied according to the patient's needs; the most common variable is potassium.

BOX 18-5   Sample Renal Diet Menu

The National Renal Diet is often used to develop diet guidelines and meal plans. The tool is useful and provides visual indicators, such as shown in the following table:

High phosphorus.

High sodium—each serving counts as 1 starch choice and 1 salt choice

High sodium—each serving counts as 1 vegetable choice and 2 salt choices

High sodium—each serving counts as 1 vegetable choice and 3 salt choices

Examples of a diet within these renal guidelines might include the following pattern, with some portions increased for individuals needing more kcal. Intake of some foods cannot be increased because of their phosphorus content; thus, the renal dietitian must individualize the plan.

Breakfast
½ cup milk (whole)—4 g protein, 120 kcal, 80 mg sodium, 100 mg phosphorus ( )
½ cup cooked oatmeal—2 g protein, 90 kcal, 80 mg sodium, 35 mg phosphorus
1 poached egg—7 g protein, 65 kcal, 25 mg sodium, 65 mg phosphorus
1 small bagel—4 g protein, 180 kcal, 160 mg sodium, 70 mg phosphorus
1 tsp margarine—trace protein, 45 kcal, 55 mg sodium, 5 mg phosphorus
2 jelly packs
Coffee
Non-dairy creamer, 1 Tbsp
2 sugar or sugar substitute packets

Lunch
¼ cup cottage cheese—7 g protein, 65 kcal, 25 mg sodium, 65 mg phosphorus
1 oz canned tuna (canned without salt)—7 g protein, 65 kcal, 25 mg sodium, 65 mg phosphorus
1 cup salad with lettuce, cabbage, shredded carrots, cucumbers—2 g protein, 50 kcal, 30 mg sodium, 40 mg phosphorus

Balsamic vinegar + 1 Tbsp olive oil—trace protein, 45 kcal, 55 mg sodium, 5 mg phosphorus
1 small dinner roll—2 g protein, 90 kcal, 80 mg sodium, 35 mg phosphorus
1 tsp margarine—trace protein, 45 kcal, 55 mg sodium, 5 mg phosphorus
2 jelly packs
1 medium tangerine—0.5 g protein, 70 kcal, 15 mg phosphorus
Hot tea
2 sugar or sugar substitute packets

Dinner
2 oz chicken, shredded for tacos—14 g protein, 130 kcal, 50 mg sodium, 130 mg phosphorus
1 flour tortilla (6″ diameter)—2 g protein, 90 kcal, 80 mg sodium, 35 mg phosphorus
¾ cup shredded lettuce, 2 Tbsp chopped onion
¼ cup salsa—1 g protein, 25 kcal, 15 mg sodium, 20 mg phosphorus
½ cup peas, cooked and prepared without salt—1 g protein, 25 kcal, 15 mg sodium, 20 mg phosphorus
Plain muffin, 1 small—2 g protein, 90 kcal, 80 mg sodium, 35 mg phosphorus
Angel food cake, 1 oz—2 g protein, 90 kcal, 80 mg sodium, 35 mg phosphorus
Sliced peaches (1/2 medium)—0.5 g protein, 70 kcal, 15 mg phosphorus
1 tsp margarine—trace protein, 45 kcal, 55 mg sodium, 5 mg phosphorus
1 cup lemonade—trace protein, 100 kcal, 15 mg sodium, 5 mg phosphorus

Snacks
10 pretzel sticks—2 g protein, 90 kcal, 80 mg sodium, 35 mg phosphorus
1 cup plain popcorn—2 g protein, 90 kcal, 80 mg sodium, 35 mg phosphorus
1 apple—0.5 g protein, 70 kcal, 15 mg phosphorus
1 cup cranberry juice cocktail—trace protein, 100 kcal, 15 mg sodium, 5 mg phosphorus

---

The average treatment lasts 3 to 6 hours and is usually performed three times per week (Figure 18-3). Hemodialysis is performed in a dialysis unit by trained staff. Patients who have received special training may assist in their own treatment.

Food and Nutrition Therapies

Individual diet prescriptions (see Table 18-2) are determined by residual kidney function, dialysate components, duration of dialysis, and rate of blood flow through the artificial kidney. The meal plan is designed, monitored, and reevaluated by the renal dietitian. Objectives are to attain or maintain good nutritional status, prevent excessive accumulation of waste products and fluid between treatments, and minimize the effects of metabolic disorders that occur.

Protein and Energy

Recommendations for protein are intended to counteract losses from dialysis, abnormalities in protein metabolism, altered albumin turnover, increased amino acid degradation, inflammation, and infection. The recommended protein intake for patients receiving hemodialysis is 1.2 g protein per kg standard body weight per day with at least 50% of the dietary protein being of high biologic value.

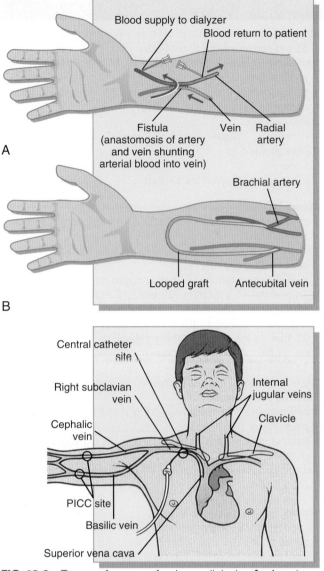

FIG 18-2 Types of access for hemodialysis. **A,** Arteriovenous (AV) fistula; **B,** artificial loop graft. (**A** and **B** from Mahan LK, et al, editors: *Krause's food & nutrition therapy*, ed 13, Philadelphia, 2012, Elsevier.)

Energy

Energy expenditure in patients undergoing hemodialysis is similar to that in healthy individuals. For adult patients younger than 60 years, daily energy intake of 35 kcal/kg of standard body weight is recommended. Obese individuals and adults older than age 60 may benefit from 30 to 35 kcal/kg.

Fat

Patients receiving hemodialysis are at risk for lipid disorders. As such, less than 10% of total kcal should be from saturated fat, and *trans* fats should be avoided. Restricting intake from fat may not be beneficial because the decreased energy intake may lead to malnutrition. It is beneficial to use fish oils and olive oil because they reduce damage from inflammatory cytokines.

Sodium and Fluid

Sodium and fluid restrictions should be individualized to manage weight gain between dialysis procedures, blood pressure, and residual renal function. The recommended intradialytic fluid gains is less than 5% of the patient's dry (nonedematous) weight. Corresponding sodium and fluid restrictions are as follows:

Fluid output >1 L (1000 mL) per day:
- 2 to 4 g (87 to 174 mEq) sodium per day
- 2 L (2000 mL) fluid intake per day

Fluid output <1 L (1000 mL) per day:
- 2 g (87 mEq) sodium per day
- 1 to 1.5 L (1000 to 1500 mL) fluid intake per day

Anuria:
- 2 g (87 mEq) sodium per day
- 1L (1000 mL) fluid intake per day.

Potassium

Dietary potassium restriction varies depending on urine output. Excretion of potassium increases as GFR declines. Generally, 2.5 g of potassium per day is well tolerated. On the other hand, patients with anuria or constipation may experience hyperkalemia. Patients with insulin deficiency or metabolic acidosis, those in a hypercatabolic state, and those being treated with beta-blockers or aldosterone antagonists may require a stricter potassium restriction.

Phosphorus and Calcium

Phosphorus is routinely restricted in patients receiving hemodialysis. High serum levels contribute to secondary hyperparathyroidism and raise the calcium-phosphorus product in the plasma. Although an intake of 12 mg/kg/day is a typical recommendation, this restriction often must be liberalized to meet protein needs. Foods high in phosphorus, such as milk, milk products, cheese, beef liver, chocolate, nuts, and legumes, are usually severely limited or avoided.

Iron and Trace Minerals

Anemia results from decreased production of erythropoietin, the hormone that stimulates bone marrow to produce red blood cells. An adequate available iron supply is necessary for normal erythropoiesis to take place. Supplementation of trace minerals is not necessary unless a deficiency is suspected or documented. Serum levels of chromium, magnesium, and other minerals should be measured at least several times a year.

Vitamin D

In renal failure, kidneys lose their endocrine function of producing calcitriol (the active form of vitamin D). Although many forms of vitamin D are available for supplementation, it is this active form that helps prevent bone disease. The active form of vitamin D is available in oral form as calcitriol (Rocaltrol) and as intravenous (IV) form for use during

FIG 18-3 Hemodialysis. Treatment is usually given for 3 to 6 hours, three times a week. (From Mahan LK, et al, editors: *Krause's food & nutrition therapy,* ed 13, Philadelphia, 2012, Elsevier.)

hemodialysis (calcitriol [Calcijex], paricalcitol [Zemplar], Hectorol).

Other Vitamins

Patients treated with hemodialysis are at risk for deficiencies of water-soluble vitamins, particularly vitamin B₆ and folic acid. The reason is twofold: poor intake and loss of the nutrients during dialysis. Supplementation of the fat-soluble vitamins A, E, and K is usually not necessary. In fact, patients treated with hemodialysis have been reported to experience vitamin A toxicity.

Role of Nursing

Phosphate binders are medications used to control serum phosphorus levels; they are given with meals. The medications of choice are calcium carbonate (Tum), calcium acetate, and sevelamer hydrochloride (Renagel).

Recombinant erythropoietin (EPO), given as epoetin alfa (Epogen), may be given intravenously during dialysis or subcutaneously just after dialysis treatment. Oral or IV iron supplementation is often necessary before EPO to replenish iron stores.

Patients who have inadequate oral intake are at risk for nutrient deficiencies and poor nutritional status. Intake can be the result of anorexia, changes in taste acuity and in food preferences (especially red meat and sweets), nausea, vomiting, or dietary limitations. When patients experience changes in taste, it may be useful to offer foods with sharp, distinct flavors to stimulate appetite (Box 18-6).

> **BOX 18-6** **Suggestions for Patients with Altered Taste**
>
> - Brush teeth and tongue 6 to 8 times per day
> - Rinse mouth with a chilled mouthwash (commercial product or water mixed with lemon juice or vinegar); or try cool black or green tea, lightly salted water, or baking soda and water before eating
> - Suck lemon wedges or hard candy before meals
> - Chew gum
> - Before meals, drink water with lemon, or eat a small amount of sherbet or fruit sorbet
> - Try cold foods that do not have strong flavors.
> - Try different or unusual flavors such as basil, oregano, rosemary, tarragon, mustard, catsup, and mint
> - For metallic taste, try using plastic utensils instead of regular silverware

Approximately one third of patients requiring hemodialysis have diabetes mellitus. Diets for these patients should incorporate the necessary renal modifications, provide consistent carbohydrate content, and facilitate glycemic control.

PERITONEAL DIALYSIS

Peritoneal dialysis (PD) removes excess fluid and waste products from blood using the peritoneal membrane as a filter. Dialysate is instilled and removed through a catheter that has been surgically placed into the peritoneal cavity. The

The peritoneal cavity is filled with dialysate, using gravity.

At the end of the exchange, the dialysate is drained into the bag, again using gravity.

FIG 18-4 Continuous ambulatory peritoneal dialysis; 20-minute exchanges usually are given four or five times a day, every day. (From Mahan LK, et al, editors: *Krause's food & nutrition therapy*, ed 13, Philadelphia, 2012, Elsevier.)

peritoneum (the lining of the abdominal cavity) is used as the dialysis membrane (Figure 18-4). Waste products cross the membrane passively from the peritoneal capillaries into the dialysate in the peritoneal cavity. The dialysate contains dextrose, which increases osmolality of the solution and facilitates removal of excess fluid. As the fluid moves from vascular space into the peritoneal cavity, osmolality of the solutions becomes equal. Toxins and excess fluids collected in the peritoneal cavity are then drained from the body through the catheter and discarded. An advantage of PD is that it is usually performed in the home.

Intermittent Peritoneal Dialysis

Intermittent peritoneal dialysis (IPD) involves infusion of approximately 2 L of dialysate instilled over 20 to 30 minutes. Dialysate is then drained by gravity, and the process is repeated over an 8- to 10-hour period four or five times per week. IPD can be performed manually or mechanically. During the time of dialysis, patients are restricted to a chair or bed. This method is not commonly used as a long-term treatment modality because of the time involvement.

Continuous Ambulatory Peritoneal Dialysis

Continuous ambulatory peritoneal dialysis (CAPD) entails infusion of dialysate in four or five "exchanges" within a 24-hour period into the peritoneum. A specific volume of dialysate is infused and allowed to dwell for approximately 4 hours. At the end of the designated time, dialysate containing waste and excess fluid is drained by gravity, and a new exchange begins. Dialysate is present 24 hours per day in the peritoneum, except for the 20- to 30-minute exchange when

dwelling dialysate is drained and fresh dialysate is instilled. Dialysis exchanges are done continuously, 7 days a week. CAPD is a reasonable procedure for adults who work outside the home and are able to complete the procedure discretely while at work.

Continuous Cycling Peritoneal Dialysis

Continuous cycling peritoneal dialysis (CCPD) is a combination of IPD and CAPD. At night, a cycler (mechanical) performs three dialysate exchanges. During the day, a fourth exchange is infused for the entire day. At bedtime, the fourth exchange is drained, and the process is started again. Although restricted to bed during nighttime infusions, patients are ambulatory during the day. Thus, CCPD is another reasonable option for working adults.

Food and Nutrition Therapies

Objectives are to (1) maintain good nutritional status while replacing albumin lost in the dialysate, (2) minimize complications of fluid imbalance, (3) minimize symptoms of uremic toxicity, and (4) minimize secondary metabolic disorders. As with hemodialysis, patients treated with PD are at risk for deficiencies of water-soluble vitamins and minerals. A daily multivitamin supplement that includes folic acid is recommended. In addition, some patients may receive recombinant EPO for correction of anemia and need iron supplementation to maximize the effectiveness of the drug.

Energy requirements for patients treated with PD are usually lower than for those receiving hemodialysis because approximately 60% of the dialysate is absorbed. Dextrose is used as an osmotic agent in PD dialysate and must be taken into consideration when energy needs are calculated.

Protein losses during PD range from 20 to 30 g per day and are reflected in slightly higher dietary protein recommendations (see Table 18-2). Serum blood urea nitrogen BUN and creatinine levels, uremic symptoms, and weight should be monitored as indicators of sufficient protein intake, and the diet should be adjusted accordingly.

During PD, sodium, potassium, and fluid are continually removed, making severe dietary restrictions unnecessary. However, it is important to remember that nutrient needs vary among patients, so individualized recommendations are still necessary.

Restriction of dietary phosphorus is critical to prevent development of osteodystrophy (defective bone development). Unfortunately, higher protein requirements for PD consequently provide high amounts of phosphorus. Therefore, severely restricting or eliminating dairy products will be necessary to control phosphorus intake; calcium supplementation is usually prescribed. Phosphorus is also controlled by prescribed phosphate binders.

Role of Nursing

All forms of PD require special training of the patient and caregiver. Anorexia, nausea, and vomiting are common signs of uremia and inadequate dialysis. Consequently, nutritional status is an important measure. The National Kidney

Foundation suggests regular and ongoing nutritional assessment of patients undergoing PD by a renal dietitian and other team members. Excessive weight gain and other factors should be carefully reviewed with each visit.

The absorption of glucose from PD dialysate presents a special challenge for patients with diabetes. Blood glucose levels and hyperlipidemia become more difficult to control. Weight gain is caused by the increased calorie load of the dialysate. Dehydration is another concern when there is excessive fluid removal and extracellular fluid volume deficits. Thus, careful monitoring of blood glucose, I&O, and weights are preventive measures in this patient population.

RENAL TRANSPLANTATION

Kidney transplantations are the second most frequent transplant operations in the United States. Approximately 9000 patients receive kidney transplants each year, and in excess of 35,000 are on waiting lists. Generally, there is a shortage of donors (see the *Cultural Considerations* box Barriers to Organ Donations).

Food and Nutrition Therapies

Pretransplantation

Nutritional status is evaluated to identify and correct deficits before surgery. Poor nutritional status is caused by blood loss, protein and nutrient loss during dialysis, the catabolism of chronic illness, anorexia and altered taste, suboptimal oral intake, and depression. Decreased visceral protein stores and body weight are common, as are deficiencies of vitamin B_6, folic acid, vitamins C and D, and iron. Nutrition therapy requires an individualized approach, as outlined in Table 18-2.

Immediately After Transplantation and Long Term

Energy needs in the immediate post-transplantation period are high (30 to 35 kcal/kg) because of stress from surgery and catabolism. These requirements decline approximately 6 to 8 weeks after transplantation, and intake should then be provided to achieve and maintain a desirable body weight. Restriction of dietary protein is not necessary. In fact, protein catabolism is increased as the result of surgery and the administration of corticosteroids for immunosuppression.

Steroid therapy may cause glucose intolerance and therefore necessitate control of total carbohydrate intake. Fats are limited if dyslipidemia occurs. Recommendations regarding sodium and potassium should be individualized for each patient. Fluids are generally unrestricted and limited only by graft function. Many drugs used postoperatively and after transplantation have the potential to influence nutritional needs and status. Careful observation of the patient may prevent problems.

Role of Nursing

Nutritional care of renal transplant recipients involves continual reassessment of nutritional goals and efficacy of therapy during the different phases of recovery. Nurses can be very

---

🌐 CULTURAL CONSIDERATIONS
Barriers to Organ Donations

In the United States, there is a shortage of organ donations from members of minority groups. This is a concern because successful organ transplantation requires some matching of genetic characteristics. Religious and cultural beliefs are often issues that promote a distrust of the medical system, misunderstandings about religious stances, and ignorance about the donation process (Irving, et al, 2012).

Two studies of African American and Hispanic American communities provide insight about some of the barriers against organ donation. The first study of African American community residents and clergy in Texas included focus groups and three cross-sectional surveys. Community residents tended not to value organ donation, considered donation incompatible with their religion viewed donation as mutilating a person's body, and felt health care professionals couldn't be trusted to properly declare death before taking organs. In contrast, the African American clergy valued the importance of organ donation in every way.

A telephone-interview survey of Hispanic Americans in Arizona suggested that predictors of willingness to be an organ donor include participating in a family discussion about organ donation, knowing someone who is willing to be a donor, and agreeing that carrying a donor card means receiving proper medical care. Barriers consist of organ donation not being discussed, discussion of donation tied to one's mortality (a topic not to be talked about), and putting oneself or family members at risk for inadequate medical care so that the health care professionals have access to organs.

Once organ donation is openly discussed, misconceptions can be addressed through educational efforts. Efforts must take into account the diversity and geographic distribution of the various cultural groups. Strategies can be implemented to create trust among members of minority groups who are currently less willing to donate organs.

Culturally appropriate interventions can be used to engage and educate minority groups, especially through religious or cultural leaders (Irving, et al, 2012).

Data from Alvaro EM, et al: Predictors of organ donation behavior among Hispanic Americans, *Prog Transplant* 15(2):149-156, 2005; Davis K, et al: Leading the flock: Organ donation feelings, beliefs, and intentions among African American clergy and community residents, *Prog Transplant* 15(3):211-216, 2005; Irving MJ, et al: Factors that influence the decision to be an organ donor: A systematic review of the qualitative literature, *Nephrol Dial Transplant* 27:2526-33, 2012.

---

helpful by discussing and reinforcing the measures that are needed. For example, the immunosuppressant drugs often cause weight gain and secondary diabetes as a long-term consequence after transplantation. Patients will need support and guidance on how to manage and cope after the procedure.

More than 80% of kidneys transplanted from cadavers still function well 1 year after surgery. Outcomes are even better for transplants from living donors. Nurses play an essential role for both sets of families and friends of the donor and the transplant recipient (see the *Personal Perspectives* box Organ Donation: Helping Families Cope).

Organ Donation: Helping Families Cope

It was such a pleasure to watch my brother-in-law, David, marry his high school sweetheart, Carol. They had dated for years and finally made the marital plunge in June of 1987. Our 3-year-old son was the ring-bearer, adorable in his little white tux which matched that of his uncle. How joyful that day was for all!

Unfortunately, a few months later on a clear, cold night in January, David had been playing cards with friends until the early morning hours. His drive home was unfamiliar, in an older part of the city where the highways were narrow and poorly marked for night driving. Evidently, he headed in the wrong direction and had to make a U-turn on the highway. When he did so, a woman on her way to work did not see him, and her car crashed into the back of his car. David's car was spun around, and he exited the car through the hatchback onto the pavement. Even though a medical helicopter was quickly called to transport him to a large, tertiary care center, it was too late. He had already experienced massive brain trauma, with a closed-head injury and extensive swelling. Unlike soft tissue, the human cranium has no natural way to expand.

David was connected to a ventilator, and the many tests began. His family had been called, which included my husband. I stayed at home with our son until he called later that day. It would be important for us to go to the hospital quickly, as signs did not show a promise for recovery. Because David was married, his wife was to make decisions for him, but the rest of us had opinions as well. His sister was a Nursing Supervisor, and I was a Registered Dietitian, so we had seen many head trauma cases. We were all ready to play a part in his recovery, however long that would take.

However, David failed all of the Glasgow Coma Scale tests and was truly "brain dead." His doctors indicated that no family decision would be necessary; they would automatically remove the life support. It was so sad to look at this beautiful young man with few signs of trauma, a newlywed less than a year. We realized that there would be no nieces or nephews to play with our children. No more holidays together, no more beach vacations or life event celebrations. No more David and Carol, no more intact family.

At some point that day, the nurses and chaplain helped us discuss organ donation. We were encouraged to touch David and say our goodbyes. Carol knew that David had signed up for organ donation, but she just could not give away his heart; it was where she "resided" in him. It would be okay for the other organs. In the midst of this terrible and painful weekend, we all knew this was the right thing to do. His organs would give others the chance to live a healthy life, even if he could not do so.

Our minister was outstanding in his love and support, discussing how we would all need to grieve a little each day and not hurry the process to "get on with our own lives." That advice and knowing that others had actually been given a second chance helped us accept that David's life had a courageous, if unexpected, purpose.

Sylvia Escott-Stump
Winterville, North Carolina

RENAL CALCULI

Renal calculi (kidney stones, urolithiasis) are a common and often recurrent urologic condition. Stone formation is more common among men than women, and approximately half of those in whom renal calculi develop have them again within 10 years. Formation of calculi depends on simultaneous occurrence of the following factors: (1) low urine volume (usually from inadequate fluid intake); (2) high urinary pH; (3) excessive urinary excretion of calcium, oxalate, uric acid, or a combination; and (4) decreased levels of substances in urine that normally inhibit stone formation (Wilkens and Juneja, 2012.).

Food and Nutrition Therapies

The type and cause of stone formation provide impetus for individualization of dietary modifications. Most calculi are composed of calcium oxalate (70% to 80%), uric acid (10%), struvite (9% to 17%), or cystine (<1%). A comprehensive diet history is essential to ascertain the extent of dietary modifications required. Dietary interventions must include generous fluid intake; Box 18-7 outlines recommendations.

Calcium Oxalate Stones

Too much calcium in the urine (hypercalciuria) is the most common identifiable cause of calcium renal calculi.

BOX 18-7 Dietary Recommendations for Renal Calculi

- Tailor diet to specific metabolic disturbance and individual dietary habits (to ensure compliance).
- Calcium restriction should be avoided. Take calcium (800-1500 mg/day).
- Limit intake of spinach, rhubarb, beets, nuts, chocolate, tea, wheat bran, and strawberries (which increase urinary oxalate excretion).
- Do not exceed recommended dietary allowance (RDA) for vitamin C for gender and age.
- Animal protein should be "restricted" to 1 g/kg body weight.
- Salt intake should be restricted to less than 2300 mg per day.
- Potassium intake should be encouraged (5 or more servings of fruits and vegetables/day).
- Include a high fluid intake to produce at least 2 L of urine per day (2-3 L intake/day).

Approximately 50% of people who form calcium stones have some type of absorptive hypercalciuria (Table 18-3). There is no need to restrict dietary calcium. Kidney stone formation is influenced more by the amount of oxalate than of calcium in the urinary tract. In fact, an adequate calcium intake

TABLE 18-3 Types and Treatment of Absorptive Hypercalciuria

TYPE	OCCURRENCE	MEDICAL TREATMENT
I	Relatively uncommon and most severe	Thiazides and orthophosphates
II	Most common and less severe	Thiazides may be prescribed
III	Also called *renal phosphate leak;* relatively rare	Oral orthophosphate therapy to correct hypophosphatemia

Data from Leslie SW: *Hypercalciuria,* n.d.. Accessed August 29, 2013, from emedicine.medscape.com/article/436343-overview.

(800-1200 mg) combined with restricted animal protein and sodium intake appears to protect against calcium stone development (Heilberg and Goldfarb, 2013).

High alcohol intake also promotes urinary excretion of calcium and should be reduced accordingly. Low intake of potassium is an additional risk factor for stone development. Potassium reduces urinary calcium excretion by causing transient sodium diuresis and increased renal phosphate absorption.

Oxalate is found primarily in foods of plant origin and is the end product of ascorbic acid metabolism. Restriction of dietary oxalate intake has been used to reduce risk of recurrence of calcium oxalate kidney stones.

Uric Acid Stones

Uric acid is a metabolic product of purines (a nitrogen-containing compound in protein). Uric acid stones are associated with acidic urine (hyperuricosuria) and gout. Allopurinol (Zyloprim) is effective in reducing high levels of uric acid. The key therapy is weight loss, plus urinary alkalinization provided by a more vegetarian diet and reduced animal protein intake (Heilberg and Goldfarb, 2013).

Cystine Stones

Cystine stones form in people with a hereditary disorder that causes the kidneys to excrete excessive amounts of the amino acid cystine (cystinuria). The goal of treatment is to reduce urinary cystine concentration. To do this, urine volume should be greater than 3 L/day, and urine should be alkalinized to a pH in the range of 6.5 to 7. Restrictions in animal protein and sodium are associated with reduced cystine production (Heilberg and Goldfarb, 2013).

Struvite Stones

Struvite stones are caused by urinary tract infections by bacteria that split urea into ammonium in urine. No specific diet is needed other than avoidance of dehydration. Surgery or lithotripsy is almost always performed.

Role of Nursing

Education is important in the treatment of renal calculi. Only a motivated and informed patient can be expected to maintain a long-term preventive program.

▌ SUMMARY

- The chief life-preserving function of the kidneys is to help maintain chemical homeostasis in the body.
- Various inflammatory, obstructive, and degenerative diseases affect the kidneys in different ways and interfere with normal functioning of nephrons that regulate products of metabolism.
- Because of glomerular damage, nephrotic syndrome results in increased urinary excretion of protein, decreased serum albumin levels, hyperlipidemia, and edema.
- Nephrotic syndrome may resist treatment and progress to renal failure. Primary goals of medical nutrition therapy are to control hypertension, minimize edema, decrease urinary albumin losses, prevent protein malnutrition and muscle catabolism, supply adequate energy, and slow the progression of renal disease.
- Acute renal failure is characterized by an abrupt loss of renal function that may or may not be accompanied by oliguria or anuria; common causes are trauma, hemorrhage, shock, nephrotoxic chemicals or drugs, septicemia, and streptococcal infection.
- Nutritional needs in ARF are determined by the underlying cause of the condition and whether dialysis is used for treatment. Patients may be hypermetabolic if renal failure was caused by trauma, burns, septicemia, or infection.

- CKD is the result of progressive, irreversible loss of kidney function. It can develop over days, months, or years. CKD always leads to retention of nitrogenous waste products and fluid and electrolyte imbalances that affect all body systems.
- Before end-stage renal failure, management focuses on slowing progression and minimizing complications of CKD.
- Once CKD progresses to renal failure, management focuses on reducing uremia with various treatment modalities: conservative management, hemodialysis, peritoneal dialysis, and renal transplantation.
- Planning renal diets requires skill in calibrating intakes of fluids, energy, protein, lipids, phosphorus, potassium, sodium, vitamins, and other minerals.
- Currently, the National Renal Diet is used to develop diet guidelines and meal plans. Individual renal diet prescriptions are based on residual kidney function, dialysate components, duration of dialysis, and rate of blood flow through the artificial kidney.
- Objectives are to attain or maintain good nutritional status, prevent or minimize symptoms of uremic toxicity and fluid imbalance between treatments, and minimize effects of metabolic disorders caused by CKD, hemodialysis, and PD.

- Nutritional care of renal transplant recipients involves continual reassessment of nutritional goals and efficacy of therapy during the different phases of care.
- Renal calculi are a common, recurrent urologic condition. Most are composed of calcium, oxalate, or phosphorus, with a small proportion made up of cystine or uric acid. Uric acid is a metabolic product of purines.

- Sufficient fluid intake has the most significant impact on reducing risk of stone formation.
- Calcium oxalate stone formation is influenced more by the amount of oxalate in the urinary tract than by the amount of calcium. Oxalate is found primarily in plant foods and is the end product of ascorbic acid metabolism.

◎ THE NURSING APPROACH

Case Study: Chronic Renal Failure

Ian, age 28, was diagnosed with end-stage renal disease (ESRD) a few months ago subsequent to glomerulonephritis. His kidneys produce very little urine or sometimes none at all, requiring Ian to receive hemodialysis treatments three times a week. He hopes for a kidney transplant, but the waiting list is long. The nurse wants to encourage him.

Assessment
Subjective (from Patient Statements)
- "I don't have any energy. I'm tired all of the time."
- "Food doesn't taste good anymore. I don't have any appetite."
- "I'm sick of trying to follow the diet the dietitian recommended. It's not worth it."
- "Why try? Dialysis will take care of any extra fluid and minerals."
- "I know what I am supposed to eat, but it's too hard. I just eat and drink what I like whenever I want to."

Objective (from Physical Examination)
- Generalized ashen skin color, pale conjunctivae, wasted appearance
- BP 162/105, pulse 92, respirations 20
- Low hemoglobin and hematocrit, high blood urea nitrogen (BUN) and creatinine
- Weight gain of 6 pounds since last hemodialysis 2 days ago
- Edema of ankles, crackles (sounds) in both lungs

Diagnoses (Nursing)
1. Excess fluid volume related to impaired renal function and excessive intake of fluid and sodium as evidenced by oliguria, weight gain of 6 pounds, ankle edema, crackles in both lungs, and BP 162/105
2. Imbalanced nutrition: less than body requirements related to anorexia, fatigue, and altered taste secondary to impaired renal function as evidenced by ashen skin, pale conjunctivae, wasted appearance, high BUN, and low hemoglobin and hematocrit
3. Noncompliance related to lack of motivation, as evidenced by "I'm sick of trying to follow the diet the dietitian recommended," "Why try? Dialysis will take care of any extra fluid and minerals," and "I know what I am supposed to eat, but it's too hard. I just eat and drink what I like whenever I want to."

Planning
Patient Outcomes
Short term (by the end of the nurse-patient interaction):
- Commits to meet with the renal dietitian to plan a diet he can follow

- Recognizes the connections among diet, effectiveness of dialysis, and feeling better
- Agrees to take charge of his health by continuing dialysis and taking prescribed medications
Long term (by 2 weeks):
- Says he is following the renal diet and feels more energetic
- No more than 1- to 2-pound weight gain per day between dialysis treatments
- BP 130/85, no ankle edema, lungs clear

Nursing Interventions
1. Refer Ian to the renal dietitian.
2. Try to motivate him to adhere to the medical plan, including medical nutrition therapy.
3. Discuss why following the renal diet is necessary and how it can help him feel better.

Implementation
1. Referred Ian to the renal dietitian.
   The renal dietitian can help individualize the complex diet according to the patient's lifestyle, health condition, and food preferences. The dietitian also can teach the patient how to apply general principles of the renal diet.
2. Explained the connections among pathophysiology, diet, and patient problems (signs and symptoms).
   A patient may be motivated to make healthy food choices if he can see a direct positive effect. Failed kidneys cannot remove fluids, electrolytes, and nitrogenous wastes. Restricting certain foods and some fluid intake can help alleviate signs and symptoms of uremia and fluid and electrolyte problems.
   a. Discussed the need to ingest adequate calories (including carbohydrates and unsaturated fats) and high biologic value proteins (soy, lean red meats, fish, chicken, eggs, and milk) to reduce urea formation.
   Nausea, anorexia, and metallic tastes may be reduced by decreasing urea production. Adequate intake of calories decreases protein catabolism, thus decreasing nitrogenous waste. High–biologic value proteins produce less urea than low–biologic value proteins (e.g., grains and cereals).
   b. Discussed the need to restrict fluids and sodium to reduce fluid retention.
   Hypertension, peripheral edema, and pulmonary edema may result from excessive fluid intake, accentuated by sodium retention. Because the heart has to work harder, heart failure may occur. Dialysis can remove some fluid, but it is more effective and better tolerated by the patient if large accumulations of fluid are not present.

THE NURSING APPROACH—cont'd

c. Discussed the need to restrict potassium to avoid problems in the heart.

Too much potassium, resulting from decreased excretion by the kidneys, can cause deadly dysrhythmias. Foods high in potassium should be avoided or limited, such as bananas, oranges, potatoes, tomatoes, and milk. Milk is often limited to ½ cup per day because it is high in both potassium and phosphorus.

d. Discussed the need to restrict phosphorus to avoid problems in the bones.

Failed kidneys cannot remove phosphorus, and dialysis does not remove phosphorus well. Phosphorus concentration in the blood is inversely related to serum calcium level, so a high level of phosphorus causes decreased absorption of calcium from the intestines. The resultant hypocalcemia stimulates the parathyroid gland to keep the serum calcium level in a safe range, and it does so by pulling calcium from the bones. This puts the patient at risk for bone fractures. Foods high in phosphorus should be limited, such as milk, cheese, nuts, legumes, beef liver, and chocolate.

3. Helped Ian plan what he can do to improve his health and nutrition.

Helping the patient take charge of his health provides a sense of control and empowerment.

a. Choose foods from the National Renal Diet.

Foods are grouped into choices by the amount of protein, calories, sodium, phosphorus, and potassium that the foods contain. The dietitian can specify the number of servings in each choice (group), allowing the patient to eat any food within the choice and still follow guidelines of medical nutrition therapy. Choices (groups) include protein, fruits and vegetables, dairy and phosphorus, bread/grains, fluid, and high-kcal foods and flavoring.

b. Download and read the pamphlet "Eat Right to Feel Right on Hemodialysis," National Institutes of Health, at http://kidney.niddk.nih.gov/KUDiseases/pubs/eatright/

The government distributes free publications to educate patients with renal failure. This pamphlet is easy to read, empowering the patient with knowledge.

c. Weigh and measure foods periodically to match recommended serving sizes.

Accuracy is needed to obtain expected results.

d. Eat small, frequent meals, spacing protein foods throughout the day.

Small, frequent meals are usually better tolerated than large meals when the patient has nausea and anorexia. Spreading proteins throughout the day helps control the amount of urea that is in the patient's body at any one time.

e. Brush teeth frequently and chew gum if desired.

Good oral care makes the mouth feel fresher, improving the taste of food. Chewing gum improves taste in the mouth and can stimulate salivary glands, providing moisture in the mouth and possibly decreasing thirst.

f. Set a target range of gaining no more than 1 to 2 pounds per day between hemodialysis treatments. Weigh self every morning, and adjust fluid and sodium intake to avoid exceeding the target.

Working toward a goal can provide motivation. Daily fluid allotment is generally 500 to 1000 mL plus the amount of urine output.

g. Make a plan for spacing out allowed fluids throughout the day, including foods that melt at room temperature or are high in water content.

Spreading out fluid intake can help control thirst. Using smaller glasses and freezing some fluids to eat like ice pops may also reduce thirst.

4. Encouraged Ian to adhere to the medical plan, including both undergoing hemodialysis three times per week and taking medications.

Hemodialysis involves circulating blood through a dialyzer (artificial kidney) to remove urea, metabolic waste products, toxins, and excess fluid. Failed kidneys cannot produce the hormone erythropoietin (necessary for red blood cell production), so anemia is common. Epoetin alfa (Epogen) is given to stimulate red blood cell synthesis. In addition, iron, B vitamins, and folic acid are usually prescribed to enhance the erythropoiesis. Failed kidneys cannot produce calcitriol (the active form of vitamin D), so it may be taken orally to promote absorption of calcium and subsequent bone formation. Usually phosphate binders (such as calcium carbonate) are prescribed by a physician and taken with each meal to facilitate fecal elimination of phosphorus.

5. Suggested involving his family and friends in meal planning.

Family support is extremely helpful. A person with renal failure often lacks energy for grocery shopping and food preparation. Families can eat similar meals with the patient, though serving sizes will probably vary.

a. Recommended purchasing a renal diet cookbook.

Recipes from a renal diet cookbook can add variety to the family meal.

b. Advised Ian to avoid salt and salt substitutes (usually potassium) and add spices such as garlic, onions, and oregano to food.

Adding spices adds flavor to foods.

6. Helped Ian write some short-term goals.

Achievement of small steps provides encouragement.

a. Asked how Ian would reward himself when he achieved each goal.

Positive reinforcement helps establish desirable behaviors.

b. Reminded him that he must stay healthy to be prepared for a possible kidney transplant.

Kidney transplants succeed best when the patient is healthy. Patients are more likely to be considered for a kidney transplantation if they are healthy and taking charge of their health.

Evaluation

Short term (by the end of the nurse-patient interaction):

• Ian stated he was willing to meet with the dietitian at the dialysis center and follow the dietitian's recommendations.

• Ian said he could see how eating the right foods and following the medical plan might make him feel better.

• He agreed to continue taking prescribed medications and getting hemodialysis.

Continued

◎ THE NURSING APPROACH—cont'd

Goals met.
The nurse planned to meet with Ian again in 2 weeks.

Discussion Questions

Ian met with the nurse for follow-up in 2 weeks. He kept a record of his weight, his urine output, and his fluid intake every day for the 2 weeks. He gained 1 to 2 pounds per day between dialysis treatments. He reported that he felt better during the days that he adhered closely to his fluid restrictions. The nurse praised him for his efforts.

1. When assessing Ian, what signs and symptoms would the nurse look for to validate improvement in fluid balance?
2. Ian said he had met with the dietitian but was still having a hard time maintaining his diet. How could the nurse motivate Ian and help him set some small, realistic goals?

？ CRITICAL THINKING

Clinical Applications*

Julia, age 40, works full time in an office and has a sedentary lifestyle. She is 5 feet 6 inches tall, has a medium frame, and weighs 125 pounds (dry weight). Her usual body weight is 132 pounds. Her appetite has not been good for the past 3 months, but it is improving. She is on hemodialysis for 3 hours, three times per week. Her urine output is approximately 500 mL/24 hours.

Her predialysis laboratory results include BUN 57 mg/dL; Na^+ 133 mEq/L; K^+ 4.7 mEq/L; Po_4 6.3 mg/dL; Ca^{2+} 9.5 mg/dL; serum albumin 3 g/dL; and ferritin 7 μg/L. Her diet prescription is 2200 kcal, 70 to 80 g protein, 2000 mg Na^+, 2000 mg K^+, 1000 mg Po_4, and 1500 mL fluid.

Julia's diet history indicates that she doesn't like meat, but does like cheese and orange juice and will occasionally overindulge on these foods. She admits to having had too much cheese and orange juice when she came in for her last dialysis. The patient is taking Nephro-Vite.

1. What is the purpose of hemodialysis?
2. How are metabolic waste products removed during dialysis?
3. Give two explanations why Julia's serum albumin levels are decreased.
4. Why is the serum ferritin often low in renal patients?
5. Why are high biologic value proteins recommended for patients with renal disease?
6. Why are water-soluble vitamin supplements (Nephro-Vite) usually prescribed for patients with renal disease?

Julia is considering trying a type of peritoneal dialysis so she won't have to go to the kidney dialysis center three times each week.

1. Explain how peritoneal dialysis works.
2. What dietary changes might need to be made if Julia switches to peritoneal dialysis?

■ WEBSITES OF INTEREST

Life Options Rehabilitation Program

www.lifeoptions.org
Helps individuals live well and long with kidney disease; includes Kidney School, an interactive, web-based kidney learning center.

National Kidney and Urological Diseases Information Clearinghouse (NKUDIC)

kidney.niddk.nih.gov
Functions as an information dissemination service of the National Institute of Diabetes and Digestive and Kidney Diseases (NIDDK).

National Kidney Center

www.nationalkidneycenter.org/
Many resources for the public and for health professionals on managing kidney health.

Renal Support Network (RSN)

rsnhope.org
Provides nonmedical services to those affected by chronic kidney disease (CKD) as a nonprofit, patient-focused, patient-run organization.

REFERENCES

Calvo MS, Uribarri J: Public health impact of dietary phosphorus excess on bone and cardiovascular health in the general population, *Am J Clin Nutr* 98:6–15, 2013.

Centers for Disease Control: *Fastats: Kidney disease*, 2012. From: http://www.cdc.gov/nchs/fastats/kidney-disease.htm. Accessed September 23, 2013.

Goraya N, et al: Dietary acid reduction with fruits and vegetables or bicarbonate attenuates kidney injury in patients with a moderately reduced glomerular filtration rate due to hypertensive nephropathy, *Kidney Int* 81:86–93, 2012.

Heilberg IP, Goldfarb DS: Optimum nutrition for kidney stone disease, *Adv Chronic Kidney Dis* 20:165–174, 2013.

National Kidney Foundation, Kidney Dialysis Outcomes Quality Initiative: *KDOQI clinical practice guidelines for peritoneal dialysis adequacy: Update 2006*, New York, 2006, National Kidney Foundation. From: www.kidney.org/professionals/ KDOQI/guideline_upHD_PD_VA/pd_intro.htm. Accessed August 29, 2013.

National Kidney Foundation, Kidney Disease Outcomes Quality Initiative: *KDOQI clinical practice guidelines for diabetes and CKD: 2012 update*, 2012. From: www.kidney.org/professionals/ KDOQI/guidelines_diabetesUp/diabetes-ckd-update-2012.pdf. Website accessed September 23, 2013.

Ruta LA, et al: High-salt diet reveals the hypertensive and renal effects of reduced nephron endowment, *Am J Physiol Renal Physiol* 298:F1384–F1392, 2010.

Wilkens KG, Juneja V: Medical nutrition therapy for renal disorders. In Mahan LK, Escott-Stump S, Raymond JL, editors: *Krause's food & nutrition therapy*, ed 13, Philadelphia, 2012, Elsevier.

---

*Courtesy Kim Dittus, PhD, RD, Syracuse University, Syracuse, NY.

CHAPTER 19

Nutrition for Neuro-Psychiatric Disorders

The brain requires a steady stream of glucose and has a protein membrane around each cell, filled with lipid. The neurotransmitters are dependent upon amino acids in the right amount and time to be effective. Thus, the healthy blood-brain barrier needs ample glucose, lipid, and proteins of the right type to work properly.

http://evolve.elsevier.com/GRODNER/FOUNDATIONS

LEARNING OBJECTIVES

- Explain the rationale for nutrition interventions that provide foods rich in certain nutrients for neurologic disorders such as Alzheimer's disease (AD), Parkinson's disease (PD), and amyotrophic lateral sclerosis (ALS).
- Identify infections, particularly food-related, after which Guillain–Barré syndrome (GBS) may occur.
- Discuss the relationship of food-related triggers to migraine occurrence.

- List two neurologic disorders for which a plant-based diet or Mediterranean dietary pattern are suggested.
- Compare and contrast the eating disorders (EDs) anorexia nervosa (AN) and binge eating disorder (BED).
- Assess the similarities of nutritional requirements for bipolar spectrum, depression, and schizophrenia.

NUTRITION IN BRAIN HEALTH

Psychiatric and metabolic disorders are linked: diabetes, hypertension, insulin resistance, metabolic syndrome, obesity, attention deficit disorders, depression, psychosis, sleep apnea, inflammation, autism, and schizophrenia (SCZ) operate through common pathways. Altered dietary precursors (tryptophan, tyrosine, and choline) affect nerve functioning, and neurotransmitters are especially affected by dietary availability. Deficiencies of vitamin B_{12}, B_6, C, or E, folic acid, iron, or zinc imitate the effects of radiation on the body by damaging DNA. The brain requires a varied diet with multiple nutrients (Figure 19-1).

Inflammatory processes, infections, and host immune responses cause chronic neurologic damage. Different pathogens directly trigger neurotoxic pathways and are risk factors for neurodegenerative Alzheimer's disease, Parkinson's disease, and amyotrophic lateral sclerosis (DeChiara, et al, 2012) (Figure 19-2). *Toxoplasma gondii* has been implicated in schizophrenia, Alzheimer's disease, Parkinson's disease, and autoimmune disorders (Carter, 2013). Neurodegeneration can also occur from herpes simplex type 1, human immunodeficiency and influenza viruses, and *Chlamydia pneumonia* (DeChiara, et al, 2012).

Prevention of malnutrition, restoration of feeding abilities, and improved nutritional quality of life are the goals. Team members will focus on the patient's overall health status, medical therapies, prescribed medicines, herbs and alternative therapies, and appropriate nutrition treatments.

NEUROLOGIC DISORDERS

Alzheimer's Disease

Alzheimer's disease involves progressive deterioration of intellect, memory, personality, and self-care. Early stages of AD manifest as memory loss, language problems, asking the same questions repeatedly, disorientation and confusion, odd behavior, lack of hygiene, loss of initiative, and personality changes. Box 19-1 provides a checklist of early signs.

Food and Nutrition Therapies

There is a positive correlation between a high intake of antioxidant foods and better cognitive function. Nutrients that raise the levels of brain catecholamines and protect against oxidative damage are critical: Foods rich in vitamins C and E, zinc, iron, copper, and selenium should be provided. Blueberries, cranberries, strawberries, kale, spinach, and coffee intake may improve cognitive function. Include vitamins B_6 and B_{12} and folate to lower elevated total homocysteine (tHcy) levels when needed.

A Mediterranean diet, omega-3 fatty acids, and light to moderate alcohol use are protective. High levels of consumption of fats from fish, vegetable oils, nonstarchy vegetables,

FIG 19-1 A mixed diet provides the nutrients needed by the brain.

BOX 19-1   Ten Warning Signs of Alzheimer's Disease

- Memory loss that disrupts daily life
- Challenges in planning or solving problems
- Difficulty completing familiar tasks at home, at work, at leisure
- Confusion with time or place
- Trouble understanding visual images or spatial relationships
- New problems with words in speaking or writing
- Misplacing things and losing the ability to retrace steps
- Decreased or poor judgment
- Withdrawal from work or social activities
- Changes in mood or personality

Data from Alzheimer's Association: *Know the 10 signs; early detection matters,* 2009. Accessed September 29, 2013, from http://www.alz.org/national/documents/checklist_10signs.pdf.

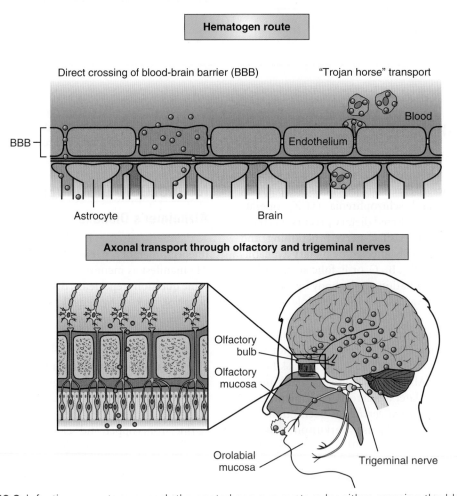

FIG 19-2 Infectious agents can reach the central nervous system by either crossing the blood–brain barrier (hematogen route) or being transported by axons of cranial nerve neurons. (Redrawn from DeChiara G, et al: Infectious agents and neurodegeneration, *Mol Neurobiol* 46:614-638, 2012.)

FIG 19-3 The Mediterranean diet is an excellent diet for the whole body, but it is especially beneficial for the brain.

low-glycemic fruits, and low levels of consumption of foods with added sugars, and moderate wine intake should be encouraged (Figure 19-3).

Application to nursing. Patients with AD are often malnourished, so assessing nutrition status is essential to providing care. As the disease progresses, the ability to recognize hunger, thirst, and satiety is impaired, and weight loss and dehydration are common. Because of forgetfulness, decreased appetite, and constant pacing, it is important to monitor intake, assist with feeding, and provide nutrition supplementation if necessary. It is also important to decrease distractions during mealtime.

Incontinence can be an issue for patients with Alzheimer's disease (Andrews, 2013). Another concern is caregiving. Depending on the stage, levels of care are more demanding. Of the seven stages of AD, stages 6 and 7 require the most assistance. Box 19-2 discusses issues of concern. The *Cultural Considerations* box Inadequate Treatment in Dementia suggests cultural issues in relation to delayed recognition and treatment.

Amyotrophic Lateral Sclerosis

Amyotrophic lateral sclerosis, also known as Lou Gehrig's disease, is a progressive degenerative motor neuron disease that destroys nerve cells from the spinal cord to the muscle cells in adults. Symptoms include muscular wasting, atrophy, difficulty speaking, drooling, loss of reflexes, respiratory infections or failure, spastic gait, and weakness. Both upper and lower motor neurons are affected, with progressive paralysis and respiratory failure. Neuromuscular respiratory failure is the most common cause of death, usually within 2 to 5 years the disease onset (Radunovic, et al, 2013).

🌐 CULTURAL CONSIDERATIONS
Inadequate Treatment in Dementia

Patients of minority groups often receive delayed diagnosis or inadequate treatment for dementia. Ethnic and racial differences in biologic risk factors, such as genetics and cardiovascular disease, may help to explain disparities in the incidence and prevalence of Alzheimer's disease (AD), whereas race-specific cultural factors may impact diagnosis and treatment. Cultural factors include differences in perceptions about what is normal aging and what is not, lack of adequate access to medical care, and issues of trust between minority groups and the medical establishment.

Racial biases are inherent in the cognitive screening tools widely used by clinicians. Controlling for literacy level has the potential to mitigate these biases. Biomarker-based diagnostic tools may be useful in further characterizing diverse populations with AD. Education and outreach are critical steps to understanding AD as it relates to diverse populations.

Data from: Chin AL, et al: Diversity and disparity in dementia: The impact of ethno-racial differences in Alzheimer disease, *Alzheimer Dis Assoc Disord* 25:187-195, 2011.

BOX 19-2   Final Stages in Alzheimer's Disease

Stage 6: Severe Cognitive Decline
People with severe cognitive decline:
- Lose awareness of recent experiences as well as of their surroundings
- Remember their own name but have difficulty with their personal history
- Distinguish familiar and unfamiliar faces but have trouble remembering the name of a spouse or caregiver
- Need help dressing properly and may, without supervision, make mistakes such as putting pajamas over daytime clothes or shoes on the wrong feet
- Experience major changes in sleep patterns—sleeping during the day and becoming restless at night
- Need help handling details of toileting (for example, flushing the toilet, wiping or disposing of tissue properly)
- Have increasingly frequent trouble controlling their bladder or bowels

Stage 7: Very Severe Cognitive Decline
People in stage 7 of Alzheimer's disease:
- Lose the ability to respond to their environment, to carry on a conversation and, eventually, to control movement; may still say words or phrases
- Experience major personality and behavioral changes, including suspiciousness and delusions (such as believing that their caregiver is an impostor) and compulsive, repetitive behavior, like hand-wringing or tissue shredding
- Tend to wander or become lost
- Need help with much of their daily personal care, including eating and using the toilet
- May also lose the ability to smile, to sit without support, and to hold their heads up
- Have abnormal reflexes, and their muscles grow rigid

Data from Alzheimer's Association. Accessed September 29, 2013, from www.alz.org/care/alzheimers-late-end-stage-caregiving.asp#food.

Food and Nutrition Therapies

ALS alters nutritional state, energy intake, and energy expenditure (Genton, et al, 2011). A genetic mutation reduces the energy supply in neurons and other cells. Respiratory failure occurs as a result of bulbar, cervical, and thoracic loss of motor neurons; inspiratory lung muscles are affected. Malnutrition occurs from elevated metabolic needs and swallowing dysfunction in the lower set of cranial nerves. This malnutrition produces neuromuscular weakness and adversely affects patients' quality of life. Maintaining a neutral energy balance prevents malnutrition and its complications and may improve physical functioning, quality of life, and survival (Genton, et al, 2011).

Application to nursing. Strategies are necessary to limit aspiration pneumonia, reduce secretions, position the patient to a maximal mechanical advantage, and provide noninvasive positive pressure ventilation. In the later stages of the disease, percutaneous endoscopic gastrostomy (PEG) feeding may be needed. However, quality of life will not necessarily improve. Individuals have the right to refuse treatments, including tube feeding. Some patients decide not to prolong their suffering. Supporting respiratory function with mechanical ventilation may improve survival and quality of life (Radunovic, et al, 2013).

Coma

Coma is the unconscious state in which the patient is unresponsive to verbal or painful stimuli. The Glasgow Coma Scale (GCS) is used to assess level of consciousness; a score of 8 or less is usually indicative of coma. Impaired consciousness or coma can occur from a stroke, head injury, meningitis, encephalitis, sepsis, lack of oxygen, epileptic seizure, toxic effects of alcohol or drugs, liver or kidney failure, high or low blood glucose levels, or altered body temperature. A *persistent vegetative state* (PVS) is a deep state of unconsciousness. PVS is not brain death. The person is still alive but unable to move or react.

Food and Nutrition Therapies

A patient in PVS does not have the ability to request or refuse treatment. The doctor determines the diagnosis of PVS. Nutrition support is associated with improved survival in patients with coma. Most patients are tube fed.

Application to nursing. Informed consent for adults with PVS is necessary. Patients will not be able to answer questions or respond to requests; thus a family member or legal guardian must be the advocate and assist with medical decisions. Understanding the patient's background and wishes allows the health team and family to make valid decisions about initiating, withholding, or withdrawing artificial nutrition and hydration. Family counseling is especially important as ethical issues come into play.

Epilepsy and Seizure Disorders

A seizure is the result of uncontrolled excessive neuronal discharges in the brain. Epilepsy involves a disturbance of the nervous system with recurrent seizures, loss of consciousness, convulsions, motor activity, or behavioral abnormalities. Seizures are classified by their clinical manifestation. A grand mal seizure involves an aura, a tonic phase, and a clonic phase. A petit mal seizure involves a momentary loss of consciousness. Overall, a single seizure does not imply epilepsy. Indeed, there are many forms of epilepsy, each with its own symptoms.

Food and Nutrition Therapies

A ketogenic diet should be considered for refractory epilepsy. In children, this diet results in short- to medium-term benefits in seizure control, comparable to that achieved with antiepileptic drugs (Levy, et al, 2012). The ketogenic diet contains 70% to 90% fat with the remainder as protein and carbohydrates. Patients consuming this high-fat diet produce ketone bodies, which boost energy production in brain tissue. Ketogenic diets increase the brain energy molecule adenosine triphosphate (ATP) as well as the levels and actions of the related endogenous inhibitory neuromodulator adenosine; both are important modulators of seizures.

A medium-chain triglyceride (MCT) diet alleviates some of the obstacles of compliance and acceptance. MCTs are quickly digested and are more ketogenic than long-chain triglycerides. Although overall caloric restriction may improve the efficacy of the ketogenic diet, the diet may slow growth. Many children find the diet difficult to tolerate (Levy, et al, 2012). An alternative diet that is not as strict uses a low–glycemic index treatment, with more liberal total carbohydrate intake.

Bone health, metabolism of vitamin D, and calcium absorption are impaired by the use of antiepileptic drugs. Problems include bone mineral density loss and double or triple the risk of fracture (Harijan, et al, 2013). Low-dose vitamin D supplementation should be prescribed, and compliance followed up.

Application to nursing. The ketogenic diet can be challenging. The patient and family members will need a great deal of support and education. Since the ketogenic diet is commonly used with children, the nurse can share ideas listed in the *Teaching Tool* box Tips for Parents about the Ketogenic Diet with parents.

Guillain–Barré syndrome

Guillain–Barré syndrome is a rare, acute inflammatory demyelinating polyneuropathy with rapidly increasing weakness, numbness, pain, and paralysis of the legs, arms, trunk, face, and respiratory muscles. The exact cause is unknown, but it often occurs a few days or weeks after infection with a respiratory illness, influenza, or *Campylobacter jejuni*. Contaminated water, undercooked poultry, and unpasteurized milk are often sources of *C. jejuni*. The bacterium resides in the epithelial layer of the human gastrointestinal route and causes mainly inflammation and diarrhea (Figure 19-4) (Nyati and Nyati, 2013).

Bloody diarrhea, fever, cramping, and headache are presenting symptoms. Older individuals are at greater risk. GBS may progress to respiratory failure, paralysis of lower

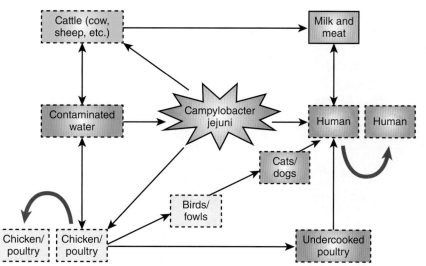

FIG 19-4 Sources and transmission of *Campylobacter jejuni*. Chicken is a natural reservoir of the *C. jejuni*. Sometimes antibodies produced against the bacterium mimic the host nerve ganglio-sides, resulting in demyelination and axonal degeneration of peripheral nerves that cause Guillain-Barré syndrome. (Redrawn from Nyati KK, Nyati R: Role of *Campylobacter jejuni* infection in the pathogenesis of Guillain-Barré syndrome: An update, *Biomed Res Int* 2013:852195, 2013.)

✸ TEACHING TOOL

Tips for Parents about the Ketogenic Diet for Epilepsy

- Most children handle the initial fasting surprisingly well because of the promise of fewer seizures.
- Getting into a routine when fixing meals should make things easier.
- Involve your child in measuring food by guiding the child while he or she places food on the gram scale.
- Your child may feel hungry (because the diet restricts calories) and may try to sneak food from the refrigerator, and even from the pet's dish. Using water with saccharin and splitting meals in half may help fight hunger pains.
- Use a salad plate to present each meal, because the smaller plate makes it look as if the child is getting more food.
- If your child loves dessert, always keep a stock of home-made cream ice pops in the freezer. These are then calculated into meal plans.
- Keep a few pre-prepared meals in small plastic containers in the fridge. Label them carefully for your older child's use if you are not home or your child goes to a friend's house.
- Cut foods into interesting shapes to make them more appealing.
- Check with your doctor about how to handle days when it's hot and your child perspires more than usual.

Data from Epilepsy Foundation. Accessed September 27, 2013, from http://www.epilepsy.com/learn/treating-seizures-and-epilepsy/dietary-therapies/ketogenic-diet

---

extremities, or quadriplegia. Patients may experience unstable blood pressure, aspiration, impaired speech, muscular pain; low-grade fever, tachycardia, and chronic urinary tract infections. With proper care, most patients recover completely.

Food and Nutrition Therapies

In patients with GBS who have dysphagia and difficulty with chewing, tube feeding may be required. In later stages of the disease, weakness or paralysis may inhibit the patient's ability to self-feed, leading to weight loss and anorexia. Discussion about safe food handling is important for prevention of this disease, including proper cooking temperatures for chicken and the use of pasteurized milk products.

Application to nursing. Sometimes ventilatory assistance is needed. Although most people recover within a few weeks

from GBS, some have residual effects for years. Some may need intensive care support followed by wheelchair assistance. No treatment has been totally effective. Patients and family members need support and education on how to manage care with for GBS.

Huntington's Disease

Huntington's disease (HD) is a progressive, fatal neurodegenerative disease characterized by chorea (involuntary, spasmodic, irregular movements), behavioral and psychiatric disturbances, and dementia (Pringsheim, et al, 2012). Prevalence is high in populations of European background (Warby, et al, 2011) (Figure 19-5).

HD generally develops between ages 30 and 50, with chorea, cerebral degeneration, cognitive decline, and speech difficulties. Behavioral changes begin 10 years before the

HD Prevalence Estimates

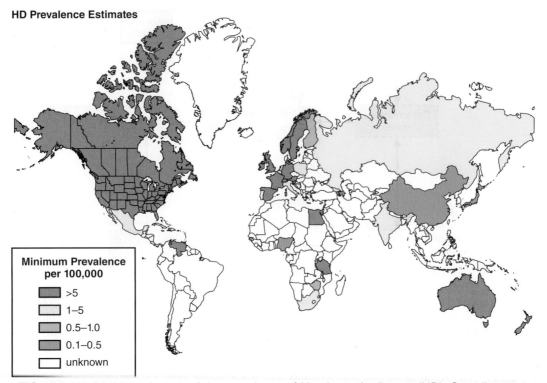

FIG 19-5 Worldwide estimates of the prevalence of Huntington's disease (HD). Overall, prevalence of this disease is much higher in European than in East Asian populations. (From Warby SC, et al: HTT haplotypes contribute to differences in Huntington disease prevalence between Europe and East Asia, *Eur J Hum Genet* 19:561-566, 2011.)

movement disorder. Unfortunately, there is no cure, and death is often a result of pneumonia, suicide, or a fall.

Food and Nutrition Therapies

Nutritional intake plays an important role in HD. Because of dysphagia and the inability to self-feed, patients are at high risk for aspiration and malnutrition. Folic acid, coenzyme Q10, and unsaturated fatty acids are important for neuroprotection. Consuming diets that deliver sugar to the blood rapidly (high glycemic index) exacerbates the symptoms; thus, calorie restriction may be of benefit (Jiang, et al, 2011). In later stages, tube feeding may be required.

Application to nursing. Eventually in the patient with HD, there is complete dependency and the need for full-time care. Remotivation therapy leads to increased self-awareness, greater self-esteem, and improved quality of life. While stem cell transplantation shows promise, it is not yet available as a treatment modality.

Migraine Headache

Migraine is a brain disorder resulting from altered sensory stimuli and trigeminal nerve dysfunction. Migraine headaches (migraines) affect millions of people in the United States. They often begin between the ages of 10 and 40 and diminish after age 50. People who are prone to migraines are at risk for stroke and should be monitored carefully.

Nausea, vomiting, and acute sensitivity to light or sound may occur with migraines, along with attacks of headache, vasospasm, and visual disturbances. Lack of food or sleep, exposure to light, and anxiety, stress, fatigue, or hormonal irregularities can set off a migraine attack. Migraines are especially common among women in their reproductive years (Smitherman, et al, 2013).

Food and Nutrition Therapies

Food allergy is common in people with migraine. Food sensitivities often occur within 24 hours after consumption of the offending food or beverage. Egg white and cow's milk are foods that may trigger migraines in sensitive individuals. It is important that testing be done before foods that are nutrient-rich are eliminated from the patient's diet.

Food elimination based on specific antibodies in patients with migraine who also suffer from irritable bowel syndrome may reduce symptoms of both disorders (Aydinlar, et al, 2013). Treatment begins with a headache-food diary and the selective avoidance of foods presumed to trigger attacks. Migraines may also be reduced with intake of fish oil and olive oil.

Application to nursing. Exercise, relaxation, massage therapy, biofeedback, adequate sleep, and other therapies can limit discomfort. Long-term prophylactic drug therapy is needed for some individuals. Patients should seek improved sleep habits, limited or moderate caffeine intake, regular exercise, and identification of provocative influences. See the *Personal Perspectives* box Thank Goodness for Menopause!

FIG 19-6 This man has multiple sclerosis and has learned to use adaptive techniques for preparing meals at home.

Multiple Sclerosis

Multiple sclerosis (MS) involves scarring and the loss of myelin sheath, the insulating material around nerve fibers. The disease causes progressive or episodic nerve degeneration and disability. The age at onset of MS is usually between 20 and 40 years. Symptoms include tingling; numbness in arms, legs, trunk, or face; double vision; fatigue; weakness; clumsiness; tremor; stiffness; sensory impairment; loss of position sense; and respiratory problems. Dysphagia, spasticity, and bladder dysfunction are also common.

Genetic factors and environmental factors play a role, as do dietary components and their interactions (Ho, et al, 2012). MS has a high incidence among Caucasians and affects women two to three times as often as men. Insufficient vitamin D_3 plays a role; persons living in colder climates and those with less sun exposure are more prone to the disease.

Food and Nutrition Therapies

Nutrition is one of the environmental factors involved in MS. A lower salt intake may be protective against inflammatory and autoimmune responses. Vitamin D deficiency has been implicated. Serum levels of the vitamin should be tested regularly.

Application to nursing. Patients with MS may have periods of remission; others may experience a progressive decline. Eventually, full dependency for many activities of daily living can occur. For some patients, a wheelchair becomes necessary. Adaptations for shopping and cooking at home will require interventions from the physical therapist, the occupational therapist, and the registered dietitian (Figure 19-6).

Myasthenia Gravis

Myasthenia gravis (MG) is an autoimmune disorder caused by autoantibodies at the neuromuscular junction that attack acetylcholine receptors. The attack prevents acetylcholine from stimulating muscle contraction. The neuromuscular junction lies beyond the protection of the blood-brain barrier and is particularly vulnerable to antibody-mediated attack.

BOX 19-3	Symptoms of Parkinson's Disease

- Tremor of hands, arms, legs, jaw, and face
- Rigidity or stiffness of limbs and trunk
- Slowness of gait and movement (bradykinesia)
- Postural or coordination difficulty
- Problems with speech
- Depression and dementia-related symptoms

Data from Parkinson's Disease Foundation: *What is Parkinson's disease?* n.d. Accessed September 29, 2013, from www.pdf.org/en/about_pd.

MG involves the thymus gland. Initially, the ocular muscles are affected, with intermittent drooping eyelids (ptosis) and double vision (diplopia). Weak voice, pneumonia or respiratory arrest, and sleep apnea are also commonly found.

Few forms of MG are congenital; most are acquired. Acquired neuromuscular junction disorders include botulism, autoimmune MG, and drug-induced MG. When MG is suspected, a Tensilon (edrophonium) test involves insertion of a small intravenous catheter through which the agent is given, blocking degradation of acetylcholine. The short-term availability of acetylcholine results in improved muscle function, often in the eye area. General immunosuppression becomes a primary treatment. Removal of the thymus gland works for some patients.

Food and Nutrition Therapies

Dysphagia is a concern in patients with MG. Other concerns requiring nutritional intervention include diabetes and thyroid conditions. Dietary alterations will be necessary.

Application to nursing. Patients with MG present with fatigue and weakness. Assistance with feeding may be required.

Parkinson's Disease

Parkinson disease is a neurodegenerative disorder that affects 1% to 2% of persons 60 years and older. Symptoms are shown in Box 19-3. Loss of dopaminergic neurons in brain will

BOX 19-4   Colorful Antioxidant-Rich Foods

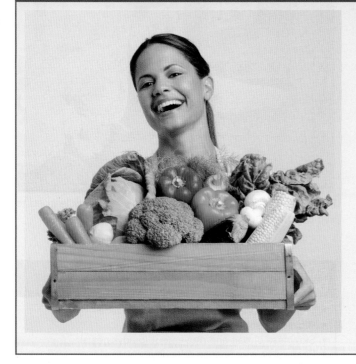

Red/Pink
Lycopene is found in tomatoes, strawberries, pink grapefruit, and watermelon.

Orange
Carotenoids are the antioxidants in carrots, mangoes, pumpkin, and sweet potatoes. They store beta carotene, which the body turns into vitamin A.

Yellow and Green
Get lutein and zeaxanthin from honeydew melon, avocados, and yellow corn. Green cruciferous vegetables such as broccoli and Brussels sprouts contain indoles.

Purple/Blue
Purple in grapes, blackberries, blueberries, and eggplant comes from anthocyanidin, which reduces inflammation. Because different foods contain different anthocyanidins, one should try to eat a range of purple and blue foods to benefit the most.

White
Garlic, onions, and cruciferous vegetables such as cabbage and cauliflower contain allium and sulforaphane. White button mushrooms have cancer-preventive properties in beta-glucan.

---

occur. Although levodopa is required, its long-term use is associated with potentially disabling motor complications. Deep brain stimulation shows promise. Medtronic, Inc. (Minneapolis, MN) offers two neurotransmitters that can be used to help control tremors: Activa RC and Activa PC.

Food and Nutrition Therapies

Genetics and oxidative stress have been implicated in PD. Adherence to a Mediterranean diet is associated with slower cognitive decline. An antioxidant-rich diet may be protective. See Box 19-4.

Application to nursing. Unintentional weight loss is common in the patient with PD, from increased energy expenditure because of tremor, dyskinesias, and rigidity. Thus, most patients require either a longer time with meals, assistance, or dysphagic dietary adaptations. Extra calories and protein may also be needed.

Stroke

A stroke or cerebrovascular accident (CVA) involves damage to a portion of the brain resulting from loss of blood supply due to a blood vessel spasm, clot, or rupture. Hypertension, smoking, diabetes mellitus, atrial fibrillation, and oral contraceptive use are key risk factors. Inflammation in the neural cells plays a central role in the pathogenesis of the disease.

Sporadic strokes can occur, but most of those have a genetic component. Transient ischemic attacks (TIAs) are brief episodes of blood loss to the brain from a clot or an embolism (Figure 19-7); 10% of people who have a TIA will have a major CVA within a year.

FIG 19-7 In the brain, transient ischemic attacks often precede a larger stroke.

Food and Nutrition Therapies

Intake of red and processed meats, refined grains, sweets, and desserts should be limited. Instead, quality protein, magnesium, and potassium from cruciferous and green leafy vegetables, citrus fruits, and carotenoids should be used. Both fish and omega-3 fatty acids seem to prevent thrombotic strokes. Thus, a plant-based diet high in fruits, vegetables, fish, and whole grains may be a wise plan.

Application to nursing. The patient who has suffered a stroke needs medical treatment within 60 minutes. Left-sided CVA affects sight and hearing most commonly, including the ability to see where foods are placed on a plate or tray. Patients with a right-hemisphere, bilateral, or brainstem CVA have significant problems with self-feeding, swallowing, and speech.

Motor deficits may occur with muscle weakness of the tongue and lips. With nerve damage, lack of coordination and sensory deficits occur, including the inability to feel food in the mouth. Cognitive deficits include difficulty sustaining attention, poor short-term memory, visual field problems, impulsiveness, aphasia, and judgment problems such as not knowing how much food to take or what to do with the food once it reaches the mouth.

PSYCHIATRIC CONDITIONS

Eating Disorders

Anorexia Nervosa

Anorexia nervosa is an eating disorder in which the patient severely rejects food, causing extreme weight loss, low basal metabolic rate, and exhaustion. AN affects 1% of teens between ages 10 and 20, especially girls. Onset peaks at 12 to 13 and 19 to 20 years of age; however, it can occur at any age. Signs include relentless pursuit of thinness, misperception of body image, and restrained eating, binge eating, or purging. The intense fear of becoming fat is not diminished as weight loss progresses and has no known physical cause.

Early detection and treatment are important. Oral symptoms, including mucosal, dental, and saliva abnormalities, are observed in the early stages. Weight is 85% or less of former weight at diagnosis, and women usually have amenorrhea and low bone density.

Many dancers, athletes, models, and entertainers struggle with an ED. Anorexic individuals are perfectionistic, overly dependent, meticulous, introverted, emotionally reserved, and socially insecure. *Emotion acceptance behavior therapy* (EABT) is a new treatment method. that emphasizes management of anorexic symptoms by increasing awareness of emotions, decreasing avoidance of emotions, and resuming valued activities and relationships outside the eating disorder (Wildes and Marcus, 2011).

Teens with ED often fake cooperation with treatment plans. These behaviors prolong treatment and can lead to malnutrition. The main concern is inadequate energy intake. The majority of patients with EDs make a full recovery with treatment. Without treatment, death may occur from cardiac arrhythmia.

Food and nutrition therapies. Enteral nutrition is the preferred route of feeding if the patient's gastrointestinal (GI) tract is functional. Tube feeding, when accepted, helps increase weight and improve cognitive and physical functioning. Higher-calorie diets instituted at admission lead to faster weight gains and shorter hospital stays. Thus, specially qualified dietitians should be involved in all levels of care of patients with EDs, including individual and group treatment programs.

Application to nursing. Feeding must be performed cautiously and in a specialized unit to avoid the refeeding syndrome. To provide assistance with the EABT, nurses may benefit from specialized training.

Binge Eating Disorder and Bulimia

Binge eating disorder (BED) involves recurrent episodes of eating in a discrete period of time an amount of food larger than most people would eat in the same time, a sense of lack of control over the eating episodes, rapid or secretive eating, guilt, and shame. Binge eating is a serious problem among some obese individuals, with weight cycling and psychologic distress. Chronic dieting may predispose vulnerable individuals to binge eating, alcoholism, or drug abuse.

Bulimia nervosa (BN) is an eating disorder in which food addiction is the primary coping mechanism. Criteria for diagnosis include recurrent episodes of binge eating, a sense of lack of control, self-evaluation unduly influenced by weight or body shape, recurrent and inappropriate compensating behavior (vomiting, use of laxatives or diuretics, fasting, excessive exercise) two times weekly for 3 months or longer. When not bingeing, individuals with BN tend to be dieting; when hungry, they may binge and purge again. Their self-worth tends to be associated with thinness. Bulimic people use food as a coping mechanism. Because disturbances in neuronal systems modulate feeding, mood, and impulse control, altered serotonin levels contribute to the disordered eating.

Food and nutrition therapies. Mindfulness-based eating awareness training (MB-EAT) involves training in mindfulness meditation and guided practices that are designed to address the core issues. Patients learn how to control responses to varying emotional states, make conscious food choices, develop an awareness of hunger and satiety cues, and cultivate self-acceptance (Kristeller and Wolever, 2011.)

Application to nursing. The team approach to BED and BN is best coordinated with the physician, the nurse, a qualified dietitian, and a mental health professional. Sometimes, an appropriate exercise program under the guidance of a physical therapist may also be offered.

Bipolar Disorder

Abnormalities in brain biochemistry and circuits are responsible for the extreme shifts in mood, energy, and functioning in bipolar affective disorders (BPADs). Bipolar disorders often develop in the late teens or early adult years, usually before age 25. In general, the later the onset of an observable mood disorder, the less severe the case. The spectrum involves depression with varying degrees of excitatory signs and symptoms. The World Health Organization reports that BPAD is the sixth leading cause of years lived with disability, worldwide.

Food and Nutrition Therapies

Adults with mood disorders are at risk for many nutrient inadequacies as well as occasional excesses. Many signaling pathways respond to hormones and nutrition. Because healthier diets protect mental health, individuals with mood disorders could benefit from nutritional interventions to improve diet quality.

Application to nursing. Anxiety disorders, post-traumatic stress disorder (PTSD), social phobia, and attention deficit hyperactivity disorders (ADHD) may be comorbidities with BPAD. For "dual diagnoses," both psychotherapy and appropriate medications are important. During the depressive phase of the illness, patients may try to self-medicate with alcohol or other substances, leading to problems with abuse or dependence. Painful physical symptoms are also common. Thus, treatment of both physical and emotional symptoms associated with mood disorders may increase a patient's chance of achieving remission.

DEPRESSION

Depression involves changes in body chemistry (neurotransmitters) because of a mix of genetics and environmental stress. Depression most frequently develops between 25 and 44 years.

Dysthymia is a chronic, moderate type of depression expressed as poor appetite or overeating, insomnia or oversleeping, low energy, fatigue, irritability, and high stress. Children and teens who have dysthymia or depression may experience frequent headaches and absences from school.

Major depressive disorder (MDD) is quite disabling. Persons with MDD have had at least one major depressive episode for 14 days or longer, and such episodes may be recurrent throughout their lives. MDD is debilitating and has a high morbidity rate. Men with the disorder often mask signs of depression by working long hours or drinking too much. Women may have depression during times of hormonal change: menstruation, pregnancy, miscarriage, the postpartum period, and menopause.

Postpartum depression (PPD) is distinctive from major depression in that it begins during pregnancy. This depression occurs in about 15% of pregnancies, negatively affecting both mother and child. Early detection and treatment are needed.

In late-life depression, older individuals experience depression along with a chronic disease such as heart disease, diabetes, or hypertension. In nursing homes, it is expected that about 50% of residents have some form of depression for which medication should be prescribed.

Food and Nutrition Therapies

Many persons with depression have a deficiency of brain serotonin. A mixed diet of protein and carbohydrate should provide adequate amounts of tryptophan, the precursor of serotonin. Painful physical symptoms are common in depressive disorders; abnormalities of serotonin and noradrenaline are strongly associated with pain perception. Monitoring of physical health, including nutrition, is an important adjunctive therapy. Folic acid and *S*-adenosylmethionine (SAMe)

are natural compounds involved with mood disorders (Papakostas, et al, 2012).

Vitamin D is another consideration; supplementation, sunlight exposure, and light therapy are often beneficial.

A mixed diet containing magnesium, calcium, selenium, zinc, omega-3 polyunsaturated fatty acids (omega-3 PUFAs), and antioxidants (coenzyme Q10, glutathione peroxidase, or zinc) will improve the functions of brain receptors. Antidepressants as well as omega-3 PUFAs and physical activity enhance neuroplasticity. Indeed, an anti-inflammatory diet protects against depression, whereas a diet rich in highly processed, refined foods may promote it.

Application to nursing. In many cases, nursing personnel may be the first to take note of depressive symptoms. Diagnosis of depression is indicated by any four of the following symptoms: *SIGECAPS*—*s*leep changes, loss of *i*nterest, inappropriate *g*uilt (hopelessness), *e*nergy decline, *c*oncentration changes, *a*ppetite changes, *p*sychomotor changes, and *s*uicidal thoughts. Prolonged sadness and unexplained crying spells, chronic irritability and agitation or anxiety, chronic pessimism or indifference, indecisiveness, social withdrawal, and unexplained aches and pains may also be present.

Some of the medications used in depression can have undesirable side effects. Older forms of monoamine oxidase inhibitors (MAOIs) may cause a hypertensive crisis when taken with foods such as aged cheeses, Chianti wine, and other tyramine-containing foods. Although treatment guidelines recommend new antidepressants as first-line therapy for patients with depression, newer MAOI formulations have improved safety and tolerability (Cohen and Sclar, 2013). Good nutrition, talk therapy, and medication are all useful, and new research suggests that acupuncture may also be of benefit (MacPherson, et al, 2013).

Schizophrenia

Schizophrenia (SCZ) is a group of disorders manifested as disordered thinking, hallucinations, delusions, apathy, social withdrawal, and mood or behavioral disturbances (delusional, catatonic, or paranoid). Delusions may involve control, persecution, grandiosity, or abnormal fears. *Hallucinations* are perceptions of an external stimulus without a source in the external world. In the resulting psychosis, the individual loses contact with reality.

Less than 1% of the population experiences SCZ, with onset generally between ages 15 and 25 years (earlier in males). There is a strong genetic component (Figure 19-8). Schizophrenia is an autoimmune disorder caused by pathogens, genes, and the immune system acting together (Carter, 2013). Viral prenatal or adult infections, toxoplasmosis, and Lyme disease may trigger susceptible genes. There are many DNA variants in the brains of individuals with SCZ.

SCZ can be either episodic or chronic. Patients often have chronic problems with substance abuse, long-term unemployment, poverty, and homelessness. When schizophrenic patients are at risk for self-harm or harm to others, hospital treatment is required. Patients with the disease have markedly

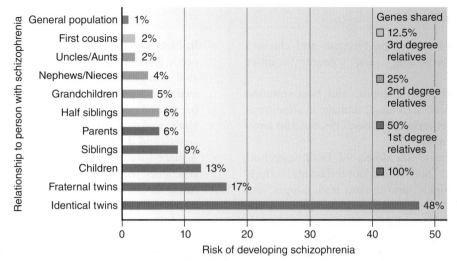

FIG 19-8 A genogram showing the heritability of schizophrenia. (Data from Schizophrenia.com: Accessed on September 30, 2013, from www.schizophrenia.com/research/hereditygen.htm.)

premature mortality, often from underdiagnosed ischemic heart disease and cancer (Crump, et al, 2013).

Food and Nutrition Therapies

Oxidative stress or injury and abnormal membrane phospholipid metabolism lead to fatty acid depletion. Antioxidant-rich foods such as lutein, zeaxanthin, selenium, and N-acetyl-cysteine (NAC), a glutathione precursor, are important considerations. Omega-3 fatty acids help lower inflammation, which is especially damaging to the brain. Low vitamin D availability during brain development interacts with susceptibility genes to alter brain development. Finally, folic acid and vitamin B_{12} are also essential for DNA to function properly.

Application to nursing. Weight gain is an adverse effect of many antipsychotic drugs. Lifestyle intervention and metformin may be suggested for antipsychotic drug–induced weight gain. Use of cannabis (marijuana) should be strongly discouraged as it promotes psychotic behavior in susceptible individuals.

Sleep Disorders

Primary insomnia occurs in 10% of the population, especially among older adults. Circadian rhythms control sleeping and waking, neurotransmitter secretion, and cellular metabolism. Short sleep duration may be related to high blood pressure, depression, and obesity. Altered circadian rhythms may also lead to the metabolic syndrome. In circadian rhythm sleep disorders, wake-sleep cycles differ from the typical pattern. Other sleep disorders are sleep apnea in which breathing is interrupted during sleep, daytime sleepiness (narcolepsy), and restless legs syndrome.

Food and Nutrition Therapies

Melatonin (MT) is formed from L-tryptophan, which plays a major role in sleep and circadian rhythm. Production of melatonin increases with darkness and drops again with light, including artificial lighting. MT production also decreases

with age. Although no specific diet has been identified for use in sleep disorders, light therapy and melatonin supplements have been pilot-tested as treatments. Weight loss and avoidance of alcohol and smoking may be used to treat mild sleep apnea.

Application to nursing. Patients with sleep disorders need support and encouragement to try natural therapies before regular use of sleeping pills, in which dependency may occur.

Night shift work has health consequences that are not always recognized. Researchers are studying the effects of "light at night," which disrupts circadian sleep-wake cycles. Disturbed wake-sleep cycles may contribute to excessive body mass index, cardiovascular diseases, diabetes, cancer, even autism. Melatonin may play a role.

Substance Abuse and Addictions

Addiction is a chronic brain disorder with compulsive and relapsing behavior. The master "pleasure" molecule of addiction is dopamine; it is triggered by heroin, amphetamines, marijuana, alcohol, nicotine, and caffeine. Abnormalities in the metabolism of dopamine, serotonin, and norepinephrine contribute to substance dependency. In some cases, antidepressant medication use alleviates the dependency.

Food and Nutrition Therapies

Addictions share some biologic pathways. Many alcoholics are malnourished, and nutrition intervention is needed to prevent liver disease. Methamphetamine (meth) users often present with poor oral hygiene, xerostomia, rampant caries (Meth mouth), and excessive tooth wear. Cocaine users may experience gastrointestinal hemorrhage. Polydrug use may alter food intake, taste preferences, and nutrient metabolism.

Application to nursing. Dysfunctional eating patterns and excessive weight gains have been observed during recovery from drug and alcohol addictions. Patients need reinforcement of new and healthier behaviors.

SUMMARY

- Dietary precursors (tryptophan, tyrosine, and choline) affect nerve functioning and neurotransmitter effectiveness.
- Inflammatory processes, infections, and host immune responses cause chronic neurologic damage in conditions such as Alzheimer's disease, Parkinson's disease, and amyotrophic lateral sclerosis.
- Nutrients that increase the levels of brain catecholamines and protect against oxidative damage include foods rich in vitamins C and E, zinc, iron, copper, and selenium.
- A Mediterranean diet is useful for Alzheimer's disease; it includes omega-3 fatty acids, light to moderate alcohol use, vegetable oils such as extra virgin olive oil, nonstarchy vegetables, low-glycemic fruits, and lower intake of foods with added sugars.
- Hunger, thirst, and satiety are impaired and lead to weight loss and dehydration in Alzheimer's disease.
- ALS manifests as muscular wasting, atrophy, difficulty speaking, drooling, loss of reflexes, respiratory infections or failure, spastic gait, and weakness. It eventually leads to progressive paralysis and respiratory failure.
- The Glasgow Coma Scale (GCS) is used to assess level of consciousness; a score of 8 or less is usually indicative of coma.
- Patients in a persistent vegetative state (PVS) require tube feeding.
- Guillain-Barré syndrome (GBS) causes weakness, numbness, pain, and paralysis of the legs, arms, trunk, face, and respiratory muscles, often following infection with a respiratory illness, influenza, or food poisoning. *Campylobacter jejuni*, a bacteria associated with GBS, is found in contaminated water, undercooked poultry, and unpasteurized milk.
- Huntington's disease (HD) is a progressive, fatal neurodegenerative disease consisting of chorea, behavioral and psychiatric disturbances, and dementia. Tube feeding is often required.
- Lack of food or sleep; exposure to light; and anxiety, stress, fatigue, or hormonal irregularities can set off a migraine attack. For some people, food allergies may be triggers, and an elimination diet may be beneficial to determine the cause(s).
- MS has a high incidence among Caucasians and affects women two to three times as often as men,; insufficient exposure to sunshine and vitamin D_3 plays a role in MS.
- In myasthenia gravis (MG), symptoms include drooping eyelids (ptosis,) double vision (diplopia), weak voice, pneumonia or respiratory arrest, and sleep apnea. Dysphagia is common.

- In Parkinson's disease, loss of dopamine in the brain will occur; levodopa is required, but its long-term use is associated with potentially disabling motor complications. Self-feeding is a problem for patients with Parkinson's disease because of tremors, and weight loss is common.
- High intake of red and processed meats, refined grains, sweets, and desserts should be discouraged after a stroke. A plant-based diet or Mediterranean diet high in fruits, vegetables, fish, and whole grains is suggested.
- Anorexia nervosa (AN) is an eating disorder (ED) in which the patient severely rejects food, causing extreme weight loss, low basal metabolic rate, and exhaustion. Emotion acceptance behavior therapy (EABT) is a new treatment method.
- Binge eating disorder (BED) involves recurrent episodes of eating in a discrete period of time an amount of food larger than most people would eat in the same time, a sense of lack of control over the eating episodes, rapid or secretive eating, guilt, and shame. Bulimia nervosa (BN) is an eating disorder with food addiction as the primary coping mechanism. Mindfulness-based eating awareness training (MB-EAT) may be useful for both conditions.
- Bipolar spectrum involves depression with varying degrees of excitatory signs and symptoms. Physical and emotional symptoms are associated with mood disorders and should be treated.
- A mixed diet of protein and carbohydrate should provide adequate amounts of tryptophan, the precursor of serotonin, for patients with depression.
- Diagnosis of depression is indicated by any four of the following symptoms, remembered with the pnemonic SIGECAPS—*s*leep changes, loss of *i*nterest, inappropriate *g*uilt (hopelessness), *e*nergy decline, *c*oncentration changes, *a*ppetite changes, *p*sychomotor changes, and *s*uicidal thoughts.
- Schizophrenia is an autoimmune disorder caused by pathogens, genes, and the immune system acting together. A nutritional diet is very important and should include sources of vitamin D, omega-3 fatty acids, and other nutrients.
- Short sleep duration may be related to high blood pressure, depression, and obesity. Altered circadian rhythms may also lead to the metabolic syndrome. Weight loss and decreased intake of alcohol may help conditions such as sleep apnea.
- Addiction is a chronic brain disorder related to dopamine; it is triggered by heroin, amphetamines, marijuana, alcohol, nicotine, and caffeine.

WEBSITES OF INTEREST

Alzheimer's Association

www.alz.org/

Provides background and tips for managing dementias; research advances; publications and resources.

National Alliance on Mental Illness (NAMI)

www.nami.org/

The nonprofit, grassroots mental health education, advocacy, and support organization for mental illness in the United States.

National Eating Disorders Association

www.nationaleatingdisorders.org/

Devoted to providing information to and assistance for individuals and family members of those suffering from eating disorders; education and research.

National Institute of Mental Health (NIMH)

www.nimh.nih.gov/health/index.shtml

The largest scientific organization in the United .States for prevention of mental disorders and the promotion of mental health.

◎ THE NURSING APPROACH

Case Study: Eating Disorder

Brenda, a 16-year-old junior student in high school, came to see the school nurse with complaints of abdominal discomfort. During the interview and examination, the nurse learned that Brenda was concerned about her friend, who had anorexia nervosa. The nurse suspected that Brenda also had some anorexic behaviors. Brenda's school record indicated she weighed 129 pounds 6 months earlier but her current weight was only 109 pounds.

Assessment

Subjective (from Patient's Statements)

- "My stomach hurts. I don't have any energy today."
- "I don't remember when my last period was. It probably was a few months ago. I am not sexually active."
- "I have not had any diarrhea or vomiting. I tend to be constipated. No one in my family has been sick."
- "I haven't eaten anything unusual. I frequently skip lunch at school. I would rather spend the time running. I exercise every day."
- "I always feel so fat."
- "I am worried about my friend Sonya, who is in the hospital with anorexia nervosa. Her mother said Sonya just about died 2 days ago. That scares me."

Objective (from Physical Examination)

- Blood pressure: 108/60; temperature: 97.4° F; pulse: 68; respirations: 14
- Height 5 feet 6 inches, weight 109 pounds
- Abdomen tender, bowel sounds hypoactive
- Appears thin, pale; skin dry, hair dull

Diagnoses (Nursing)

1. Imbalanced nutrition: less than body requirements related to regular exercise and insufficient intake of food as evidenced by 84% ideal body weight, 16% weight loss in 6 months, feels fat, skips meals, abdominal discomfort, loss of menstruation, constipation, fatigue, dull hair, and BP 108/60
2. Disturbed body image related to body distortion as evidenced by "I always feel so fat."
3. Fear related to severe consequences of anorexia nervosa as evidenced by concern for anorexic friend and "that scares me."

Planning

Patient Outcomes

Short term (at the end of this visit):

- Brenda will agree to see a physician for a physical examination and lab tests.
- Brenda will agree to eat small meals frequently throughout the day and to return to the school nurse once a week to report eating and activity and to check weight.

Long term (in 4 months):

- Gradual weight gain, preferably about 1 pound per week
- Develop a regular eating pattern
- Return of menstrual periods, energy, shiny hair
- No abdominal pain and no constipation

Nursing Interventions

1. Express concern for Brenda's friend and state observations that Brenda has some danger signs of poor nutrition.
2. Contact parents regarding the need for Brenda to get follow-up medical care and professional care.

Implementation

1. Expressed concern for Brenda and her friend. Conveyed a nonjudgmental attitude and praised Brenda for seeking help from the school nurse.
   Establishing trust facilitates open discussion about health concerns.
2. Assessed Brenda's knowledge of possible consequences of anorexia nervosa and its treatment, and then corrected misunderstandings.
   Fear may be a motivating factor for behavioral changes. Full information may lead to wiser choices.
3. Told Brenda that she needs to see a physician to determine the cause of her discomfort and evaluate her general health.
   A medical doctor can assess her health, determine a diagnosis, and prescribe care.
4. Related the nurse's observations of Brenda's health to poor nutrition and emphasized benefits of healthy eating.
   It is common for people with anorexia nervosa to deny eating problems and to not associate health difficulties with poor nutrition. Striving for desirable physical characteristics (e.g., shiny hair) and comfort (e.g., lack of constipation) may motivate behavior changes.

Continued

◎ THE NURSING APPROACH—cont'd

5. Gave her a chart indicating normal weights for adolescents her height and showed her how her weight was much lower than expected.

    An individual who has distorted body image may see a more accurate picture of personal weight when comparing own weight to the expected weight on the chart.

6. Helped Brenda set goals to avoid further weight loss and helped her identify possible changes she could make in her lifestyle.

    Involving the individual in planning contributes to empowerment and a sense of control. Small steps may be needed to reach desired changes.

7. Suggested eating small portions of nutrient-dense foods more frequently, including whole grains, milk, fruits, and vegetables.

    Low intake of calories may initially be necessary to prevent refeeding syndrome. Because of early satiety, food intake should be spread throughout the day. These foods will provide nutrients needed for normal metabolism and function, and fiber and adequate water will help reduce constipation. Quantities may be increased gradually.

8. Asked Brenda to visit the nurse once a week for several weeks. Asked her to keep a food and activity record for the next week and to bring it to the school nurse.

    Frequent monitoring of weight helps track improvement (or lack of improvement) and helps an individual to be accountable. Food records can be used for praise of positive eating

when accompanied by stable weight or weight gain. Imbalance of activity versus food may aid discussion and further planning.

9. Telephoned Brenda's parents to invite them to come for a discussion of possible health problems for Brenda and to advise them of the need for medical follow-up and counseling.

    Parents have the responsibility to protect the health of their children and seek medical care as needed. They may not be aware of eating problems. Should the physician diagnose anorexia nervosa, a referral can be made for counseling.

Evaluation

Short term (at the end of the visit):

* Brenda said she would see a doctor.
* She reluctantly agreed to record her food intake and activity for 1 week and return to see the school nurse each week for a few weeks.

Short-term goals met.

Discussion Questions

1. What foods might be acceptable to Brenda for frequent small meals?
2. How can the nurse know whether Brenda's food diary is an honest recording of food and fluids she actually consumed?
3. What would be a reasonable weight gain for Brenda at the end of 1 month?

💡 CRITICAL THINKING

Alzheimer's Disease

Joe, age 70, was diagnosed with Alzheimer's disease 5 years ago and is currently residing with his daughter Joni. Joni recently noticed that her father has lost 5 pounds unintentionally in the past month. She is worried about her father's health and decides to bring him in for an exam. Joni reports that Joe is distracted at meal times, forgets to eat, and often paces around the house. Joe is 5 feet 9 inches and weighs 185 pounds.

1. What can Joni do to decrease distractions at meal time?
2. What suggestions do you have to prevent further weight loss?
3. Joni is worried that she may develop Alzheimer's disease. What foods may protect against this disease?

REFERENCES

Andrews J: Maintaining continence in people with dementia, *Nurs Times* 109:20–21, 2013.

Aydinlar EI, et al: IgG-based elimination diet in migraine plus irritable bowel syndrome, *Headache* 53:514–525, 2013.

Carter CJ: Toxoplasmosis and polygenic disease susceptibility genes: Extensive *Toxoplasma gondii* host/pathogen interactome enrichment in nine psychiatric or neurological disorders, *J Pathog* 2013:965046, 2013.

Cohen LJ, Sclar DA: MAOIs: Issues in treatment adherence and rates of treatment failure, *J Clin Psychiatry* 74:e02, 2013.

Crump C, et al: Comorbidities and mortality in persons with schizophrenia: A Swedish national cohort study, *Am J Psychiatry* 170:324–333, 2013.

DeChiara G, et al: Infectious agents and neurodegeneration, *Mol Neurobiol* 46:614–638, 2012.

Genton L, et al: Nutritional state, energy intakes and energy expenditure of amyotrophic lateral sclerosis (ALS) patients, *Clin Nutr* 30:553–559, 2011.

Harijan P, et al: Vitamin D deficiency in children with epilepsy: Do we need to detect and treat it? *J Pediatr Neurosci* 8:5–10, 2013.

Ho SL, et al: Vitamin D and multiple sclerosis, *Crit Rev Food Sci Nutr* 52:980–987, 2012.

Jiang M, et al: Neuroprotective role of Sirt1 in mammalian models of Huntington's disease through activation of multiple Sirt1 targets, *Nat Med* 18:153–158, 2011.

Kristeller JL, Wolever RQ: Mindfulness-based eating awareness training for treating binge eating disorder: the conceptual foundation, *Eat Disord* 19:49–61, 2011.

Levy RG, et al: Ketogenic diet and other dietary treatments for epilepsy, *Cochrane Database Syst Rev* (3):CD001903, 2012.

MacPherson H, et al: Acupuncture and counselling for depression in primary care: A randomised controlled trial, *PLoS Med* 10:e1001518, 2013.

Nyati KK, Nyati R: Role of *Campylobacter jejuni* infection in the pathogenesis of Guillain-Barré syndrome: An update, *Biomed Res Int* 2013:852195, 2013.

Papakostas GI, et al: L-methylfolate as adjunctive therapy for SSRI-resistant major depression: results of two randomized, double-blind, parallel-sequential trials, *Am J Psychiatry* 169:1267–1274, 2012.

Pringsheim T, et al: The incidence and prevalence of Huntington's disease: A systematic review and meta-analysis, *Mov Disord* 27:1083–1091, 2012.

Radunovic A, et al: Mechanical ventilation for amyotrophic lateral sclerosis/motor neuron disease, *Cochrane Database Syst Rev* (3):CD004427, 2013.

Smitherman TA, et al: The prevalence, impact, and treatment of migraine and severe headaches in the United States: A review of statistics from national surveillance studies, *Headache* 53:427–436, 2013.

Warby SC, et al: HTT haplotypes contribute to differences in Huntington disease prevalence between Europe and East Asia, *Eur J Hum Genet* 19:561–566, 2011.

Wildes JE, Marcus MD: Development of emotion acceptance behavior therapy for anorexia nervosa: A case series, *Int J Eat Disord* 44:421–427, 2011.

Nutrition in Cancer and HIV/AIDS

The nutritional status of patients with cancer, human immunodeficiency virus (HIV), and acquired immunodeficiency syndrome (AIDS) is challenged by manifestations not only of the disease but also by the ramifications of treatment.

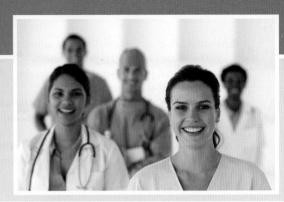

http://evolve.elsevier.com/GRODNER/FOUNDATIONS

LEARNING OBJECTIVES

- Describe common characteristics of cancer and AIDS in terms of their effects on the gastrointestinal (GI) tract, on which nutrition therapy focuses.
- List local or systemic effects of cancer that increase risk of malnutrition or cancer cachexia.
- Discuss the individualized nature of nutrition support in the management of cancer and the benefits that may result

- Summarize the multiple factors that lead to malnutrition in HIV/AIDs.
- Explain the basis of interventions to achieve the goals of HIV nutrition therapy.
- Identify indicators that are key to effective nutrition support and related medical therapies for cancer and HIV/AIDS.

MEDICAL STRESS AND WELLNESS

The nutritional status of patients with cancer, HIV infection, and AIDS is challenged by manifestations of the disease and by the complex treatments. Nutrition therapy focuses on reducing these effects and supporting patients through the side effects of treatment. The goal of maintaining good nutritional status is to improve survival rates, reduce treatment side effects, and improve the quality of life.

Consider the effects of these disorders on the dimensions of health. The *physical health* dimension challenge is to halt or minimize the malnutrition and wasting that are often associated with symptoms or treatments. A person must maintain optimal nutrient intake while also dealing with serious illness, requiring *intellectual health* to comprehend the many different treatments. Facing possible death from AIDS or cancer stresses *emotional health;* nurses need to be sensitive to the emotional burden patients and families are experiencing. *Social health* may be compromised because prejudice or fear of HIV/AIDS and cancer will affect personal and professional relationships. *Spirituality* and deep faith can provide the inner strength to heal. *Environmental health* is implicated because patients who have cancer or HIV infection are at high risk for foodborne illness and superimposed infections.

NUTRITION ASSESSMENT IN CANCER AND HIV/AIDS

The initial step in assessing nutritional risk for cancer or HIV/AIDS is to evaluate anthropometric data. Comparison of current body weight with the client's usual body weight is more crucial than comparison with an "ideal" body weight. Any unexplained weight loss should be noted, but weight loss greater than 10% in 6 months is considered to put the client at risk. Calculation of *body mass index (BMI)* also estimates nutrition risk. A calculated BMI of less than 18 is associated with malnutrition and may be associated with increased mortality. Muscle depletion is also significant. Patients who experience involuntary weight loss and muscle depletion share a poor prognosis, regardless of overall body weight (Martin, et al, 2013).

Note that using only weight loss in the assessment may be misleading. *Bioelectrical impedance analysis (BIA)* has been successfully used to evaluate changes in lean body mass. If BIA is not available, a calculation of upper-arm muscle area can be useful in providing a baseline measurement with which the client can be monitored over time. Other measures such as transferrin value are not applicable because of possible bone marrow suppression.

Dietary assessment may be evaluated by 24-hour recall, food frequency, or food diary. Careful attention should be made to gastrointestinal (GI) function, the presence of steatorrhea and diarrhea, and any other physical symptoms that might interfere with adequate oral intake. In addition, vitamin and mineral status should be monitored closely. Deficiencies may evolve not only from suppressed oral intake but also the increased requirements for certain micronutrients. Research has studied the effects of supplementation but has not identified specific benefits. Indeed, the message continues to be "choose wisely and eat nutritious foods rather than using supplemental nutrients." Whole or natural foods can easily be promoted over refined and highly processed foods.

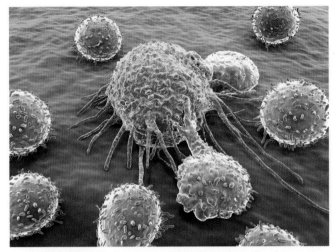

FIG 20-1 Early stage of cancer cell replication.

TABLE 20-1 **Estimated New Cancer Cases by Sex, United States, 2013**		
Men	Prostate	238,590
	Lung and bronchus	118,080
	Colorectal	73,680
	Urinary bladder	54,610
	Melanoma	45,060
	Kidney/renal pelvis	40,430
Women	Breast	232,340
	Lung and bronchus	110,110
	Colorectal	69,140
	Uterine corpus	49,560
	Thyroid	45,310
	Non-Hodgkin's lymphoma	32,140

Data from American Cancer Society: *Cancer facts and figures 2013*, 2013. Accessed October 1, 2013, from www.cancer.org/acs/groups/content/@epidemiologysurveilance/documents/document/acspc-036845.pdf.

CANCER

Cancer cells differ from normal cells in several ways. These characteristics may involve any or all of the following: (1) uncontrolled cellular reproduction occurs, in which cells become independent of normal growth signals; (2) cells contain abnormal nucleus and cytoplasm; and (3) the mitosis rate generally increases (Figure 20-1). The nuclei of the cells may be abnormally shaped and have clearly abnormal chromosomes. This process is called **carcinogenesis**. In carcinogenesis, cells receive sustained signaling to proliferate and evade growth suppressors while also resisting normal cell death (Hanahan and Weinberg, 2011).

The abnormalities in cell replication occur in several stages: initiation, promotion, and progression. *Initiation* of the process results in a mutation of deoxyribonucleic acid (DNA). Inflammation, physical and chemical agents, or exposure to microorganisms may initially cause the mutation in a genetically susceptible individual. The second phase is when the replication of the mutated cell is *promoted* and abnormal cell growth results. Factors that have been identified in some malignancies are estrogen, testosterone, nitrates, cigarette smoke, and alcohol. The third stage is the *progression* of the abnormal cells outside the original location of the cell.

The rate of tumor growth depends on characteristics of both the host and the tumor. Host factors may include age, sex, genetics, nutritional status, the presence of other diseases, hormone production, and immune function. Tumor factors include where the tumor is located and its access to adequate blood supply. The increased blood supply is referred to as a form of *angiogenesis*.

Cancer remains a leading cause of mortality in the United States. Cancer is the second leading cause of death, accounting for more than 550,000 deaths each year. Most diagnoses of cancer occur in older individuals, with almost two thirds in people older than 65 years. The most common types of cancer are lung, prostate, breast, and colorectal (Table 20-1). The National Cancer Institute encourages cancer prevention by following these guidelines:

FIG 20-2 Targets of reactive oxygen species (ROS) in tumorigenesis. ROS can both suppress and promote the transformation, survival, proliferation, invasion, inflammation, angiogenesis, and metastasis of tumor cells.

- Not smoking cigarettes or using other tobacco products
- Limiting daily alcohol intake (one drink for women, two for men)
- Eating five or more daily servings of fruits and vegetables
- Eating a low-fat diet
- Maintaining or reaching a healthy weight
- Being physically active
- Protecting skin from excessive sunlight.

Scientists estimate that 50% to 75% of all cancer deaths can be linked to human behaviors and lifestyle factors. **Reactive oxygen species** (ROS) are produced in the body and play a major role in various cell-signaling pathways; stress, tobacco, environmental pollutants, radiation, viral infection, diet, and bacterial infection are promoters of ROS (Gupta, et al, 2012). ROS have both cancer-suppressing and cancer-promoting actions, making them a paradox (Figure 20-2).

Although ROS activate various transcription factors that promote tumor cell proliferation and invasion, angiogenesis, and metastasis, they have also been implicated in the chemo-preventive and antitumor action of nutraceuticals derived from fruits, vegetables, spices, and other natural products used in traditional medicine (Gupta, et al, 2012). Indeed, nutrition factors are considered one of the important environmental and lifestyle factors in the etiology and prevention of cancer.

For example, antioxidants in the diet may protect the cell from DNA mutation, but high use of supplements is problematic (see the Critical Thinking section, p. 430, "Food: A Pharmaceutical Agent?").

Cancer Diagnosis and Cachexia

With more than 100 variations, cancer affects many individuals in the United States. The physiologic response to malignancy is different for each specific tumor type, but there are general nutrition risk factors that may apply. Physical impairment because of the location of the tumor, the extent of tumor involvement, metabolic changes, and the use of cancer drugs all put the patient at increased risk for malnutrition or wasting syndrome.

Cancer cachexia is a complex syndrome with anorexia that results in severe wasting of lean body mass and weight loss; it affects about half of patients with cancer (Suzuki, et al, 2013). Cytokines are proteins that, in small amounts, assist in the communication between cells of the immune system. These cytokines, such as interleukins, interferons, and tumor necrosis factor (TNF), drive the weight loss, anorexia, hypermetabolism, wasting of skeletal muscle mass, and increased levels of lipid breakdown. Cachexia may be present at the beginning stages of tumor development, even before actual weight loss is observed.

The best treatment of cachexia is a multifactorial approach, including a trial of medications such as appetite stimulants, cytokine inhibitors, steroids, nonsteroidal anti-inflammatory drugs, branched-chain amino acids, and omega-3 fatty acids (Suzuki, et al, 2013). Aggressively approaching nutrition support as a major component of medical care can assist with minimizing these nutritional complications. It is also essential to gain the support of family and friends during this time (see *Personal Perspectives* box Behind the Cancer Headlines).

Nutrition and Cancer Treatments

Maintenance of nutritional status during cancer treatment may accomplish the following:
- Decrease the risk of surgical complications.
- Ensure that patients are able to meet increased energy and protein requirements.
- Help repair and rebuild normal tissues damaged by antineoplastic therapy.
- Promote an increased tolerance to therapy.
- Assist in promoting an enhanced quality of life.

Surgery

Treatment for many malignancies (in particular solid tumors) includes surgical resection of the tumor. This route of

---

👤 PERSONAL PERSPECTIVES
Behind the Cancer Headlines

News about the latest cancer therapies is often in the headlines. Information about cancer is readily available on the Internet. What are not as easily accessible are the experiences of individuals whose lives are touched by cancer. Following is a compilation of comments from individuals of varying ages in my life or people whom I've met.

Michele Grodner
Montclair, NJ

- My mother was in the late stages of a malignant brain tumor, but my brother just couldn't bear the thought of putting "his mother" in a nursing home. Instead, he had her stay with him and his family, setting up a bed in their family room. Within a few days, when she could no longer control her bowels, he found himself sponge bathing his 75-year-old mother who hardly knew where she was. He then understood that he could no longer care for her.
- My friend Karen fought the good fight against breast cancer. For 9 years she battled but lost. When she was first diagnosed, she came to see each of us (her neighbors) to tell us in person. I felt honored. I think it was her way of making it real, of announcing it to the world. She learned everything there was to know about every kind of treatment. Several times she traveled to the Dominican Republic for controversial stem cell treatments, riding through the countryside in a rickety van with others in search of medical miracles. The cancer spread, but so did Karen's spirit. Perhaps the miracle of Karen's spirit was to show us how to struggle against disease while still enjoying life.
- Barbara said she didn't want to hold her newborn grandson because she was too weak, but I think it was because she knew that her cancer had spread and she didn't want to become too attached to the baby.
- My uncle's case was complicated. What with inoperable bladder and prostate cancer, high blood pressure, anemia, and advancing Parkinson's disease, there was a lot to consider. One day his oncologist told him that "there are no more treatments available for your cancer" and that he (the oncologist) was going on vacation for 2 weeks. Fortunately, my uncle, guided by my aunt, immediately found a new oncologist who prescribed a different treatment protocol. My uncle is now in remission.

---

treatment can allow for diagnosis, resecting a solid tumor, preventing spread (metastasis) of the malignancy, or reducing the size of the tumor to alleviate pain. The nutritional consequences of surgery depend on the type and extent of the surgical resection. Resections of any portion of the GI tract can alter nutrition intake and nutrient absorption.

Energy and protein requirements may need to be increased to promote optimal wound healing postoperatively. Malabsorption tends to be the primary nutritional problem with procedures involving the GI tract. Unless small bowel resection is extensive, the adaptability of the small intestine may prevent the occurrence of major clinical problems. Many patients with cancer enter surgery already experience malnutrition, raising the risk for complications. For example, more

TABLE 20-2 Nutritional Side Effects of Cancer Surgery

SITE OF SURGERY	SIDE EFFECT
Head and neck	Impaired chewing and swallowing
Esophagectomy	Diarrhea, steatorrhea, esophageal stenosis
Vagotomy	Gastric stasis, diarrhea, fat malabsorption
Gastrectomy	Dumping syndrome; hypoglycemia; malabsorption; possible deficiencies of iron, calcium, vitamin B_{12}, and fat-soluble vitamins
Pancreatectomy	Type 1 diabetes mellitus; possible malabsorption of fats, protein, fat-soluble vitamins, minerals
Small bowel resection	Possible malabsorption of many nutrients; depends on extent and site of surgery
Ileostomy	Sodium and water losses, vitamin B_{12}, malabsorption, fat malabsorption, bile salt diarrhea

Data from Academy of Nutrition and Dietetics: *The complete resource kit for oncology nutrition (online access)*, n.d. Accessed October 1, 2013, from www.eatright.org/shop/product.aspx?id=6442477212.

than 60% of patients with malignancies affecting the head and neck enter surgery malnourished. Additionally, any problems associated with surgery (Table 20-2) will be further complicated if the patient receives subsequent radiation therapy and chemotherapy.

Chemotherapy

Most chemotherapy protocols involve a combination of agents. Chemotherapy agents include alkylating agents, antimetabolites (folate antagonists), purine/pyrimidine antagonists, anthracyclines, platinum antitumor compounds, antibiotics, nitrosoureas, mitotic inhibitors, cytokines, biologic response modifiers, monoclonal antibodies, immunotherapeutic agents, hormones, and enzymes. These agents act by inhibiting one or more steps of DNA synthesis in the rapidly proliferating cells that are characteristic of the malignant cell or by enhancing the host's immune system to improve the response to therapy. Using a combination of medications that interrupt the cancer process in different ways allows for maximum effect with the fewest side effects.

Cells of the bone marrow and those lining the GI tract tend to be susceptible to damage from chemotherapy because of their rapid turnover rate. The effect on these cells accounts for many of the side effects: nausea, vomiting, diarrhea, inflamed mucous membranes of the mouth (mucositis), hair loss, and immunosuppression. The severity and manifestation of the side effects depend on the particular chemotherapy agent, dosage, duration of treatment, rates of metabolism, accompanying drugs, and individual tolerance. These symptoms can lead to malnutrition through a variety of mechanisms: anorexia; nausea; vomiting; mucositis; cardiac, renal,

or liver injury (toxicity); and new food aversions. Nutritional implications of chemotherapeutic agents are summarized in Table 20-3.

Radiation Therapy

Radiation therapy uses ionizing radiation to kill cells by altering the DNA of the malignant cells. This alteration interferes with the factors controlling replication. Irradiation is used to treat tumors that are sensitive to radiation exposure or that cannot be surgically resected. Irradiation also can be used to reduce tumor size so that a successful surgical resection can occur. Though technology has allowed for significant specificity in the use of radiation therapy, some normal cells within the treatment range may also be damaged, causing hair loss, mucositis, and vomiting and diarrhea.

Nutritional problems vary according to the region or area of the body irradiated, dose, and whether radiation therapy is used in combination with surgery or chemotherapy. Complications may develop during radiation treatment or may become chronic and progress even after treatment is completed.

Irradiation sites that usually result in nutrition problems include the head and neck, the abdomen and pelvis (GI tract), and the central nervous system (CNS). Irradiation at any of the three sites may cause anorexia, nausea, and vomiting. In the head and neck, problems include difficulty with ingestion, stomatitis, esophageal mucositis, loss of taste sensation, and changes in the production of saliva. Side effects of radiation therapy of the abdomen and pelvis alter the GI tract (radiation enteritis), reducing digestion and absorption of nutrients because of the development of diarrhea and steatorrhea, malabsorption, ulceration, bowel damage, or obstruction.

Bone Marrow or Stem Cell Transplantation

Bone marrow or stem cell transplantation is used to treat certain hematologic malignancies (acute and chronic leukemia and some forms of lymphoma) as well as in adjunct therapy for solid tumors such as breast cancer.

When bone marrow transplantation (BMT) is used as the treatment of a solid tumor, the patient's own bone marrow is harvested and saved before the initiation of chemotherapy or radiation therapy. The patient then receives high-dose chemotherapy and possibly total body irradiation to eradicate the cancer. The patient's bone marrow is then infused as an autologous "rescue" from the effects of both chemotherapy and irradiation. For hematologic malignancies, a patient receives bone marrow from a genetically matched (allogeneic) donor or in some cases from a twin (syngeneic) donor. In a stem cell transplantation, stem cells are removed from a newborn baby's umbilical cord immediately after birth and are stored until needed for a transplant.

The ability to maintain adequate oral intake is difficult because of the nausea, vomiting, and mucositis that are associated with such high-dose therapies. Parenteral nutrition is a standard protocol, but maintaining some oral or enteral nutrition is important to promote health of the small intestine.

TABLE 20-3 Nutritional Implications of Chemotherapeutic Agents

DRUG CLASSIFICATION	SELECTED EXAMPLES	ACTIONS	NUTRITIONAL IMPLICATIONS
Alkylating agents	Cisplatin Hexamethylmelamine Dacarbazine	React with susceptible deoxyribonucleic acid (DNA) sites	Anorexia, nausea, vomiting, mucositis/stomatitis
Antibiotics	Bleomycin Doxorubicin Dactinomycin	Bind to DNA and inhibit cell division, interfere with ribonucleic acid (RNA) transcription	Anorexia, nausea, mucositis/ stomatitis, diarrhea; some may cause decreased calcium and iron absorption
Antimetabolites	Methotrexate 5-Fluorodeoxyuridine 5-Fluorouracil	Inhibit a stage of DNA synthesis	Anorexia, nausea, vomiting, diarrhea, mucositis, abdominal pain, intestinal ulceration; some may cause decreased absorption of vitamin B_{12}, fat, and xylose
Hormones	Prednisone Tamoxifen Diethylstilbestrol	Alter cell metabolism to cause unfavorable tumor growth	Corticosteroids: sodium and fluid retention, hyperglycemia, gastrointestinal upset, osteoporosis (calcium losses), negative nitrogen balance Estrogens: nausea, vomiting, anorexia, hypercalcemia
Enzymes	Asparaginase	Delay DNA and RNA synthesis by inhibiting protein synthesis (deprive cells of asparagine)	Anorexia, nausea, hyperglycemia, pancreatitis, azotemia (uremia), weight loss
Plant alkaloids	Vinblastine Vincristine	Inhibit mitosis	Nausea, vomiting, constipation, diarrhea, abdominal pain
Biologic response modifiers	Interferon Interleukin	Modify host biologic response to tumor	Nausea, vomiting, anorexia, weight change (increase or decrease)

Data from Academy of Nutrition and Dietetics: *The complete resource kit for oncology nutrition (online access)*, n.d. Accessed October 1, 2013, from www.eatright.org/shop/product.aspx?id=6442477212.

Immunosuppression, due to the antineoplastic regimens and BMT, puts the patient at high risk for infection by bacterial and fungal pathogens. Pathogens can be commonly found in the environment, including fresh fruits and vegetables that ordinarily do not present a hazard to healthy persons (Table 20-4). A *low-bacteria, "neutropenic"* diet is used in a few institutions. Food safety guidelines include avoiding undercooked meats and eggs, ensuring that raw fruits and vegetables are washed well and/or are peeled (including salads and garnishes), and following sanitation guidelines for food preparation and storage. Frequent monitoring of nutritional intake and encouragement to take in adequate nutrition are essential in the care of immunosuppressed patients (Box 20-1).

A major complication that may occur with an allogeneic BMT is graft-versus-host disease (GVHD), which is best described as reverse rejection. In this case, the grafted tissue or organ recognizes the host's cells as foreign and attacks them. GVHD may result in multiple organ damage, but the skin, GI tract, and liver are of particular concern. The nutritional management for GVHD may require intense therapy for several years after transplantation.

Food and Nutrition Therapies

Patients with cancer are at high risk for malnutrition; thus, recognition of the clinical signs and symptoms and early treatment may prevent the consequences. The

Patient-Generated Subjective Global Assessment (PG-SGA) screening tool allows for early identification of patients who have a nutrition deficit or who are at risk for one when treatment is initiated (Figure 20-3).

Nutritional interventions will be tailored to support the energy and protein needs of the patient so that body stores can be maintained, and then, as symptoms arise, interventions can be introduced to maximize nutritional intake. Nutrition should be an essential component of every treatment plan for the patient with cancer. Table 20-5 summarizes interventions used in treating these symptoms. The following are goals for nutrition therapy:

- Maintenance of weight and lean body mass within the established goal range through consumption of adequate energy and protein or with appropriate nutritional support
- Adequate hydration, as measured by clinical and physical assessment
- Adequate energy and protein intakes to perform activities of daily living
- Use of appropriate and safe complementary nutrition therapies

Altered Taste

Many patients with cancer describe alterations in their ability to taste foods. These alterations relate to changes in or

Text continued on p. 423

TABLE 20-4 Common Foods: Lower-Risk Options for Safety in Immunosuppressed Patients

TYPE OF FOOD	HIGHER-RISK	LOWER-RISK	TIP(S)
Meat and poultry	Raw or undercooked meat or poultry	Meat or poultry cooked to a safe minimum internal temperature	Use a food thermometer to check the internal temperature
Seafood	Any raw or undercooked fish, e.g., sushi or ceviche Refrigerated smoked fish Precooked seafood, such as shrimp and crab	Smoked fish and precooked seafood heated to 165° F Canned fish and seafood Seafood cooked to 145° F	
Milk	Unpasteurized milk	Pasteurized milk	
Eggs	Foods that contain raw eggs: Caesar salad dressings, homemade raw cookie dough or eggnog*	At home: Use pasteurized eggs/egg products when preparing recipes that call for raw eggs Away from home: Ask whether pasteurized eggs were used	Most premade foods from grocery stores, such as Caesar dressing, premade cookie dough, and packaged eggnog, are made with pasteurized eggs
Sprouts	Raw sprouts (alfalfa, bean, or any other sprout)	Cooked sprouts	
Vegetables	Unwashed fresh vegetables, including lettuce/salads	Washed fresh vegetables, including salads	
Cheese	Soft cheeses made from unpasteurized milk, such as: – Feta – Brie – Camembert – Blue-veined cheese – Queso fresco	Hard cheeses Processed cheeses Cream cheese Mozzarella Soft cheeses that are clearly labeled "made from pasteurized milk"	
Hot dogs and deli meats	Hot dogs, deli meats, and luncheon meats that have not been reheated	Hot dogs, luncheon meats, and deli meats reheated to steaming hot or 165° F	Reheat hot dogs, deli meats, and luncheon meats before eating them, because the bacteria *Listeria monocytogenes* grows at refrigerated temperatures; this bacterium may cause severe illness, hospitalization, or even death Reheating these foods destroys the dangerous bacterium, making these foods safe to eat
Patés	Unpasteurized, refrigerated patés or meat spreads	Canned patés or meat spreads	

Food Safety.gov: *Food safety for persons with chronic illnesses,* n.d. Accessed October 1, 2013, from www.foodsafety.gov/poisoning/risk/chronicillnesses/.

BOX 20-1 Food Safety for Immunosuppressed Patients

Safe food handling can help to decrease a person's risk of foodborne illness. People with weakened immune systems must take extra caution to avoid putting themselves at risk of becoming infected by a foodborne pathogen. The following precautions help avoid such infections:

Shopping
- Shop for groceries when you can take food home right away; do not leave food sitting in the car.
- Avoid cans of food that are dented, leaking, or bulging.
- Do not purchase food in cracked glass jars.
- Ensure that safety buttons on metal lids are down and do not make a clicking noise when pushed. Make sure that tamper-resistant safety seals are intact.
- Avoid food in torn or punctured packaging.
- Pick up perishable foods (e.g., meat, eggs, milk) last.

- Place packaged meat, poultry, or fish in separate plastic bags to prevent meat juices from dripping onto other groceries or other meats.
- Make sure the "sell by" or "use by" date has not passed.
- Do not buy any food that has been displayed in any unclean or unsafe manner (e.g., meat allowed to sit outside refrigeration, cooked shrimp displayed next to raw shrimp).
- When ordering in the deli department, make sure the clerk washes his or her hands between handling raw food and cooked food.

Storage
- Keep your refrigerator and freezer clean.
- Use a refrigerator thermometer to make sure the temperature inside is 40° F or below.
- Make sure the temperature inside the freezer is 0° F.

Continued

BOX 20-1   Food Safety for Immunosuppressed Patients—cont'd

- On arriving home from the store, immediately refrigerate and freeze appropriate foods.
- Leave eggs in their carton; do not place in refrigerator door.
- Store raw meat, poultry, and fish on the bottom shelf of the refrigerator; prevent their juices from dripping onto other foods. Raw ground meat, poultry, and fish may be stored for 1 or 2 days; other red meat may be stored for 3 to 5 days.
- Store canned foods and other shelf-stable products in a cool, dry place. Avoid hot garages and damp basements.

Preparation
- Wash hands before, during, and after food preparation and service.
- Use plastic or glass surfaces for cutting raw meat and poultry. Use a separate cutting board for preparing other foods, such as fruits, vegetables, and bread.
- Wash cutting boards with hot, soapy water after each use. All cutting boards (except those that are made with laminated wood) can be washed in the dishwasher.
- After handling raw meat, poultry, and fish, wash hands, work surfaces, and utensils with hot, soapy water.
- Wash all fruits and vegetables before cutting, cooking, or eating them raw.
- Defrost frozen food in a bowl in the refrigerator or microwave it. Cook food immediately after thawing.
- Use different utensils and dishes for cooked foods from those used for raw foods.
- Wash kitchen towels and cloths often in hot water in a washing machine.
- A sanitizing solution can be made with one teaspoon of liquid chlorine bleach mixed with one quart of water. Use solution on countertops and other work surfaces. Do not rinse. Allow surface to air-dry.

Cooking
- Keep hot foods hot at 140°F or higher and cold foods cold at 40°F or lower.
- Do not leave perishable foods out for more than 2 hours.
- Promptly refrigerate or freeze leftovers in shallow containers or wrapped tightly in bags.
- Use leftovers within 3 or 4 days.
- When reheating foods in the microwave, cover and rotate or stir foods once or twice during cooking. The food should be steaming hot.
- Do not eat foods past their expiration date.
- Follow the handling and preparation instructions on product labels to ensure top quality and safety.

Meat, Poultry, and Fish
- Do not eat raw or undercooked meat.
- Cook all meat and poultry until it is no longer pink in the middle.
- Fish should be cooked until flaky, not rubbery.
- The temperature inside the meat should be higher than 165°F.
- Cook poultry to an internal temperature of 180° to 185°F.
- Cook fish to 160°F.
- Do not eat stuffing cooked inside poultry. Instead, cook stuffing separately to 165°F.
- Cook only shellfish that are closed. Discard any shellfish that do not open during cooking.

Dairy
- Eat or drink only pasteurized milk or dairy products.

Eggs
- Cook eggs until the yolk and white are solid, not runny.
- Do not eat foods that may contain raw eggs, such as Caesar salad dressing and raw cookie dough.
- If eating fried eggs, be sure eggs are fried on both sides.

Fruits and Vegetables
- Raw fruits and vegetables are generally safe to eat if washed carefully first.
- Discard any fruits or vegetables with mold.
- Wash fruits and vegetables under cool running water.
- Do not let cut fruits or vegetables sit unrefrigerated.
- Discard the outermost leaves of a head of lettuce or cabbage.

Water
- Do not drink water straight from lakes, rivers, streams, or springs.
- Always check with your local health department and water company to learn whether they have issued any special notices for people with weakened immune systems.
- Water bottles and ice trays should be cleaned with soap and water before use.

Other
- Home canned foods: Use within 1 year of canning. Cook food for 10 minutes before eating.
- Commercially canned foods: Safe to eat without any further cooking.
- Condiments: Use a clean utensil when dipping into jars. Keep jars refrigerated. Do not use homemade mayonnaise.
- Baby food: Use a clean utensil to remove amount needed from jar. Store opened jars in the refrigerator.

Dining Away from Home
- Avoid the same foods that you would at home (e.g., raw meats, undercooked eggs).
- If the food arrives undercooked, send it back.
- Avoid foods that may contain raw eggs, such as Caesar salad dressing and uncooked sauces such as Hollandaise.
- If you are not sure about the ingredients in a dish, ask your waiter before you order.
- Do not order any raw or lightly steamed fish or shellfish, such as oysters, clams, mussels, sushi, or sashimi.

Traveling
- Do not eat uncooked fruits and vegetables unless you can peel them.
- Avoid salads.
- Eat cooked foods while they are still hot.
- Boil all water before drinking it.
- Drink only canned or bottled drinks or beverages made with boiled water.
- Steaming hot foods, fruits you peel yourself, bottled and canned processed drinks, and hot coffee or tea should be safe.
- Talk with your health care provider about other advice on travel abroad.

Adapted from Caring4cancer: *Food safety during cancer treatment*, 2010. Accessed October 1, 2013, from www.caring4cancer.com/go/cancer/nutrition/eatingwell/food-safety-during-cancer-treatment.htm.

Scored Patient-Generated Subjective Global Assessment (PG-SGA)

Patient ID Information

History (Boxes 1-4 are designed to be completed by the patient.)

1. Weight *(See Worksheet 1)*

In summary of my current and recent weight:

I currently weigh about _____ pounds
I am about _____ feet _____ tall

One month ago I weighed about _____ pounds
Six months ago I weighed about _____ pounds

During the past two weeks my weight has:

☐ decreased $_{(1)}$ ☐ not changed $_{(0)}$ ☐ increased $_{(0)}$

Box 1 [_____]

2. Food Intake: As compared to my normal intake, I would rate my food intake during the past month as:

☐ unchanged $_{(0)}$
☐ more than usual $_{(0)}$
☐ less than usual $_{(1)}$
    I am now taking:
    ☐ *normal food* but less than normal amount $_{(1)}$
    ☐ little solid food $_{(2)}$
    ☐ only liquids $_{(3)}$
    ☐ only nutritional supplements $_{(3)}$
    ☐ very little of anything $_{(4)}$
    ☐ only tube feedings or only nutrition by vein $_{(0)}$

Box 2 [_____]

3. Symptoms: I have had the following problems that have kept me from eating enough during the past two weeks (check all that apply):

☐ no problems eating $_{(0)}$
☐ no appetite, just did not feel like eating $_{(3)}$

☐ nausea $_{(1)}$ ☐ vomiting $_{(3)}$
☐ constipation $_{(1)}$ ☐ diarrhea $_{(3)}$
☐ mouth sores $_{(2)}$ ☐ dry mouth $_{(1)}$
☐ things taste funny or have no taste $_{(1)}$ ☐ smells bother me $_{(1)}$
☐ problems swallowing $_{(2)}$ ☐ feel full quickly $_{(1)}$
☐ pain; where? $_{(3)}$ _____
☐ other** $_{(1)}$ _____

** Examples: depression, money, or dental problems

Box 3 [_____]

4. Activities and Function: Over the past month, I would generally rate my activity as:

☐ normal with no limitations $_{(0)}$
☐ not my normal self, but able to be up and about with fairly normal activities $_{(1)}$
☐ not feeling up to most things, but in bed or chair less than half the day $_{(2)}$
☐ able to do little activity and spend most of the day in bed or chair $_{(3)}$
☐ pretty much bedridden, rarely out of bed $_{(3)}$

Box 4 [_____]

Additive Score of the Boxes 1-4 [_____] A

The remainder of this form will be completed by your doctor, nurse, or therapist. Thank you.

(Optional for completion by clinicians)

5. Disease and its relation to nutritional requirements *(See Worksheet 2)*

All relevant diagnoses (specify) _____

Primary disease stage (circle if known or appropriate)   I   II   III   IV   Other _____

Age _____

Numerical score from Worksheet 2 [_____] B

6. Metabolic Demand *(See Worksheet 3)*

Numerical score from Worksheet 3 [_____] C

7. Physical *(See Worksheet 4)*

Numerical score from Worksheet 4 [_____] D

Global Assessment *(See Worksheet 5)*

☐ Well-nourished or anabolic (SGA-A)
☐ Moderate or suspected malnutrition (SGA-B)
☐ Severely malnourished (SGA-C)

Total PG-SGA score

(Total numerical score of A+B+C+D above) [_____]

(See triage recommendations below)

Clinician Signature _____   RD RN PA MD DO Other ___   Date _____

Nutritional Triage Recommendations: Additive score is used to define specific nutritional interventions including patient & family education, symptom management including pharmacologic intervention, and appropriate nutrient intervention (food, nutritional supplements, enteral, or parenteral triage). First line nutrition intervention includes optimal symptom management.

0-1   No intervention required at this time. Re-assessment on routine and regular basis during treatment.
2-3   Patient & family education by dietitian, nurse, or other clinician with pharmacologic intervention as indicated by symptom survey (Box 3) and laboratory values as appropriate.
4-8   Requires intervention by dietitian, in conjunction with nurse or physician as indicated by symptoms survey (Box 3).
≥ 9   Indicates a critical need for improved symptom management and/or nutrient intervention options.

© FD Ottery, 2001. Used with permission.   email: fdottery@btgc.com or noatpres1@aol.com

FIG 20-3 Patient-Generated Subjective Global Assessment (PG-SGA) of nutritional status. (Copyright FD Ottery, 2001.)

Continued

Worksheets for PG-SGA Scoring © FD Ottery, 2001. Used with permission.

Boxes 1-4 of the PG-SGA are designed to be completed by the patient. The PG-SGA numerical score is determined using
1) the parenthetical points noted in boxes 1-4 and 2) the worksheets below for items not marked with parenthetical points. Scores for
boxes 1 and 3 are additive within each box and scores for boxes 2 and 4 are based on the highest scored item checked off by the patient.

Worksheet 1 - Scoring Weight (Wt) Loss

To determine score, use 1 month weight data if available. Use 6 month data only if there is no 1 month weight data. Use points below to score weight change and add one extra point if patient has lost weight during the past 2 weeks. Enter total point score in Box 1 of the PG-SGA.

Wt loss in 1 month	Points	Wt loss in 6 months
10% or greater	4	20% or greater
5-9.9%	3	10 -19.9%
3-4.9%	2	6 - 9.9%
2-2.9%	1	2 - 5.9%
0-1.9%	0	0 - 1.9%

Score for Worksheet 1 [ ]
Record in Box 1

Worksheet 2 - Scoring Criteria for Condition

Score is derived by adding 1 point for each of the conditions listed below that pertain to the patient.

Category	Points
Cancer	1
AIDS	1
Pulmonary or cardiac cachexia	1
Presence of decubitus, open wound, or fistula	1
Presence of trauma	1
Age greater than 65 years	1

Score for Worksheet 2 = [ ]
Record in Box B

Worksheet 3 - Scoring Metabolic Stress

Score for metabolic stress is determined by a number of variables known to increase protein & calorie needs. The score is additive so that a patient who has a fever of > 102 degrees (3 points) and is on 10 mg of prednisone chronically (2 points) would have an additive score for this section of 5 points.

Stress	none (0)	low (1)	moderate (2)	high (3)
Fever	no fever	>99 and <101	≥101 and <102	≥102
Fever duration	no fever	<72 hrs	72 hrs	> 72 hrs
Corticosteroids	no corticosteroids	low dose (<10mg prednisone equivalents/day)	moderate dose (≥10 and <30 mg prednisone equivalents/day)	high dose steroids (≥30 mg prednisone equivalents/day)

Score for Worksheet 3 = [ ]
Record in Box C

Worksheet 4 - Physical Examination

Physical exam includes a subjective evaluation of 3 aspects of body composition: fat, muscle, & fluid status. Since this is subjective, each aspect of the exam is rated for degree of deficit. Muscle deficit impacts point score more than fat deficit. Definition of categories: 0 = no deficit, 1+ = mild deficit, 2+ = moderate deficit, 3+ = severe deficit. Rating of deficit in these categories are *not* additive but are used to clinically assess the degree of deficit (or presence of excess fluid).

Fat Stores:

orbital fat pads	0	1+	2+	3+
triceps skin fold	0	1+	2+	3+
fat overlying lower ribs	0	1+	2+	3+
Global fat deficit rating	**0**	**1+**	**2+**	**3+**

Fluid Status:

ankle edema	0	1+	2+	3+
sacral edema	0	1+	2+	3+
ascites	0	1+	2+	3+
Global fluid status rating	**0**	**1+**	**2+**	**3+**

Muscle Status:

temples (temporalis muscle)	0	1+	2+	3+
clavicles (pectoralis & deltoids)	0	1+	2+	3+
shoulders (deltoids)	0	1+	2+	3+
interosseous muscles	0	1+	2+	3+
scapula (latissimus dorsi, trapezius, deltoids)	0	1+	2+	3+
thigh (quadriceps)	0	1+	2+	3+
calf (gastrocnemius)	0	1+	2+	3+
Global muscle status rating	**0**	**1+**	**2+**	**3+**

Point score for the physical exam is determined by the overall subjective rating of total body deficit.

No deficit	score = 0 points
Mild deficit	score = 1 point
Moderate deficit	score = 2 points
Severe deficit	score = 3 points

Score for Worksheet 4 = [ ]
Record in Box D

Worksheet 5 - PG-SGA Global Assessment Categories

Category	Stage A	Stage B	Stage C
	Well-nourished	Moderately malnourished or suspected malnutrition	Severely malnourished
Weight	No wt loss OR Recent non-fluid wt gain	~5% wt loss within 1 month (or 10% in 6 months) OR No wt stabilization or wt gain (i.e., continued wt loss)	> 5% wt loss in 1 month (or >10% in 6 months) OR No wt stabilization or wt gain (i.e., continued wt loss)
Nutrient Intake	No deficit OR Significant recent improvement	Definite decrease in intake	Severe deficit in intake
Nutrition Impact Symptoms	None OR Significant recent improvement allowing adequate intake	Presence of nutrition impact symptoms (Box 3 of PG-SGA)	Presence of nutrition impact symptoms (Box 3 of PG-SGA)
Functioning	No deficit OR Significant recent improvement	Moderate functional deficit OR Recent deterioration	Severe functional deficit OR recent significant deterioration
Physical Exam	No deficit OR Chronic deficit but with recent clinical improvement	Evidence of mild to moderate loss of SQ fat &/or muscle mass &/or muscle tone on palpation	Obvious signs of malnutrition (e.g., severe loss of SQ tissues, possible edema)

Global PG-SGA rating (A, B, or C) = [ ]

FIG 20-3, cont'd

TABLE 20-5 Nutritional Approaches to Nutrition-Related Problems in Cancer and Cancer Therapy

PROBLEM	RECOMMENDATIONS
Loss of appetite/early satiety	Eat frequent small meals, increase kcal/protein content of foods, use high-protein/high-kcal supplements, eat foods cool or at room temperature, avoid excess fat, exercise regularly if tolerated, limit liquids at mealtime; appetite may be best in the morning
Diarrhea*	Eat frequent small meals, eat foods cool or at room temperature, increase fluid intake, eat and drink slowly, decrease fiber intake, avoid excess fat, avoid gas-forming foods, limit liquids at mealtime, avoid highly seasoned foods, limit beverages containing caffeine and alcohol; trial avoidance of lactose may be helpful; take antidiarrheal medication per physician order
Nausea and vomiting	Eat frequent small meals, avoid strong odors, eat foods cool or at room temperature, increase fluid intake, eat and drink slowly, avoid excess fat, limit liquids at mealtime, avoid highly seasoned foods, rest after meals with head elevated, take antiemetic medication per physician order
Chewing and swallowing difficulties	Eat frequent small meals, increase kcal/protein content of foods, use high-protein/high-kcal supplements, eat food cool or at room temperature, increase fluid intake, eat and drink slowly, add sauces and gravy to soften and moisten foods, avoid highly seasoned foods, alcohol, tobacco, and commercial mouthwashes; coarse-textured and acidic foods may irritate
Constipation	Increase fluid intake, increase fiber intake, exercise regularly if tolerated; stool softener and/or laxative may be necessary
Abdominal gas	Eat and drink slowly, decrease fiber intake, avoid excess fat, avoid gas-forming foods, exercise regularly if tolerated, limit lactose if not tolerated
Dry mouth	Increase fluid intake, add sauces and gravy to soften and moisten foods, try using tart foods or sugar-free hard candy to stimulate saliva, avoid alcohol, tobacco, and commercial mouthwash
Taste/smell alterations	Eat food cool or at room temperature, increase fluid intake, use seasonings to enhance flavors, avoid cooking odors, try alternative protein sources for meat aversion

*Diarrhea secondary to malabsorption, dumping syndrome, or other causes may require different treatment modalities.
Data from Academy of Nutrition and Dietetics: *The complete resource kit for oncology nutrition (online access)*, n.d. Accessed October 1, 2013, from www.eatright.org/shop/product.aspx?id=6442477212.

destruction of the oral mucosa, the systemic presence of tumor byproducts, changes in the quantity or quality of saliva, inadequate mouth care, or drugs. It is appropriate for patients with cancer to avoid those foods that taste bad to them. However, alternate food choices may be required to maintain adequate nutrient intake. Eating foods that are tart or spicy may enhance overall intake.

Anorexia

Anorexia is loss of appetite, generally caused by changes in taste and smell; decreased transit time and subsequent, early satiety; opportunistic infections; therapy and medication side effects; pain; and emotional and psychologic effects. Early education of the patient with cancer on the role of nutrition in treatment is essential to promote adequate nutritional intake. The nutrient density of food must be stressed. Small, frequent meals, the use of high-kcal supplements, and a pleasant eating environment can help.

Nausea and Vomiting

Nausea and vomiting may result from delayed transit time, hypercalcemia or central nervous system involvement, medications, or anxiety. Cold foods without odor tend to be best tolerated when the patient experiences nausea and vomiting.

Hormonal Cancers

Diets rich in vegetable fiber may be associated with a small reduction in risk for breast cancer (Ferrari, et al, 2013),

whereas a high carbohydrate intake increases risk (Romieu, et al, 2012). High intake of refined carbohydrates may also promote prostate cancer (Drake, et al, 2012). For both cancers, weight reduction can be safely recommended in patients who are overweight.

Lung Cancer

Nutritional supplements should be avoided. In particular, beta carotene and vitamin E should be avoided because they may actually enhance progression of lung cancer (Mondul, et al, 2013).

Skin, Renal, and Urinary Tract Cancers

Plant-based and fiber-rich diets high in vegetables, fruit, and whole grains are recommended to prevent cancer and associated conditions, such as obesity, hypertension, and diabetes (Daniel, et al, 2013). In addition, improved vitamin D status significantly affects expression of genes that have a wide variety of biologic functions in more than 160 pathways linked to cancer (Hossein-Nezhad, et al, 2013).

Application to nursing. Support of patients with cancer must be individualized. Prognosis should be considered to appropriately adjust the aggressiveness of the intervention (supportive, adjunctive, and definitive). Nurses play a key role in helping patients cope with the issues associated with cancer treatment. Patients should be educated on what to expect from their treatment regimen in order to decrease fear and anxiety.

The first line of treatment for nausea and vomiting is adequate and aggressive antiemetic therapy. It is essential to give medication 60 to 90 minutes before meals to ensure effectiveness. Patients are at risk for dehydration, so fluid intake should be monitored.

Behavioral strategies such as guided imagery and relaxation techniques are useful for some individuals. Medications such as megestrol (Megace) and dronabinol (Marinol) have been used successfully to stimulate appetite in patients with cancer. Excellent mouth care is also essential.

HIV INFECTION AND AIDS

In 1983 the human immunodeficiency virus was isolated as the cause for acquired immunodeficiency syndrome. A retrovirus injects its ribonucleic acid (RNA) into the target cell and then transcribes the RNA into DNA using a reverse transcriptase enzyme. Target cells for HIV include the T4 or CD4 lymphocytes, B lymphocytes, monocytes, macrophages, and other cells of the immune system. Currently, there are two major strains of HIV. HIV-1 is commonly found in the United States, whereas HIV-2 is the most common strain found on the African continent.

HIV is a bloodborne and sexually transmitted infection. It is transmitted through contact with contaminated blood, semen, vaginal secretions, and breast milk. HIV also crosses the placenta from the mother to the baby. Approximately 40 million people throughout the world have HIV infection, and they are concentrated in southern and eastern African countries. In sub-Saharan Africa, AIDS is the leading cause of death. In the United States nearly a million people live with HIV infection, primarily minority populations, women, and youth.

As many as 1 billion copies of HIV can be made in 1 day, and several generations can exist in just hours. The initial infection with HIV may involve symptoms such as fever and malaise. Antibodies are produced against the virus and are detectable within 2 to 4 months of exposure. Screening technology (enzyme-linked immunosorbent assay [ELISA]) allows for rapid testing for HIV infection but is followed with tests to confirm the presence of HIV antibodies.

The replication of the infected cell results in a steady depletion of the CD4 cell count, causing a severe depression of immune function and increasing the risk for opportunistic infections and malignancies (Table 20-6). The progression from HIV to AIDS varies for each person and may not be evident for several years. The two major prognostic factors for HIV are the CD4 cell count and the measurement of plasma HIV RNA (viral load for HIV). The diagnosis of AIDS includes the positive antibody test result for HIV, a CD4 cell count of less than $200/mm^3$ or less than 14% of the total white blood cell count, and the clinical diagnosis of 1 of 25 AIDS-defining diseases.

There has been significant progress in treatment of HIV and AIDS over the past decade with the use of drug combinations for highly active antiretroviral therapy (HAART). The goal of these treatment regimens is to maintain a low viral load.

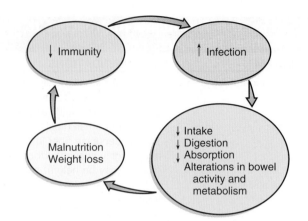

FIG 20-4 Vicious circle of malnutrition and AIDS. (From Rolin Graphics.).

Malnutrition in HIV/AIDS

Malnutrition has been documented in all stages of HIV infection. Most nutritional problems coincide with the incidence of high viral loads, opportunistic infections, and the development of viral resistance. With the evolution of HAART, nutritional problems have shifted to include more chronic disease issues such as hyperlipidemia, insulin resistance, and diabetes mellitus. In infected individuals who do not have access to these medication regimens and in people who choose not to use them, malnutrition is still common.

AIDS-related wasting syndrome consists of involuntary weight loss of greater than 10% of body weight in 1 month with the presence of chronic diarrhea, weakness, or fever for more than 30 days in the absence of a concurrent illness or condition. Malnutrition in HIV and AIDS is multifactorial, as shown in Figure 20-4. Altered nutrient intake, weight loss and body composition changes, physical impairment, endocrine disorders, metabolic changes, malabsorption, the presence of opportunistic infections, psychosocial issues, and economic conditions all contribute (see Table 20-6).

Malnutrition and weight loss are important predictors of both morbidity and mortality from AIDS. Thus, nutrition is a crucial element of medical care, not simply an alternative or adjunct therapy. Nutrition is one area in which clients can exert some control over their medical care. It is critical to begin interventions early. The first step should be education about the role of nutrition. Emphasizing the benefits of maintaining nutritional status such as repair and building of tissue, preserving lean body mass and GI function, minimizing fatigue, and improving quality of life are important components (see the *Teaching Tool* box Maximizing Food Intake in HIV/AIDS).

Food and Nutrition Therapies
Altered Nutrient Intake

Anorexia or loss of appetite is a frequent symptom of altered nutrient intake. Economic availability of adequate food supplies cannot be forgotten and often may be the most difficult problem to solve. Strategies for coping with loss of appetite are listed in Table 20-5.

TABLE 20-6 Clinical and Nutritional Complications of Acquired Immunodeficiency Syndrome

NEOPLASMS, PARASITES, OPPORTUNISTIC INFECTIONS	CLINICAL AND NUTRITIONAL PRESENTATION
Neoplasms	
Kaposi's sarcoma	Oral, esophageal lesions
Lymphoma: Burkitt's, immunoblastic	Dependent on primary site—diarrhea and malabsorption possible if gastrointestinal (GI) tract involved
Protozoa/Parasites	
Cryptosporidium spp.	Watery diarrhea, malabsorption, nausea, vomiting, abdominal pain, cholecystitis, pancreatitis
Pneumocystis jiroveci	Pneumonia
Toxoplasmosis	Fever, headache, confusion
Entamoeba histolytica; Entamoeba coli; Giardia lamblia; Acanthamoeba	Diarrhea, nausea, vomiting, loss of appetite
Bacteria	
Mycobacterium avium complex (MAC)	Fever, diarrhea, malabsorption, anorexia
Legionella	Pneumonia
Salmonella	Fever, abdominal pain and cramping, diarrhea
Listeria	Diarrhea, abdominal pain, fever
Shigella	Bloody diarrhea, abdominal pain, fever
Fungi	
Candida albicans	Thrush, stomatitis, esophagitis
Cryptococcus	Meningitis, nausea, vomiting, fever, dementia
Aspergillosis	Pneumonia
Coccidioidomycosis	Pneumonia, fungemia
Histoplasmosis	Fever, pneumonia
Viruses	
Cytomegalovirus (CMV)	Depends on site of infection—entire GI tract can be involved with diarrhea, nausea, and vomiting
Herpes simplex	Painful blisters—symptoms depend on site of infection

Data from Centers for Disease Control and Prevention: 1993 Revised classification system for HIV infection and expanded surveillance case definition for AIDS among adolescents and adults, *MMWR Recomm Rep* 41(RR-17):1-19, 1992. Accessed October 1, 2013, from www.cdc.gov/mmwr/preview/mmwrhtml/00018871.htm.

✳ TEACHING TOOL

Maximizing Food Intake in HIV/AIDS

Clients dealing with the chronic effects of human immunodeficiency virus/acquired immunodeficiency syndrome (HIV/AIDS) may have difficulty consuming enough kcal to meet physiologic requirements. Home health care nurses can teach the following strategies to clients and their caregivers improve calories and protein intake without necessarily expanding the volume of food:

- Substitute nutrient-dense, high-calorie foods and beverages for low- or no-kcal foods and beverages: milk or shakes instead of coffee or tea; 100% fruit juice for sugar-free drinks.

- Increase the number or size of feedings daily. Offer five or six small meals/snacks.
- Fortify foods with kcal and protein-containing ingredients. Add skim milk powder to milk, shakes, gravies, and hot cereals.
- Use high-calorie condiments. Add butter/margarine to hot cereals, vegetables, and starches.
- Modify diet according to tolerances. Try cold or room-temperature foods, bland or salty foods; avoid greasy and sweet foods and liquids between meals.
- Add kcal-containing supplements as needed.

Data from Fields-Gardner C, et al: *Living well with HIV and AIDS,* American Dietetic Association: Chicago, 2003.

Body Composition and Weight Changes

Patients with HIV/AIDS may experience weight loss and changes in body composition. Weight loss appears to occur not only from fat stores but also from lean body mass. This phenomenon is not as easily explained. Acute weight loss differs from chronic weight loss not only in its etiology but also in the type of energy stores that are depleted. Chronic weight loss, as seen in malnutrition, is often accompanied by a decrease in metabolic rate and a reliance on fat stores for energy. Acute weight loss, such as seen in stress, is

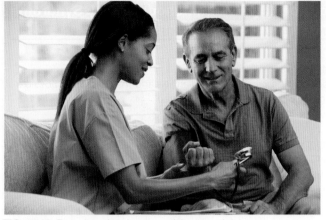

FIG 20-5 Regular checkups and home visits are necessary for managing acquired immunodeficiency syndrome.

accompanied by an increase in metabolic rate, a reliance on glucose as fuel, and a depletion of lean body mass. These changes in body composition and weight loss are commonly seen in the wasting syndrome and often coincide with increases in viral load. Regular checkups are important to evaluate changes in status (Figure 20-5).

Endocrine and Metabolic Disorders

Hypogonadism, which is common with this disease, is associated with fatigue, decreased libido, loss of muscle mass, muscle weakness, impotence, and loss of body hair. The associated fatigue contributes not only to decreased appetite but also to impaired ability to prepare and consume meals. Loss of lean body mass is a prominent feature. Adrenal insufficiency may contribute to changes in appetite, loss of fuel storage, and alterations in metabolism. It is unclear, though, whether any of these abnormalities is a causal factor in the development of malnutrition in HIV.

Exercise

Regular aerobic exercise and resistance training have been suggested to assist with lipid abnormalities, the fat redistribution syndrome, and other body composition changes noted in patients with HIV and AIDS. Recommendations should be individualized and initiated slowly after receiving a physician's approval. Benefits may include the following:
- Increased muscle volume, strength, functional capacity, and quality of life
- Decreased abdominal fat
- Prevention of glucose abnormalities and reduced insulin sensitivity
- Better circulation
- Improved bone density

Fat Redistribution Syndrome (Lipodystrophy)

HIV-associated lipodystrophy syndrome (HALS) is a known side effect of HAART. HALS is associated with both body composition changes (lipoatrophy, lipohypertrophy) and metabolic alterations (dyslipidemia, glucose intolerance, diabetes, hypertension, endothelial dysfunction, and atherosclerosis), which may occur singly or in combination and are associated with an increased risk of CVD (Loonam and Mullen, 2012).

A Mediterranean-style diet and supplementation with omega-3 polyunsaturated fatty acids have been found to be effective in improving HALS (Loonam and Mullen, 2012).

Malabsorption

Malabsorption can be a result of (1) opportunistic infections that damage the GI tract, (2) the effects of malnutrition on villus height and enterocyte function, and (3) the disease itself. In patients with HIV-related diarrhea, *steatorrhea* has been noted. Treatment of the underlying cause, if possible, is crucial.

Restriction of fat and lactose is common. Lactose-free supplements and supplements containing medium-chain triglycerides (Advera, Alitraq, Peptamen, Lipisorb) are frequently prescribed. Additionally, probiotics and prebiotics, as well as glutamine and arginine, either in enteral products or given separately, have been used to assist in malabsorption syndrome and diarrhea. Careful attention must be given to ensure adequate caloric and protein intake when fat and lactose, important energy and protein sources, must be restricted.

Physical Impairment

Nausea, vomiting, mouth and esophageal lesions, and impaired dentition are all frequent problems. They may be a result of opportunistic infections such as candidiasis and gingivitis or of side effects of antiretroviral therapy, prophylactic treatment to prevent opportunistic infections, and medication for the management of pain. Determining the causes of impaired intake is crucial to a successful intervention (see Table 20-5).

Prevention of Foodborne Illness

Prevention of a foodborne illness is a crucial component of nutrition therapy and nutrition education for people with HIV and AIDS. As CD4 cell counts fall, clients are at higher risk for infections from foods. Nutrition education should focus on safe methods for food purchasing, preparation, and storage.

Cryptosporidium infections can be life threatening and may lead to chronic, debilitating diarrhea. Infectious outbreaks have been linked to water sources. This protozoan is resistant to chlorination, and recent documentation of infections has led to recommendations that people with AIDS and HIV monitor their water sources. Suggestions have been made to avoid all public tap water and to drink only filtered water or water that has been boiled for 1 minute (Box 20-2). Fruits and vegetables can be cleaned with a mixture of 20 drops of 2% iodine in 1 gallon of water to prevent contamination.

Wasting and Malnutrition—A Vicious Circle

Malnutrition and wasting in patients with HIV and AIDS create a vicious circle that can be fatal. Interventions must be provided early. Research has shown promise concerning the

---

BOX 20-2   Safe Water for Immunosuppressed Patients

Immune system functioning may be diminished because of the effects of chemotherapy drugs, drugs used to prevent organ-transplant rejection, and HIV-AIDS. Because public water quality and treatment vary throughout the United States, always check with the local health department and water utility for any special notices about the use of tap water by immunocompromised persons. Heating water at a rolling boil for 1 minute kills Cryptosporidium. After the boiled water cools, put it in a clean bottle or pitcher with a lid, and store it in the refrigerator. Use the water for drinking, cooking, or making ice. Water bottles and ice trays should be cleaned with soap and water before use. Additional measures include filtering water or using commercially bottled water.

When traveling to developing nations, poor water treatment and food sanitation are a consideration. Raw fruits and vegetables, tap water, ice made from tap water, unpasteurized milk or dairy products, and items purchased from street vendors might be contaminated. Processed carbonated (bubbly) drinks in cans or bottles are probably safe, but drinks made at a fountain might not be because they are made with tap water.

Adapted from Centers for Disease Control, accessed June 10, 2014 at http://www.cdc.gov/parasites/crypto/gen_info/prevent_ic.html

---

BOX 20-3   Evaluation of Complementary and Alternative Therapies

Because currently there are no cures for some cancers and human immunodeficiency virus/acquired immunodeficiency syndrome (HIV/AIDS), patients with these diseases are potential victims for unproven or fraudulent health and nutrition therapies. High doses of vitamins and minerals can actually result in toxicities that are potentially harmful. Complementary and alternative therapies not only may be extremely costly but also may interfere with current medical treatments, putting the patient at even more risk. For example, microbial growth in herbal supplements may pose a risk of opportunistic infections in immunosuppressed patients.

The National Center for Complementary and Alternative Medicine (NCCAM) at the National Institutes of Health provides the structure for evaluating complementary and alternative therapies. Currently, a number of clinical studies have been or are being conducted to assess the value of complementary and alternative therapies for such disorders such as cancer and HIV/AIDS. Questionable practices or products may be reported to the following sources:

- Federal Trade Commission (FTC) Bureau of Consumer Protection; regional FTC office; chief postal inspector, US Postal Service; editor or station manager of media outlet where advertisement appeared; regional U.S. Food and Drug Administration (FDA) office; state attorney general; state health department; local Better Business Bureau; congressional representative; local or state professional society; local hospital (if practitioner is a staff member); state licensing board; local district attorney
- National Council Against Health Fraud (www.ncahf.org); Consumer Health Information Research Institute; local, state, or national professional or voluntary health groups

---

efficacy of nutrition interventions. Conducting nutrition assessment and providing counseling have enabled patients to maintain or gain weight. Health care teams can treat the nutritional problems of HIV and AIDS with multiple and complementary modes of therapy (see Box 20-3).

Application to nursing. Prevention of dehydration and effective monitoring of intake and output are required in patients with HIV/AIDS. Fluid losses may be high in the patient with diarrhea.

HAART uses combinations of fusion inhibitors, integrase inhibitors, nucleoside/nucleotide reverse transcriptase inhibitors, non-nucleoside reverse transcriptase inhibitors, and protease inhibitors. Adherence to the regimen is difficult because of the number and the complexity of medications that must be taken daily. Drug resistance can develop if adherence is not maintained. Side effects of these medications include nausea, vomiting, diarrhea, and other metabolic changes.

Anorexia may be caused by the HIV infection, the presence of other opportunistic infections, fatigue, or fever, or may be a medication side effect. Physical impairment from mucositis, esophagitis, pain, nausea, and vomiting affects the client's ability to ingest adequate nutrients. Depression, loneliness, fear, anxiety, and other psychosocial issues can play a significant role in the client's desire to eat.

Medications can be prescribed to assist with anorexia and body composition changes. Megestrol acetate (Megace), dronabinol (Marinol), oxandrolone (Oxandrin) or oxymetholone, testosterone, dehydroepiandrosterone (DHEA), and recombinant human growth hormone (r-hGH) have all been used with this population. Dronabinol has been shown to improve appetite, mood, and nausea, resulting in weight maintenance. Side effects include euphoria, dizziness, and impaired thinking. Oxandrolone is an oral analog of testosterone that increases lean body mass, elevates mood, and improves libido. DHEA and human growth hormone (r-hGH) have been used to improve lean body mass with a decrease in abdominal adiposity.

The ingestion of food along with certain medications may affect the absorption of that drugs, and vice versa. Examples are as follows:

Efavirenz (Sustiva): Avoid taking with high-fat meals.

Lopinavir (Kaletra) + ritonavir (Norvir): Moderate-fat meals increase availability of capsules; take with food.

Saquinavir (Invirase): Take this protease inhibitor within 2 hours of a meal containing high-fat foods or a large snack containing carbohydrate, protein, or fat.

Ritonavir (Norvir): If this protease inhibitor is consumed with a meal, it may decrease the abdominal cramping and diarrhea that is common when this drug is initially prescribed. These symptoms usually disappear within 8 weeks.

Indinavir (Crixivan): This protease inhibitor should be taken on an empty stomach. A meal can be eaten 1 hour after the drug is taken or 2 hours before. Some patients may find it necessary to eat a small snack with the drug, but fat should be avoided.

Effective treatment requires a multidisciplinary approach based on collaboration of all health care team members, including the nurse and dietitian. Early recognition and intervention for nutritional risk factors are keys to effective nutrition support and related medical therapies (see the *Cultural Considerations* box AIDS, HIV, and Ethnic Issues of Healing and Medicine: Lessons From Tuskegee).

🌐 CULTURAL CONSIDERATIONS

Acquired Immunodeficiency Syndrome, Human Immunodeficiency Virus, and Ethnic Issues of Healing and Medicine: Lessons from Tuskegee

As we attempt to "heal" our patients, we need to understand history to fully comprehend the perspective of the patients with whom we work. During the middle of the twentieth century (1932-1972), a medical study called the Tuskegee Experiment followed the course of syphilis among African American men from a poor county in Georgia. When the study began, there was no known cure for syphilis, but shortly into the study, penicillin was recognized as an effective drug against the ravages of this sexually transmitted disease. Nonetheless, such treatment was withheld from the men participating in this study, and most were followed to their deaths, which may or may not have been from syphilis-related causes. The study did not end until the 1070s after the men, their wives, and children were exposed and suffered the consequences of a serious systemic disease that could have been cured with inexpensive penicillin. Many people believe that the reason such an unethical protocol was allowed to continue was because the study population was poor and African American.

In 1973, a class action lawsuit for the individuals and family members affected by the study was filed by the National Association for the Advancement of Colored People (NAACP). A $9 million settlement was awarded and distributed among those affected. In 1997, President Clinton issued a formal apology on behalf of the U.S. government.

Application to nursing. Knowledge of such past mistreatments provides an understanding of current bias against government-sponsored medical treatment. By understanding our history, we can provide education about the ethical medical treatments available now.

Data from Chadwick A: *Remembering Tuskegee,* Washington, DC, July 25, 2002, National Public Radio. Accessed November 27, 2013, from www.npr.org/templates/story/story.php?storyId=1147234.

▌ SUMMARY

- The disorders cancer and AIDS are characterized by wasting and malnutrition, caused by the effect of the disorders or the secondary consequences of treatment on the GI tract.
- Nutrition therapy focuses on identifying at-risk patients, preventing malnutrition, and reducing the effects of treatment.
- Local or systemic effects of the cancer combined with antineoplastic therapy put the patient with cancer at increased risk for development of malnutrition or cancer cachexia through a variety of mechanisms: anorexia, nausea, vomiting, mucositis, organ injury (toxicity), and learned food aversions.
- Nutrition support must be individualized and is an essential component of the total management of cancer.
- With the provision of adequate nutritional support, patients with cancer may have a decreased risk of surgical complications.

- Nutrients are needed to rebuild normal tissues that have been affected by antineoplastic therapy to have a higher tolerance to therapies.
- AIDS, caused by the retrovirus HIV, leads to the breakdown of the immune system, opportunistic infections, or enteropathy.
- Malnutrition in HIV/AIDS is multifactorial and includes decreased nutrient (food) intake, malabsorption, and altered metabolism.
- Goals of HIV nutrition therapy are individualized, and interventions are based on nutritional status, cause(s) of malnutrition, infections, and complications.
- Early recognition of and intervention for HIV nutritional risk factors and indicators are keys to effective nutrition support and related medical therapies.

◎ THE NURSING APPROACH

Case Study: Cancer and Chemotherapy

Sophia, age 35, is visiting the nurse practitioner for a follow-up visit related to her breast cancer treatment. She has been receiving chemotherapy and radiation therapy for the past month after having a lumpectomy of the right breast.

Assessment
Subjective (from Patient Statements)
- "I've been really sick from the chemo. It makes me feel nauseated all the time, and often I vomit right after the treatment."
- "I've lost 5 pounds since starting the chemotherapy and radiation treatments."
- "It's hard to eat very much because my mouth is sore."
- "I'm too tired to do any cooking."

Objective (from Physical Examination)
- Height 5 feet 6 inches, weight 119 pounds
- Temperature 98.8°F
- Mouth inflamed, tongue appears red and raw; white raised patches on tongue and oral mucosa

Diagnoses (nursing)
1. Risk for imbalanced nutrition: less than body requirements related to nausea, fatigue, and impaired oral mucous membranes as evidenced by the loss of 5 pounds in the past month
2. Risk for infection related to immunosuppression secondary to chemotherapy

Planning
Patient Outcomes
Short term (by end of this visit):
- Sophia will describe ways she can improve her overall comfort and increase her food intake.
- She will agree to obtain resources about coping with chemotherapy from American Cancer Society.

Long term (by follow-up visit in 1 month):
- Lesions in mouth will be diminished, and Sophia will be able to eat with less discomfort.
- Sophia will maintain or increase weight.
- No signs of infection.

Nursing Interventions
1. Discuss measures to improve comfort and increase food intake.
2. Provide Sophia with resources for information about cancer and chemotherapy.

Implementation
1. Recommended small, frequent meals rather than large meals.
   Small meals are usually easier to tolerate than large meals when the gastrointestinal system is altered. Antineoplastic medications kill cancer cells because they divide rapidly. However, chemotherapy also kills normal cells that divide rapidly, involving the gastrointestinal system, bone marrow, and hair. Commercial nutritional supplements should be consumed between meals rather than with meals, in order to reduce satiety at mealtime.
2. Discussed ways to reduce nausea and vomiting.
   It is best to avoid foods with strong odors. If that is not possible, staying out of the kitchen and having someone else do the cooking may reduce nausea. Room deodorizers also may be helpful. Fried foods are harder to digest, so they should be avoided or minimized.
3. Stressed the importance of eating a well-balanced diet, using nutrient-dense foods. Also suggested eating favorite foods and taking a vitamin supplement.
   A well-balanced diet, including high-protein and high-kcal foods, will provide nourishment and energy to fight cancer, enable better toleration of chemotherapy, promote healing, and prevent infection. Choosing favorite foods may stimulate appetite.
4. Encouraged Sophia to prioritize her activities and to rest before meals.
   When energy is limited, an individual should do the most important activities first. When rested, a patient is more willing to expend energy to eat.
5. Encouraged Sophia to ask for help with shopping and meal preparation.
   Family members, friends, or church groups may provide assistance so that the patient's energy can be conserved and healing can take place.
6. Discussed oral care and treatment for mouth sores.
   Stomatitis (inflammation of the mouth) is a common side effect of chemotherapy. Good oral care with a soft toothbrush and flossing will reduce infection and the likelihood of damage to the oral mucosa. Frequent mouthwashing with baking soda and water help sores heal by shifting the pH to a less acidic environment. Mouthwashes with alcohol should be avoided because they irritate the mucosa.
7. Administered viscous lidocaine and Nystatin swish-and-swallow.
   Use of viscous lidocaine before eating may numb the sore mouth, decreasing discomfort and allowing the patient to eat. When immunosuppression is present, infection from Candida albicans (yeast infection, called thrush) often occurs; Nystatin swish-and-swallow may be prescribed for treatment.
8. Discussed bacterial precautions regarding food.
   Chemotherapy often causes a low white blood cell count, so the patient or food preparer should wash hands thoroughly with soap and water before preparing food and before eating. Cutting boards for meats should be designated and kept separate from cutting boards for other foods.
   No raw fruits and vegetables should be consumed, and commercially bottled water is safer than tap water. Foods need to be well cooked and must be kept hot until eaten. Leftovers need refrigeration and should be eaten within 24 hours.
9. Wrote some suggestions for improving eating while Sophia is receiving chemotherapy.

Continued

THE NURSING APPROACH—cont'd

When the patient has a sore mouth, soft, bland, cool, or lukewarm food and drinks should be consumed. Avoid tart, salty, acidic (citrus fruits and tomatoes), spicy, coarse, dry, and scratchy foods. Also avoid caffeine, alcohol, and tobacco. Such foods could cause irritation of the mucous membranes, adding to the damage done by the chemotherapy.

10. Encouraged Sophia to download patient information about *Nutrition for the Person with Cancer During Treatment* (2014), from the American Cancer Society (at http://www.cancer.org/treatment/survivorshipduringandafter treatment/nutritionforpeoplewithcancer/nutritionforthe personwithcancer/index).
Specific information about nutrition before, during, and after treatment is provided free. Especially helpful is the section in the pamphlet entitled "Managing Eating Problems Caused by Surgery, Radiation, and Chemotherapy." Education promotes empowerment.

Evaluation

Short term (by the end of this visit):
- Sophia committed to try methods designed to increase her comfort and food intake.
- She agreed to get resources from American Cancer Society. Goals met.

Discussion Questions

At a follow-up visit in 1 month, Sophia said her mouth was feeling better and she was able to eat somewhat more easily. She said that she still had problems with nausea and no energy. Her weight was stable, and she had no signs of infection. She said the information from American Cancer Society had been very helpful.

1. How could the nurse encourage Sophia and help her to set some small, realistic goals?
2. What high-calorie and nutrient-dense foods would you recommend for Sophia?

? CRITICAL THINKING #1*

Food: A Pharmaceutical Agent?

Over the past 20 years, epidemiologic researchers have consistently found that people who eat greater amounts of whole grains, fruits, and vegetables have lower rates of cancer. These foods contain hundreds of compounds called *phytochemicals* (specific chemicals found in plants) that are not strictly nutrients. Some families of plants have more than others, but none of the phytochemicals is found in animal foods. Phytochemicals include antioxidants such as vitamin C; flavonoids, flavanols, flavanones, isoflavones; catechins, epicatechins; anthocyanins, anthocyanidins, proanthocyanidins; isothiocyanates; carotenoids; allyl sulfides, polyphenols, and phenolic acids (American Cancer Society, 2013).

Most health professionals believe that the whole plant is probably more important than the sum of its nutrients and chemical components. More benefits are derived from nutrients and phytochemicals by eating foods rather than swallowing supplements. Clients may question why they shouldn't just take specialized supplements of phytochemicals if we know their actions:

1. Where do these foods fit in the phytochemical categories: blueberries? Onions and garlic? Green tea? Citrus fruits?

Broccoli? Check out websites and see what your patients find when they search.
2. How will you explain the benefits of fruits and vegetables to your patients?
3. What foods will you begin to include in your own diet?
4. No one food causes cancer, and no one food can prevent it. Describe a cancer-preventive diet that could be accepted by children, teens, adults, and seniors. Include several days of menus with a breakfast, lunch, and dinner option.

? CRITICAL THINKING #2

Clinical Applications

Minnie, age 20, is a college student with an uneventful medical history and no significant illness. After finals, she came down with the flu and has felt run-down ever since. She has also had a persistent low-grade fever since the flu. She was admitted to the hospital for dehydration and fever of unknown origin. Laboratory tests show that she has gonorrhea. Minnie confides in you that she has recently started having unprotected sex with a new male partner. She agrees to be screened for human immunodeficiency virus (HIV) and signs the informed consent form for the doctor. The results show that she is HIV positive, and the doctor immediately starts her on a combination of HAART. She is 5 feet 6 inches tall and weighs 120 pounds on admission. Her usual weight is 130 pounds.

1. What side effects from HAART might Minnie encounter?
2. How will they affect her nutritional status?
3. What suggestions do you have to help Minnie prevent further weight loss?

---

*Data from the following websites, accessed October 1, 2013, American Cancer Society: *Phytochemicals*, 2013. Accessed October 1, 2013, from http://www.cancer.org/treatment/treatmentsandsideeffects/complementaryandalternativemedicine/herbsvitaminsandminerals/phytochemicals; Fruits and Veggies—More Matters. Accessed October 1, 2013, from http://www.fruitsandveggiesmorematters.org/; and Produce for Better Health Foundation: *Creating demand for fruits and vegetables*, n.d. Accessed October 1, 2013, www.pbhfoundation.org/.

WEBSITES OF INTEREST

American Institute for Cancer Research

http://www.aicr.org

Offers excellent resources and reviews of research regarding nutrition and cancer prevention.

HIV/AIDS Dietetic Practice Group (Academy of Nutrition and Dietetics)

http://www.hivaidsdpg.org

Provides excellent links for information on HIV/AIDS, caregivers, and organizations offering medical nutrition therapy and food outreach programs.

National Cancer Institute (NCI)

www.cancer.gov

Makes available CancerNet (a cancer database on treatment, screening, prevention, and clinical trials), cancerTrials (clinical trials information center), and CANCERLIT (a bibliographic database).

REFERENCES

Daniel CR, et al: Intake of fiber and fiber-rich plant foods is associated with a lower risk of renal cell carcinoma in a large US cohort, *Am J Clin Nutr* 97:1036–1043, 2013.

Drake I, et al: Dietary intakes of carbohydrates in relation to prostate cancer risk: A prospective study in the Malmö Diet and Cancer cohort, *Am J Clin Nutr* 96:1409–1418, 2012.

Ferrari P, et al: Dietary fiber intake and risk of hormonal receptor-defined breast cancer in the European Prospective Investigation into Cancer and Nutrition study, *Am J Clin Nutr* 97:344–353, 2013.

Gupta SC, et al: Upsides and downsides of reactive oxygen species for cancer: The roles of reactive oxygen species in tumorigenesis, prevention, and therapy, *Antioxid Redox Signal* 16:1295–1322, 2012.

Hanahan D, Weinberg RA: Hallmarks of cancer: The next generation, *Cell* 144:646–674, 2011.

Hossein-Nezhad A, et al: Influence of vitamin D status and vitamin D3 supplementation on genome wide expression of white blood cells: A randomized double-blind clinical trial, *PLoS ONE* 8:e58725, 2013.

Loonam CR, Mullen A: Nutrition and the HIV-associated lipodystrophy syndrome, *Nutr Res Rev* 25:267–287, 2012.

Martin L, et al: Cancer cachexia in the age of obesity: Skeletal muscle depletion is a powerful prognostic factor, independent of body mass index, *J Clin Oncol* 31(12):1539–1547, 2013.

Mondul AM, et al: Metabolomic profile of response to supplementation with β-carotene in the Alpha-Tocopherol, Beta-Carotene Cancer Prevention Study, *Am J Clin Nutr* 98:488–493, 2013.

Romieu I, et al: Dietary glycemic index and glycemic load and breast cancer risk in the European Prospective Investigation into Cancer and Nutrition (EPIC), *Am J Clin Nutr* 96:345–355, 2012.

Suzuki H, et al: Cancer cachexia—pathophysiology and management, *J Gastroenterol* 48(5):574–594, 2013.

GLOSSARY

A

absorption the process by which substances pass through the intestinal mucosa into the blood or lymph

Academy of Nutrition and Dietetics formerly known as The American Dietetic Association; sets standards of education and expectations for registered dietitians/nutritionists (RDN) and for dietetic technicians, registered (DTRs). The new credential for registration may be stated as RD or RDN, as selected by the individual practitioner

acanthosis nigricans hyperpigmentation and thickening of the skin into velvety irregular folds in the neck and flexural areas

Acceptable Macronutrient Distribution Range (AMDR) intake range for an energy source associated with reducing chronic disease risk while supplying adequate essential nutrients

acesulfame K a synthetically produced non-nutritive sweetener

acetyl coenzyme A (acetyl CoA) important intermediate byproduct in metabolism formed from the breakdown of glucose, fatty acids, and certain amino acids

acupuncture the use of fine needles to open blockages of the flow of Qi, or life force, and thus restore balance

acute respiratory failure (ARF) sudden absence of respirations, with confusion or unresponsiveness caused by obstructive airflow or failure of the pulmonary gas exchange mechanism

acute tubular necrosis (ATN) sudden death of cells in the small tubules of the kidneys as a result of disease or injury

adaptive thermogenesis energy (or heat released) used by the body to adjust to changing physical and biologic environments

adenosine triphosphate (ATP) an energy-rich compound used for all energy-requiring processes in the body

Adequate Intake (AI) the approximate level of an average nutrient intake, determined by observation of or experimentation with a particular group or population that appears to maintain good health

adipocytes cells specialized for storage of fat

adipose tissue stored form of fat (mainly triglycerides) in the body

ADIME acronym for *a*ssessment, nutrition *d*iagnosis, *i*mplementation, and *m*onitoring-*e*valuation

adrenocorticotropic hormone (ACTH) an adrenal cortex hormone that stimulates secretion of more hormones

aerobic glycolysis the conversion of glucose to ATP for energy when oxygen is available

aerobic pathway a form of energy production that depends on oxygen and increases the use of fat

aerophagia swallowing of air, usually the result of eating with the mouth open, followed by belching, gastric distress, or flatulence

alcoholic cirrhosis associated with chronic alcohol abuse; accounts for 50% of all cases; also called Laënnec's cirrhosis

aldosterone a hormone secreted by the adrenal gland in response to sodium levels in kidneys; affects kidneys to balance fluid levels as needed

allogeneic transplant between different individuals who are not genetically identical

alternative medicine healing practices that replace conventional medical treatment

alternative sweeteners nonnutritive sweeteners (or artificial sweeteners) synthetically produced to be sweet tasting but to provide no nutrients and few, if any, kcal; aspartame, saccharin, acesulfame K, and sucralose are alternative sweeteners

Alzheimer's disease a progressive, degenerative disorder that attacks the brain's nerve cells, or neurons, resulting in loss of memory, thinking and language skills, and behavioral changes.

amenorrhea absence of a menstrual period in a woman of reproductive age; a condition that may occur with anorexia nervosa

amino acid pool the assortment of amino acids available to cells

amino acid score a simple measure of an amino acid composition of a food as compared with a reference protein; based on the limiting amino acid

amino acids organic compounds containing carbon, hydrogen, oxygen, and nitrogen

aminopeptidase an intestinal peptidase that releases free amino acids from the amino end of short-chain peptides

amyloidosis a disorder characterized by accumulation of waxy starchlike glycoprotein (amyloid) in organs and tissues, affecting their function

anaerobic glycolysis the conversion of glucose to pyruvate to provide energy in the absence of oxygen

anaerobic pathway a form of energy production that does not require oxygen

anaphylaxis a severe immune system response to an allergen

anencephaly a congenital defect in which the brain does not develop; death may occur shortly after birth

angina pectoris chest pain that often radiates down the left arm and is frequently accompanied by a feeling of suffocation and impending death

anorexia nervosa a mental disorder characterized by self-imposed starvation; may include binge-eating episodes associated with bulimic behaviors

antidiuretic hormone (ADH) a hormone secreted by the pituitary gland in response to low fluid levels; affects kidneys to decrease excretion of water; also called vasopressin

antineoplastic therapy substance, procedure, or measure that prevents the proliferation of malignant cells; usually chemotherapy, radia-tion therapy, surgery, biologic response modifiers, or bone marrow transplantation

antioxidant a compound that guards other compounds from damaging oxidation

anuria excretion of less than 250 mL urine every 24 hours

appetite desire for food

ariboflavinosis a group of symptoms associated with riboflavin deficiency

aromatherapy use of extracts or essences of herbs, flowers, and trees in the form of essential oils to support health and well-being

arteriosclerosis thickening, loss of elasticity, and calcification of arterial walls, resulting in decreased blood supply to tissues

ascites abnormal intraperitoneal accumulation of fluid containing large amounts of protein and electrolytes, usually resulting in abdominal swelling, hemodilution, edema, and/or decreased urinary output

aspartame a nonnutritive sweetener formed by the bonding of the amino acids phenylalanine and aspartic acid

asthma a chronic respiratory disorder characterized by airway obstruction due to excessive mucus production and respiratory mucosal edema; may be triggered by infection, cold air, vigorous exercise, stress, or inhalation of environmental allergens or pollutants

ataxia muscle weakness and loss of coordination

atherosclerosis development of lesions (also called fatty streaks) in the intima of arteries; during aging the lesions develop into fibrous plaques that project into the vessel lumen and begin to disturb blood flow

athetoid purposeless weaving motions of the body or extremities

atonic lacking normal muscle tone

autoantibodies self-antibodies produced in the pancreas; these include autoantibodies to islet cells, to insulin, and to glutamic acid decarboxylase (GAD65)

autologous transplantation in which the organ or tissue is from the same individual (oneself)

Ayurveda a system of healing focusing on diet and herbal remedies that emphasizes the use of body, mind, and spirit to prevent and treat disorders

B

basal metabolism the amount of energy required to maintain life-sustaining activities for a specific period

beikost (*BYE-cost*) supplemental or weaning foods

beriberi a severe chronic deficiency of thiamine characterized by muscle weakness and pain, anorexia, mental disorientation, and tachycardia

beta cells insulin-producing cells situated in the islets of Langerhans of the pancreas

bezoars physical obstacles created by tangles of fibrous material in the gastrointestinal (GI) tract that may cause dangerous obstructions of the tract

bile a substance that emulsifies fats to aid the digestion of lipids; produced by the liver and stored in the gallbladder

biliary atresia a congenital condition in which the major bile duct is blocked, limiting the availability of bile for fat digestion

biliary cirrhosis cirrhosis associated with obstruction of biliary drainage or biliary disorders; accounts for 15% of all cases of the disease

binge-eating disorder (BED) a mental disorder characterized by frequent binge-eating behaviors, not accompanied by purging or compensatory behaviors; commonly called compulsive overeating

bingeing losing control when eating, resulting in the consumption of excessive amounts of food; often stress-related

bioelectric impedance analysis (BIA) a method using a mild electric charge to estimate lean body mass to determine body fat composition

biofeedback the use of special devices to convey physiologic information to enable a person to learn how to consciously control medically important functions

biologic value a method to determine the quality of food protein by measuring the amount of nitrogen kept in the body after digestion, absorption, and excretion

body mass index (BMI) a measure that describes relative weight for height and is significantly correlated with total body fat content

bolus a masticated lump or ball of food ready to be swallowed

branched-chain amino acids (BCAAs) leucine, isoleucine, and valine; important in metabolism of lean body mass

bulimia nervosa a mental disorder characterized as the binge-and-purge syndrome; includes experiencing repetitive food binges accompanied by purging or compensatory behaviors

C

cachexia general ill health and malnutrition, marked by weakness and emaciation

calcitonin a hormone that reacts in response to high blood levels of calcium; released by the special C cells of the thyroid gland

calcitriol active vitamin D hormone that raises blood calcium levels

calcium rigor a condition of hardness or stiffness of muscles when blood calcium levels are too high

calcium tetany a condition of spasms and nerve excitability when blood calcium levels are too low

cancer uncontrolled growth of cells that tend to invade surrounding tissue and metastasize to distant body sites

carbohydrates organic compounds composed of carbon, hydrogen, and oxygen

carboxypeptidase a pancreatic protease that hydrolyzes polypeptides and dipeptides into amino acids

cardiac cachexia unintentional severe weight loss caused by heart disease

carcinogenesis the process of cancer production

cardiac decompensation impaired cardiac output (reasons not entirely understood)

cardiovascular endurance the ability of the body to take in, deliver, and use oxygen for physical work

cerebrovascular conditions affecting the blood supply of the brain; a cerebrovascular accident is another term for a stroke

cheilosis inflammation of the mucous membrane of the mouth and lips (angular stomatitis) caused by deficiencies of riboflavin and other B vitamins

chemical digestion the chemical altering effects of digestive secretions, gastric juices, and enzymes on food substance composition

chiropractic manipulation a manipulation modality addressing the ties between body structure (particularly of the spine) and function and how those ties affect the maintenance and return to health

cholecystectomy surgical removal of the gallbladder, performed to treat cholelithiasis and cholecystitis

cholecystitis acute inflammation of the gallbladder associated with pain, tenderness, and fever

cholecystokinin (CCK) a hormone secreted by the small intestine that initiates pancreatic exocrine secretions, acts against gastrin, and activates the gallbladder to release bile

choledocholithiasis gallstones in the common bile duct

cholelithiasis presence of stones in the gallbladder

chronic dieting syndrome a lifestyle inhibited or controlled by a constant concern about food intake, body shape, or weight that affects an individual's physical and mental health status

chronic hunger a continual experience of undernutrition, often related to food insecurity

chronic obstructive pulmonary disease (COPD) a progressive and irreversible condition identified by obstruction of airflow, chronic bronchitis, asthma, and emphysema (also called chronic obstructive lung disease)

chylomicrons the first lipoproteins formed after absorption of lipids from food

chyme a semiliquid mixture of food mass

chymotrypsin a pancreatic protease that hydrolyzes polypeptides into dipeptides

***cis* fatty acids** *cis* indicates the configuration of the double bond in a natural oil

coenzyme a substance that activates an enzyme

colic sharp visceral pain

colostomy surgical creation of an artificial anus on the abdominal wall by incising the colon and bringing it out to the surface; may be single-barreled (one opening) or double-barreled (distal and proximal loops open onto the abdomen)

colostrum the fluid secreted from the breast during late pregnancy and the first few days

postpartum; contains immunologically active substances (maternal antibodies) and essential nutrients

complementary and alternative medicine (CAM) a cluster of medical and health care approaches, methods, and items not associated with conventional medicine; also called integrative medicine

complementary medicine non-Western healing approaches used at the same time as conventional medicine

complete protein protein containing all nine essential amino acids

complex carbohydrates polysaccharides of starch and fiber

component puréeing each food item is pureed separately (food thickeners may be added to help maintain consistency), then presented in a manner that resembles the original product (e.g., a pork chop can be pureed, then molded into a pork-chop shape and served)

comprehensive nutritional assessment a procedure conducted by dietetic professionals to determine appropriate medical nutrition therapy based on the identified needs of the patient

congestive heart failure (CHF) circulatory congestion resulting in the heart's inability to maintain blood supply adequate to meet oxygen demands

constipation straining to pass hard, dry stools; slow movement of feces through colon

conventional insulin therapy consists of (1) one or two daily injections of insulin, including mixed intermediate and rapid-acting insulins; (2) daily self-monitoring of urine or blood glucose; and (3) education about diet and exercise

cor pulmonale an abnormal cardiac condition characterized by hypertrophy of the right ventricle as a result of hypertension of the pulmonary circulation

coronary artery disease (CAD) term used for several abnormal conditions that may affect the arteries of the heart and have various pathologic effects, especially reduction in flow of oxygen and nutrients to the cardiac tissue

Crohn's disease an inflammatory disorder that involves all layers of the wall of the small or large intestine or both; is associated with stricture formation, fistulous tracts, and abscesses

cystic fibrosis a genetic disorder in which excessive mucus is produced, primarily affecting respiratory airways; also limits fat absorption in the digestive system; most common among white populations

D

Daily Values (DVs) a system for food labeling composed of two sets of reference values: reference daily intakes (RDIs) and daily reference values

deamination a process through which an amino acid group breaks off from an amino acid molecule, resulting in molecules of ammonia and keto acid

denatured   a change in the shape of protein structures caused by heat, light, acids, alcohol, or mechanical actions

densitometry   underwater weighing

diabetes mellitus   a disorder of carbohydrate metabolism characterized by hyperglycemia and caused by either defective or deficient insulin

diabetic ketoacidosis (DKA)   a potentially life-threatening complication in patients with diabetes mellitus (usually type 1) resulting from a shortage of insulin and producing acidic ketone bodies

dialysate   dialysis solution

dialysis   a procedure that involves diffusion of particles from an area of high to lower concentration, osmosis of fluid across the membrane from an area of lesser to greater concentration of particles, and the ultrafiltration or movement of fluid across the membrane as a result of an artificially created pressure differential

diarrhea   frequent passing of loose, watery bowel movements

diet-induced thermogenesis/thermic effect of food (TEF)   an increase of cellular activity when food is eaten

diet manual   the reference (usually in a three-ring binder or on computer) that describes the rationale and indications for using a specific diet, lists the allowed and restricted foods, and provides sample menus

dietary fiber   carbohydrates (polysaccharides) and lignin in plant foods that cannot be digested by humans

Dietary Reference Intakes (DRIs)   dietary standards including Estimated Average Requirement (EAR), Recommended Dietary Allowance (RDA), Adequate Intake (AI), and Tolerable Upper Intake Level (UL)

dietary standards   a guide to adequate nutrient intake levels against which to compare the nutrient values of foods consumed

dietary supplements   substances consumed orally as an addition to dietary intake

Dietetic technicians, registered   Dietetic technicians, registered (DTRs), are trained in food and nutrition and are an integral part of the health-care and foodservice management teams. DTRs have met the following criteria: completion of at least a two-year degree from an accredited institution, supervised practice, and a national examination through the Accreditation Council for Education in Nutrition and Dietetics (ACEND) of the Academy of Nutrition and Dietetics

digestion   the process through which foods are broken down into smaller and smaller units to prepare nutrients for absorption

digestive system   a series of organs that functions to prepare ingested nutrients for digestion and absorption

dipeptidase   an intestinal peptidase that completes the hydrolysis of proteins to amino acids

disaccharides   a sugar formed by two single carbohydrate units bound together; sucrose, maltose, and lactose are disaccharides

disease prevention   the recognition of a danger to health that could be reduced or alleviated through specific actions or changes in lifestyle behaviors

diverticula   pouchlike herniations protruding from the muscular layer of the colon

diverticulitis   inflammation of one or more diverticula

diverticulosis   the presence of diverticula

dry beriberi   thiamine deficiency affecting the nervous system that produces paralysis and extreme muscle wasting

dumping syndrome   contents from the stomach empty too rapidly into the duodenum, causing symptoms profuse sweating, nausea, dizziness, and weakness

durable power of attorney   a legal document in which a competent adult authorizes another competent adult to make decisions for him/her in the event of incapacitation

dyslipidemia   an abnormal amount of lipid (cholesterol, fatty acids) in the blood

dysphagia   the inability to swallow normally or freely or to transfer liquid or solid foods from the oral cavity to the stomach; may be caused by an underlying central neurologic or isolated mechanical dysfunction

E

eating disorders   a group of behaviors fueled by unresolved emotional conflicts, symptomized by altered food consumption

edema   excess accumulation of fluid in interstitial spaces caused by seepage from the circulatory system

edentulous   toothless

eicosapentaenoic acid (EPA)   the main omega-3 fatty acid in fish

elemental formulas   solutions that provide ready-to-absorb basic nutrients, requiring minimal digestion

emetics   substances that cause vomiting

emulsifier   a substance that works by being soluble in water and fat at the same time

endogenous   originating from within the body or produced internally

endometrium   mucous membrane of the uterus

end-stage renal disease (ESRD)   the kidneys can no longer function properly; also known as the 5th or final stage in chronic kidney disease

enrichment   returning nutrients that were lost during processing to their original levels in foods

enzyme-linked immunosorbent assay (ELISA)   a test that uses color change and antibodies to detect the presence of a substance, usually an allergen, in the bloodstream

enteral nutrition   administration of nourishment via the gastrointestinal (GI) tract

enteritis   infection of the small intestine caused by a virus, bacteria, or protozoa

ergogenic aids   drugs and dietary regimens believed by some (but not proven) to increase strength, power, and endurance

esophageal varices   large and swollen veins at the lower end of the esophagus that are especially vulnerable to ulceration and hemorrhage, usually the result of portal hypertension

esophagitis   inflammation of the lower esophagus

essential amino acids (EAAs)   amino acids that cannot be manufactured by the human body

essential fat   certain components of body fat that are essential for life

essential fatty acids (EFAs)   polyunsaturated fatty acids that cannot be made in the body and must be consumed in the diet

essential or primary hypertension   elevated blood pressure for which the cause is unknown

Estimated Average Requirement (EAR)   the amount of a nutrient needed to meet the basic requirements of half the individuals in a specific group; the basis for setting the RDAs

Estimated Energy Requirement (EER)   dietary energy intake predicted to maintain energy balance in a healthy adult of a defined age, weight, and level of physical activity consistent with good health

exocrine glands   glands that secrete chemicals into ducts that release into a cavity or to the surface of the body, such as salivary glands (mouth) and the liver (gallbladder)

exogenous   originating outside the body or produced from external sources

extracellular fluids   all fluids outside cells including interstitial fluid, plasma, and watery components of body organs and substances

F

faith healing   healing by invoking divine intervention without the use of conventional or surgical therapy

fatty infiltration   accumulation of fat (triglycerides) in the liver

feeding relationship   the interactions or patterns of behaviors that surround food preparation and consumption within a family

fetal alcohol syndrome (FAS)/fetal alcohol spectrum disorder (FASD)   a disorder caused by maternal alcohol consumption during pregnancy that produces a range of specific anatomic and central nervous systems defects in the fetus

flatus   intestinal gas

flexibility   the ability to move muscles to their full extent without injury

fluid volume deficit (FVD)   the state in which a person experiences vascular, cellular, or intracellular dehydration

fluid volume excess   the state in which a person experiences increased fluid retention and edema

fluorosis   a condition of mottling or brown spotting of the tooth enamel caused by excessive intake of fluoride

food allergy   the overreaction to a food protein or other large molecule that produces an immune response

food choice   the specific foods that are convenient to choose when we are actually ready to eat

food intolerance   an adverse reaction to a food that does not involve the immune system

food preferences the foods we choose to eat when all foods are available at the same time and in the same quantity

fractionation administration of radiation therapy in smaller doses over time rather than in a single large dose; minimizes tissue damage

functional foods foods or ingredients in a food that have potentially positive health effects beyond basic nutrition

G

galactosemia an autosomal recessive disorder resulting in an inability to metabolize galactose and lactose milk products

gastrin a hormone secreted by stomach mucosa that increases the release of gastric juices

gastroesophageal reflux (GER) return of gastric contents into the esophagus that results in a severe burning sensation under the sternum; commonly called heartburn

gastroesophageal reflux disease (GERD) a syndrome of chronic or recurrent return of gastric contents into the esophagus that results in a severe burning sensation under the sternum and possibly nausea, belching, cough, or hoarseness

gastrointestinal (GI) tract the main organs of the digestive system that form a tube that runs from the mouth to the anus

gerontology the study of aging

gestational diabetes mellitus (GDM) a form of diabetes occurring most commonly after the 20th week of gestation

glomerulonephritis inflammation of the glomerulus of the kidney, characterized by proteinuria, hematuria, decreased urine production, and edema

glossitis inflammation of the tongue

glucagon a pancreatic hormone that releases glycogen from the liver

glucocorticoid an adrenal cortex hormone that affects food metabolism

gluconeogenesis the process of producing glucose from fat and protein

glycemic index the level to which a food raises blood glucose levels compared with a reference food

glycemic load the total glycemic index effect of a mixed meal or dietary plan; calculated by sum of products of glycemic index for each of the foods multiplied by amount of carbohydrate in each food

glycogen carbohydrate energy stored in the liver and muscles

glycogenesis the process of converting glucose to glycogen

glycogenolysis the process of converting glycogen back to glucose

glycolysis the conversion of glucose to carbon compounds

glycosylated hemoglobin (A1C) a substance (glycohemoglobin) formed when hemoglobin combines with some of the glucose in the bloodstream

goiter enlargement of the thyroid gland caused by iodine deficiency

graft-versus-host disease (GVHD) a complication that can occur after a stem cell or bone marrow transplantation in which the newly transplanted donor cells attack the transplant recipient's body as if it were a foreign substance; GVHD is more common in transplants where the donor and recipient are unrelated

H

hard water water containing high amounts of minerals such as calcium and magnesium

health the merging and balancing of five physical and psychologic dimensions of health: physical, mental, emotional, social, and spiritual

health literacy the ability to understand basic health concepts and apply them to one's own health decisions

health promotion strategies used to increase the level of health of individuals, families, groups, and communities

healthy weight weight that allows comfortable physical movement, without undue food restrictions, excessive exercise or experience of weight-related associative disorders

heme iron dietary iron found in animal foods of meat, fish, and poultry

hemochromatosis a hereditary disorder of iron metabolism characterized by excessive dietary iron absorption and deposition of iron in body tissues

hemodialysis a procedure to remove impurities or wastes from the blood in treating renal insufficiency by shunting the blood from the body through a machine for diffusion and ultrafiltration and then returning it to the patient's circulation

hemodilution dilution of the blood

hemoglobin oxygen-transporting protein in red blood cells

hemosiderosis a condition in which too much iron is stored in the body

heparinized use of an antithrombin factor to prevent intravascular clotting

hepatic coma neurophysiologic symptom of extensive liver damage caused by chronic or acute liver disease

hepatic encephalopathy a type of brain damage caused by liver disease and consequent ammonia intoxication

hepatotoxic potentially destructive to liver cells

hiatal hernia herniation of a portion of the stomach into the chest through the esophageal hiatus of the diaphragm

high-fructose corn syrup (HFCS) corn syrup processed to contain an increased proportion of fructose, producing sweetness similar to or higher than that of sugar (sucrose)

high-density lipoproteins (HDLs) lipoproteins that carry fats and cholesterol from body cells to the liver and are made of large proportions of proteins

high-quality protein a food containing the best balance and assortment of essential and nonessential amino acids for protein synthesis

homeopathic medicine an alternative medical system through which a small amount of a diluted substance is prescribed to relieve symptoms for which the same substance, given in larger amounts, will cause the same symptoms

homeostasis a state of physiologic equilibrium produced by a balance of functions and of chemical composition within an organism

hormones substances that act as messengers between organs to cause the release of needed secretions

hunger a physiologic need for food

hydrogenation breaking a double bond on a fatty acid carbon chain and saturating it with hydrogen

hydroxyapatite a natural mineral structure of bones and teeth

hyperbilirubinemia a neonatal condition of excessively high levels of bilirubin (red bile pigment) leading to jaundice, in which bile is deposited in tissues throughout the body

hypercaloric containing more than 1 kcal/mL

hypercholesterolemia total blood cholesterol levels greater than 200 mg/dL; greater than normal amounts of cholesterol in the blood; may be reduced or prevented by avoiding saturated fats

hyperemesis gravidarum severe and unrelenting vomiting in the second trimester of pregnancy or vomiting that severely interferes with the mother's life; a serious condition usually requiring intravenous replacement of nutrients and fluids

hyperglycemia elevated blood glucose level (>120 mg/dL)

hyperosmolar abnormally increased osmolarity

hyperplasia an increase in the number of cells occurring during the growth spurts accompanying normal development

hypertension (HTN) an average systolic blood pressure >140 mm Hg or a diastolic pressure >90 mm Hg (or both)

hypertonic having greater concentration of solute than another solution

hypertrophy an increase in the size of cells

hypoglycemia blood glucose levels that are below normal values

hypogonadism a deficiency in the secretory activity of the ovary or testis

hyponatremia low blood sodium level

hypophosphatemia low serum phosphorus level

hyporeflexia a neurologic condition characterized by weakened reflex reactions

hypoxia lack of oxygen to the cells

I

iatrogenic inadvertently caused by treatment or diagnostic procedures

idiopathic steatorrhea fat malabsorption caused by unknown causes

ileostomy in a patient with entire colon and rectum removed, surgical formation of an opening of the ileum onto the surface of the abdomen, through which fecal matter is emptied

incidental (indirect) food additives substances that inadvertently contaminate processed foods

incomplete protein proteins lacking one or more of the essential amino acids

insensible perspiration water lost invisibly through evaporation from the lungs and skin

insoluble dietary fibers dietary fibers that do not dissolve in fluids

insulin a hormone produced by the pancreas that regulates blood glucose levels

integrative medicine merging of conventional medical therapies with CAM modalities for which safety and efficacy, based on scientific data, have been demonstrated

intensive insulin therapy consists of (1) administration of insulin more than three times daily (injection or pump) with dosage adjusted according to results of self-monitoring of blood glucose performed at least four times daily, (2) dietary intake, and (3) anticipated exercise

intentional (direct) food additives substances purposely added during manufacturing to food products

interstitial fluid fluid between the cells containing concentrations of sodium and chloride

intracellular fluid fluid within the cells composed of water plus concentrations of potassium and phosphates

intrinsic factor a substance produced by stomach mucosa that is required for vitamin B_{12} absorption

irradiation a procedure by which food is exposed to radiation that destroys microorganisms, insect growth, and parasites that could spoil food or cause illness

ischemic deficient supply of blood to a body part (as the heart or brain) that is due to obstruction of the inflow of arterial blood

isotonic having the same concentration of solute as another solution, therefore exerting the same amount of osmotic pressure as that solution

K

keratomalacia a condition caused by vitamin A deficiency in which the cornea becomes dry and thickens from the formation of hard protein tissue

ketone bodies a breakdown product of fatty acid catabolism

ketosis a condition in which the absence of plasma glucose results in partial oxidation of fatty acids and the formation of excessive amounts of ketones

Kt/V Kt/V is a calculation used to quantify hemodialysis and peritoneal dialysis treatment adequacy. K= dialyzer clearance of urea; t = dialysis time; V = volume of distribution of urea, approximately equal to patient's total body water

kwashiorkor malnutrition in children caused by a lack of protein in spite of adequate energy consumption

L

lactation the production of breast milk

lacto-vegetarian dietary pattern a food plan consisting of only plant foods plus dairy products

lifestyle a pattern of behaviors

limiting amino acid the essential amino acid or amino acids that incomplete proteins lack

linoleic acid an essential polyunsaturated fatty acid with the first double bond located at the sixth carbon atom from the omega end

linolenic acid an essential polyunsaturated fatty acid with the first double bond located at the third carbon atom from the omega end

lipogenesis anabolism (synthesis) of lipids

lithotripsy extracorporeal shock wave lithotripsy (ESWL), a noninvasive technique whereby high-intensity shock waves cause fragmentation of gallstones from a device outside the body

locus of control the perception of one's ability to control life events and experiences

low birth weight weighing less than 5.5 pounds (2500 g) at birth

low-density lipoproteins (LDLs) lipoproteins that carry fats and cholesterol to body cells and that are made of large proportions of cholesterol

M

macrophages cells that are able to surround, engulf, and digest microorganisms and cellular debris; big scavenger cells

macrosomia abnormally large body size in a newborn infant

macrovascular pertaining to larger blood vessels found in the aorta, coronary arteries, limbs, and brain

major minerals essential nutrient minerals required daily in amounts of 100 mg or higher

malnutrition an imbalanced nutrient and/or energy intake

marasmus malnutrition in children caused by a severe lack of energy (kcal) intake

MCT fats (oils) specialized modular formulas made of medium-chain triglycerides that do not require pancreatic lipase or bile for digestion and absorption; they are absorbed directly into the portal vein (like amino acids and monosaccharides) rather than through the lymphatic system like other lipids

mechanical digestion the crushing and twisting effects of teeth and peristalsis that divide foods into smaller pieces

medical nutrition the use of specific nutrition services to treat an illness, injury, or condition

medical nutrition therapy legal definition of nutrition therapy provided by a registered dietitian for Medicare clients (pre-renal failure, diabetes only)

meditation a self-directed technique of relaxing the body and calming the mind

megacolon massive, abnormal dilation of the colon that may be congenital, toxic, or acquired

menopause the end of menstruation due to the cessation of ovarian and follicular function

metabolism a set of processes through which absorbed nutrients are used by the body for energy and to form and maintain body structures and functions

metastasis the spread of malignant cells to other sites from the original tumor location

microcephaly abnormal smallness of head with brain underdevelopment

monosaccharides a sugar composed of a single carbohydrate unit; glucose, fructose, and galactose are monosaccharides

monounsaturated fatty acid a fatty acid containing a carbon chain with one unsaturated double bond

mucosa the inside gastrointestinal muscle tissue layer composed of mucous membrane

mucositis inflammation of mucous membranes

multifactorial phenotype a characteristic that is the product of numerous genetic and environmental factors

multiple organ dysfunction syndrome (MODS) the progressive failure of two or more organ systems (e.g., the renal, hepatic, cardiac, or respiratory systems) at the same time

muscular strength and endurance the ability of the muscles to perform hard or prolonged work

muscularis a thick layer of muscle tissue surrounding the submucosa

myocardial infarction (MI) occlusion of a coronary artery; sometimes called heart attack

myoglobin oxygen-transporting protein in muscle

N

naturopathic medicine the use of the body's natural healing forces to recover from disease and to achieve wellness; it incorporates techniques from Eastern and Western traditions

nephrosclerosis necrosis of the renal arterioles, associated with hypertension

nephrotoxic toxic or destructive to a kidney

night blindness the inability of the eyes to readjust from bright to dim light caused by vitamin A deficiency

nitrogen-balance studies measurement of the amount of nitrogen entering the body compared with the amount excreted

nocturia excessive urination at night

nonessential amino acids (NEAAs) amino acids manufactured by the human body

nonheme iron dietary iron found in plant foods

nutrients substances in foods required by the body for energy, growth, maintenance, and repair

nutrition the study of essential nutrients and the processes by which nutrients are used by the body

nutritional genomics a science studying the relationship between human genome, nutrition and health; how food affects genes and how genetic differences affect response to dietary intakes

Nutrition Care Process a systematic approach to providing high quality nutrition care by registered dietitians; includes steps of Assessment, Nutrition Diagnosis, Intervention, Monitoring and Evaluation

nutrition therapy the provision of nutrient, dietary, and nutrition education needs based on a comprehensive nutritional assessment to treat an illness, injury or condition; definition may be dictated by state laws licensing registered dietitians (RDs)

nutritional risk the potential to become malnourished because of primary (inadequate intake of nutrients) or secondary (due to disease or iatrogenic effects) factors

nutritional support although commonly used in reference to enteral and parenteral nutrition delivery systems, can refer to any nutrition intervention used to minimize patient morbidity, mortality, and complications

nutritionist a professional who has completed a master's or doctoral degree in foods and nutrition

O

oliguria less than 400 mL urine excretion every 24 hours

osmolality concentration of electrically charged particles per kilogram of solution

osmotic diarrhea diarrhea-associated water retention in the large intestine resulting from an accumulation of nonabsorbable water-soluble solutes

osteodystrophy defective bone development associated with disturbances in calcium and phosphorus metabolism and renal insufficiency

osteomalacia an adult disorder due to vitamin D or calcium deficiency and characterized by soft, demineralized bones

osteopathic medicine an approach based on the assumption that the systems of the body function together and that diseases stem from the musculoskeletal system

osteoporosis a multifactorial disorder in which bone density is reduced and remaining bone is brittle, breaking easily

overnutrition consumption of too many nutrients and too much energy in comparison with Dietary Reference Intake levels

ovo-lacto vegetarian dietary pattern a food plan consisting of only plant foods plus dairy products and eggs

oxygen debt the amount of oxygen required to clear lactic acid buildup from the body

oxytocin a hormone that initiates the uterine contractions of labor and has a role in the ejection of milk in lactation

P

pancreatitis inflammation of the pancreas; may be acute or chronic

parathormone a hormone that raises blood calcium levels; secreted by the parathyroid gland in response to low blood calcium levels

parenteral nutrition administration of nutrients by a route other than the gastrointestinal (GI) tract, usually intravenous

pellagra the deficiency disorder of niacin characterized by diarrhea, dermatitis, and dementia

pepsin a gastric protease

pepsinogen the inactive form of pepsin

percutaneous endoscopic placement (PEG) placing a feeding tube into stomach via the esophagus and then drawing it through the abdominal skin using a stab incision

perimenopause the time before menopause during which hormonal, biologic, and clinical changes begin to occur

peripheral vascular disease (PVD) condition affecting blood vessels outside the heart, characterized by a variety of signs and symptoms such as numbness, pain, pallor, elevated blood pressure, and impaired arterial pulsations. Causative factors include obesity, cigarette smoking, stress, sedentary occupations, and numerous metabolic disorders

peristalsis the rhythmic contractions of muscles causing wavelike motions that move food down the gastrointestinal tract

peritoneal dialysis (PD) a dialysis procedure performed to correct an imbalance of fluid or electrolytes in the blood or other wastes by using the peritoneum as the diffusible membrane

pernicious anemia inadequate red blood cell formation caused by a lack of intrinsic factor in the stomach with which to absorb vitamin B_{12}

phenylketonuria (PKU) a genetic disorder in which the body cannot break down excess phenylalanine

phospholipids lipid compounds that form part of cell walls and act as fat emulsifiers-physical activity any body movement produced by skeletal muscles that results in energy expenditure

physical fitness the limits on the actions that the body is capable of making

phytochemicals nonnutritive substances in plant-based foods that appear to have disease-fighting properties

pica a condition characterized by a hunger and appetite for nonfood substances

plaque deposits of fatty substances, including cholesterol, that attach to arterial walls

polydipsia excessive thirst

polymeric formulas solutions that provide intact nutrients (e.g., whole proteins and long-chain triglycerides) that require a normally functioning gastrointestinal tract

polyphagia excessive hunger and eating

polysaccharide a carbohydrate consisting of many units of monosaccharides joined together; starch and fiber are food sources, and glycogen is a storage form in the liver and muscles

polyunsaturated fatty acid (PUFA) a fatty acid containing two or more double bonds on the carbon chain

polyuria excessive urination

portal hypertension increased blood pressure in the portal circulation caused by

compression or occlusion in the portal or hepatic vascular system

postischemic injury after decreased blood supply to a body organ or part

postnecrotic cirrhosis associated with history of viral hepatitis, improperly treated hepatitis, or hepatic damage from toxic chemicals

postprandial occurring after a meal

preeclampsia a sudden rise in arterial blood pressure accompanied by rapid weight gain and marked edema during pregnancy; also known as pregnancy-induced hypertension

primary or essential hypertension elevated blood pressure for which the cause is unknown; often a genetic component

prolactin a hormone responsible for milk synthesis

proteases protein enzymes

protein efficiency ratio (PER) a method to determine the quality of food protein by comparing weight gain with protein intake

protein-energy malnutrition (PEM) malnutrition caused by the lack of protein, of energy, or both

proteins organic compounds formed from chains of amino acids

Q

Qi gong a modality of traditional Chinese medicine that merges breathing regulation, movement, and meditation to increase the flow of Qi, or life force, in the body

quality of life (QOL) the general well-being of an individual

R

reactant a substance that enters into and is altered during a chemical reaction

Reactive oxygen species chemically active compounds containing oxygen; they may cause chronic inflammation and tissue damage over time

recombinant erythropoietin (EPO) recombinant human erythropoietin; drug used to treat anemia by replacing erythropoietin for patients with chronic renal failure who do not produce this hormone in adequate amounts

Recommended Dietary Allowance (RDA) the level of nutrient intake sufficient to meet the needs of almost all healthy individuals of a life stage and gender group

recumbent measures measurements taken while the subject is lying down or reclining

refeeding syndrome physiologic and metabolic complications associated with reintroducing nutrition (refeeding) too rapidly to a person with protein-energy malnutrition; can include malabsorption, cardiac insufficiency, congestive heart failure, respiratory distress, convulsions, coma, and perhaps death

refined grains grains that contain only some of the edible kernel

regional enteritis a form of inflammatory bowel disease more commonly called Crohn's disease

registered dietitian/nutritionist (RDN) a professional trained in foods and the management of diets (dietetics) who is credentialed by the Commission on Dietetic Registration of the Academy of Nutrition and Dietetics; credentialing is based on completing a bachelor of science degree from a U.S. accredited program, receiving clinical and administrative supervised practice, and passing the national registration examination

reiki an energy therapy based on the belief that healing the patient's spirit also heals the physical body

renal transplantation the transfer of a kidney from one person to another

respiratory distress syndrome (RDS) a respiratory disorder identified by insufficient respiration and abnormally low levels of circulating oxygen in the blood

respiratory quotient (RQ) ratio of CO_2 exhaled to O_2 inhaled; depending the net metabolic needs of the body, the ratio ranges from 0.7 to 1 and averages around 0.8; carbohydrate metabolism produces an RQ of 1; protein metabolism, an RQ of 0.8; and fat metabolism, an RQ of 0.7.

retrovirus a ribonucleic acid (RNA) virus that becomes integrated into the deoxyribonucleic acid (DNA) of a host cell during replication; human immunodeficiency virus (HIV) is a retrovirus

rickets a childhood disorder caused by vitamin D or calcium deficiency and leads to insufficient mineralization of bone and tooth matrix

S

saccharin a nonnutritive sweetener

saliva the secretions of the salivary glands of the mouth

saturated fatty acid a fatty acid with carbon chains completely saturated or filled with hydrogen

scurvy extreme vitamin C deficiency disorder characterized by inflammation of connective tissues, gingivitis, muscle degeneration, bruising, and hemorrhaging as the vascular system weakens

secondary hypertension elevated blood pressure for which the cause can be identified

secretin a hormone secreted by the small intestine that causes the pancreas to release bicarbonate to the small intestine

segmentation the forward and backward muscular action that assists in controlling food mass movement through the gastrointestinal tract

senescence older adulthood

sepsis systemic infection

serosa the outermost layer of the gastrointestinal wall; made of serous membrane

set point a natural level (of some characteristic) that the body regulates or defends

simple carbohydrates monosaccharides and disaccharides

sleep apnea disorder in which breathing stops for short periods during sleep

small for gestational age (SGA) having a lower birth weight than expected for the length of gestation

soft water water filtered to replace some of the minerals with sodium

soluble dietary fibers dietary fibers that dissolve in fluids

solute a substance dissolved in another substance

solvent the liquid in which another substance (the solute) is dissolved to form a solution

somatic protein skeletal muscle protein

somatostatin a hormone produced by the pancreas and hypothalamus that inhibits insulin and glucagons

spina bifida a congenital neural tube defect caused by the incomplete closure of the fetus's spine during early pregnancy; may involve incomplete development of brain, spinal cord, and/or their protective coverings, resulting in a range of disabilities

steatorrhea presence of excess fat in the feces

stem cell transplantation a procedure that replaces a person's faulty stem cells with healthy ones from blood or bone marrow

sterols fatlike class of lipids that serve vital functions in the body

stomatitis inflammation of mucous membranes of the mouth

storage fat layers and cushions of fat providing stored energy and protection from extremes of environmental temperatures; also protects internal organs against physical trauma

submucosa a layer of connective muscle tissue under the mucosa

sucralose a nonnutritive sweetener, suitable for cooking, that provides no energy

sugar alcohols nutritive sweeteners related to carbohydrates that provide 2 to 3 kcal/g; sorbitol, mannitol, and xylitol are sugar alcohols, also called sugar replacers

syngeneic genetically and immunologically compatible transplant from an identical twin

systemic lupus erythematosus (SLE) a chronic autoimmune inflammatory disease affecting many systems of the body; pathophysiology includes severe vasculitis, renal involvement, and lesions of the skin and nervous system

T

tachycardia rapid beating of the heart

teratogen an agent capable of producing a malformation or a defect in the unborn fetus

The Joint Commission (TJC) a United States-based nonprofit organization that accredits more than 20,000 health care organizations using a peer review process for quality of care

therapeutic touch an energy therapy based on facilitating energy flow in and around the body

thermic effect of food (TEF)/diet-induced thermogenesis an increase of cellular activity when food is eaten

third space (third spacing) a condition in which fluid shifts from the blood into a body cavity or tissue from which it is no longer available as circulating fluid

thrombosis an abnormal vascular condition in which a blood clot (thrombus) develops within a blood vessel

thrombus blood clot

thyrotoxicosis iodine-induced goiter

Tolerable Upper Intake Level (UL) the level of nutrient intake that should not be exceeded to prevent adverse health risks

trace minerals essential nutrient minerals required daily in amounts of 20 mg or less

trans **fatty acids** fatty acids with unusual double-bond structures caused by hydrogenated unsaturated oils

tricarboxylic acid (TCA) cycle cellular reactions that liberate energy from fragments of carbohydrates, fats, and protein; also called the Krebs cycle

triglycerides the largest class of lipids found in food and body fat; composed of three fatty acids and one glycerol molecule

trypsin the primary pancreatic protease

type 1 diabetes mellitus (T1DM) a form of diabetes mellitus in which the pancreas produces no insulin at all

type 2 diabetes mellitus (T2DM) a form of diabetes mellitus in which the pancreas produces some insulin that is defective and unable to serve the complete needs of the body

U

ulcerative colitis (UC) an inflammatory bowel disease confined to the mucosa of any or all of the large intestine

undernutrition consumption of insufficient energy or nutrients based on Dietary Reference Intake values

unrefined grains grains prepared for consumption containing all edible portions of kernels; also known as whole grains

urea product of ammonia conversion produced during deamination

uremia excessive amounts of urea and other nitrogenous waste products in the blood

uremic toxicity buildup of toxic waste products (urea and other nitrogenous waste products) in the blood; symptoms include anorexia, nausea, metallic taste in the mouth, irritability, confusion, lethargy, restlessness, and pruritus (itching)

V

vegan dietary pattern a food plan consisting of only plant foods

very low-calorie diets (VLCDs) usually defined as diets containing 800 kcal/day or less

very low-density lipoproteins (VLDLs) lipoproteins that carry fats and cholesterol to body cells and are made of the largest proportions of cholesterol

villi fingerlike projections on the walls of the small intestine that increase the mucosal surface area

visceral fat fat that is within the abdominal cavity

visceral proteins proteins other than muscle tissue; for example, internal organs and blood

vitamins essential organic molecules needed in very small amounts for cellular metabolism

vomiting reverse peristalsis

W

wasting syndrome an involuntary weight loss of more than 10% in 1 month with the presence of either chronic diarrhea, weakness, or fever for more than 30 days in the absence of a concurrent illness or condition

wellness a lifestyle enhancing our level of health

Wernicke-Korsakoff syndrome cerebral form of beriberi that affects the central nervous system

wet beriberi thiamine deficiency with edema affecting cardiac function by weakening of heart muscle and vascular system

whole-grain products food items made using unrefined grains

Wilson's disease a rare, inherited disorder of copper metabolism in which copper accumulates slowly in the liver and is then released and taken up in other parts of the body; as copper accumulates in red blood cells, hemolysis and hemolytic anemia occur

X

xerophthalmia a condition caused by vitamin A deficiency with symptoms ranging from night blindness to keratomalacia; may result in complete blindness

INDEX

Page numbers followed by "f" indicate figures, "t" indicate tables, and "b" indicate boxes.

Dietary Reference Intakes (DRIs): Recommended Dietary Allowances and Adequate Intakes, Total Water and Macronutrients Food and Nutrition Board, Institute of Medicine, National Academies

LIFE STAGE GROUP	TOTAL WATER^a (L/d)	CARBOHYDRATE (g/d)	TOTAL FIBER (g/d)	FAT (g/d)	LINOLEIC ACID (g/d)	α-LINOLENIC ACID (g/d)	PROTEIN^b (g/d)
Infants							
0 to 6 mo	0.7*	60*	ND	31*	4.4*	0.5*	9.1*
6 to 12 mo	0.8*	95*	ND	30*	4.6*	0.5*	**11.0**
Children							
1-3 y	1.3*	**130**	19*	ND^c	7*	0.7*	**13**
4-8 y	1.7*	**130**	25*	ND	10*	0.9*	**19**
Males							
9-13 y	24*	**130**	31*	ND	12*	1.2*	**34**
14-18 y	3.3*	**130**	38*	ND	16*	1.6*	**52**
19-30 y	3.7*	**130**	38*	ND	17*	1.6*	**56**
31-50 y	3.7*	**130**	38*	ND	17*	1.6*	**56**
51-70 y	3.7*	**130**	30*	ND	14*	1.6*	**56**
> 70 y	3.7*	**130**	30*	ND	14*	1.6*	**56**
Females							
9-13 y	2.1*	**130**	26*	ND	10*	1.0*	**34**
14-18 y	2.3*	**130**	26*	ND	11*	1.1*	**46**
19-30 y	2.7*	**130**	25*	ND	12*	1.1*	**46**
31-50 y	2.7*	**130**	25*	ND	12*	1.1*	**46**
51-70 y	2.7*	**130**	21*	ND	11*	1.1*	**46**
> 70 y	2.7*	**130**	21*	ND	11*	1.1*	**46**
Pregnancy							
14-18 y	3.0*	**175**	28*	ND	13*	1.4*	**71**
19-30 y	3.0*	**175**	28*	ND	13*	1.4*	**71**
31-50 y	3.0*	**175**	28*	ND	13*	1.4*	**71**
Lactation							
14-18	3.8*	**210**	29*	ND	13*	1.3*	**71**
19-30 y	3.8*	**210**	29*	ND	13*	1.3*	**71**
31-50 y	3.8*	**210**	29*	ND	13*	1.3*	**71**

NOTE: This table (take from the DRI reports, see www.nap.edu) presents Recommended Dietary Allowances (RDA) in **bold type** and Adequate Intakes (AI) in ordinary type followed by an asterisk (*). An RDA is the average daily dietary intake level; sufficient to meet the nutrient requirements of nearly all (97-98 percent) healthy individuals in a group. It is calculated from an Estimated Average Requirement (EAR). If sufficient scientific evidence is not available to establish an EAR, and thus calculate an RDA, an AI is usually developed. For healthy breastfed infants, an AI is the mean intake. The AI for other life stage and gender groups is believed to cover the needs of all healthy individuals in the groups, but lack of data or uncertainty in the data prevent being able to specify with confidence the percentage of individuals covered by this intake.

^{a}Total water includes all water contained in food, beverages, and drinking water.
^{b}Based on g protein per kg of body weight for the reference body weight, e.g., for adults 0.8 g/kg body weight for the reference body weight.
^{c}Not determined.

SOURCE: *Dietary Reference Intakes for Energy, Carbohydrate, Fiber, Fat, Fatty Acids, Cholesterol, Protein, and Amino Acids* (2002/2005) and *Dietary Reference Intakes for Water, Potassium, Sodium, Chloride, and Sulfate* (2005). The report may be accessed via www.nap.edu.

Dietary Reference Intakes (DRIs): Tolerable Upper Intake Levels, Vitamins Food and Nutrition Board, Institute of Medicine, National Academies

LIFE STAGE GROUP	VITAMIN A (µg/d)^a	VITAMIN C (mg/d)	VITAMIN D (µg/d)	VITAMIN E (mg/d)^{b,c}	VITAMIN K	THIAMIN	RIBOFLAVIN	NIACIN (mg/d)^c	VITAMIN B$_6$ (mg/d)	FOLATE (µg/d)^c	VITAMIN B$_{12}$	PANTOTHENIC ACID	BIOTIN	CHOLINE (g/d)	CAROTENOIDS^d
Infants															
0 to 6 mo	600	ND^e	25	ND	ND	ND	ND	ND	ND	ND	ND	ND	ND	ND	ND
6 to 12 mo	600	ND	38	ND	ND	ND	ND	ND	ND	ND	ND	ND	ND	ND	ND
Children															
1-3 y	600	400	63	200	ND	ND	ND	10	30	300	ND	ND	ND	1.0	ND
4-8 y	900	650	75	300	ND	ND	ND	15	40	400	ND	ND	ND	1.0	ND
Males															
9-13 y	1,700	1,200	100	600	ND	ND	ND	20	60	600	ND	ND	ND	2.0	ND
14-18 y	2,800	1,800	100	800	ND	ND	ND	30	80	800	ND	ND	ND	3.0	ND
19-30 y	3,000	2,000	100	1,000	ND	ND	ND	35	100	1,000	ND	ND	ND	3.5	ND
31-50 y	3,000	2,000	100	1,000	ND	ND	ND	35	100	1,000	ND	ND	ND	3.5	ND
51-70 y	3,000	2,000	100	1,000	ND	ND	ND	35	100	1,000	ND	ND	ND	3.5	ND
> 70 y	3,000	2,000	100	1,000	ND	ND	ND	35	100	1,000	ND	ND	ND	3.5	ND
Females															
9-13 y	1,700	1,200	100	600	ND	ND	ND	20	60	600	ND	ND	ND	2.0	ND
14-18 y	2,800	1,800	100	800	ND	ND	ND	30	80	800	ND	ND	ND	3.0	ND
19-30 y	3,000	2,000	100	1,000	ND	ND	ND	35	100	1,000	ND	ND	ND	3.5	ND
31-50 y	3,000	2,000	100	1,000	ND	ND	ND	35	100	1,000	ND	ND	ND	3.5	ND
51-70 y	3,000	2,000	100	1,000	ND	ND	ND	35	100	1,000	ND	ND	ND	3.5	ND
> 70 y	3,000	2,000	100	1,000	ND	ND	ND	35	100	1,000	ND	ND	ND	3.5	ND
Pregnancy															
14-18 y	2,800	1,800	100	800	ND	ND	ND	30	80	800	ND	ND	ND	3.0	ND
19-30 y	3,000	2,000	100	1,000	ND	ND	ND	35	100	1,000	ND	ND	ND	3.5	ND
31-50 y	3,000	2,000	100	1,000	ND	ND	ND	35	100	1,000	ND	ND	ND	3.5	ND
Lactation															
14-18 y	2,800	1,800	100	800	ND	ND	ND	30	80	800	ND	ND	ND	3.0	ND
19-30 y	3,000	2,000	100	1,000	ND	ND	ND	35	100	1,000	ND	ND	ND	3.5	ND
31-50 y	3,000	2,000	100	1,000	ND	ND	ND	35	100	1,000	ND	ND	ND	3.5	ND

NOTE: A Tolerable Upper Intake Level (UL) is the highest level of daily nutrient intake that is likely to pose no risk of adverse health effects to almost all individuals in the general population. Unless otherwise specified, the UL represents total intake from food, water, and supplements. Due to a lack of suitable data, ULs could not be established for vitamin K, thiamin, riboflavin, vitamin B$_{12}$, pantothenic acid, biotin, and carotenoids. In the absence of a UL, extra caution may be warranted in consuming levels above recommended intakes. Members of the general population should be advised not to routinely exceed the UL. The UL is not meant to apply to individuals who are treated with the nutrient under medical supervision or to individuals with predisposing conditions that modify their sensitivity to the nutrient.

^{a}As preformed vitamin A only.
^{b}As α-tocopherol; applies to any form of supplemental α-tocopherol.
^{c}The ULs for vitamin E, niacin, and folate apply to synthetic forms obtained from supplements, fortified foods, or a combination of the two.
^{d}β-Carotene supplements are advised only to serve as a provitamin A source for individuals at risk of vitamin A deficiency.
^{e}ND = Not determinable due to lack of data of adverse effects in this age group and concern with regard to lack of ability to handle excess amounts. Source of intake should be from food only to prevent high levels of intake.

SOURCES: *Dietary Reference Intakes for Calcium, Phosphorous, Magnesium, Vitamin D, and Fluoride* (1997); *Dietary Reference Intakes for Thiamin, Riboflavin, Niacin, Vitamin B$_6$, Folate, Vitamin B$_{12}$, Pantothenic Acid, Biotin, and Choline* (1998); *Dietary Reference Intakes for Vitamin C, Vitamine E, Selenium, and Carotenoids* (2000); *Dietary Reference Intakes for Vitamin A, Vitamin K, Arsenic, Boron, Chromium, Copper, Iodine, Iron, Manganese, Molybdenum, Nickel, Silicon, Vanadium, and Zinc* (2001); and *Dietary Reference Intakes for Calcium and Vitamin D* (2011). These reports may be accessed via www.nap.edu.